THE ART OF
NATURAL
FAMILY PLANNING

Fourth Edition
Tenth Printing

John F. Kippley and Sheila K. Kippley

Foreword by Konald A. Prem, M.D.

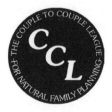

The Couple to Couple League International, Inc.
P.O. Box 111184
Cincinnati, OH 45211-1184, USA

Fourth Edition
        Tenth printing: 20,000, April 2005
        Previous printings: 103,000 (1996-2004)
        Previous editions: 279,000 (1972-1996)

Cataloging data
        L.C. 94-069471
        Dewey 613.94

Kippley, John F. and Kippley, Sheila K.
The Art of Natural Family Planning
Foreword by Konald A. Prem. M.D.
        1. Natural Family Planning   2. Birth Control
        3. Breastfeeding   4. Sexual Morality

ISBN 0-926412-13-2

All net proceeds from the sale of this book support the work of the Couple to Couple League International, Inc. The League is a not-for-profit organization that helps couples with the successful practice of natural family planning.

For further information
        The Couple to Couple League
        P.O. Box 111184
        Cincinnati OH 45211-1184
        U.S.A.
        (513) 471-2000
        Orders only: (800) 745-8252
        FAX: (513) 557-2449
        E-Mail: ccli@ccli.org
                Note: When contacting the League via e-mail, *if you request a response* please include your name, complete address, and phone number. Frequently the office includes an appropriate brochure or form requesting more information as part of the response.
        Website: www.ccli.org

Note: The national office cannot accept collect phone calls from anyone, nor can it provide counseling to non-members. Please see the Membership section in the "Introduction" for information about obtaining and maintaining membership. The 800-number is only for orders.

Local teachers' names and phone

Table of Contents

Foreword

There is no question about it: Natural Family Planning has come of age. It is therefore with great pleasure that I introduce the Fourth Edition of *The Art of Natural Family Planning.*

Throughout the history of man, a natural but limited form of child spacing has been available through long term breastfeeding. However, the introduction of bottlefeeding deprived most Western mothers of this natural form of baby spacing. Today, only two groups of women still enjoy a time of prolonged postpartum infertility: 1) those in cultures which continue the practice of nursing described in this book as "ecological breastfeeding," and 2) those who have learned this practice despite the lack of cultural support. On the average, such a nursing pattern may provide 18 to 30 months spacing between births. Since it is scientifically well established that maternal breastmilk is the best infant food, I am pleased that the Fourth Edition has an expanded treatment of the advantages of breastfeeding and how to do ecological breastfeeding.

However, most couples today seek to regulate conception beyond the possibilities offered by breastfeeding alone, and many are interested in natural methods. The first real help for those interested in natural family planning (NFP) became available in the 1930s through the independent research of Doctors Kyusaku Ogino in Japan and Hermann Knaus in Austria. As you will read later in this book, they developed systems known as "calendar rhythm." Because their systems did not sufficiently consider the various forms of menstrual irregularity experienced by many women, more than a few couples were disillusioned by repeated surprise pregnancies. Although the reasons for these "system-failures" are now better understood, calendar rhythm is no longer recommended by teachers of natural family planning. It is still recognized, however, for what it was: the first natural family planning system in the history of mankind based upon scientific study and oriented toward an educated awareness of fertility.

The efficiency of natural family planning was aided immensely by the discovery that the hormone progesterone, produced by the ovary after ovulation, causes an easily measured elevation of the waking body temperature which persists until menstruation. Observations of other signs led to the development of the sympto-thermal method of natural family planning; these signs include changes in the quantity and the qualities of cervical mucus, physical changes in the cervix, and ovulation pain or Mittelschmerz. During the 1950s and 1960s, I assisted many couples to develop a high degree of proficiency using these signs for family limitation. Published studies referred to in this manual have shown that well instructed and motivated couples can use the sympto-thermal method with an efficiency comparable to or better than most of the unnatural methods except sterilization and the original high dose birth control Pill.

Even in the 1990s, the question remains for many couples, "Where can we learn about natural family planning?" Medical school training traditionally focuses on the diagnosis and treatment of disease. When it comes to "family planning," the emphasis is on drugs, internal devices, and surgery—matters requiring medical expertise. Being natural, healthy, and not requiring any medical expertise, natural family planning is rarely mentioned in medical schools.

The neglect of NFP in the health care professions led interested married couples and physicians in the 1960s to organize teaching teams to instruct interested married couples outside the traditional medical setting. In 1971, John and Sheila Kippley asked me for help to establish the Couple to Couple League, a volunteer organization to provide effective teaching of natural family planning on a nationwide and then international basis. In addition, they saw the need for an authoritative instruction manual. I was pleased to cooperate in both of these projects and allowed them to use many informative fertility graphs I had collected over more than 20 years of interest and experience with the sympto-thermal method.

The normal way to learn NFP combines formal classes such as those taught by the Couple to Couple League with the personal study of an authoritative manual. However, many couples do not have the opportunity to attend classes. While a book is no substitute for adequate personalized instruction, this manual can be used for self-instruction in geographic areas where formal classes are not yet available. Married couples and physicians alike will find it an indispensable aid to the successful practice of natural family planning.

Konald A. Prem, M.D.
Professor Emeritus
Department of Obstetrics and Gynecology
University of Minnesota

Acknowledgements

This Fourth Edition of *The Art of Natural Family Planning* represents a significant revision from the Third Edition which the Couple to Couple League published from 1984 to 1996. It is not just a revision of the Third Edition; it also includes and revises *The Home Study Guide to Natural Family Planning*, published by CCL since 1988, and the *Practical Applications Workbook* published separately by CCL since the early Seventies.

The current edition is a group effort. First, it includes two chapters written by others. We want to thank Thomas A. McGovern, M.D., for writing Chapter 13 dealing with Effectiveness; the subject is complex and we are highly grateful for his making this technical subject accessible to non-technical readers. We also thank Paul Weckenbrock, R.Ph., for writing Chapter 35 that deals with the technical subject of pharmaceutical drugs and their effects on the fertility cycle. Medical illustrator Erin Browne provided five drawings, and for these we are grateful.

Second, in preparation for the Fourth Edition, we received significant help from our advisors and fellow teachers of natural family planning. Previous editions were reviewed by Konald A. Prem, M.D., primarily for bio-medical correctness; this edition was reviewed not only by Dr. Prem but also by a number of advisors and NFP teachers for readability, insight and different perspectives. Everyone had at least a few suggestions for improvement; some had many. Certainly they all contributed to making this a better book than it would have been otherwise. We want to thank Jeff Brand, Dominic Cerrato, William Corey, Mary Durbin, Mark Hayden, Kim Hardey, M.D., Linda Kracht, Joy Kondash, M.D., Robert Laird, Mary Schmiesing, Kris Severyn, R.Ph., and Douglas Touchet. Their reviews of various chapters were truly helpful. On the technical side, Keith O. Bower efficiently put all the charts into the computer, a task that neither of us was prepared to tackle.

We have a very special thanks to those who reviewed the entire text under the constraints of deadlines—Paul Busam, M.D., Sherry Hartz, Clifford and Jean Kreifels, Konald A. Prem, M.D., David Prentis, Marilyn Shannon, and Ann and Christopher Wolfe, Ph.D. We greatly appreciate such labors of love and their many thoughtful suggestions.

Once a manuscript is written, even on modern word processing equipment, it has to be further manipulated to put it into the final version for printing. We are most grateful to Ann Gundlach, CCL's publications editor, for her extremely able assistance in getting the copy ready for publication and for her patience in dealing with changes. Finally, the text has to be proofread, and we are certainly grateful to Ginny Niehaus, CCL's head secretary, for her able proofing and suggestions for readability.

John and Sheila Kippley

Part I

Introduction
and
Basics

Introduction

Natural Family Planning is usually abbreviated as **NFP**.

Part I of this book contains the basic NFP information you need to post-pone pregnancy. Part III is important for the long-term practice of NFP. Part IV is of special interest to those who are seeking pregnancy.

Reading and workbook schedule

If you are attending the regular CCL course of four meetings spaced a month apart, please follow this schedule:

Between Meetings I and II: Read Chapters 15, 1 through 10, and 17. Do the Low and High Temperature lines on Workbook Charts 4, 5, 6, 7 and 9. Skip Chart 8. Note Peak Day on Charts 2-9.

Between Meetings II and III: Read Chapters 11 through 22 plus 31. In Workbook Charts 3-9, do the "End of Phase I" line. Look at Charts 1-5.

Between Meetings III and IV: Read Chapters 23 through 28. Look at Workbook Charts 6-10.

After Meeting IV: Do the rest of the Workbook charts.

If any of the situations covered in Chapters 29 - 35 as indicated in the Table of Contents apply to you, be sure to read those chapters, too. Feel free to ask your teachers to clarify anything that isn't clear.

If you are teaching yourself through the *CCL Home Study Course,* try to do a chapter every day or two. In that way, you will learn the basics in about two weeks to a month, and you will complete the course in approximately one or two months.

If you are **coming off the Pill,** be sure to read Chapter 29 right away. However, the details of what to do may not make much sense until you have also completed Chapters 1 through 6.

If you have a history of **irregular cycles,** take an early look at Chapters 21 and 31. They will, of course, make more sense after you have completed Chapters 1 through 9.

Finding a subject

This book has 38 chapters dealing with different subjects. To find a particular subject, we suggest first using the Table of Contents, then Chapter 15, and then the Index.

Natural Family Planning

Natural Family Planning (or NFP) is a system in which you become aware of the fertile and infertile times of your menstrual cycle, and you act accordingly. If you want to avoid pregnancy, you have marital relations only during the infertile times. If you want to become pregnant, through NFP you know the best days in each cycle for seeking pregnancy.

There is also a non-systematic form of NFP that we call "ecological breastfeeding." This is the world's original form of Natural Family Planning. Here we want to make only three points: 1) True ecological breastfeeding *does* space babies; the average is about two years apart. 2) Cultural breastfeeding generally has no spacing effect. 3) Some couples use only ecological breastfeeding for natural spacing between babies. We describe this in detail in Chapters 23 - 25.

NFP: the scientific method

You may recall from your grade school or high school introduction to science this definition of the scientific method: "The systematic observation and recording of recurring events." That's what NFP is all about, and that's why we can say that **modern NFP is truly a scientific method of family planning.** In this book, you will learn how to make systematic observations of your own bodily signs of fertility and infertility and how to make simple recordings.

If you want to avoid pregnancy, Natural Family Planning requires chaste abstinence during the fertile time. NFP excludes using a condom, diaphragm, sponge, spermicidal foam, or withdrawal during the fertile time for three reasons: 1) All of these methods have their own surprise pregnancy rates that are higher than the rates for modern NFP. 2) Contraceptive intercourse during the fertile time may confuse the normal signs of fertility. 3) According to 19 centuries of Christian teaching, it is immoral to use unnatural methods of birth control. (You will read about contraceptive surprise pregnancy rates in Chapters 1 and 13 and about moral questions in Chapters 16-19.)

Is NFP easy to learn and use?

The practice of natural family planning is so easy to learn and use that a basic set of rules can be written on the two sides of a business card like this:

To ACHIEVE Pregnancy

1. Abstain from Cycle Day 1 until you have the more-fertile mucus.

2. Have marital relations every other day up through Peak Day plus 2.

3. Keep taking your waking temperature. A thermal shift of 21 days provides you with a 99% probability that you are pregnant.

4. To estimate your due date, determine the first day of sustained thermal shift, subtract seven days, and add nine months.

To AVOID/POSTPONE Pregnancy

1. Phase I ends on Cycle Day 6, providing you are still mucus-dry and have not had cycles shorter than 26 days in the last two years. Abstain beginning with Cycle Day 7.

2. Phase III begins on the evening of Peak Day plus 4 cross-checked by 3 days of full thermal shift after Peak Day.

You won't understand these rules right now, but take a look. You will notice that the reason you don't understand them is very simple: you don't understand the terminology and the shorthand phrases. For example,

"Phase III" means "the postovulation infertile time of the cycle, the phase of the cycle when progesterone is naturally suppressing ovulation." Even that sentence contains some shorthand, for "cycle" means the female menstrual cycle, the time from the beginning of one menstruation up through the day before the beginning of the next menstruation. If you read that last sentence a couple of times, you will quickly understand why we have to use some shorthand phrases.

The brief rules on the "To Avoid/Postpone Pregnancy" side of the business card summarize part of our system. Experience suggests that most married couples can use those brief and simple rules in most of their fertile cycles even though those rules are conservative.

So why do we have a whole book instead of a business card?

First, we want to help you, especially if you are one of those who might find the above rules difficult to apply to your own cycle pattern. Some of our other rules provide a better fit in some cases; others are more liberal in certain situations.

Second, you need to learn the terminology. However, that's quite easy and doesn't take many of the following pages.

Third, most people like you who can read also like to understand what's going on to cause the changes in a woman's menstrual cycle. You don't have to know these things, but most people, husbands as well as wives, find it helpful.

Fourth, take a look at the Table of Contents. You will see that this book takes you step by step into the practice of Natural Family Planning. You will notice some chapters that explain the various reasons for choosing and sticking with NFP; you will learn about the good effects that NFP can have on your marriage. Then you will see chapters that answer special questions such as these: "What if I'm coming off the Pill?" "What if my cycles are irregular in one way or another?" "What if we don't get pregnant right away when we want to?" "What should I do after I've had a baby?" "Will breastfeeding affect the return of my fertility?" "How do I use NFP when I'm going through pre-menopause?" And more. Our experience of teaching Natural Family Planning since 1971 shows that some of these questions will most likely be very important to you in the future if not today.

Why is NFP like tying your shoelaces?

What is simpler and more automatic than tying your shoelaces? Yet, imagine what you would have to do to explain in writing and diagrams how to tie your shoelaces. Wouldn't it look complicated? So it is with learning NFP. The initial concept is very simple—just learning how to determine the fertile and infertile times of the cycle. Then as you get into the details, it might start to look complicated. Once you've learned it, it's simple again. Just like having learned to tie your shoelaces.

Who should learn NFP?

EVERY engaged or married man and woman should learn NFP even if they intend to let their babies come as they may. Any couple may meet some sort of health problem that would indicate they should postpone pregnancy for a time.

Every married couple should learn the kind of breastfeeding that spaces babies about two years apart—on the average.

Every health care professional should learn the facts about modern NFP and "ecological breastfeeding." They need to be able to distinguish between the calendar rhythm of the 1930s and what informed couples use today. They need to know the huge difference between "cultural breastfeeding" that has little or no baby-spacing effects and "ecological breastfeeding" that has important spacing effects.

Every minister and priest owes it to the couples they counsel to learn not just the how-to-do-it of NFP but also the moral and religious principles that are involved. They should understand why experienced counselors call NFP "marriage insurance." More on those subjects in chapters 17 - 19.

Who should <u>use</u> NFP?

Every married couple who have a sufficiently serious reason to postpone pregnancy should practice NFP. The toughest part of NFP, once you let God into your decision-making process, is answering this question: "Is the Lord calling us to have another baby now or is He calling us to postpone pregnancy for the present?" Or, "Do we or don't we have a sufficiently serious reason to postpone pregnancy?" We have tried to provide a balanced approach to planning, prudence and Providence in Chapter 16.

Every husband and wife should give very serious consideration to the world's oldest form of NFP—ecological breastfeeding—because it provides so many health and emotional benefits to their baby; it also provides a natural spacing between their babies. More on that in Chapters 23 - 25.

Note on usage and pronouns

For easy reading, the biological sections of this book address a woman; for example, "Observe your cervical mucus . . ." However, to get the real benefits of NFP, it is important for husbands to read these sections, too. Babies and doctors are referred to as "he" simply to avoid the awkward "he or she" and to clearly distinguish the wife/mother from the doctor and baby.

Smaller print like this will be used for little stories to illustrate a point. It is also used for things you don't really have to know for the practice of NFP, generally more technical things. If you find the small print paragraphs confusing, just skip them.

The Couple to Couple League

The Couple to Couple League International, Inc. is a non-profit organization that helps couples build healthy marriages through the practice of Natural Family Planning. The League was founded in 1971 by the authors of this manual, John and Sheila Kippley, with the great and gracious help of Konald A. Prem, M.D., professor of obstetrics and gynecology at the University of Minnesota School of Medicine. The League's principal activity is teaching engaged and married couples how to practice NFP. It does this in the context of the Christian Tradition regarding marital love, sexuality and family. The League has become the largest provider of NFP services in America. It teaches regular NFP classes in many parts of the United States and in a growing number of other countries. It has developed the *CCL Home Study Course* for those couples who cannot attend the regular NFP course.

We started the first series of classes in a school library in Shoreview, Minnesota, a suburb north of St. Paul. At the appointed hour, the only people in the room were Dr. Konald A. Prem—our medical advisor, one man who was there to check us out, and ourselves. With queasy stomachs, we reconsidered our decision to start promptly at eight o'clock, and within ten minutes about 30 people filled the room. The League was born.

From the very beginning, we have used essentially the same teaching program—four two-hour meetings spaced a month apart, the cross-checking Sympto-Thermal Method of NFP, ecological breastfeeding, and all of this in the context of the Christian Tradition regarding marital chastity. To be sure, there have been all sorts of minor changes, but the teaching experience of over 20 years has confirmed those initial decisions.

Membership

If you are taking the CCL course of four classes or are enrolled in the *CCL Home Study Course*, you are automatically a member. If you are not, see "How do I become a member" below.

What do you get out of your membership?

The membership benefit that you will notice the most is the *CCL Family Foundations* which will come to your home every other month. Many members tell us that this magazine is the only thing they read cover to cover as soon as it arrives in the mail. It summarizes recent health research related to fertility—and sometimes broader areas. Other features include columns on natural parenting, developments in natural family planning, challenges to young parents, a vibrant "Letters" section, and much more. In short, it's so informative that you may want to keep back issues, and it's interesting, well written, and thought provoking.

As a member, you can use CCL's *counseling* services. First, contact your local CCL Teaching Couple; they are trained for this. Sometimes they will refer you to CCL Headquarters. If you are unable to reach any nearby CCL teachers, contact CCL Headquarters directly. The staff at CCL Headquarters are not physicians. They will be able to answer most true NFP-related questions (as contrasted with medical diagnosis), and in certain cases they will call upon the expertise of the CCL Medical Advisory Board.

As a member, you can also derive *satisfaction* from knowing you are helping the pro-chastity work of the Couple to Couple League. You are already aware of the many serious consequences of unchastity today. You hear regularly about the epidemic levels of sexually transmitted diseases including the deadly AIDS. The high rates of out-of-wedlock pregnancy, marital unhappiness, and divorce are other consequences of unchastity. The League is working to change attitudes and to encourage a rebirth of chastity. Your support helps this work to make progress.

*The CCL website — **www.ccli.org** — provides a convenient way to find a nearby CCL Teaching Couple. If you e-mail or write CCL Headquarters, please provide your current address, phone, and member number. (For the latter, see the mailing label on your **CCL Family Foundations** magazine.)*

How do I become a member?

If you are not enrolled in a regular CCL NFP course or in the CCL *Home Study Course*, one easy way to become a member is to phone CCL headquarters to charge your membership to VISA, MasterCard or Discover. CCL Headquarter's order number is 800-745-8252. You can also become a member via the CCL website at **www.ccli.org** by using a credit card.

Another way is to send a note requesting membership information to CCL, P.O. Box 111184, Cincinnati OH 45211, or via e-mail at *ccli@ccli.org*.

The yearly membership contribution is roughly equal to the cost of a one month supply of the Pill in the United States.

Why the Moral/Religious Dimension?

The services of the League are open to all regardless of religious affiliation or conviction, but that doesn't mean that we teach NFP without moral and religious convictions.

First, we believe that God is the Author of nature; He is the one who put together in the marriage act what we call "making love" and "making babies."

We believe that what Jesus taught about marriage applies also to the marriage act: "What God has put together, let no one take apart" (Mt 19:6). It is also God, the Sacred Author of nature, Who made woman in such a way that she is fertile for only about 25% of her menstrual cycle and generally infertile for slightly more than a year while doing ecological breastfeeding. It is God who in his providence has allowed us to learn in the 20th century about woman's alternating fertility and infertility—and about Natural Family Planning—at the same time that other medical advances greatly increased the population survival rate. NFP is truly God's way of spacing babies.

Second, we believe in being open with you whether you agree with us or not. For better or for worse, you know where we are coming from. Can you say the same about most people who write about family planning and other aspects of sexual behavior?

Third, in the long run, your moral/religious convictions guide your decisions about sexual behavior.

Please note: NFP does **not** mean Not For Protestants. You don't have to be Catholic to have strong moral/religious convictions that it's wrong to use unnatural methods of birth control. Protestant leaders at one time thoroughly condemned such practices. Luther called them a form of sodomy, Calvin called them a form of homicide, and John Wesley taught that those who used preventive measures would lose their souls if they didn't repent. The U. S. anti-contraceptive laws of the 19th century were passed by essentially Protestant legislatures for a basically Protestant America. If this is news to you, don't blame yourself. It's been one of the best kept secrets of the 20th century (along with the "secret" of NFP). You will learn a lot more in Chapters 18 and 19.

At the Last Supper, Jesus prayed for unity among his disciples (John 17:20-23). We hope that greater understanding of the Christian Tradition regarding sex, love, marriage, and birth control will dissolve some of the barriers among Christians and even between Christians and Jews and other non-Christians.

Can you get support?

Yes, you can get both technical and psychological support, and you might need the latter just as much as the former. In the contraception and abortion culture of the West, many NFP users find themselves in a lonely position. The League provides an opportunity for couples to share concerns, friendship and values in an atmosphere of love and support.

Your first line of support is your local CCL teacher, even if you could not attend classes and are taking the *CCL Home Study Course.* Teachers are supported by the staff at the CCL headquarters, and the Headquarters staff are supported by the CCL Medical Advisory Board.

Your next line of regular support is the *CCL Family Foundations*, a mini-magazine sent to all members every other month. It provides tremendous psychological support as well as keeping you up-to-date on matters related to the practice of NFP.

You can gain a third level of support by joining or forming a CCL chapter to promote and teach NFP. Teachers are needed in every community, and the opportunity to promote the concept of NFP is unlimited. Contact CCL Headquarters for local contacts in your community.

NFP works well in three ways.

1) It helps many couples of low fertility to achieve much desired pregnancies.

2) It works extremely well to avoid or postpone pregnancy.

3) Best of all, it helps couples to build stronger marriages. Since NFP is God's way of spacing babies, it only makes sense that if you follow God's ways, your marriage will be more like the community of love that God and you want it to be.

Statement of Teaching Philosophy

In this book you will learn how to practice the Sympto-Thermal Method (STM) of Natural Family Planning. This is a universal system because it uses all the common indicators of fertility and infertility in cross-checking ways. Some NFP programs or books teach only one sign of fertility (usually the mucus sign) and only one way of observing that sign. People sometimes ask us: "Why do you teach the temperature sign along with the mucus? Wouldn't it be simpler just to teach one sign?"

We have two reasons for teaching the Sympto-Thermal Method.

The practical reason

The practical reason is this: it may be easier to **teach** only one sign of fertility, but many couples find it much easier to **learn** and to **use** at least two signs in a cross-checking way. Look at it this way: it's certainly easier to build a unicycle than to build a bicycle or a tricycle, but which is easier to learn to use?

The philosophical reason

Good philosophy is concerned with expanding the true freedom of the human person. *Learning the full Sympto-Thermal Method expands your freedom to choose among several morally legitimate choices.*

We do not care what natural method of family planning you use once you are well experienced. That is truly your choice. However, you can choose only what you know about. You can choose to use the signs in a cross-checking way only when you learn what each sign is and how to use it.

We strongly recommend that you **learn** the full Sympto-Thermal Method instead of just a single-sign system whether that be mucus-only or temperature-only. By actually using all the signs for a few cycles, you can then make a decision based on your own experience. You will be free to choose to use two or three signs in a cross-checking way or you can choose to use a single-sign approach. In this manual you will learn the cross-checking rules; you will also learn the single-sign rules.

It never hurts to know more, even if you decide to use less.

We believe that by teaching you the full Sympto-Thermal Method of Natural Family Planning and Ecological Breastfeeding, we are giving you the best, the most wholesome, and the most effective means of NFP known today.

1

Why NFP?
The Practical Reasons

Section I of this chapter gives some of the practical reasons for using Natural Family Planning to avoid or postpone pregnancy. When you look at NFP just as a method of family planning, you can see it as an inexpensive, safe, healthy, and highly effective method of "birth control."

Natural Family Planning is also much more than that. It is a means of fertility awareness that encourages husbands and wives to love each other through communication and self-control during times of abstinence. "Building healthy marriages through natural family planning" is the CCL motto based on years of experience.

Because sexuality affects every aspect of our lives, so does NFP. Therefore we go beyond the pragmatic and address several major life issues in Part III of this book. In Chapter 16 you may be pleased or challenged to find a discussion about family planning in the lives of those who believe in a provident God. In Chapter 17 you will learn how NFP can be a real marriage builder. Finally, in Chapters 18 and 19 you will find some of the moral and religious reasons for choosing only NFP.

It is obvious that we cannot say everything at once. We start with this chapter on down-to-earth reasons for deciding to use only the natural methods of family planning once you determine that you have a sufficient reason to postpone pregnancy.

This chapter has two major sections. The first describes the practical reasons to choose NFP; the second section points out some hardheaded reasons not to use the unnatural methods.

Section I: Why Use NFP?

In this section, the emphasis is on the *positive* reasons for choosing NFP when you need to avoid pregnancy. However, some of these reasons require us to make brief references to various unnatural methods.

NFP: Safe, Healthy, and Effective

The Couple to Couple League publishes a leaflet and a short videotape both titled *NFP: Safe Healthy and Effective.* The birth control professionals tell us that these are the main features people want in their method of family planning, and they are solid reasons for choosing NFP.

Why is NFP safe?

In the practice of Natural Family Planning, you simply observe the signs of fertility and infertility that God built into female human nature. What could be more safe and in tune with nature?

Natural Family Planning uses no birth control drugs or devices. Every drug has potential side effects, and you should not take a drug product unless it is necessary to cure or relieve something that's wrong with you. But your fertility is a normal process, not a disease. Birth control chemicals are at best unnecessary drugs.

You may not appreciate how safe NFP is for you personally until you understand the risks of chemical birth control (the Pill, implants, and injections) and invasive devices (the IUD). You may think that whatever birth control chemicals are being sold now are perfectly safe. Not so. More about that later, but for now just remember that the drug companies have consistently claimed great safety for every birth control drug that has appeared since 1960. It's generally only when they come out with a "new generation" of the Pill that they admit the problems of the "old" Pill. Keep also in mind that most intrauterine devices (IUDs) have been taken off the American market because of health-related lawsuits. Lastly, you should be aware that some physicians have linked chemical spermicides with birth defects.

Why is NFP healthy?

The practice of Natural Family Planning promotes good health in two ways.

1. With NFP charting, you will quickly find out if you have a more or less normal cycle pattern. A truly abnormal cycle pattern is an indication that something might be wrong. Some cycle irregularities may indicate dietary problems or low thyroid activity. Occasionally a woman detects a more serious disorder just by changes in her charting, and thus she is able to seek medical help much sooner. Sometimes it's as simple as improving your nutrition or getting your weight into a better balance with your height. (See Chapter 31, "Cycle Irregularities.") At other times it might be something serious.

One young couple was married just a few months. She felt fine, but her cycle just went on and on and on. A medical examination revealed cancer of the thyroid gland. The cancerous gland was successfully removed; she took a simple drug to make up for the absence of the gland, and she returned to extremely regular cycles.

2. The practice of NFP encourages better nutrition. We have been amazed at how poorly some young women eat, and for them this is a real benefit. With the practice of NFP, you become more aware of your state of health and well being. By learning more about your fertility, you will be encouraged to make sure that you and your family are getting proper nutrition. Good nutrition is so important for so many aspects of your menstrual-fertility cycle that CCL publishes *Fertility, Cycles and Nutrition.* The author, Marilyn Shannon, has an advanced degree in human physiology, is a teacher of NFP, and has done extensive counseling related to fertility, nutrition, and NFP. For further information, see "Resources" at the back of this book.

Natural Family Planning is highly effective for achieving pregnancy, and it is even more effective for avoiding pregnancy.

● Achieving pregnancy

If you and your husband are like most young couples, you think that you are highly fertile. Most likely you are. However, approximately 20% of couples today have problems achieving pregnancy when they want to. If there is a true, permanent physical reason that makes either you or your spouse infertile, then NFP can't help. But if you are a couple who simply have low mutual fertility, then the fertility awareness of NFP can be of great help. Be assured that many couples of low fertility achieve pregnancy within six months simply with the cost-free, low-tech, fully natural approach of NFP fertility awareness. Sometimes spouses have to make some minor changes in a few behaviors including exercise and nutrition, but nothing extraordinary is required. More on that in Chapters 20, 21 and 22 which focus on achieving pregnancy, especially for couples of marginal fertility.

● Avoiding pregnancy

How effective is Natural Family Planning when used to avoid pregnancy? The short answer is this: The Sympto-Thermal Method of Natural Family Planning can be used at the 99% level of effectiveness to postpone or avoid pregnancy.

You may find that hard to believe, especially if you've read typical articles about birth control in various women's magazines. Back in the mid-1970s, there was similar skepticism at the birth control branch of the U.S. Department of Health, Education and Welfare (HEW, now called HHS for Health and Human Services). At the time there were frequent claims that the mucus-only approach called the Ovulation Method (OM) was simpler and superior in every way to the Sympto-Thermal Method (STM). Mr. Larry Kane, the executive director of the Human Life Foundation, persuaded HEW to run a study to compare the two methods. We call it the Los Angeles study.

Please note: The Los Angeles study was **not** designed to find out how effective each method could be under the best of conditions with the best of teachers. It was designed only to compare the two different systems working under the same conditions. If you want more detail, you can read the scientific report in a 1981 issue of the *American Journal of Obstetrics and Gynecology*.[1]

No method failures. If you have a serious reason to avoid pregnancy, you can take heart from this sentence in the scientific report: "There were no method failures in the STM group."[2] "Method failures" refer to unplanned pregnancies among couples who followed the rules; the "STM group" were those couples using the Sympto-Thermal Method.

In the Couple to Couple League we do not claim the 100% method effectiveness found by this well-designed study. In a very large group, sooner or later an unexplained pregnancy will be found. However, this study and others give us very solid grounds for saying that adequately instructed couples can practice the Sympto-Thermal Method at the 99% level of effectiveness.

There's much more to say about the overall subject of effectiveness. For example, how do you measure effectiveness? When couples have unplanned pregnancies, what rules do they most commonly *not* follow? To explain these matters, we have to get more technical. If you want, you can study these things in Chapters 13 and 14. The truth is this: study after study has shown that when couples follow the Sympto-Thermal rules, they can and do achieve a 99% level of effectiveness in avoiding pregnancy.

How effective is NFP?

Our conviction is this:
Every couple who have difficulty achieving pregnancy should completely implement the low-tech, natural approach for six to twelve months before seeing a fertility specialist.

Ecological breastfeeding is another part of Natural Family Planning that is rarely described accurately in the media. We explain this subject in Chapters 24 and 25. Here we will only affirm that the *right kind* of nursing—which we call *ecological* breastfeeding—**does** normally space babies. However, *cultural* breastfeeding generally does not delay the return of postpartum fertility.

Other Practical Reasons

Besides the Big Three—Safe, Healthy, and Effective, there are a number of other very practical advantages of Natural Family Planning. We review them in alphabetical order.

Easy to learn

When you attend NFP classes taught by the Couple to Couple League, you learn enough at the first class to enable you to practice NFP right away. Assuming you are married, you don't need to wait a full cycle; you learn enough at the first class to know when you are in Phase III that very first cycle. By the time you finish the second meeting a month later, you know how to apply the Phase I rules. (Phase I = pre-ovulation infertility; Phase II = the fertile time; Phase III = postovulation infertility.)

If you are teaching yourself through the *CCL Home Study Course*, try to do one lesson every other day. In that way, you can finish all the basics within a month and most of the course within two months.

We know from the vast experience of the Couple to Couple League: ordinary couples learn the techniques of NFP very easily.

Easy to use

Most couples are able to use the Sympto-Thermal Method of NFP without further counseling after two or three cycles of experience. They tend to settle down with just a couple of the rules instead of using all the options. In other words, for their cycle-to-cycle use of NFP, they really could write the rules they use on both sides of a business card as we did in the "Introduction."

To be sure, once in a while you may have a strange looking chart, and that's why our volunteer teachers give you their telephone number. Write their phone number in your manual so you don't lose it. If you run into something out of the ordinary, call your teachers. Keep in mind that their professional training is mostly about applying the standard rules in out of the ordinary situations. However, the main point is this: most of the time you will have normal cycles, and you will find it very easy to apply the rules of NFP.

We are not saying that it is always easy to practice chaste abstinence. Ordinarily, however, the amount of abstinence is generally less than the abstinence practiced by many Orthodox Jews for around 3,000 years.

Write your Teaching Couple's name and phone number on the copyright page of this manual.

Leviticus 15:19 called for abstinence for seven days during menstruation; in addition, Leviticus 15:28 was frequently interpreted as adding an additional seven days. We understand that while the actual interpretation is left up to individual rabbis, it has been a common practice to have the couple resuming relations after 12 to 14 days of abstinence—at the most fertile time of the cycle. This part of the Jewish Law appears to have been designed to build up the children of Abraham as fast as possible.

"Ecology" has to do with interrelationships in nature. The term came into common use in the 1960s when people began to realize that the run-off of farmland chemicals was having devastating effects on wildlife. They began to realize that the application of scientific knowledge to one problem could upset the balance of nature and create other and greater problems.

If there's a difference between "ecology" and "environment," it is this: "ecology" tends to mean specific relationships while "environment" tends to refer to the big picture.

At any rate, if you want to live with nature and if you believe that nature has the last word, you have one more excellent reason for using only the natural methods of spacing babies. If someone is concerned about eating healthy foods, wouldn't it be highly inconsistent for her to be polluting her body with powerful birth control chemicals? If someone is concerned about the lives of trees and birds and baby seals, shouldn't he or she be much more concerned about the lives of human babies still within their mothers' wombs?

A sentence that borrows from the language of baseball says it all: "Nature bats last."

Note also that long lasting solutions to basic ecological and environmental problems depend upon people like you and us practicing self-control—such as not wasting water and other natural resources, recycling, not dumping chemicals on the ground, and so forth. The acceptance of self-control as the key to solving problems of ecology and the environment should help us to accept the role of self-control in dealing with any problems of population—whether in our own homes or in the bigger picture, whether those problems are real or imaginary.

Esthetic

Esthetics refers to the beauty or "pleasing-ness" of something. Natural family planning leaves the marital embrace in its natural beauty. On the other hand, contraceptive condoms, diaphragms, foams and jellies, and sponges have definite esthetic problems. They make it extremely obvious to the couple that they are interfering with the natural character of the act; some of them also interrupt a certain spontaneity of the spouses' lovemaking. Couples who are really serious about avoiding pregnancy with these methods use two or three of them together. Former users of these methods have told us that when they used a condom and a diaphragm with spermicidal jelly, they felt as if they were girding up for war, not love.

The Pill did not introduce birth control to the West. Almost all the early Sixties' users of the Pill were married couples who were tired of the barrier forms of contraception. Yet the Pill itself has an esthetic problem: it reduces sexual desire in 14% to 50% of women who use it.[3]

Inexpensive

When we were writing this in 1993-1994, women were paying $17.00 to $21.00 *per month* for the Pill, and the most used Pill was the most expensive. NFP is extremely inexpensive by comparison.

Lifelong

As you go through married life, you will go through different stages regarding your fertility. There may be times when you think the Lord is telling you that you should be postponing pregnancy; at other times, you may recognize that He is calling you to try to achieve pregnancy. After the birth of a baby, the way you feed your baby will have a tremendous impact on when

The combination of extended breastfeeding and no birth control chemicals is your best protection against breast cancer. (More in Chapter 24.)

your fertility returns. (Very briefly, "ecological breastfeeding" spaces babies on the average of two years apart without any fertility awareness or periodic abstinence. More about that in Chapters 23 - 25.) Eventually you will reach the time of decreasing fertility called *pre*-menopause, and then menopause when you stop ovulating. Natural family planning is there to help you in each stage of your fertile lifetime.

In addition, the combination of extended ecological breastfeeding and not using birth control hormones is your best protection against breast cancer. The combination of using NFP and not resorting to tubal sterilization is your best hope for entering your menopausal years with healthy female organs. And your female organs **are** important beyond your child-bearing years.[4]

Reversibility

Natural family planning is immediately reversible. You simply change your timing to change from postponing to achieving pregnancy. This is truly the Lord's way.

On the other hand, the Pill manufacturers warn against seeking pregnancy for three months after stopping the Pill. (They don't want lawsuits alleging birth defects due to using their birth control chemicals.) And we wish you could read the letters that come our way from couples who seriously regret their previous decision to have a tubal ligation or vasectomy! (See these topics in Section II of this chapter.)

Variety

Natural family planning is not just one method. There are two basic "methods" for spacing babies. One is ecological breastfeeding. It doesn't require any fertility awareness or periodic abstinence. Instead it generally provides months and months of breastfeeding infertility; on the average it spaces babies about two years apart.

The other method is periodic abstinence. Within this overall method, you can use different systems (even though they are called "methods") to identify the fertile time.

Section II: The Unnatural Methods — Why Not to Use Them

The term "Unnatural Methods" covers a wide variety of methods and practices. By the way, we didn't invent the phrase. In the early part of the 20th century, the bishops of the Church of England used the term "unnatural methods" for contraceptive behaviors.

The most fundamental reason not to use unnatural forms of birth control is that it is immoral to use any unnatural form of birth control. Why such actions are wrong is the subject of Chapters 18 and 19. Here we simply affirm that such actions are against the nature of the human person as God has created us and against the nature of the marital embrace that God has given us.

"Ha!" some will say. "There they go, dragging God into the picture. I just want hard facts." We will deliver them.

You may think we are stretching the point; what person reading this book or taking a course on Natural Family Planning would ever consider using abortion for birth control? We wish there were none, but we remember the experience of one of our girls in a religion class at a Catholic high school. The subject of the day was abortion. The teacher made her case against it. There was discussion. The teacher finished the case for respecting human life, and she asked how many of the students were against abortion. All raised their hands. Then she described a difficult situation; the unplanned pregnancy would interfere with the expectant mother's career plans. She asked, "How many of you would have an abortion in this case?" Almost half the class raised their hands in the affirmative! She should have told them that they needed to repent and to confess the sin of murder, but she said nothing.

The reality is that in the United States 26.4% of abortions are committed by married women.[5] Some may use abortion as their primary form of birth control. However, most have relied on one of the unnatural forms of birth control, experienced an unplanned pregnancy, and then resorted to abortion as "backstop" birth control.

The reality is that 35% of abortions in the United States are committed by women between the ages of 20 and 24, and another 19% by women aged 25-29.[6] That's a little over half. Young women who have their eyes on a career or higher education may be particularly tempted to kill their unborn babies, and the women who read this manual are not exempt from the temptations of our day.

● Risks to health and life

Some women die in the process of having a licensed physician kill their babies in what is called "safe and legal" abortion. Other women suffer medical complications which they may notice either immediately or later. For example, if the abortionist perforates a woman's uterus or does something else to cause significant bleeding or infection, she will know it right away, and without emergency medical treatment she may die. On the other hand, the damage done by the abortionist may not be evident at the time. However, its healing may leave so much scar tissue that she will be unable to conceive or carry a baby when she wants to.

Abortion increases the risk of **breast cancer**. "Over 20 studies indicate that women who abort their first pregnancy have a much higher risk . . . almost double. . . of developing cancer. . . With 2 or more abortions, there is a 3-4 fold increase."[7]

● Psychological damage

It's called "post-abortion syndrome." The tough and hard teenager matures and develops a conscience. The girl who was more or less forced by her parents to kill her baby cannot be forced by them to forget her child. The young woman who was lied to about a "blob of tissue" comes to recognize how she was deceived by others—or how she deceived herself. She comes to realize that she killed her baby. The career woman starts asking herself, "Why?"

Each year thereafter as she sees children about the age her child would be, she wonders what her child would have been like, what talents he or she would have developed, what sort of love they might have exchanged.

The psychological damage done by abortion is so widespread that a national organization has developed for women to help each other and to witness to the evil of abortion. For further information, contact WEBA (Women Exploited by Abortion) listed in "Resources."

Why not use the Pill?

We cannot understand why any well-informed woman would ever use the Pill, Norplant or Depo-Provera.

Entire books have been written on why not to use the Pill.[8] In 1993 the Couple to Couple League published a 64-reference pamphlet on the Pill that we will be happy to share with you. (Just send a self-addressed stamped business-size envelope, and we'll send it free. If you do not send a SASE, we have to use time and stationery, so please send a minimum of two dollars and we'll send you three copies. Be sure to ask for "The Pill" by Paul Weckenbrock.)

Without repeating all the detail, we can say that the evidence is strong that the Pill increases your risk of **breast cancer.** One study found that Swedish women who took the Pill in the 1960s had a five times greater rate of breast cancer than non-users.[9]

In the scientific community almost everyone agrees that there's a statistical link between the Pill and **cervical cancer.** However, the picture is clouded because cervical cancer is also linked with several other factors. These include beginning sexual intercourse at an early age, having multiple sexual partners, smoking cigarettes, the hygiene of her sexual partners, and the transmission of the human papillomavirus. At the same time, almost everyone admits that the Pill has contributed enormously to sexual promiscuity among young women, thus increasing the likelihood of fornicating early in life and with multiple partners.

Liver tumors in younger women (15 to 40) were almost unheard of before the common use of the Pill. In the mid-Eighties, a study by the American College of Surgeons' Commission on Cancer found "a large peak in the 26-to-30-year age group which corresponds with the increased use of oral contraceptives in this age group."[10]

Blood clotting defects are the most common source of problems caused by the Pill; women using the Pill have a 3 to 11 times increased risk of developing blood clots.[11] A blood clot in the brain can cause a stroke; in the heart it can cause a heart attack; in the lungs it is called a pulmonary embolism and can be fatal. In the arteries serving the eye, it is called a retinal thrombosis and can cause loss of vision and even total blindness.

The risk of fatal **heart attacks** is approximately twice as great among users of the current low-dose Pill compared to non-users.[12] The risk of a fatal **brain hemorrhage** is 1.4 times higher among Pill users than among non-users. Among women who smoke and use the Pill, there's a 12-fold increase in fatal heart attacks and a 3.1-fold increase in fatal brain hemorrhage.[13]

There are a number of other side effects, some minor, some more severe. Here's a partial list.

> Headaches, migraines, mental depression (even to the point of suicide and/or suicidal tendencies), a decrease or loss of sexual drive, abdominal cramps, bloating, weight gain or loss, and water retention; nausea and vomiting (in about 10% of users); symptoms of PMS, vaginitis and vaginal infections, changes in vision (temporary or permanent blindness, and an intolerance to contact lenses); gall bladder disease: and either temporary or permanent infertility, when discontinuing the Pill, in users with previous menstrual irregularities or who began the drug before full maturity. . . Consult the *Physicians' Desk Reference* at your public library or consult with your pharmacist for a more complete list of the Pill's harmful effects.[14]

Quite frankly, we cannot understand why any informed woman would ever take the Pill for birth control — or for any reason. We cannot understand why any husband who loves his wife and understands the health hazards of the Pill would allow his wife to use it if he has anything to say about it.

Sure, you might never get hit badly by the Pill. Then again, you could be like the 1963 Miss America, Jackie Townsend. Everything was going her way. Then it happened at age 28. According to the *Washington Post*:

> It was the morning after Thanksgiving 1970 when the fairy-tale bubble of Townsend's existence burst. She'd had a stroke doctors believed was induced by a single month on the Pill. (Her suit against the drug manufacturer was settled out of court.)[15]

● Abortifacient properties of the Pill

Every form of chemical birth control has the power to cause early abortions. This applies to every form of the Pill, to implants such as Norplant, and to injections such as Depo-Provera.

Some cause more early abortions than others. For example, the **RU-486** drug is openly touted as an abortion pill.

The abortifacient properties of the progestin-only (or progestogen-only) **mini-Pill** are openly admitted. According to the FDA,

> The primary mechanism through which [the progestogen-only pill] prevents conception is not known, but progestogen-only contraceptives are known to alter the cervical mucus, exert a progestational effect on the endometrium, interfering with implantation, and in some patients, suppress ovulation.[16]

Practical experience has demonstrated that even though cervical mucus is thickened by progesterone, coitus on days of less-fertile, thick mucus close to ovulation can still cause pregnancy. Therefore, in plain language the above FDA statement means that the mini-Pill rarely suppresses ovulation. The primary birth control action of the mini-Pill is to shrivel up the inner lining of the uterus so that a newly conceived baby cannot implant.

Scientists have known since 1957 that the **combined Pill** (synthetic estrogen and progesterone) has a triple threat mechanism for birth control: 1) it suppresses ovulation, 2) it thickens cervical mucus which renders sperm migration more difficult, and 3) it changes the endometrium to make it hostile to implantation. Today, we know that the Pill also affects the Fallopian tubes and the corpus luteum in ways which help its abortifacient potential.

The number of early abortions caused by hormonal birth control may well exceed the number of surgical abortions each year.

Interestingly, pro-abortion organizations have no hesitancy about admitting the abortifacient potential of the Pill. For example, one pro-abortion organization advertised that a Human Life Amendment would ban IUDs (probably true) and the Pill (probably false because its actions are more ambiguous). The people who have trouble admitting the abortifacient potential of the Pill are doctors who prescribe the Pill but call themselves pro-life.

The reality is that although the combined Pill probably suppresses ovulation in 95% of cycles, a tremendous number of early abortions can occur among that other 5%. A "breakthrough ovulation" rate of 4.7% was reported in 1984.[17] Applying that rate to the 13.8 million American women on the Pill in the early 1990s would yield 648,000 ovulations *per cycle*. However, not every ovulation results in pregnancy. The probability of conception occurring for a couple not using anti-conception devices (condom, diaphragm, and spermicides) is at least 25%[18] in any given cycle among normally fertile couples of average sexual activity, and it ranges up to 68% for couples who have relations every day during the fertile time.[19] Let's use the lower rate of 25%. That means that those 648,000 ovulations would result in 162,150 new human lives conceived each cycle. That's 1,945,800 each year, almost all of whom would be denied implantation and thus be aborted. That exceeds the annual number of surgical abortions in the United States.

Back in the 1960s, breakthrough ovulation rates were estimated between 2% and 10%. Even if you use the lowest estimated rate (which we think is probably too low considering the lower dosages and the mini-Pill) you will still calculate over 800,000 early abortions from the Pill alone, about half as many as from surgical abortion in the United States.

Let's try to put this in perspective. Imagine a computerized "Russian roulette" pistol that would fire a live bullet only 2 out of every 100 trigger-pulls—on the average. However, it could be the first pull or it could be the hundredth. Would you fire such a pistol at your spouse? at your baby? If it went off, would you not expect to be convicted of murder or manslaughter? Would you expect a jury to accept your argument that most of the time your playing Russian roulette this way didn't hurt anyone? In a similar way, the moral judgment of the Pill must be that it is an abortifacient. It has the potential to cause an early abortion in any woman in any cycle even though it may suppress ovulation most of the time. This holds true even when the Pill is prescribed as medicine to relieve a medical condition.

Why not use Norplant and Depo-Provera?

Norplant is a device implanted in a woman's body. Depo-Provera is a long-lasting injection. Both Norplant and Depo-Provera use the same or similar progestin that is used in both the combination Pill and the progestin-only Pill. (Progestin is a synthetic form of progesterone.) They carry the same risks of side effects caused by the progestin in the various forms of the Pill. They have the same abortifacient properties seen in the progestin-only mini-Pill. The big difference is the manner of delivery.

The Norplant chemical is delivered from several small tubes that are inserted in a woman's arm. It is more expensive and much more difficult to have these removed than to have them inserted; some women are left permanently scarred.

The delivery of Depo-Provera is by injection. Once the shot has been given, there is no turning back from all of its effects until the chemicals have been completely metabolized or broken down by the body. This takes a minimum of three months. According to reports, it takes from 4 to 31 months, with an average of 10 months, from the date of the last injection to the time when fertility returns and pregnancy can be achieved.[20, 21]

We think it is fair to say that these drugs were developed primarily for use on unwary teenagers and third-world women. How convenient for birth control clinics to insert tubes and tell a teenager she is safe and free to be as promiscuous as she cares to be because she can't get pregnant for three to five years! (How many teenagers would accept these drugs if they were told that women gain an average of 8.1 pounds after two years of such "treatment" and 13.8 pounds after four years?[22]) Pity the poor women in developing countries who are sometimes pressured into using various unnatural forms of birth control. They're much worse off than women in the developed countries because they don't have the medical support needed when they suffer the inevitable side effects. Heavy bleeding from a shot of Depo-Provera? "Too bad," say the birth controllers.

It is hard to believe that free Americans would use these things, but they do. Shortly after Depo-Provera went on the U.S. market (it was banned for years), we began to hear from women who wanted to switch from it to NFP. Certainly it can be done, but with the lasting effects of the injection, it may take some time before they experience normal cycles. The advantage of NFP that we called "Reversibility" takes on a whole new meaning considering the long lasting effects of these chemicals.

If you ever hear of anyone who is considering using these birth control chemicals, try to stop her. What we said at the end of the section above ("Why not use the Pill?") applies even more strongly to these.

● Risks to health and life

For the most part, the Intra-Uterine Device (IUD) has been taken off the market in the United States. Why? Enough women suffered damages to health and some lost their lives to infections caused by their IUDs. For example, the A. H. Robins Co. manufactured the Dalkon Shield, a supposedly safe IUD. In 1985, lawsuits for medical injuries caused by its IUD drove Robins into bankruptcy. Please note: the United States Food and Drug Administration fully approved that IUD. FDA approval obviously did not guarantee that women could use the device without serious risks to health and life.

> "Robins distributed about 4.5 million Dalkon Shields in the United States and abroad before taking the device off the market in 1974. Robins paid about $520 million to settle 9,400 of some 15,000 Dalkon Shield lawsuits before seeking bankruptcy protection." However, it was not until June 16, 1989, that a federal judge "approved the bankruptcy reorganization of A. H. Robins Co. including $2.5 billion for women who claim they were injured by the company's Dalkon Shield."[23]

A determined woman can still get an IUD in the United States, but she has to sign a legal document 12 times, releasing the manufacturer from all liability for any problems it may cause her.[24]

● Abortifacient actions

Since the mid-1970s, there has been general agreement that the primary action of the IUD is to prevent a newly conceived human life from implanting in the uterus.[25] When a drug or device prevents the implantation of a newly conceived human life, it has to be classified as an abortifacient, something causing an abortion.

However, in the late 1980s a challenge was raised. Did IUDs that give off chemicals operate in the same way? Or did they act more often to prevent conception instead of preventing implantation? The answer is not clear-cut, especially for those IUDs that give off copper ions or synthetic progesterone. Do IUDs kill sperm? A World Health Organization report inferred that IUDs kill some sperm—but not all. "Spermatozoa can migrate to the fallopian tubes in some cases but are less likely to reach the site of fertilization in the same numbers as in control women. The fertilizing capacity of these spermatozoa has not been determined."[26] The same report noted that some researchers have found human chorionic gonadotropin (hCG) in IUD users in the luteal phase of the cycle.[27] The hormone hCG is secreted by the very young embryo and is detectable as early as 9 days after ovulation.

One article argued for some sort of pre-conception effect, but it also noted this: "The finding of two eggs undergoing destruction by macrophages in women using a CopperT device" supported a different hypothesis. Translation: If those were *fertilized* eggs, the destruction would be an early abortion action.[28]

The conclusion is this. The only debate is whether the abortifacient action of the IUD is its *primary* method of operation. As the WHO report states, "It is unlikely that any single mechanism accounts for the antifertility effect of IUDs."[29] The weight of the evidence suggests that for *inert* IUDs—those are the ones that do not emit chemicals—the primary action remains abortifacient. The chemical producing IUDs may have some anti-sperm effects. However, there is no question that all IUDs may act as abortifacients anywhere from most of the time to at least some of the time. Therefore, the moral judgment has to be that the IUD is an abortifacient.

Why not use barrier methods?

The barrier methods are those which provide a physical or chemical barrier to prevent sperm from reaching the ovum. They include, in alphabetical order: cervical cap, condom-male, condom-female, diaphragm, foams and jellies, and sponge.

The *pragmatic* reasons for not using the various barrier methods are the same as those given by those who promoted the Pill back in the 1960s and even today.

1) Barrier methods are messy.

2) Barrier methods generally heighten the contraceptive intent right at the time of intercourse. Many spouses believe that marital intercourse is a gift of God, and barrier contraception makes it obvious that they are rejecting the natural consequences of that gift.

3) Most of them interfere with the natural progression of the marital embrace.

4) For some, condoms reduce the pleasure of the act.

5) All the barrier methods have problems with effectiveness.

These are the reasons or the experiences that motivated the mass migration from the barrier methods to the Pill in the early 1960s. However, research has discovered more serious problems.

Life and health. The most serious problem with barrier methods is an increased risk of miscarriage if pregnancy occurs. "Women who inadvertently become pregnant while using spermicidal contraceptives suffer about twice the rate of miscarriages in the first three months of pregnancy as other women, according to researchers at Temple University and the New Jersey School of Osteopathic Medicine."[30]

Another serious problem: spermicidal foams and jellies may cause **birth defects.** This allegation was made in the medical literature in 1981, challenged, and reaffirmed by those who made it.[31] In January 1985, "U.S. District Court Judge Marvin Shoob said Ortho Pharmaceutical Corp., which makes Ortho-Gynol Contraceptive Jelly, knew its product could cause birth defects and was negligent for not warning its users." The court awarded a judgment of $5,100,000 to the parents of an unplanned pregnancy child born with birth defects.[32]

Some spouses have **allergic reactions**, ranging from mild to serious, to the latex used in condoms[33] and to the chemicals used in spermicidal foams and jellies. Some women may suffer toxic shock syndrome from the sponge if they leave it in place too long. Diaphragms may increase the risk of urinary tract infections due to the pressure they put on the bladder when they are left in place too long.

Here's another indication that Nature has the last word: "Women who rely on birth control methods, such as condoms and diaphragms, that prevent semen from reaching the uterus are more than twice as likely to develop one of the most serious complications of pregnancy as are their counterparts who had been repeatedly exposed to sperm from the prospective father."[34] The complication is called **preeclampsia** or "toxemia of pregnancy" and "is the third-ranking cause of pregnancy-related death, following infection and hemorrhage."

The University of North Carolina research group found that repeated exposure to the sperm of her husband helped to prime the mother's immune system. Without this exposure, according to that research group, a woman tends to develop a reaction against her own baby in the uterus. However, certain proteins in the husband's semen signal the woman's body to produce antibodies that do not attack the fetus but instead protect the fetus from antibody attack and perhaps even stimulate certain cells in the fetus to grow. Lastly, "The researchers stressed that the results of their studies apply only to repeated exposure to semen from the father of the fetus, not from other men."

The practice of withdrawal has been known since the beginning of recorded biblical history. It was the infamous "sin of Onan" described in Genesis 38:6-10. "And what he did was displeasing in the sight of the Lord, and He slew him also" (v.10). From a practical point of view, it has some problems with effectiveness, and some practitioners find it frustrating.

The "etc." (in the sidebar heading) refers to anal and oral copulation. When we wrote the first edition of this book in 1972, it didn't even cross our minds to mention sexual perversities. However, over the years, some books dealing with sexuality have openly recommended anal and oral copulation as substitutes for natural marital relations. When these acts are performed by homosexuals, they are called sodomy. When performed by spouses, they are called marital sodomy.

From a strictly practical viewpoint, they are as unhealthy for spouses as they are for homosexuals. Anal copulation is highly unsanitary, and the rectal tissues tear and bleed easily. The rectum was never intended for such purposes. Oral copulation may be less unsanitary, but it can quickly transfer genital infections to the mouth. Furthermore, many, and perhaps most, women find it psychologically demeaning. This is "kinky sex," the sort of thing for which some men pay prostitutes. However, we suspect that most wives want to be full partners in the marital embrace, not vehicles for kinky sex. They want love, and kinky sex is lust.

We are not writing about oral-genital contact that is foreplay to the normal marriage act. However, such contact still carries the possibility of transferring infections from mouth to genitalia and vice versa.

There are two kinds of sexual sterilization: tubal ligation for women and vasectomy for men. There are two very practical reasons not to get sterilized: risks to health and life, and unwanted permanence.

● Post-tubal ligation syndrome
The health problems of tubal ligations are so common that doctors have a new phrase: "post-tubal ligation syndrome." A syndrome isn't a disease by itself; rather, it's a combination of various troublesome signs that are associated with a disorder. This syndrome is not at all uncommon. Two authors described their review of the medical literature: "The incidence of complications was 22% to 37%, with symptoms of dysfunctional uterine bleeding, dysmenorrhea [painful periods], dyspareunia [pain during intercourse] and pelvic pain. This group of symptoms has been called the post-tubal-ligation or post-sterilization syndrome."[35]

To bring that rather sophisticated language down to earth, read the following letter a couple wrote us; it describes a variety of problems that acquaintances told them in casual conversations.

> We have talked with five women who have been sterilized by tubal ligation within the last five years. They all suffer gynecological problems that were not present until after they had their tubals.
>
> Two of the women have been hospitalized; laparascopic exams revealed endometriosis. They both have heavy bleeding and severe cramping, and are being treated with medication that costs them $140 for a 90 day supply. The side effects from the medication has caused one of the women (age 32) to take several leaves of absence from her job. The second woman (age 25) has

to stay in bed because of nausea and sleepiness caused by the medication. Their doctors have told them a hysterectomy may be the only relief in sight.

Two other women complain about having more severe cramping at menstruation than before their tubals. They both freely admit having feelings of remorse over the thought of never having more children. Their ages: 24 and 31.

The fifth woman had a hysterectomy because of problems after the tubal and is still having complications. Her age: 32.[36]

And from a published autobiographical account:

Rollin was opposed to the ligation, but I had the so-called "band-aid" operation, anyway. ("It's my body and my decision," I had parroted.) No one else opposed this surgery at all, quite the opposite, in fact. The very first effect of this, as in an abortion, was relief. That relief didn't last long. Ensuing hormonal imbalance caused a deep, prolonged depression. In fact, as I later learned, my estrogen level dropped to a menopausal level, literally overnight. I gained a lot of weight in a very short time, another common side effect. My mind was confused; and I was filled with irrational resentment. There was abdominal pain for months after the surgery, probably caused by the nitrous oxide gas that was used to inflate my abdomen for surgery. Periods became so heavy that twice I was hospitalized for excessive hemorrhaging, another common but seldom publicized side-effect. At the age of thirty, I was forced by deteriorating health to have a hysterectomy.[37]

Women, don't ever have your tubes tied! The odds are extremely low that you will die on the operating table, but there is a good possibility you'll have increased "female problems."

That sort of reporting is called "anecdotal" and is sometimes scoffed at by medical professionals. However, those personal stories are confirmed by professional observation and by studies. Vicki Hufnagel, a Los Angeles obstetrician-gynecologist, has written that she rarely performs tubal ligations anymore because of the suffering she has seen in women who have had them. "My patients have to fight me for this form of birth control and fight hard."[38] According to Hufnagel,

Three theories explain why these problems occur:
1. Tubal ligation destroys the blood supply to the ovaries.
2. Certain types of tubal sterilization procedures are more likely to result in endometriosis.
3. An increase in the blood pressure within the ovarian artery can create an estrogen-progesterone imbalance.[39]

Hufnagel is an ardent opponent of unnecessary hysterectomy as is indicated by the title of her book, *No More Hysterectomies*. She opposes tubal ligation because the result may be a hysterectomy—which has its own serious problems, both short term and long term.

● Ectopic pregnancies

An ectopic pregnancy is one in which the newly conceived human life takes up residence in the fallopian tube (and very rarely someplace else like the ovary or the abdomen). A tubal pregnancy is always fatal for the developing baby; if the tube ruptures, the bleeding can be fatal to the mother if it is not controlled. The woman who has a tubal ligation and later becomes pregnant has a much higher chance of having an ectopic pregnancy than if she had not been sterilized. Why? The microscopic-sized sperm manage to get by the place where the fallopian tube was blocked, but the much larger conceptus cannot do so.

How often does this occur? Pregnancies after a tubal ligation are rare, but they occur often enough so that statistics on post-tubal ectopic pregnancies are available. "The rate of ectopic pregnancies in sterilized women ranges from 4% to 64% of pregnancies, depending upon the procedure used."[40] The ectopic rate among non-sterilized women is only 0.5% to 1% of pregnancies.[41] The electro-coagulation technique, popular because it can be done by laparoscopy, appears to have about a 50% ectopic rate when pregnancies occur.[42] In addition, the risk of a tubal pregnancy is higher than normal after tubal reversal surgery.

● Premenstrual Syndrome (PMS)

According to Dr. Katharina Dalton, a pioneer researcher into the causes of PMS, "Premenstrual syndrome often increases in intensity following tubal ligation."[43] This is most likely because tubal ligation reduces a woman's level of progesterone. "The average progesterone value of the tubal ligation group was significantly lower than that of a control group."[44]

● Delayed reactions

If your friend or relative has recently had a tubal ligation and is telling you that everything is just fine, wish her good luck. There is good evidence that many of the women who will suffer from the post-tubal-ligation syndrome may not experience the bad effects until two years or more after being sterilized. "At follow-up intervals longer than 2 years, the tubal sterilization group had significantly increased risks of abnormal menstrual cycles and combinations of two or more adverse menstrual outcomes."[45] The longer the follow-up on sterilized women, the higher the rates of problems. M.V. Muldoon reported that of 374 patients who were followed for at least 10 years after tubal ligation, 43% needed further gynecological treatment and 25% had major gynecological surgery [read hysterectomy].[46]

● Risks from the surgery itself

Tubal ligation surgery is not risk free. H.P. Dunn, M.D., has noted that "every operation carries the risk of hemorrhage or infection. Sterilization by laparoscopy involves blowing up the abdominal cavity with nitrous oxide gas, introducing a small telescope, and dividing the tubes with diathermy [cauterization by heat]. Some patients have died from cardiac failure during the inflation procedure. Others have suffered wounds of the bowel, bladder, and large blood vessels. Even intra-abdominal explosions have occurred." He also notes that "the 14 days after childbirth are the worst, not the best, time to have any operation."[47] Dr. Dunn repeated these same warnings in a more extended format 15 years later.[48]

● Unwanted permanence

For all practical purposes, the woman who has her tubes tied has to consider that she is permanently sterile. This doesn't mean that there isn't any hope at all that she cannot have it reversed. However, it would be completely irresponsible for anyone to suggest that she could have a tubal ligation and then have her fertility restored with certainty. A number of physicians do reversal surgery, but it is difficult and expensive. Success cannot be guaranteed. However, if this applies to you, you can check out the pregnancy-achieving success rate of different physicians who perform this surgery. We have heard of at least one surgeon who will waive his personal fee, but there are still operating room costs, etc. You can write our office for a list of physicians who have been recommended for this service.

● Psychological effects

Back in the Sixties, a Californian who knew his ethnic community well warned us about sterilization. He told us that he had never known a family in which one of the spouses had been sterilized that didn't start to fall apart. The author of the personal account of her sterilization and subsequent hysterectomy related above continues:

> Thereafter, Rollin and I seldom talked about the operation or what had led up to it. We seldom talked at all. We became very touchy about "slights"; we were impatient and sometimes rude to each other; we were often filled with self-pity. Despite a steady and comfortable income, we quarreled constantly about money. We became stressed and tense. Our fears for the children's safety became exaggerated to the point of panic; we were terrified that we would lose one of these precious, irreplaceable lives. We lost our sense of humor and seemed to bicker over everything. He began to lose respect for me and I for him. Aversion to intimacy began to develop. Life became a horrid burden to us both, each secretly resenting and blaming the other.

By the way, the preceding couple did manage to get things worked out but only after much pain and a profound religious conversion.

Women, don't ever get your tubes tied! The odds are extremely low that you will die on the operating table, but there are very good odds that you will have increased problems as previously discussed. Beware of the pressure that some doctors will put on you to have a tubal ligation. They may even argue that it's better for you to risk the post-tubal problems than for your husband to get sterilized—because vasectomy is linked to prostate cancer which can kill him while a tubal ligation may leave you merely miserable!

Why not have a vasectomy?

Probably no method of birth control has been promoted as so safe, so simple, so permanent, so risk-free as vasectomy. Medical columnists in the daily papers have regularly assured the general public about the safety of vasectomy. And how simple! Just make a little incision in the scrotum and cut the vas deferens, the tube that carries sperm to the prostate gland where it would normally mix with other fluids for ejaculation.

Critics were ignored. Dr. H.J. Roberts, an award winning specialist in internal medicine, tried to blow the whistle in 1968. In men only in their 20s and 30s he was finding medical problems generally associated only with older men, and among these young men, the "only common denominator was vasectomy."[50] These problems included "unexplained thrombophlebitis, prolonged fever, generalized lymph node enlargement . . . recurrent infection, various skin eruptions, acute multiple sclerosis, [and] liver dysfunction. . ."[51] In 1979 he published an entire book on the subject, *Is Vasectomy Safe?*, because of his concern that vasectomy causes all sorts of medical problems. At least some of these are related to the fact that vasectomy may affect a man's autoimmune system.[52] Undeterred by what he calls "Vasectogate: the information blackout," Dr. Roberts published a second and much shorter book that is apparently getting much better response.[53]

● Prostate cancer

Two studies published in 1993 in the *Journal of the American Medical Association* brought national attention to the health problems of vasectomy. Both studies showed that vasectomy greatly increases the risk of developing prostate cancer. One study showed a 66% to 85% greater risk,[54] and the other showed the increased risk to run from 56% to 106%.[55] Interestingly, two other studies had been published in 1990 pointing out this danger. One showed increased risks of 1.7 times (70%) at any age and 2.2 times (120%) for men who had been sterilized for 13-18 years.[56] The second reported that the relative risk of prostate cancer ranged from 3.5 to 5.3 times that of the control groups.[57]

This was a big-time warning because prostate cancer is the second leading cause of men dying from cancer. The educated estimate is that 132,000 men were diagnosed with prostate cancer and 32,000 men died from it in 1991.[58] Apparently gone forever are the years when vasectomy was described as free of all known risks.

● Less dramatic effects

We think men ought to be just as concerned about the less dramatic potential damages to health that Dr. Roberts describes in his writings. After a vasectomy, the testicles continue to make millions of sperm each day, but they can't be released in the normal fashion during marital relations or nocturnal emission. Instead they enter the body by leakage. Once there, the body reacts as if the sperm were foreign bodies. This is called an auto-immune response, and about 50% of vasectomized men develop sperm antibodies. Dr. Roberts and others think that the effects on a man's immune system cause a host of problems though they do not claim definitive proof. This book is not the place to review these, but the headings in one chapter of his 1993 book indicate what Roberts and others have seen and think are (or may be) related to vasectomy: thrombophlebitis, pulmonary embolism, infection, arthopathy (arthritis), narcolepsy, multiple sclerosis, migraine and related headaches, hypoglycemia, allergic manifestations, emotional disturbances, impaired sexual function, kidney stones, angina pectoris and heart attack, tumors and cancer.[59]

We cannot settle a legitimate debate about whether vasectomy was a contributing cause in each case where linkage is suspected. However, we are very confident in saying that the more you investigate these matters, the more you will become convinced that once again nature has the last word. An editorial in the *British Medical Journal* put it this way:

> It is a sound guiding principle of surgery never to disturb the function of a normal structure except as may be necessary for the effective treatment of a related disorder. Consequently, whereas vasectomy may be appropriate in the treatment of an established urogenital disease to prevent the spread of infection, its performance in a healthy man for a purpose other than for the protection of his own health is difficult to reconcile with the traditions that normally guide clinical judgment.[60]

● Reversals

Reversals of vasectomies are possible. They are quite expensive, and the return of normal fertility cannot be guaranteed. Reversal effectiveness can vary significantly depending upon the damage done by the vasectomy physician and the skill of the reversal physician. Many insurance plans will pay for tubal ligations and vasectomies but will not pay for the reversals.

A few Christian physicians will waive their fees for vasectomy reversals. However, the patient must still pay the anesthesia and hospital fees. For a short list, send a self-addressed stamped business-size envelope to CCL requesting the vasectomy reversal list.

Summary

The Lord has made us in wonderful ways. Natural family planning is founded upon respect for the ways of the Lord. The unnatural methods of birth control are based on two erroneous assumptions: 1) that it is morally permissible to take apart what God has joined together in the marriage act and 2) that man knows nature better than God.

Each and every modern form of contraceptive birth control has come with the approval of the medical establishment with the promise that "this is perfectly safe." Each one of them—IUD, Pill, chemical implants and injections, tubal ligation and vasectomy—is a testimony to the ignorance and/or arrogance of those who have made such statements. The financial success of each of these indicates the gullibility of consumers who have believed that chemicals or a bit of surgery would solve basic human and marital problems.

The real answer to these problems is not a Pill but a Person, Jesus. To be sure, He never teaches that love is easy. Instead, He teaches that true love is the way of the daily cross (Lk 9:23). Countless millions have found that it is true that his yoke is easy and his burden is light, that He really does give you rest for your soul (Mt 11:29-30).

In short, to adopt again the slogan from American baseball, nature bats last. It is bad medical practice to contradict mother nature by performing surgery that has no health benefit but has significant risks. If you have truly serious reasons to avoid pregnancy—perhaps even life-threatening or health-threatening reasons, the sensible choice is NFP. Why compound existing problems by adopting unnatural methods of birth control which themselves can threaten both health and life?

When you are convinced that it would not be morally responsible for you to deliberately seek pregnancy (or at least you are convinced that the Lord is not calling you to seek pregnancy), the only moral answers are 1) complete abstinence or 2) natural family planning.

Additional readings

You will find additional information in the following brochures and booklet available from CCL.

"Dear Healthcare Provider"
"The Deadly After-Effect of Abortion: Breast Cancer"
"The Pill: How does it work? Is it safe?"
"Tubal Ligation: Some Questions and Answers"
"Vasectomy: Some Questions and Answers"
Birth Control and Christian Discipleship, pages 12-15

● Additional readings packet

All the brochures and booklets referred to here and at the end of other chapters are contained in the "Additional readings packet." See "Resources" at the end of the book to order the packet and other materials.

Self-Test Questions: Chapter 1

1. True_____ False_____   Every drug has potential side effects and should not be taken except to cure or relieve some disease or abnormality.

2. True_____ False_____   Fertility is a normal process, not a disease.

3. True_____ False_____   A woman can achieve a better sense of changes in her own health through the fertility awareness of NFP.

4. True_____ False_____   A study conducted by the U. S. Department of Health, Education and Welfare in the late 1970s found zero surprise pregnancies among couples who followed the rules for the Sympto-Thermal Method in that study.

5. Name the two basic methods of natural family planning:
   a)_____
   b)_____

6. The combination Pill (estrogen-progesterone) works in the following three ways to achieve its birth control effects:
   a)_____
   b)_____
   c)_____

7. Because every form of the Pill can be acting in any cycle to prevent the implantation of a week-old new human being in the uterus, it is called an _____.

8. The IUD has been mostly taken off the American market because the manufacturers fear

   _____.

9. A conservative estimate of the number of early abortions from the Pill each year is
   _____ in the United States alone.

10. True_____ False_____   A woman can learn to observe and understand her natural signs of fertility and infertility while using the Pill.

11. True_____ False_____   There are no risks to health associated with the barrier devices and chemicals.

12. The combination of the problems associated with tubal ligations is called _____
    _____ _____.

13. Several studies have shown men who have a vasectomy have a significantly higher risk of developing _____ cancer.

14. What slogan adapted from baseball applies well to the many problems associated with the attempts to destroy personal fertility? _____

Answers to self-test
1. True   2. True   3. True   4. True   5. a) Ecological breastfeeding b) periodic abstinence   6. a) to suppress ovulation b) to thicken cervical mucus c) to deny implantation of the new life in the uterine wall   7. abortifacient   8. lawsuits related to damages to health   9. 1,945,800   10. False   11. False   12. post-tubal ligation syndrome   13. prostate   14. Nature bats last.

References

(1) Maclyn E. Wade, Phyllis McCarthy, et al., "A random prospective study of the use-effectiveness of two methods of natural family planning," *Am. J. Ob and Gyn* 141:4 (15 Oct 1981) 368-376.

(2) Wade, 374.

(3) J.W. Long, M.D., *The Essential Guide to Prescription Drugs* (New York: Harper and Row, 1990) 719.

(4) See Vicki Hufnagel, M.D., *No More Hysterectomies* (New York: Penguin, 1989) for a strong case for keeping the female organs and their contribution to postmenopausal health. Hufnagel is apparently unacquainted with NFP, but she opposes sterilization because of its unhappy effects known generally as the post-tubal ligation syndrome.

(5) Andrew Hacker, *U/S: a statistical portrait of the American people* (New York: Viking, 1983) 63. The statistic is based on reports from 31 states reporting marital status of women having abortions.

(6) Hacker, 63. Statistic is based on 37 states reporting age of aborting women.

(7) J.C. Willke, M.D., *The Deadly After-Effect of Abortion: Breast Cancer* (Cincinnati: Hayes Publishing, 1993) brochure.

(8) For example: Morton Mintz, *The Pill: An Alarming Report* (Boston: Beacon Press, 1970); Natalie S. Greenfield, *"First Do No Harm . . .": A dying woman's battle against the physicians and drug companies who misled her about the hazards of THE PILL* (New York: Two Continents Publishing, 1976); Barbara Seaman and Gideon Seaman, M.D., *Women and the Crisis in Sex Hormones* (New York: Rawson, 1977) chapter 7-11.

(9) Olsson H., Borg A., Femo M., Moller T.R., Ranstam J., "Early oral contraceptive use and premenopausal breast cancer—A review of studies performed in Southern Sweden," *Cancer Detection Prevention* 15:4 (1991) 265-271.

(10) K. Hume, "The Pill and Cancer," *Linacre Quarterly,* 52:4 (1985) 305-306.

(11) "Demulen," *Physicians' Desk Reference,* (1993) 2254.

(12) M. Thorogood, J. Mann, M. Murphy, M. Vessey, "Is oral contraceptive use still associated with an increased risk of fatal myocardial infarction? Report of a case-control study," *Br J Ob Gy,* 98 (1991) 1245-1253.

(13) Thorogood, M., Vessey, M., (1990). An epidemiologic survey of cardiovascular disease in women taking oral contraceptives. *Am J Obstet Gynecol* 163 (1) pt 2, 274-281.

(14) Paul Weckenbrock, *The Pill: How does it Work? Is it Safe?* (Cincinnati: Couple to Couple League, 1993) 8.

(15) Sandy Rovner, "Healthtalk: Here she is, heart to heart," *The Washington Post,* 7 May 1982, D5.

(16) Food and Drug Administration, "Oral Contraceptive Drug Products," *Federal Register* 43:21 (31 January 1978) 4224.

(17) "We are close to lowest steroid dosage in the Pill," *News and Views,* 30 November 1984. Excerpts from the second annual meeting of the Society for the Advancement of Contraception, Jakarta; ed. W. Korteling (West Orange, NJ: Organon International).

(18) C. Tietze, "Differential fecundity and effectiveness of contraception," *Eugenics Review* 50 (1959) 231. Thirty percent of couples discontinuing contraception achieved pregnancy in the very first cycle thereafter. Cited in C. Tietze, "Probability of pregnancy resulting from a single unprotected coitus," *Fertility and Sterility* (1960) 485-488.

(19) J.C. Barrett and J. Marshall, "The risk of conception on different days of the menstrual cycle," *Population Studies* 23 (1959) 455-461. The authors calculated the probabilities of conception based on coital frequency as follows: once per week = .14;; every sixth day = .17; every fifth day = .20; every fourth day = .24; every third day = .31; every second day = .43; and every day = .68.

(20) R.A. Hatcher et al., *Contraceptive Technology 1990-1992,* 15th rev. ed. (New York: Irvington, 1990) 327.

(21) "Medroxyprogesterone contraceptive injection," *Facts and Comparisons* (St. Louis: Facts and Comparisons, January 1993 insert), 108o.

(22) *Facts and Comparisons,* Weight changes, 108o.

(23) "Robins plan gets court OK," 17 June 1989, *The Cincinnati Post,* 6B.

(24) Alza Corporation, *Progestasert® Patient Information* (1987).

(25) Thomas W. Hilgers, M.D., "The Intrauterine Device: Contraceptive or Abortifacient?" *Marriage and Family Newsletter,* 5:1, 2, 3 (January-March 1974). Hilgers did this research paper with 129 references while a resident on Obstetrics and Gynecology, Mayo Graduate School of Medicine (University of Minnesota), Rochester, Minnesota. At the time of his research, the chemical releasing IUDs were too new to have been the subject of much research, so Hilgers studied the research on inert IUDs. He specifically noted the research of those who found that the presence of an IUD "does not prevent the ascent of sperm to the site of fertilization" and that "no one has described contrary results"(9). Further, "There is no evidence that the IUD consistently prevents fertilization"(9). His conclusion: "In light of current, accepted medical definitions of contraception, abortifacient, pregnancy, conception and abortion, the conclusion is that the primary action of the IUD must be classed as abortifacient."

(26) World Health Organization Scientific Group, *Mechanism of action, safety and efficacy of intrauterine devices* (Geneva: WHO, 1987) WHO Technical Report Series, Number 753.

(27) WHO, 15.

(28) Frank Alvarez, M.D., et al., "New insights on the mode of action of intrauterine contraception devices in women," *Fertility and Sterility* 49:5 (May 1988) 770.

(29) WHO, 68.

(30) *The Cincinnati Enquirer,* 24 November 1983, E-2. The newspaper story reported an article in a current issue of *Family Planning Perspectives,* a Planned Parenthood publication.

(31) Hershel Jick, A.M. Walker, et al., "Vaginal spermicides and congenital disorders," *JAMA* 245:13 (3 April 1981) 1329-1332.

(32) *The Cincinnati Enquirer,* 23 January 1985, A-2.

(33) Joyce Price, "Condoms can also be hazardous to health," *The Washington Times* 1 November 1989. Reports an article by James S. Taylor, M.D. in *Journal of the American Academy of Dermatology* (November 1989) about severe allergic reactions to the latex in condoms and gloves.

(34) William Booth, "Pregnancy disorder tied to condoms, diaphragms," *Washington Post* (8 December 1989) A-3. Reports on the work of Hillary Klonoff-Cohen described in *JAMA,* 8 December 1989.

(35) Joel T. Hargrove and Guy E. Abraham, "Endocrine profile of patients with post-tubal-ligation syndrome," *Journal of Reproductive Medicine* 26:7 (1981) 359.

(36) G. and K. Folzenlogen, personal correspondence, 30 October 1987. Edited slightly for brevity.

(37) Ruth D. Lasseter, "Sensible Sex," *Why Humanae Vitae was Right: A Reader*, ed. Janet Smith (San Francisco: Ignatius Press, 1993) 488. First appeared in *Homiletic and Pastoral Review* 92:11 (Aug-Sept 1992) 19-31.

(38) Hufnagel, 228.

(39) Hufnagel, 228.

(40) Hatcher, R.A., et al., *Contraceptive Technology 1990-1992*, 15th rev. ed. (New York: Irvington, 1990) 402.

(41) Hatcher, 403.

(42) Hatcher, 403.

(43) Katherine Dalton, *Once a Month: the original premenstrual syndrome handbook* (Claremont CA: Hunter House, 1990) 33, 110.

(44) Frank Alvarz-Sanchez, Sheldon J. Segal, et al., "Pituitary-ovarian function after tubal ligation," *Fertility and Sterility* 36:5 (Nov. 1981) 607, reporting on the research done by Radwanska, Berger and Hammong, *Obstet Gynecol* 54:189, 1979.

(45) Frank DeStefano, Jeffrey A. Perlman, Herbert B. Peterson, and Earl L. Diamond, "Long-term risk of menstrual disturbances after tubal sterilization," *Am J Obstet Gynecol* 152 (1985) 835.

(46) M.J. Muldoon, "Gynaecological illness after sterilization," *British Medical Journal* (8 Jan 1972) 84-85.

(47) H.P. Dunn, "Unexpected sequellae of sterilization," *International Review of Natural Family Planning* 1:4 (Winter 1977) 318.

(48) H.P. Dunn, M.D., *The Doctor and Christian Marriage* (New York: Alba House, 1992) 84-85.

(49) Lasseter, 488.

(50) H.J. Roberts, "Voluntary sterilization in the male," *British Medical Journal* (17 August 1968) 434.

(51) Roberts, 434.

(52) H.J. Roberts, *Is Vasectomy Safe: Medical, Public Health, and Legal Implications* (West Palm Beach: Sunshine Academic Press, 1979) 95.

(53) H.J. Roberts, *Is Vasectomy Worth the Risk? A Physician's Case Against Vasectomania*, (West Palm Beach: Sunshine Sentinal Press, 1993) 19-31, plus personal correspondence dated 20 May 1993.

(54) Edward Giovannucci, Alberto Ascherio and four others, "A prospective cohort study of vasectomy and prostate cancer in US men," *JAMA* 269:7 (17 Feb 1993) 873.

(55) Giovannucci, 878.

(56) Curtis Mettlin, Nachimuthu Natarajan, and Robert Huben, "Vasectomy and prostate cancer risk," *Am Journal of Epidemiology* 132:6 (1990) 1056.

(57) Lynn Rosenberg, Julie R. Palmer, and four others, "Vasectomy and the risk of prostate cancer," *Am Journal of Epidemiology* 132:6 (1990) 1051. The relative risk of prostate cancer was 3.5 times that of a cancer control group and 5.3 times that of a non-cancer control group.

(58) Giovannucci, 873.

(59) Roberts, (1993) "Some observed medical problems after vasectomy," 53-72.

(60) Editorial, "Sterilization in Man," *British Medical Journal* 1 (1966) 1554.

2

Getting Started with Temperatures

In this chapter you will learn how to take and record your waking temperature. In Chapter 5 you will learn how to interpret your temperature pattern. You can learn **why** your waking temperature goes up after ovulation in Chapter 9 dealing with hormones and your fertility. If you want to know more about your entire menstrual-fertility cycle at any time in these early lessons, feel free to jump ahead to Chapter 9 and then return.

The method of Natural Family Planning that you are learning is called the "Sympto-Thermal Method"—abbreviated as STM. The "sympto" refers to the fertility signs you get from your cervix and cervical mucus. The "thermal" refers to fertility signs you get from changes in your waking temperature.

Right now we want to give you a very brief overview of what you will learn in Chapter 9. Your menstrual-fertility cycle is controlled by chemical signals called hormones; these are secreted by certain internal organs. The big event of every cycle is ovulation, the release of an egg from one of your ovaries. The hormone estrogen is dominant before ovulation; the hormone progesterone is dominant after ovulation. Estrogen causes your cervix to secrete a mucus discharge; it causes some physical changes in your cervix; and estrogen generally causes your waking body temperature to be a bit lower before ovulation. Progesterone causes your cervical mucus to dry up and disappear; it reverses the physical changes in the cervix; and progesterone causes your body temperature to go up after ovulation. On the average, your temperatures stay up for about two weeks after ovulation, and they generally start to come down just before or when your period starts.

Terminology

We will gradually introduce the special terms we use. Toward the back of the book, there is a "Glossary of Terms" that defines every technical word or phrase used in this book and in scientific talk about fertility. You can also use the Index to find where the terms are used.

Fertile time: The time of the female cycle when sexual intercourse can result in pregnancy.

Infertile time: The times of the cycle when pregnancy will not occur.

Phase I: The infertile time before ovulation.

Phase II: The fertile time before and immediately after ovulation.

Phase III: The infertile time after ovulation.

What does the temperature sign tell you?

Your body temperature rises slightly after ovulation. You take your waking temperature to get a positive, easily seen sign that tells you when you are in the infertile time after ovulation. It will take you a while to learn your mucus and cervix patterns, but in just a few minutes you can become an expert at taking and recording your temperature, so we're starting with the temperature sign first.

At this point you need a basal temperature thermometer. We will assume you have the digital thermometer you got at the CCL classes or in the *CCL Home Study Course.*

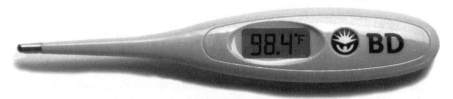

Figure 2.1
A Digital Thermometer

How to care for your thermometer

Your digital thermometer will last for years and years if you care for it properly. So will a good mercury thermometer.

● **How to clean it.** It is not necessary to clean your thermometer when you take your temperature by mouth or vaginally. The bacteria from those areas die after a few hours contact with air. If you take your temperature rectally, clean the thermometer after every use. Also clean it before changing temperature-taking methods.

If you clean your thermometer at any time, use a cloth moistened with cool or lukewarm water.

● **How to store it.** Store your digital thermometer in its original container.

Store it away from direct sunlight and other sources of heat. Never leave it on top of a radio, a radiator, or in front of a heat vent.

Keep it out of the reach of children. The best place may be at the back of your top dresser drawer.

● **When traveling.** Excessive heat will reduce the battery life of your digital thermometer. Therefore, when you travel during warm weather, be sure to keep your thermometer away from excessive heat. Never leave it in a car's glove compartment or in luggage stored in a car's trunk. Just keep it in your purse, and don't leave your purse in direct sunlight or in a closed car that's being parked for any amount of time.

How to take your temperature by mouth

Press the "On" button. Place the silver probe under your tongue, keep your lips closed, and take it for about one minute. The BD model beeps slowly while it is operating and then gives three rapid beeps when the reading is completed. If you are at home, do this now, sit down for a couple of minutes, and keep reading this chapter.

Helpful hint: If your bedroom is **cold** in the morning, your thermometer will also be cold, and it might cause a temporary cool spot under your tongue and give you a false low reading. Warm up a cold thermometer probe by holding the probe between your thumb and forefinger for about 30 seconds. Then place it in the usual place under your tongue.

If your mouth is dry when your wake up in the morning, be sure to work up some saliva before putting the thermometer under your tongue.

See "Some common questions" later in the chapter for other ways to take your temperature.

● Special notes

1. If you take your temperature orally, never have anything to drink or smoke shortly before taking your temperature. On the other hand, a glass of water at 4:30 a.m. isn't going to affect your mouth temperature at 6:30 a.m.

2. Don't fall asleep while taking your temperature.

Temperature taking: at what time?

Take your temperature **at the same waking time** each morning.

Why should you take your temperature at the same waking time? What you are measuring is your "basal body temperature" (abbreviated as BBT). That's the temperature of your body at rest, uninfluenced by activity or food or liquids.

Your body temperature normally rises and falls in a regular 24 hour cycle. Its low point is during the very early hours of the morning when you are normally sleeping, and it starts to go up about the time you normally wake up. **It continues to rise at the rate of about 1/10 of one degree Fahrenheit each half hour** until it reaches your normal high temperature when you are active, generally around 98.6° F., and it does this even when you stay in bed. (Hereafter we refer to Fahrenheit degrees as F.) This cycle of temperatures going up and going down each day and night is called the **circadian rhythm.** You take your temperature at the same waking time each day to get it at the same point in this daily cycle. (Of course, the rising rate of 1/10 of one degree per half hour and the normal high temperature of 98.6° are averages, and they may not hold true in any particular case.)

If you cannot take your temperature at the same time, taking it a half-hour earlier or later generally won't affect your waking temperature too much, but more than that will probably affect it one way or the other.

If you take your temperature more than one-half hour earlier or later than usual, make an "x" in the "Disturbances" row in the top section of the chart (see Figure 2.2) and write the actual time on the vertical temperature line for that day.

Q. If I usually take my temperature at 7:00 a.m., what might it be if I take it at 9:00 a.m.?

A. Your temperature two hours later than usual would probably be 4/10 of one degree F. higher than it was at the normal time, and that could interfere with the proper interpretation of your temperature pattern. That's why it's important to take your temperature at the same waking time each morning during the fertile time. (See Chapter 32, Figure 32.1 for contrasting 7:00 and 9:00 temperatures.)

Q. I work different shifts. When should I take my temperature?

A. Normally, take it when you awake after your longest and best rest of the 24 hour day. For more information, see "Shift work" in Chapter 5.

Temperatures: what day to start?

Do you have to take your temperature every day and at the same time each day throughout the cycle?

The short answer is "No." But something more needs to be said.

The fundamental key to the accurate interpretation of your temperature pattern is an accurate and sufficiently complete record of your daily waking temperatures.

The best way is this: Take your temperature every morning when you wake up, making sure that you have the **same waking time each day during Phase II.** If you find it is a chore to take your temperature every morning during the entire cycle, you can cut back during the early part of Phase I and during Phase III.

Always start taking your temperature 1) as soon as your menstrual period ends or 2) by Cycle Day 6 at the latest, whichever comes first. In other words, if your period lasts only four days, start taking your waking temperature on Day 5. If your period lasts more than five days, start taking your temperature on the morning of Day 6 at the latest.

There is ordinarily no great need to keep taking your temperatures once you are in Phase III, but we assure you that there are occasional unusual cycles in which it is very helpful to have the complete temperature record.

We strongly *recommend* that you keep a complete daily record for at least your first six cycles. We strongly *suggest* that you keep a daily record every cycle as we have done for years. Many of us find it easier to take the temperature every day than to have an off and on routine. You do **not** need to take your temperatures at the same waking time during early Phase I and during Phase III.

How to read your temperature

When the digital thermometer is done registering a temperature, there is usually a "completion" beep or some other indicator that it is finished. Read the directions for whichever thermometer you have purchased and be sure to follow them. The temperature will be shown in the display window. If you have just taken your temperature and have a pen or pencil handy, write down the date, time and the reading right here: _____. This record will be a souvenir 10 or 20 years from now.

How to prepare your chart

Open your personal chart booklet titled *Daily Observation Charts.* Remember when your most recent menstruation began. Count the first day of that menstruation as Cycle Day 1, and write that day of the week and month in the boxes for Day 1. Then fill in the "Day of the week" and the "Day of the month" rows all across the top of the chart or at least up to Cycle Day 30.

For example, let's say that today is Monday, April 24, and you remember that your period started on Saturday, April 15. In this example, you would write a S for Saturday in the box for Cycle Day 1 in the "Day of the week" row and a 15 in the "Day of the month" row right underneath it. Monday, April 24, would be Cycle Day 10.

If you are unsure when your last period started, make a guess, and pick a starting point for today's recordings. Your next chart will be your first complete cycle.

Record your temperature by placing a dot at the proper place on the vertical line for that day. Notice that in the CCL Daily Observation Charts, the horizontal temperature-degree lines are 2/10 of one degree F. apart. Also, they represent the even tenths: 97.4°, 97.6°, 97.8°, etc. If your temperature is an odd tenth such as 97.5°, place the dot midway between 97.4° and 97.6°. See Figure 2.2. Double-check your reading and recording, and store the thermometer in a safe place.

How to record your temperature

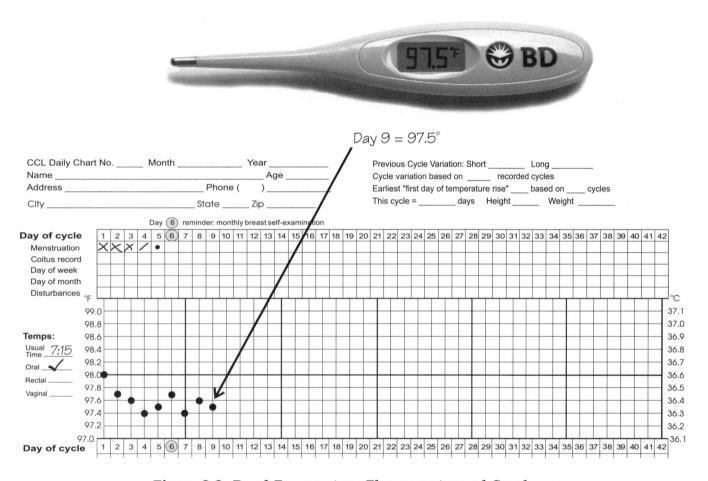

Figure 2.2 Basal Temperature Thermometer and Graph

You or your husband can record your temperature right after taking it, or either one of you can do it later. The digital display will hold the temperature until you turn the thermometer off, and some will hold this recording in a memory until another recording is made. Do not depend too much on this feature. When you press the "On" button of the B-D thermometer, your last reading appears — but only for three seconds. Then it's lost. So it's a good idea to record your temperature soon after you take it.

27   *Getting Started with Temperatures — 2*

Some common questions

This question is more or less obsolete because the digital thermometer is so fast — about one minute. Who minds an extra minute in bed?

If you use a mercury thermometer and the reading is right between two lines on the thermometer, consistently use the lower reading when recording the temperature on the chart.

Q. Is there more than one way to take my temperature?

A. Yes. You can take your temperature orally, vaginally or rectally. Our experience in the Couple to Couple League is that the vast majority of women get excellent results with oral temperatures. Day-to-day temperatures are never perfectly even, but if you get a truly irregular pattern with oral temperatures, perhaps your mouth is sometimes too dry or you are occasionally dozing off and letting your mouth open. If so, you might be better off with vaginal or rectal temps. (European experience suggests that if you have to use a mercury fever thermometer, you will get more reliable results with vaginal or rectal temperatures.) Of those two methods, the advantage of vaginal temps is that you would not have to wash the thermometer after each use.

Do not switch temperature-taking methods during the cycle. Vaginal and rectal temperatures are generally higher than oral temperatures. Make any switch at the beginning of the cycle.

If you select the vaginal or rectal method, do not insert it too deeply. With vaginal temps, insert it about two inches and be careful not to insert it into the urethra. For rectal temps, insert it also about two inches.

Q. Do I have to stay in bed while I take my temperature?

A. The general rule is to stay in bed so that your body temperature is not affected by activity. What better time for your morning prayers?

However, if you take your temperature by mouth, you may not have to stay in bed. Dr. Edward Keefe, who invented the Ovulindex mercury thermometer, had a woman do an experiment for him: she first took her temperature while staying in bed, then got up and exercised vigorously for three minutes. She took her temperature again and found no difference in the two readings.

Caution: Be careful if you take your temperature while doing light activity. When you have a thermometer in your mouth, don't brush your hair or pull a sweater over your head.

Q. If I get up during the night, will my waking temperature be affected?

A. Light activity such as taking care of a child during the night will not affect your normal waking temperature. Even if you are up quite a bit during the night, your waking temperature will usually be undisturbed if you have been able to get a good hour's rest or sleep before taking your temperature. However, if your temperature should be unexpectedly way up, make an "X" in the "Disturbance" row on your chart, and ignore that disturbed temperature when you interpret your temperature pattern.

B. Can I use a glass mercury thermometer?

A. Yes. The glass mercury thermometer was the gold standard for basal thermometers from 1948 to 2000. About that time, it became increasingly difficult for CCL to obtain and distribute a high quality glass mercury thermometer. A glass thermometer using a non-mercury substance did not prove satisfactory for us.

If you prefer the glass mercury thermometer, try to use only a **basal** temperature thermometer, not just a fever thermometer. Glass basal thermometers are usually manufactured to higher standards and are easier to read than glass fever thermometers. (Basal thermometers record only from 96.0° F. to 100° F. with an expanded, easy-to-read scale.)

Fellow husbands: Marital love and sexuality involve both husband and wife, and so should Natural Family Planning. When you cooperate willingly, NFP really does help to build your marriage. On the other hand, if you refuse to help, it sends a negative message to your wife. The easiest way to be involved is to help with the temperature taking and recording and then to help with interpretation of the chart. Your cooperation will mean a lot to your wife.

Here's how. In the evening place the thermometer on your dresser or night-stand—someplace where you can reach it easily when the alarm goes off in the morning.

When the alarm goes off, give your wife the thermometer. Make sure she's awake. If you stay in bed and she starts to snore or breathe like she's asleep, wake her up again. If her mouth is open, she will get a combination of body temperature and room temperature, and that's not what you want.

A personal suggestion: Use this minute or so to say your morning prayers. If you haven't done that in years, what better time to start than now?

After the completion beep, ask your wife for the thermometer, and record the temperature. Then store the thermometer in a safe place.

On weekends in late Phase I and during Phase II during our fertile years, I set the alarm for our usual wake-up time, got the temperature taken, and then recorded it when I got up. On weekends in early Phase I and in Phase III, we didn't set the alarm; we simply took the temperature when we woke up.

All of this is so simple and such a little price to pay for such important information that I have a hard time understanding why some people think daily temperature-taking is a big chore. The only thing hard about it is waking up, and we all have to do that anyway. Your willing cooperation is an easy way to show interest, involvement, and love to your wife.

Chapter 2: Self-Test Questions

1. Phase I refers to _____ .

2. Phase II refers to _____ .

3. Phase III refers to _____ .

4. True____   False____   Ovulation is followed by a slight rise in your regular waking temperature.

5. True____   'False____   The purpose of taking your temperature is to have a positive sign of being in postovulation infertility.

6. True____   False____   You should take your waking temperature at the same time each day—at least during the fertile time.

7. True____   False____   Some women do not have to stay in bed to get accurate waking temperatures.

8. True____   False____   Normally, the husband should prepare the thermometer at night, give it to his wife in the morning, and record the temperature.

For more on charting, see Chapter 4.

Answers to self-test
1. Pre-ovulation infertility 2. The fertile time 3. Postovulation infertility 4. True 5. True 6. True 7. True 8. True

3

Getting Started with Mucus

In this chapter, you will learn how to observe and chart your cervical mucus. You will also learn how to interpret or classify your cervical mucus discharge as less-fertile or more-fertile on a daily basis. In Chapter 7 you will learn how to interpret your overall mucus *pattern*. In Chapter 9, you will learn more about **why** your mucus comes, changes in its quality, and then disappears. If you want to know more about how your menstrual-fertility cycle works—and why, jump ahead and do Chapter 9, and then come back here.

For the present, we will repeat what we said in Chapter 2. Your menstrual-fertility cycle is controlled by chemical signals called hormones. The hormone **estrogen** is dominant before ovulation. It is secreted by follicles in your ovaries and helps to prepare you for ovulation and possible pregnancy. Of special interest: this pre-ovulatory estrogen causes your cervix to secrete a mucus discharge; increased estrogen increases the water content of your cervical mucus, and that makes it become slippery and stretchy. Sometimes a high level of estrogen makes your mucus so watery that it won't stretch any more, but it still gives you definite feelings of wetness.

What does the mucus sign tell me?

In normal cycles your cervical mucus is a very positive sign that you are fertile. It is the sign of greatest interest to couples who are seeking pregnancy, but the mucus sign—and its absence—is also of great help to couples seeking to avoid pregnancy.

● **Terminology**
Labia. The lips of the vagina. In this chapter we refer to the outer labia.
Mucus patch. The days from the first day of your mucus discharge up through Peak Day.
Peak Day. The last day of the more-fertile mucus before the drying-up process begins. (You will learn the distinction between less-fertile and more-fertile types of mucus in Chapter 7.)
Vulva. The external parts of the vagina including the outer labia or lips where you make the external mucus observation.

Where does this mucus come from?

Cervical mucus comes from glands or crypts in the wall of the cervix. The cervix is the narrow, lower end of your uterus or womb. ("Cervix" is the Latin word for "neck.") The lower opening of the cervix is the mouth of the cervix, and it is called by the Latin name for mouth—"os" (pronounced ohss with a long O sound). When the mucus begins to thin out a bit, it begins to flow out of the cervical os into the vagina. Then it flows through the vagina and onto the outer lips or vulva.

What does cervical mucus look like and how does it feel?

You can compare your cervical mucus to your nasal mucus. If you blow your nose when you don't have a cold, you may get nothing at all, or you may get some rather thick and tacky mucus. If you touch that mucus on your handkerchief or tissue, it might stick to your finger, but when you lift your finger, it will quickly break. If you have a cold, your nasal mucus will have a higher water content; it usually stretches quite easily. When you have a "runny nose," that's because the high water content in your nasal mucus makes it very fluid. Sometimes your nasal mucus gets so watery that it starts to drip like a leaky faucet. It's so watery that it won't stretch, and it gives you a feeling of wetness around your nostrils. This is very annoying, and drug companies make much money selling us products to dry up our nasal mucus when we have a cold.

Your cervical mucus also has different appearances. When your mucus discharge first starts in each cycle, it tends to be thick or tacky. If you touch it, it won't stretch very far. Tacky mucus separates immediately when you try to stretch it. Then the mucus becomes more fluid and stretchy. Typically it will cling to your fingers and stretch anywhere from a half-inch to three or four inches, sometimes even five inches. As your cervical mucus becomes more fluid, it will also give you feelings of wetness and slipperiness at the outer lips of the vagina. Sometimes cervical mucus becomes so watery that it won't stretch anymore, but you will notice definite feelings of wetness on the outer lips.

When your cervical mucus is fluid, runny and stretchy, it is very much like fluid, runny and stretchy nasal mucus. It is also very much like raw egg white.

Figure 3.1 illustrates changes in the stretchiness of cervical mucus—from the beginning to the end of the mucus patch in a typical fertility cycle.

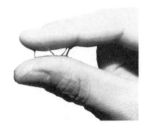

Tacky

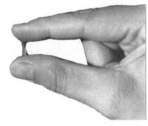

Less Stretchy

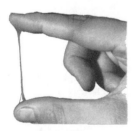

Very Stretchy

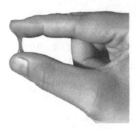

Less Stretchy

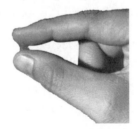

Tacky, Drying Up

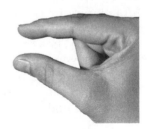

Nothing

Figure 3.1   Changes in Mucus Stretchiness

We can't say for sure how much mucus you will have because the quantity varies from woman to woman. A few women have such a heavy flow of mucus that they have to wear a pantiliner; at the other extreme, a few women have a hard time finding anything. However, if you are like the vast majority of women, you will have enough cervical mucus to notice it easily (but probably not so much that you find it bothersome).

If you are typical, you will notice a small amount when your mucus discharge is first starting; then you will notice a larger quantity as it becomes more fluid and stretchy. Finally, it tapers off and disappears.

● Scanty mucus

If your mucus discharge is very scanty every day during your mucus patch, you may have a deficiency in your nutrition. Vitamin A can increase both the quantity and the quality of cervical mucus. A friend mentioned she had a very scanty mucus discharge; we suggested eating more foods rich in vitamin A. She began eating a couple of carrots daily and reported mucus with a five inch stretch! Vitamin A is necessary for the proper functioning of all the mucus membranes in your body, including those in your cervix. On the other hand, *excessive* vitamin A is toxic and also can harm unborn babies.*

Good nutrition is important for your overall health and for the proper functioning of your fertility cycle. We get into this more in Chapter 31, "Cycle Irregularities," especially the section on Help for irregular cycles. For right now we will say that you might do yourself and your family a great favor by reading—and applying—*Fertility, Cycles and Nutrition* by Marilyn Shannon. Publication information is provided in "Resources" toward the end of this book.

Certain **medicines** such as antihistamines can also affect your cervical mucus. The general principle is that if a medicine can reduce mucus in your nose or lungs, it may have a somewhat similar effect upon your cervical mucus. It probably won't eliminate your cervical mucus during your fertile time, but it may reduce the quantity, stretchiness, and feelings of lubrication. This is not a universal experience, but be aware of this possibility if you have to take such medicines. (See Chapter 35.)

You can observe your cervical mucus in different places and in different ways. We use the word "observe" to mean "check it," "feel it," "see it," or "notice it."

First, you can observe your cervical mucus in two places: 1) *externally* on the outer lips of the vagina or 2) *internally* at the cervical os. In this chapter you will learn how to make the **external observations**. In Chapter 8 you will learn how to make the internal observations.

Second, you have two ways to make your external observations:
1) by wiping with toilet tissue paper;
2) by being aware of sensations at the vulva.

---

* Kenneth J. Rothman and five others, "Teratogenicity of high vitamin A intake," *The New England Journal of Medicine* 333:21 (23 Nov 95) 1369 ff. plus editorial by Godfrey P. Oakley and J. David Erickson. Practical advice was given in the editorial: "Woman who are, or who might become, pregnant should avoid consuming daily supplements containing more than 8,000 I.U. of vitamin A and should consume liver and liver products only in moderation because they contain large amounts of vitamin A." They also recommended consuming 0.4 mg of folic acid daily.

How much cervical mucus will I have?

A personal note from Sheila. When I first was learning the mucus sign, I thought I had very scant mucus. I felt I would never have enough to learn the sign well. However, that turned out to be just inexperience, and within a short time I did learn to make the mucus observations and to evaluate them. Don't become discouraged if your initial experience is like my own.

Where and how can I observe my cervical mucus?

The dyes and chemicals in colored and perfumed toilet paper can irritate some women and cause a confusing vaginal discharge.

1. Use white, unscented toilet paper. Fold it instead of crumpling it.

2. Wipe yourself from front to back, and concentrate on the feelings. Do this either before or after urination, whichever works best for you. However, if you typically have only scanty mucus, try to make your wiping observation both before and after urination until your mucus discharge is well established. The urination itself may remove a small amount of mucus.

As you wipe, be attentive. Does it feel positively dry? That indicates that there's no mucus at the vulva. If you have "dry" observations all day, chart a **D** for dry on your Daily Observation Chart.

Does it feel slippery? Did the tissue glide through as if well lubricated? Those feelings tell you that cervical mucus is present at the vulva, and you would record **SL** for slippery on your chart.

Does it feel *neither* dry nor slippery when wiping? Be sure to check the tissue paper for any signs of mucus.

3. Look at the tissue paper. Do you see any mucus? If you do **not** see any mucus, and if your wiping sensation was neither dry nor slippery, chart an **N** for "Nothing."

If you **do** see mucus on the toilet tissue, then you have mucus at the vulva.

Give it the touch test. Touch it and pull your finger away gradually.

If it doesn't stretch at all, chart an **M** on your Daily Observation Chart (if you didn't find something more stretchy during the day). "M" is the symbol of last resort. You know you have mucus, but you can't describe it as tacky or stretchy.

If you can stretch the mucus from the tissue paper, chart it with a **T** for tacky if it breaks right away or stretches up to a half-inch. Chart an **S** for stretchy if it stretches more than a half-inch.

Q. What if I don't have any feelings of lubrication but see just a bit of shininess on the tissue paper. Should I regard that as cervical mucus or can I regard it as a "dry" observation?

A. We encourage the internal observation (see Chapter 8) to clarify such a situation. If you find no mucus at the cervical os *and* have no feelings of lubrication at the vulva, *then* you can interpret a bit of shininess as "nothing"—**N**. If you don't make the internal observation, then interpret shininess as mucus, and chart it with an **M**.

To use these feelings or sensations, you simply need to concentrate on becoming aware of them. To develop this sort of awareness, you will probably have to think about it very frequently for the first few cycles. Then it will become more or less "second nature."

● **How to notice sensations at the vulva**

You have already learned how to pay attention to feelings of slipperiness when you wipe yourself before or after urination. (See Item 2 above.) You may also notice feelings of lubrication or wetness at the vulva at other times. These are also important; chart them as **W** for wet or **SL** for slippery. Note: **SL** refers only to sensations of slipperiness at the vulva. It does not refer to the slipperiness of the mucus between your fingers.

● **Developing mucus awareness**

Compare "mucus awareness" with other forms of awareness. When you brush your teeth after eating, you have a feeling of clean teeth. You can notice how distinctly different this is from the feeling of "dirty" teeth, especially when you finish a meal with sweets instead of a raw apple, some other fresh fruit, or celery and carrot sticks. You are certainly aware of the difference between dry, clean skin and sweaty, sticky skin simply by feeling.

The same holds true for mucus awareness. For example, you can feel the difference between oil and water without looking. You can develop the same awareness of the different feelings at the vulva when you wipe yourself and even at other times.

At first you may think that you have no mucus, but you can most likely develop this awareness with initial effort, good charting, and persistence. When you get some experience with mucus awareness, you may suddenly notice the feelings of wetness while doing ordinary day to day activities. Chart such feelings with a **W** on your Daily Observation Chart.

Clothes can make a difference. To have accurate sensations of vaginal wetness, wear cotton underpanties and loose outer clothing. Synthetic fiber underpanties (e.g., nylon and polyester) are basically non-absorbent and can produce vaginal feelings of wetness completely unrelated to your cervical mucus. In warm weather, such non-absorbency can also contribute to the persistence of vaginal yeast infections. Tight slacks, shorts, and jeans can also cause problems with mucus observations.

● When to start

Start to make your external observations at least by Cycle Day 6 even if you still have some spotting. If your period ends sooner, start right after menstruation. If you have a history of short cycles—25 days or less, start the mucus observations as soon as your heavy flow is over.

● How often during the day?

Make the external wiping observation before or after each urination and bowel movement during Phase I and Phase II. A few women who experience a scanty mucus flow say that their best observation comes after a bowel movement.

Strictly speaking, you can omit these observations during Phase III **if** you are using the temperature sign along with the mucus. However, if you do **not** use the temperature cross-check, you must make careful mucus observations every day of the cycle. (You will learn the reasons for this when you study the double-mucus-patch situation in Chapter 27 on irregular mucus patterns.)

Classify all types of mucus as either 1) less-fertile mucus or 2) more-fertile mucus. There is no such thing as "infertile" mucus.

The **less-fertile** types are these:
1) Tacky or sticky mucus.
2) Ambiguous mucus. This is cervical mucus that doesn't have any of the characteristics of the more-fertile types, and yet it's not tacky or sticky either. It is "just there" and you can't say much more about it.

Mucus that is opaque or yellowish will generally be a less-fertile mucus, but do not base your interpretation completely on either of these two qualities.

Please note: "less-fertile" does **not** mean "infertile." Before ovulation, normally you must consider the less-fertile mucus as a sign that you have started your fertile time.

The **more-fertile** types are these:
1) Anything that stretches more than one-half inch; (S).
2) Anything that produces feelings of slipperiness (SL) or wetness (W)) at the vulva.
3) "Clear" mucus (C) and generally "Cloudy" mucus (CL).

If your menstruation is shorter than usual, you __might__ ovulate earlier than usual. Be sure to start your observations as soon as your period stops.

How should I interpret my cervical mucus?

How should I chart my cervical mucus?

In this chapter, you have already learned most of the symbols to use for charting your mucus. In alphabetical sequence, here's the complete list of symbols that appear on the CCL Daily Observation Chart.

C   Clear. Generally a more-fertile mucus.

CL   Cloudy. Generally a more-fertile mucus.

D   Dry. Feelings of dryness on the external labia.

M   Mucus. The symbol of last resort. You notice something but cannot be more specific. Use **only** for a less-fertile mucus.

N   Nothing. No mucus felt or seen; no clear feelings of either dryness or lubrication.

O   Opaque. The opposite of clear.

P   Peak Day; not a mucus observation but an interpretation.

S   Stretchy and raw egg-white mucus. Generally stretches more than 1/2 inch. A more-fertile mucus.

SL   Slippery. Feelings of lubrication or slipperiness on vulva. A more-fertile mucus.

SR   Seminal residue from marital relations.

T   Tacky or sticky. Stretches up to 1/2 inch. A less-fertile mucus.

W   Wet. Feelings of wetness on outer lips of vagina—the external labia. **Note well:** You will always notice wetness in the vagina when you make the internal observations. Use the **W** symbol **only** for the feelings of external wetness. A more-fertile mucus.

Y   Yellowish.

Use **T** and **M** for the less-fertile types of mucus.

Use **C**, **CL**, **S**, **SL**, and **W** for the more-fertile types of mucus.

Use +, ++, and +++ for relative quantity; a good amount, a large amount, and a very large amount.

Record length of stretch in inches such as 1/2" or 2".

Note on Stretchy and Tacky mucus. The more-fertile Stretchy mucus *generally* stretches more than one-half inch. However, if the maximum stretch of a woman's mucus at the most fertile time was only 3/4 of an inch, then a stretch of 1/2 inch would also indicate more-fertile mucus.

● **When to chart your mucus**

At the end of each day, remember what you felt or saw when you made your observations. Write one or more of the symbols in the box for that day. Some days you will notice more than one type of mucus, so use more than one symbol. For example, you might notice some ambiguous **M** mucus early in the day and then some **T** mucus later on. The next day it might start out as **T** and turn to **S** by evening.

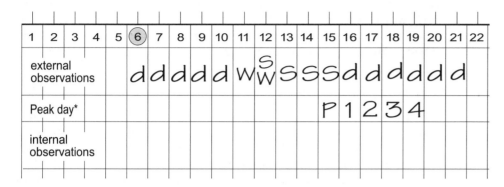

1	2	3	4	5	6	7	8	9	10	11	12	13	14	15	16	17	18	19	20	21	22
external observations	d	d	d	d	d	W	ᔆW	S	S	S	d	d	d	d	d						
Peak day*											P	1	2	3	4						
internal observations																					

Figure 3.2 External Mucus Charting

Figure 3.2 shows five dry days after menstruation stopped. On Cycle Day 11, feelings of wetness are recorded; on Day 12, she noticed feelings of wetness and was able to stretch the mucus more than a half-inch. The mucus patch ended with Cycle Day 15. The external mucus patch was five days long from start through finish.

● **Daily charting**

Be sure to record something for every day in Phase I and Phase II. It is part of your wifely communication with your husband to record accurately your mucus signs of fertility and infertility. Blank spaces are a form of non-communication. If you notice definite feelings of dryness, chart it. That's a very important sign. If you notice nothing, neither sensations of wetness or dryness or any mucus on the tissue paper, you can record it either as a **D** for Dry or as an **N** for Nothing.

Getting started

You can start making your mucus observations the next time you go to the bathroom. If you are in the fertile time, you will most likely notice some signs of mucus; if you are in the infertile times, you will most likely notice either the dry sensations or nothing at all. Be sure to record whatever you notice.

You have already figured out where you are in your cycle and have filled out the days of the week and month on your chart. **Chart** any observations you make today in the proper box for external observations, and keep doing that for the rest of the cycle.

How to make your mucus more fluid

If your cervical mucus never stretches beyond a half-inch nor becomes like raw egg white, and if your mucus never produces distinct feelings of wetness, your mucus may not be reaching a normal state of fluidity. Cervical mucus that stays thick and impedes normal sperm migration can be a cause of infertility. There are several things you can do to try to increase the fluidity of your cervical mucus.

1. Make sure you are drinking enough water. The health care people would like us to drink six to eight glasses of water each day. Compare your

intake, and if it's too far from that, drink more water for general health; it might also help the quality and quantity of your mucus.

2. Eat foods that are rich in vitamin A. This was mentioned in "Scanty mucus" early in this chapter.

3. If you are seeking pregnancy, try an expectorant medication containing guaifenesin. More on this in Chapter 21.

Should I douche?

A douche in general is any stream of water, frequently containing medicine, applied to a body part. In our context, it refers to a vaginal washing.

Should you douche? No. The vagina is a self-cleaning organ. Furthermore, a douche will wash away cervical mucus and other normal, healthy secretions. It will thus interfere with normal mucus observations and may contribute to infertility.

For cleanliness during menstruation, be sure to change your pads frequently. We suggest using tampons only for the rare occasion. Experience reported to us suggests that the regular use of tampons can cause changes in the cells of the cervix.

In this chapter, you have learned how to make and record your external mucus observations, and you have learned how to classify mucus as less-fertile and more-fertile. In Chapter 7 you will learn how to interpret your mucus pattern in terms of the fertile and infertile times of the cycle.

Self-Test Questions: Chapter 3

1. True____ False____ You should make your external observations each time you urinate.

2. A _____ feeling when you wipe indicates no mucus at the vulva.

3. A feeling of _____ when you wipe is a sign that cervical mucus is present.

4. When cervical mucus is stretchy, it is similar to _____ _____ _____.

5. The changes from tacky to stretchy to watery cervical mucus can also be compared to similar changes in _____ mucus.

6. True____ False____ You must start to make and record your mucus observations as soon as your menstrual flow ends or by Cycle Day 6 at the latest (even if you should still be spotting on Day 6).

7. If your period ends on Cycle Day 4, you should start making your mucus observations and recordings on _____‚_____.

8. True____ False____ Underpanties made from synthetic fabrics such as nylon and polyester can produce feelings of wetness that may confuse your mucus awareness, especially in warm weather.

9. True____ False____ Tight pants can confuse your mucus observations.

10. True____ False____ What you eat and drink—including medications—can affect the quantity and the quality of your cervical mucus.

11. The presence of cervical mucus before and around ovulation is a sign of being

_____.

12. Mucus that is tacky or sticky is called the _____ _____ type of mucus.

13. List three characteristics of the more-fertile mucus:
   a. _____
   b. _____
   c. _____

Answers to self-test
1. True 2. dry 3. slipperiness or lubrication 4. raw egg white 5. nasal 6. True 7. Cycle Day 5 8. True 9. True 10. True 11. fertile. 12. less-fertile 13. feelings of lubrication or wetness//stretchy//clear

4

Charting

Chart well, and you will find it is easier to interpret your mucus and temperature patterns. Use the chart developed by the Couple to Couple League (Figure 4.1). It's a convenient way to record the information you need, and it's a uniform way to convey the data CCL counselors need to assist you when you want help. This chapter explains how to use each part of the CCL Daily Observation Chart.

Daily CCL Chart No.____

Write a "1" in this space when you start your NFP charting, and add one for each succeeding cycle. If you have charted a number of cycles on some other chart form, start the CCL chart with your carry-forward number.

CCL Daily Chart No. _____ Month _____ Year _____

Name _____ Age _____

Address _____ Phone ( ) _____

City _____ State _____ Zip _____

Month and year

Write in the time covered by this cycle. Write in both months when your cycle overlaps two months, for example, November-December. Write in the year; this seems too obvious right now, but if someone else is looking at it later, it will be necessary. Again, if this cycle overlaps December and January, be sure to write in both years, for example, *Month:* December-January; *Year:* '96-'97.

Name, address, phone

This information is important when you submit a chart to your NFP teacher or other counselors.

Please write your telephone number on all charts you hand in at NFP classes. Your CCL teachers will promptly review your chart. If they see anything that indicates a possible misunderstanding or problem, they will want to call you immediately. This is part of their follow-up service to you.

Chart notations

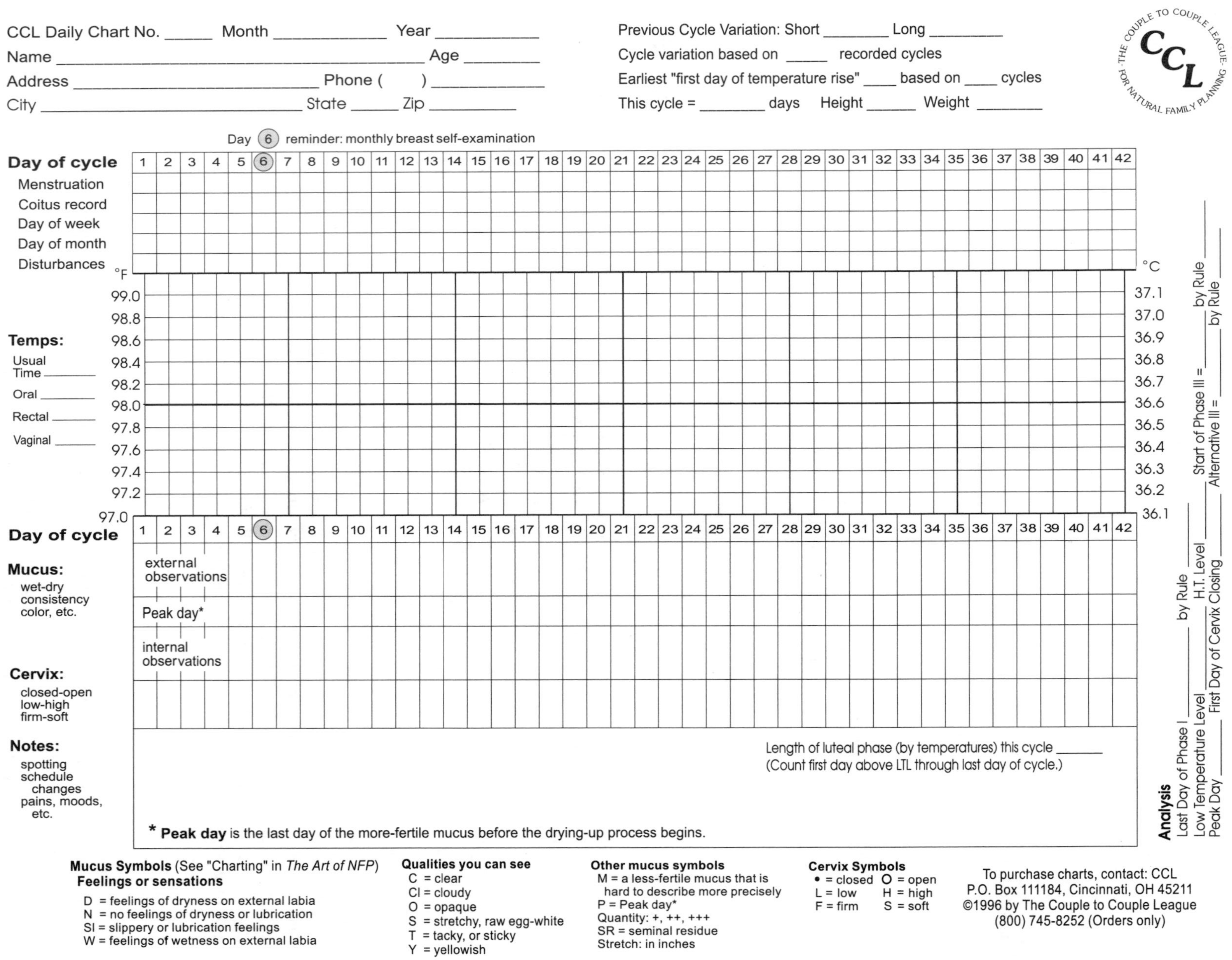

CCL Daily Chart No. _____ Month _____ Year _____
Name _____ Age _____
Address _____ Phone ( ) _____
City _____ State _____ Zip _____

Previous Cycle Variation: Short _____ Long _____
Cycle variation based on _____ recorded cycles
Earliest "first day of temperature rise" _____ based on _____ cycles
This cycle = _____ days Height _____ Weight _____

Analysis

Last Day of Phase I _____ by Rule _____
Low Temperature Level _____ H.T. Level _____
Peak Day _____ First Day of Cervix Closing _____

Start of Phase III = _____ by Rule _____
Alternative III = _____ by Rule _____

Day ⑥ reminder: monthly breast self-examination

Day of cycle 1 2 3 4 5 ⑥ 7 8 9 10 11 12 13 14 15 16 17 18 19 20 21 22 23 24 25 26 27 28 29 30 31 32 33 34 35 36 37 38 39 40 41 42
Menstruation
Coitus record
Day of week
Day of month
Disturbances

°F
99.0
98.8
98.6
98.4
98.2
98.0
97.8
97.6
97.4
97.2
97.0

°C
37.1
37.0
36.9
36.8
36.7
36.6
36.5
36.4
36.3
36.2
36.1

Temps:
Usual
Time _____
Oral _____
Rectal _____
Vaginal _____

Day of cycle 1 2 3 4 5 ⑥ 7 8 9 10 11 12 13 14 15 16 17 18 19 20 21 22 23 24 25 26 27 28 29 30 31 32 33 34 35 36 37 38 39 40 41 42

Mucus:
wet-dry
consistency
color, etc.

external observations

Peak day*

internal observations

Cervix:
closed-open
low-high
firm-soft

Notes:
spotting
schedule
changes
pains, moods,
etc.

Length of luteal phase (by temperatures) this cycle _____
(Count first day above LTL through last day of cycle.)

* **Peak day** is the last day of the more-fertile mucus before the drying-up process begins.

Mucus Symbols (See "Charting" in *The Art of NFP*)
Feelings or sensations
D = feelings of dryness on external labia
N = no feelings of dryness or lubrication
Sl = slippery or lubrication feelings
W = feelings of wetness on external labia

Qualities you can see
C = clear
Cl = cloudy
O = opaque
S = stretchy, raw egg-white
T = tacky, or sticky
Y = yellowish

Other mucus symbols
M = a less-fertile mucus that is
    hard to describe more precisely
P = Peak day*
Quantity: +, ++, +++
SR = seminal residue
Stretch: in inches

Cervix Symbols
● = closed O = open
L = low H = high
F = firm S = soft

To purchase charts, contact: CCL
P.O. Box 111184, Cincinnati, OH 45211
©1996 by The Couple to Couple League
(800) 745-8252 (Orders only)

Figure 4.1 The CCL Daily Observation Chart (about 80% normal size)
Please note: The CCL Daily Observation Chart is copyrighted.
Convenient booklets of these charts are available from CCL Headquarters and local chapters.

Previous Cycle Variation: Short and Long

Here you keep track of your shortest and longest cycle in the last two years. If you have records showing that your shortest cycle was 28 days and your longest cycle was 34 days, you would write 28 in the *Short* space and 34 in the *Long* space. If you have a cycle in the future that is shorter or longer than these, change the "cycle variation" numbers in your subsequent charts.

Previous Cycle Variation: Short _____ Long _____

Cycle variation based on _____ recorded cycles

Earliest "first day of temperature rise" ____ based on ____ cycles

This cycle = _____ days   Height _____ Weight _____

Cycle variation based on _____ recorded cycles

Here you write the number of cycles that form the basis for the record of your shortest and longest cycles. Do you have only three recorded cycles on which to base this range? Then write "3" in this space. Do you have records of two years of cycles? Then write the appropriate number of cycles which will probably be between 24 and 27.

If you have been keeping records on some other chart or form, use those records to determine your previous cycle variation and the number of cycles you used to find that variation.

Earliest "first day of temperature rise" based on _____ cycles

The earliest first day of temperature rise above the Low Temperature Level in the last 12 cycles is recorded for using the Doering end-of-Phase I rule described in Chapter 26. Keep track of the earliest first day of upward thermal shift in your last 6 to 24 cycles. See "The Doering system," in Chapter 26.

This cycle = _____ days

Here you write the length of your current cycle when it is finished. A cycle begins with the first day of menstruation and ends on the last day before your next menstruation.

Height and weight

Write here your height and your current weight. This data is useful to counselors if you experience some forms of cycle irregularity.

Day of cycle

Start a new chart on the first day of your period. Day 1 is the first day of menstruation. The chart provides for 42 cycle days; for longer cycles, use a second chart and change the numbers to start with 43, etc.

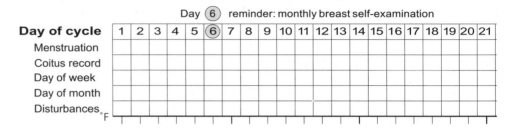

Menstruation

Write an **X** for days of heavy flow, a **/** for days of light flow, and a dot (•) for days of spotting. When your *next* period starts, write another **X** on this chart for the first day of *that* period. Then write the number of the last cycle day before your next period started in "This cycle = _____ days." For example, if your next period starts on November 6 which is Day 29 of this cycle, write an **X** in the menstruation row for Day 29. The cycle on this chart would have ended on Day 28. Write 28 in the space "This cycle = _____ days" as in this example. November 6 is Day 1 of your next cycle and chart.

This cycle = _28_ days

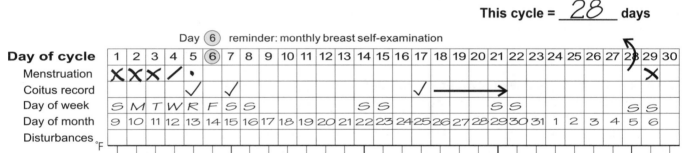

Coitus record

Coitus (ko-ee-tus) is the Latin word for intercourse. It fits better on the chart and if your kids find the chart in your dresser drawer, they probably won't know what it means.

Make a check mark for each instance of coitus in Phase I and Phase II and for the first coitus in Phase III. If you should experience an unplanned pregnancy, a counselor needs that information if he or she is to help you understand why. You may want to make such marks for the rest of Phase III, but such information is not needed by counselors.

You will learn how to determine the end of Phase I, the length of Phase II, and the start of Phase III in Chapters 10, 11, and 12 dealing with the NFP rules.

If you submit your chart for counseling, please indicate if the coitus record is complete or incomplete by writing "record complete" or "record incomplete" on this line. In the example above, the arrow starting on Day 18 indicated additional unrecorded acts of marital relations.

Day of week/Day of month

Fill in these spaces beginning with the first day of menstruation. If your period starts before midnight of a given day, that day is Cycle Day 1. If your period starts after midnight, then write the date of the new day in the column for Cycle Day 1. Some couples write in each day of the week using "R" for Thursday; others just mark Saturday and Sunday.

Disturbances

Use these spaces to mark any sort of disturbance that might affect your temperature recordings. This is explained more fully in Chapter 5, "How to interpret your temperature pattern."

The temperature graph

The left hand edge is the line for Day 1; the other darker vertical lines are at weekly intervals—Days 7, 14, 21, 28, 35, and 42.

The horizontal lines indicate the temperature levels. The Fahrenheit scale (F.) is at the left hand edge of the graph; the Celsius or centigrade scale (C.) is at the right hand edge. Each line represents a difference of 2/10 of one degree F. from the next line or 1/10 of one degree C.

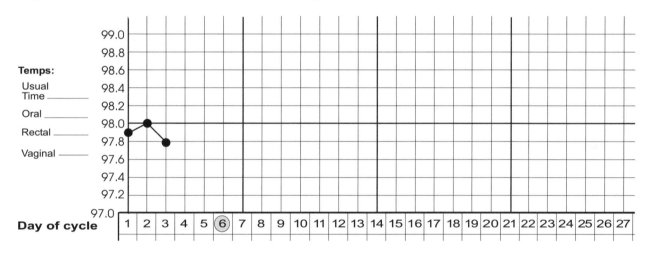

Record your temperatures directly **on** the vertical lines, **not** between them. (Follow the example given in the illustration above.) If your temperature is an even tenth such as 97.8°, record it at the intersection of the vertical "Day" line and the horizontal "degree" line for 97.8° as on Day 3 in the example above. If your temperature is an uneven tenth such as 97.9°, record it half way between the "even tenth" lines, as on Day 1 in the example above.

Temps

Write the "usual time" when you normally take your waking temperature. Check (✓) your method of temperature taking—oral, rectal, vaginal.

If you have any questions about how and when to take your temperature, review Chapter 2, "Getting started with temperatures."

Day of cycle

The "Day of cycle" line below the temperature graph is identical to the one above it; it is printed a second time simply for easy reference.

Mucus notations

Beginning with the end of menstruation, record your mucus observations each day in the proper place. Use the upper row of spaces for your external observations; use the lower row for your internal observations.

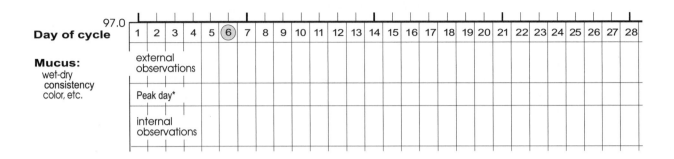

Try to use the standard charting symbols given at the bottom of the chart. If you have to use some other symbol of your own, be sure to explain it to any counselor you may ask for help. The standard symbols are as follows in alphabetical sequence:

C   Clear. Generally a more-fertile mucus.

CL   Cloudy. Generally a more-fertile mucus.

D   Dry. Feelings of dryness on the external labia.

M   Mucus. The symbol of last resort. You notice something but cannot be more specific. Use **only** for a less-fertile mucus.

N   Nothing. No mucus felt; no real feelings of dryness.

O   Opaque. The opposite of clear.

P   Peak Day; not a mucus observation but an interpretation.

S   Stretchy, raw egg-white mucus. Generally stretches more than 1/2 inch. A more-fertile mucus.

SL   Slippery. Feelings of lubrication or slipperiness on labia. A more fertile mucus.

SR   Seminal residue from marital relations.

T   Tacky. Stretches up to 1/2 inch. A less-fertile mucus.

W   Wet. Feelings of wetness on outer lips of vagina—the external labia. **Note well:** You will always notice wetness in the vagina when you make the internal observations. Use the **W** symbol **only** for the feelings of *external* wetness. A more-fertile mucus.

Y   Yellowish.

Use **T** and **M** for the less-fertile types of mucus.

Use **C**, **CL**, **S**, **SL**, and **W** for the more-fertile types of mucus.

Use +, ++, and +++ for relative quantity: a good amount, a large amount, and a very large amount.

Record length of stretch in inches such as 1/2" or 2" etc.

Peak day

Mark a **P** in the space for the Peak day of mucus. Then number the following spaces 1, 2, 3, and 4 for the first four days of drying up of the mucus. Remember: you cannot determine the Peak day until after one or two days of drying up.

Peak day definition

This definition appears in the lower left-hand corner of the "Notes" box at the bottom of the chart. ***Peak day** is the last day of the more-fertile mucus before the drying-up process begins.* A more precise definition: Peak day is the last day on which you observe the more-fertile mucus even if you observe it only once that day.

If there are several days of the more-fertile mucus, Peak day is the **last** day of that more-fertile mucus patch.

If you have a large quantity of stretchy mucus followed by another day or so of feelings of wetness, which is definitely a more-fertile mucus, Peak day is simply the **last** day of whatever "more-fertile" mucus you observe in that mucus patch.

Cervix notations

For the open-closed notation, use circles of varying sizes ranging from a dot to one that is as wide as the space on the chart.

For the firm-soft notation, use **F** and **S**.

For the low-high observation, use **L** and **H**.

You can combine the low-high and the open-closed notations by using circles of different sizes and at different heights in the spaces as we show in Figure 4.2.

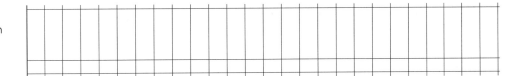

Cervix:
closed-open
low-high
firm-soft

Notes

Use the blank **Notes** space to write explanations for any "disturbances" marked near the top of the chart. Note anything else that may be helpful in understanding your fertility pattern in this cycle such as breastfeeding, coming off the Pill, cold, flu, medications, etc.

Notes:
spotting
schedule
changes
pains, moods,
etc.

* **Peak day** is the last day of the more-fertile mucus before the drying-up process begins.

47

Length of luteal phase

This notation space is at the right side of the "Notes" section at the bottom of the chart. For a temperature-based luteal phase count, start with the first day above the Low Temperature Level (LTL) through the last day before your next period. This information is helpful for analyzing certain cycle patterns and for applying the 21 Day end-of-Phase-I rule. See Figures 4.2 and 4.3.

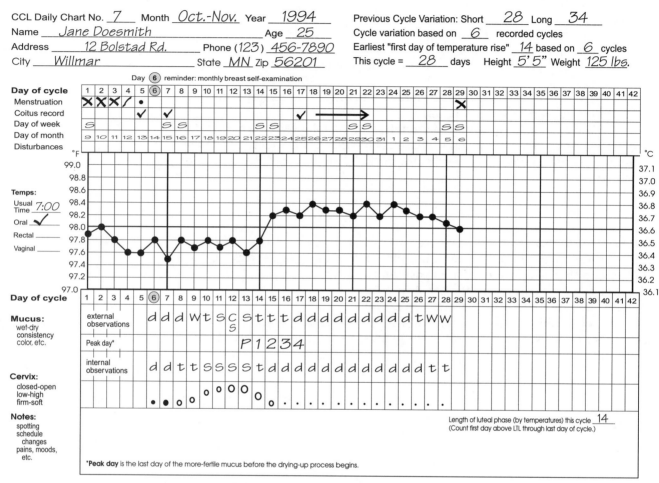

Figure 4.2 A Complete Data Chart

Other notations

● **Phase division lines**

In the above example, Phase I ended on Day 7 and Phase II started on Day 8. In this example, to mark the Phase division lines, draw the vertical Phase I/II division line freehand by starting **between** the boxes for Days 7 and 8 at the top of the graph. When you get down to the temperature section, draw it **between** the temperature lines for Day 7 and Day 8; then between the boxes at the bottom for Days 7 and 8; then between the "mucus boxes" at the bottom of the chart. It's a lot easier to see how to do it by looking at Figure 4.3 than by reading about it.

In Figure 4.2, Cycle Day 16 is the last *complete* day of Phase II. Phase III starts on the evening of Cycle Day 17. Use a pencil and draw the vertical Phase II/III division line from top to bottom between the recording spaces for Days 16 and 17.

● Low Temperature Level

You will learn how to determine the Low Temperature Level in Chapter 5, "How to interpret your temperature pattern." (Generally, you set it by the normal, undisturbed high temperatures on the six days just before the upward thermal shift begins.) Draw this horizontal line on your chart; it makes it easier for you to see the upward shift and to determine the start of Phase III.

● High Temperature Level

You draw this horizontal line 4/10 of 1° F. above the Low Temperature Level. (More on this in Chapter 5.) Drawing this line helps you to interpret the temperature pattern more easily.

There are no self-test questions for Chapter 4.

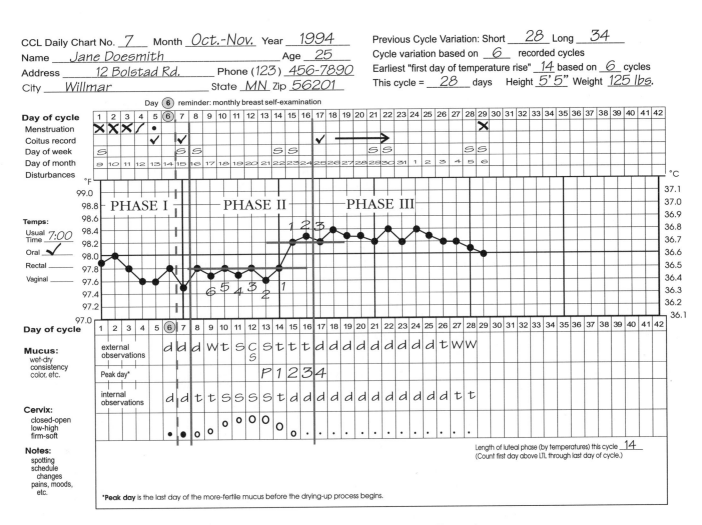

Figure 4.3   Chart 4.2 with Interpretation Lines

Preparing Your Charts for Review

You can get the best assistance from your instructors by doing a complete job of recording your observations.

In the regular classes, have each of your first three charts reviewed by your instructor. In small classes, CCL teachers rely on you to bring to class your *Daily Observation Charts* booklet. In larger classes, they may give you duplicate chart sets and ask you to leave one copy with them at each of the last three meetings.

If you are taking the *CCL Home Study Course,* use the three sets of duplicate charts. Send the white copy to CCL Headquarters at the end of each of your first three cycles. For a more permanent record of those cycles, copy them into your booklet of *Daily Observation Charts.*

The following instructions will make more sense after you have completed your first regular NFP class or the first 12 lessons of the CCL Home Study Course (or the first 12 chapters of this manual).

1. Record how far your mucus stretches, if at all, during these first cycles. The length of stretch is much more helpful in our review than just the **S** notation.

2. Draw a backslash (\) to separate the last day of the pre-shift six temperatures from the first day of the "3 above the previous 6" temperatures. Number your pre-shift six temperatures.

3. Draw in the horizontal lines for the Low Temperature Level and the High Temperature Level.

4. Determine, to the best of your ability as a beginner, the last day of Phase I and the first day of Phase III.

5. Draw a vertical line to separate the last day of Phase I from the first day of Phase II. Draw another vertical line to separate the last full day of Phase II from the day on which Phase III begins. Start your phase division line between the "Cycle day" boxes at the top of the graph; draw it downward between the temperature lines, and finish it between the "Cycle day" boxes at the bottom of the temperature graph.

6. Record any special circumstances such as coming off the Pill, the use of any other hormonal medication, etc. Note if you are breastfeeding and the age of the baby.

7. Indicate the last two acts of coitus in Phase I, any or all in Phase II, and the first in Phase III. However, if you consider this an invasion of privacy, just tell us so, and we will work with whatever data you provide. Also, note whether you were seeking to avoid/postpone or achieve pregnancy during this cycle.

8. If you are attending the regular CCL course, bring your *Daily Observation Charts* booklet to class for review by your instructor couple.

9. If you are taking the *CCL Home Study Course,* send the white copy of the duplicate chart set to CCL Headquarters. See additional details in *The Home Study Guide.*

10. Keep your charted records for at least two years. We *suggest* that you keep your completed *Daily Observation Charts* booklets indefinitely. Who knows, 25 years from now you may want to share the charted cycles of the conceptions of your children.

5

How to Interpret
Your Temperature Pattern

In Chapter 9 you will learn more about the hormones that affect your fertility. Here we can briefly mention that after ovulation a higher level of progesterone stops all subsequent ovulations in that cycle and causes your basal body temperature to rise slightly. The purpose of taking your waking temperatures is to detect that upward shift in temperatures.

Preview

The **basic principle** is this: three waking temperatures that are sufficiently above the previous six temperatures tell you that you are in Phase III, provided that the temperatures on those days are cross-checked by the drying-up of the cervical mucus.

The **standard procedure** for determining the start of Phase III involves three steps:
1) you have three normal temperatures above the previous six temperatures;
2) those temperatures are enough above the previous six temperatures;
3) the elevated temperature pattern is cross-checked by the drying-up of the cervical mucus.

From the examples in this book and soon from your own experience, you will find that not every upward shift in temperatures looks the same. Therefore, we have given labels to three different types.

You will also find some variety in the way the temperature pattern and the mucus dry-up pattern cross-check each other. Therefore we have different rules to determine the earliest beginning of Phase III.

First we define the terminology that we use and different types of temperature patterns. Then we will go step by step through the process of interpreting a typical temperature pattern.

Terminology

● **Valid temperature**. A waking temperature that is **not disturbed** by sickness, late temperature taking, or other factors that can affect your waking temperature. Also called a **normal** or **undisturbed** temperature. "Normal" here does *not* refer to an average midday non-fever temperature of about 98.6° F.

- **Consecutive temperatures.** Valid thermal shift temperatures normally have to be on consecutive days—no missed or disturbed temperatures.

- **Phase III.** The infertile time of the cycle after ovulation.

- **Pre-shift six** or pre-shift six temperatures. These are the last six normal, low-level temperatures immediately before the beginning of the upward shift in temperatures. These are the six temperatures you use to set the "Low Temperature Level."

  Occasionally it appears as though you may choose two different sets of pre-shift six temperatures. If this happens, choose the one which includes Peak Day. If neither set includes Peak Day, choose the set which is closest to Peak Day. If both sets include Peak Day, choose the one which ends closest to Peak Day.

- **Low Temperature Level.** Abbreviation: **LTL**. This is the lower level from which you measure the upward shift. You set it at the level of the highest valid (undisturbed) temperature among the pre-shift six. (The LTL tends to remain fairly consistent from one cycle to the next.)

- **Thermal shift.** The upward shift of three or more temperatures from the Low Temperature Level to the High Temperature Level.

- **High Temperature Level.** Abbreviation: **HTL**. This is the higher level of temperatures after the thermal shift. You set it 4/10 of 1° F. above the Low Temperature Level. That is, you simply add 4/10 of one degree F. to the lower level, even if all the elevated temperatures are higher than that.

Standard thermal shift patterns

Next we want to define three different kinds of thermal shifts. You may think we are trying to complicate things, but that's not the case. We are just being realistic. There *are* different patterns. We are simply providing labels for three different kinds of rising temperature patterns you might experience. (*For additional, irregular, and less common patterns*, see Chapter 28, "Irregular temperature patterns.")

- **Full thermal shift.** This is the strongest form of thermal shift.

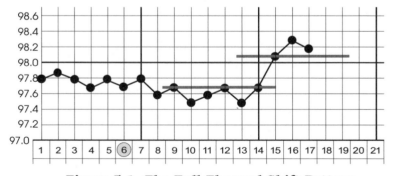

Figure 5.1 The Full Thermal Shift Pattern

A full thermal shift consists of three undisturbed temperatures on **consecutive** days that are **all** at least a full **4/10** of 1° F. above the Low Temperature Level (LTL).

● **Strong thermal shift.** This is the next strongest form of thermal shift.

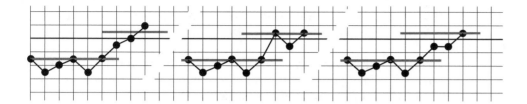

Figure 5.2 The Strong Thermal Shift Pattern: Three Examples

A strong thermal shift consists of three undisturbed temperatures on **consecutive** days that follow this pattern:

1. The first temperature is at least **2/10** of 1° F. above the Low Temperature Level;

2. The second temperature is at least **2/10** of 1° F. above the Low Temperature Level;

3. The **last** temperature is at least **4/10** of 1° F. above the Low Temperature Level.

● **Overall thermal shift.** This is the weakest thermal shift pattern.

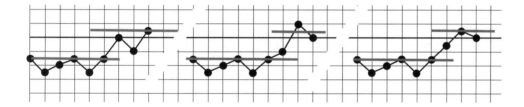

Figure 5.3 The Overall Thermal Shift Pattern: Three Examples

An overall thermal shift consists of at least three undisturbed temperatures that follow this pattern:

1. Each temperature is at least **1/10** of 1° F. above the Low Temperature Level;

2. The temperatures are in a rising or elevated pattern;

3. At least one of them reaches the normal High Temperature Level of 4/10 of 1° F. above the Low Temperature Level. The last temperature does not have to be at the HTL as it does in the full and strong thermal shifts.

The standard evaluation procedure

You will find it's much easier to evaluate a temperature pattern in practice than it is to read about it. Follow the standard procedure for interpreting your temperature pattern by asking—and answering—three questions.

1. Do I have a group of three temperatures that are above the previous six temperatures? When you can answer "Yes," you can set the low and high levels. See "Is there an upward shift" just below Figure 5.4.

2. Are these temperatures **enough** above the lower level to constitute a standard thermal shift pattern? See "A *sufficient* thermal shift?" below Figure 5.4.

3. Is this thermal shift cross-checked by a sufficient number of days of drying-up of the mucus?

Get a pencil and let's see how that works out in practice with Figure 5.4.

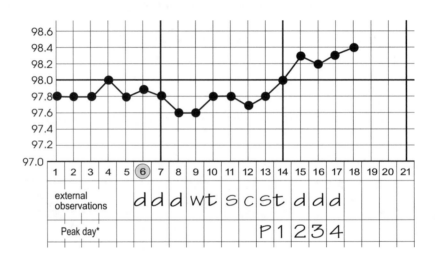

Figure 5.4 Setting the LTL and the HTL

1. Is there an upward shift?

First, cover up all the temperatures except Day 1. (Your right thumb will do well.) Now start to uncover them one at a time. As you do that, ask yourself the first basic question: **Do I see three temperatures above the previous six** temperatures? When you get out to Day 16, you can answer, "Yes. Days 14, 15, and 16 are above the previous six temperatures."

Next, **set the Low Temperature Level** by asking and answering two more questions: 1) What are the pre-shift six temperatures? and 2) What is the highest temperature among the pre-shift six?

To determine the pre-shift six, draw a backslash line (\ ) about one inch long between the last lower temperature and the first of the three rising temperatures. Thus, draw that line between the temperatures on Days 13 and 14. Now count back six starting with Day 13 and number them backwards. That is, put a 1 under day 13, a 2 beneath Day 12, etc., until you write a 6 under Day 8. The pre-shift six temperatures are Days 8 through 13 in this example.

To determine the Low Temperature Level (LTL), you ask yourself, "What is (or are) the highest undisturbed temperature (or temperatures)

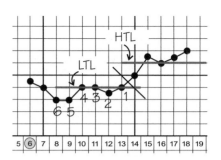

among the pre-shift six?" In this example, the temperatures on Days 10, 11, and 13 are the highest undisturbed temperatures among the pre-shift six; they set the LTL at 97.8° F. Draw a freehand horizontal line at the 97.8° level so that it covers the pre-shift six, goes through the normal high temperatures, and extends to the right for another four days or so. (Don't use a ruler.)

To determine the High Temperature Level (HTL), add 4/10 of 1° F. to the LTL level and draw another freehand horizontal line. In this example you would draw it at the 98.2° level.

2. A *sufficient* thermal shift?

Now ask yourself: Are the first three rising temperatures **enough** above the LTL to fulfill the requirements for a standard thermal shift pattern (and then for a Phase III rule)? Do the temperatures on Days 14, 15 and 16 fit one of the standard thermal shift patterns? Check out the patterns above once again. You will find that the temperatures on Days 14, 15, and 16 fulfill the requirements for a "strong thermal shift." If you drew your LTL line at 97.8° and your HTL line at 98.2°, this is easy to see.

What if you wanted to wait until your temperature pattern was a "full thermal shift"? What are the first three days that fit that definition? For a full thermal shift, the temperatures must be at or above the HTL on three consecutive days. Days 15, 16 and 17 fulfill that requirement. Number the days of **full** thermal shift. In this case, put a 1 above Day 15, a 2 above Day 16, and a 3 above Day 17.

● **Shaving high temperatures.** Sometimes you will find a temperature pattern in which one or two temperatures in the pre-shift six are so high that you never find a thermal shift that "fits," that is, that meets the requirements for one of the three standard thermal shift patterns. Yet, when you just *look* at the shift, it is obvious that there has been a shift from a lower level to a higher level of temperatures. In some cases we can "shave down" one or two of the high pre-shift six temperatures to the next highest level to get a proper fit. The rules for doing this are explained in Chapter 6, "Shaving Temperatures."

3. Is there a cross-check from the mucus sign?

We haven't explained how to interpret the mucus pattern yet, so this is getting a bit ahead of ourselves. However, you need to realize from the beginning that the essence of the Sympto-Thermal Method is the cross-check between the different signs of fertility and infertility.

Different thermal shift patterns require different cross-checks from the mucus sign. The most conservative rule (Rule C) requires four days of drying-up to cross-check three days of full thermal shift. Two days is the minimum number of days of drying-up required for any STM rule, and this applies only to Rule K. (More on this in Chapter 10, and more liberal rules in Chapter 12.)

In Figure 5.4, Day 13 is Peak Day, and the temperatures on Cycle Days 15, 16, and 17 are 3 days of full thermal shift after Peak day. This combination fulfills the mucus and temperature requirements for Rule C.

Certain things that have nothing to do with your fertility and infertility can cause your waking temperature to be elevated. We call these "explainable false rises." When these happen, just ignore them. Such false rises generally fall into the following categories:

1. Fever or some lesser illness such as a bad cold or a sore throat. However, sometimes you can have a cold and have a normal temperature.

2. Alcohol the night before. Generally one drink will have no effect.

3. Late temperature taking. See page 58 for the effects of changes in Daylight Saving Time.

Explainable false rises

The important thing is this: if you have an out-of-line temperature and there is reason to believe it is disturbed, note the disturbance.

Years ago, Sheila had an apparent three-day thermal shift, but she was sure that ovulation had not occurred since she had mucus during that "false" shift. Then she remembered: on each of those mornings our five-year-old had crawled into bed to snuggle with mommy for a couple of hours before her normal temperature-taking time. She reasoned that the child's close presence must have given additional warmth to her body. After all, we are measuring small amounts of change.

4. Time zone changes. Traveling from the East to the West has the effect of taking your temperature one hour later than usual for each time zone if you take it at the same clock time—like the change to Daylight Savings Time in the fall. Going from the West to the East has the effect of taking your temp one hour earlier than usual for each time zone—like the change to Daylight Savings in the spring. So if you traveled from New York to California, your waking temperature would be three hours later if you used the same clock time. The effect lasts about as long as jet lag—about two or three days. If you are right at the end of Phase II, you may want to use the Daylight Savings procedure (page 58) to minimize these effects.

5. Unaccustomed chill or heat. If the furnace stops working on a cold winter night in Minnesota, that could lower your body temperature. A change in the temperature setting of an electric blanket or a waterbed can certainly affect your body temperature. Even unaccustomed and prolonged snuggling might have an effect.

6. Grossly insufficient rest. Most of the time, getting up once or twice during the night won't affect your waking temperature. However, if you are up most of the night with a sick child or don't get to bed until 2:30 a.m. (and your normal waking time is 6:00 a.m.), or for some other reason just don't get any sleep during the night, don't be surprised if you have an elevated waking temperature. Treat it as a disturbed temperature and ignore it.

● **How to treat explainable false rises**

Write an "x" in the disturbance row for that day, and explain it in the Notes section of the chart. Ignore explainable false rises in setting your Low Temperature Level. If possible, go back for one or two more undisturbed temperatures so that you will have six valid temperatures to set your Low Temperature Level. Sometimes you will have to "shave" the temperatures farthest to the left because the pre-shift six temperatures are frequently a bit lower than the earlier temperatures. (The higher estrogen on the days just before ovulation has a slight temperature depressing effect.) However, sometimes you have to be satisfied with a "pre-shift five."

Unexplained rises

In some cycles, you might have one or two irregular high temperatures among the pre-shift six that cannot be explained by the above causes. Here's how to treat unexplained false rises.

1. When did it occur? Ignore any unexplained high temps that occur before the pre-shift six.

2. Does the questionable temperature among the pre-shift six make any difference? That is, have the thermal shift temperatures risen to a level at least 4/10 of 1° F. above *it*? If so, just count it among the pre-shift six.

3. If there are one or two unexplained high temps among the pre-shift six that interfere with a normal interpretation of an otherwise obvious thermal shift, shave them to the next highest level using the shaving rules in Chapter 6. If there are three unexplained high temperatures, try "averaging" as explained in Chapter 6.

A few women may regularly have an upward thermal shift pattern that is less than the normal shift of at least 4/10 of 1° F. If you are one of them, you can learn to interpret such rises *in conjunction with* the other signs of fertility and infertility. You can still use the Sympto-Thermal Method successfully.

Draw a horizontal line **just above** the pre-shift six temperatures and **below** at least three (or four) temperatures that make up the weaker thermal shift. Draw a vertical line between the last day of the pre-shift six and the first day of rising temperatures. You now have a cross with the thermal shift temperatures in the upper right hand section.

Now use this thermal shift to cross-check four days of mucus dry-up and perhaps the closing of the cervix. You see an example of this in Figure 5.5.

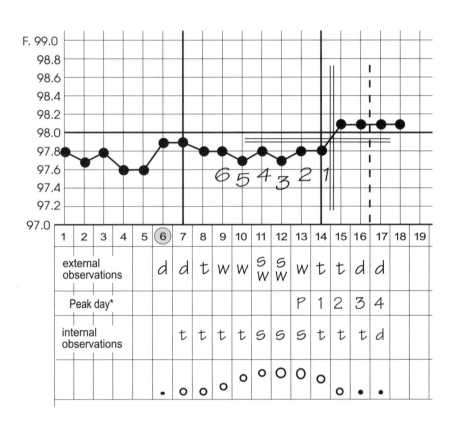

Figure 5.5 Thermal Shift of 3/10 of 1° F.

In Figure 5.5 we accepted a thermal shift of only 3/10 of 1° F. above the LTL as a sufficient cross-check on the four days of mucus dry-up.

A shift of only 2/10 of 1° F. would be extremely unusual. An NFP teacher would want to see two or three consecutive charts before accepting that as normal for you or anyone else. (The authors have *never* seen a shift of only 2/10 of 1° F.)

Generally, when you use the shaving principle correctly, you almost never have to accept a thermal shift of less than the normal amount—4/10 of 1° F. above the LTL.

Daylight saving changes

If you live where Daylight Saving Time is used, the changes have the effect of your taking your temperature an hour later in the fall and an hour earlier in the spring if you use the same clock time every morning. If you are in Phase I or Phase III, there's no problem. If you are in Phase II when the time changes and want the most accurate temperatures during the transition, follow these patterns which assume a 6:00 a.m. usual wake-up time:

● In the fall

In the fall, the change back to Standard Time has the effect of getting you up an hour LATER. That means that your temperatures at the same "clock time" are likely to be a bit higher for the first two or three days after the change. This process will minimize those changes; it assumes a regular 6:00 a.m. wake-up time.

Friday   6:00 a.m. Daylight Saving Time

Saturday   6:20 a.m. Daylight Saving Time

Set your clock back one hour before you go to bed Saturday night.

Sunday   5:40 a.m. Standard Time

Monday   6:00 a.m. Standard Time

● In the spring

In the spring of the year, the change to Daylight Saving Time has the effect of getting you up an hour EARLIER. Your temperatures taken at the same clock time might be lower after the start of Spring Daylight Saving Time, but this offers no problem as far as false high readings are concerned. However, if you are in Phase II and want the most accurate temperatures during the transition, follow this pattern—which also assumes a usual 6:00 a.m. waking time.

Friday   6:00 a.m.   Standard Time

Saturday   5:40 a.m.   Standard Time

Set your clock ahead one hour before you go to bed Saturday night.

Sunday   6:20 a.m.   Daylight Saving Time

Monday   6:00 a.m.   Daylight Saving Time

Shift work

Two questions arise if you have to work evening or night shifts.

1. When should you take your temperature if you work evening or night shifts? A general rule: take your temperature when you awake from your longest and best rest of the 24 hour day. For other options, see the next sub-section, "What to do."

2. Will working *different* shifts affect your temperature pattern? There is no universally valid answer to this question. The reason it *might* affect your temperature pattern is the circadian rhythm; review that subject in Chapter 2.

It seems to depend on how often you change from one sleeping time to another. For example, a substitute nurse changed shifts almost every day and took her temperature when she awoke from her best sleep time each day. Her temperature pattern was classic with an unmistakable sharp rise right after

Peak Day. We think her system may have been so consistently irregular that the circadian rhythm never had a chance to settle in, so to speak.

On the other hand, if your system is well established on one shift and you change to another, don't be surprised if the effect is something like time zone changes or changing back and forth from Daylight Saving Time to Standard Time.

● **What to do**

1. Be consistent and precise with your mucus observations. You should make the external observation at each urination whether you are at home or at work, and you can make the internal observation at home before you go to bed.

2. Use **Rule B** because it puts the most emphasis or reliance on the four-day drying-up process. (Rule B is explained in Chapter 12.) If your work schedule changes close to ovulation, you may be using primarily your mucus sign to determine the start of Phase III. In some cases you might be looking for just enough of a three-day temperature rise to assure you that you are not experiencing the double mucus patch described in Chapter 27, "Irregular Mucus Patterns."

3. Be your own scientist. When your schedule changes during Phase III, notice what effect it has on your temperature pattern. During Phase III, any big change when you change schedules and sleeping patterns is not caused by a change in hormones.

4. Be scientific and experiment with the best time for taking your temperatures. For one or two cycles, take them at two or three different times each day and record each reading in a different color. Suggested times:

a) when you wake up from your best sleep for that day;

b) before you go to bed

c) at some other same-clock-time when you are not too active and have not just finished eating or drinking.

At the end of a complete cycle, you will have two or three different colored temperature patterns on the same chart. Compare them with your mucus and/or cervix patterns to see which one gives you the truest picture.

Note well: If you use the "before you go to bed" temperature patterns, always require four days (not just three) of upward thermal shift to cross-check the drying-up pattern. All the rules have been developed with morning waking temperatures, and evening temperatures sometimes go up a day before the morning temperatures.

Workbook exercises

Toward the center of this book, right after Chapter 15, you will find a workbook section. This contains 24 charts to help you learn how to apply principles and rules to different situations. Each one illustrates a rule or some special point of interest.

Use a pencil and have an eraser handy. You don't need a ruler; freehand is better.

Read the instructions below; then turn to the workbook section and identify these four items **on each of the first five charts**:

1) the pre-shift six

2) the Low Temperature Level (LTL)

3) the High Temperature Level (HTL)

4) the first three days of **full** thermal shift. For right now, ignore the overall and strong thermal shift patterns.

Workbook Chart 1 is done for you; just make sure you understand *why* Days 9 through 14 make up the pre-shift six, *why* the LTL is set at 97.6°, etc.

When you start to work on Workbook Chart 2, use your right thumb to uncover one temperature at a time, starting from the left. Keep asking yourself the first basic question: "Do I see three temps that are consecutively above the previous six?" Once you do, draw a one-inch backslash between the last of the previous six lower temps and the first of the rising temps. That makes it much easier to do the proper numbering and line drawing.

Then ask yourself the second basic question: "Are those rising temperatures *enough* above the pre-shift six to make up a *full* thermal shift?

Number the pre-shift six temperatures. Draw horizontal lines to indicate the LTL and the HTL. Number the temperatures that make up the full thermal shift.

Do this for Charts 2-5. Check your answers in the workbook answer sheets that are located in the back of the workbook. Work just one chart at a time and check your answers; that way, if you make a mistake, you won't make it a habit.

Self-Test Questions: Chapter 5

1. The hormone _____ causes a woman's waking or basal temperature to rise slightly.

2. The thermal shift is a rise from a lower level to a _____ level.

3. The usual amount of thermal shift is _____ of 1° Fahrenheit.

4. The six temperatures just before the start of the thermal shift are called the _____ temperatures.

5. The Low Temperature Level (LTL) is the _____ _____ of temperatures from which you measure the upward shift.

6. You determine the Low Temperature Level from the _____ _____ readings among the pre-shift six temperatures.

7. The Low Temperature Level tends to remain fairly _____ from one cycle to the next.

8. Connect the temperature dots in all the graphs on the next page.

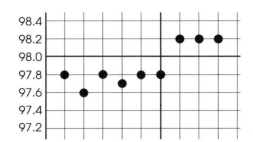

The above pattern is called a _____ thermal shift pattern.

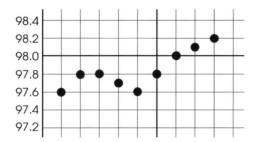

9. Draw your LTL and HTL lines. The above pattern is called a _____ thermal shift.

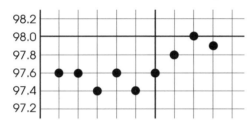

10. Draw your LTL and HTL lines. The above pattern is called a _____ thermal shift.

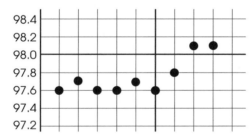

11. Draw your LTL and HTL lines. The above pattern is called a _____ thermal shift.

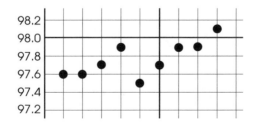

12. To get a fit in the above pattern, we would have to use the _____ principle.

Answers
1. progesterone 2. higher 3. four-tenths (4/10) 4. pre-shift six 5. lower level 6. normal high 7. consistent
8. full 9. strong 10. overall 11. overall 12. shaving

6

Shaving Temperatures

Occasionally you may have a temperature pattern something like the one in Figure 6.1 below.

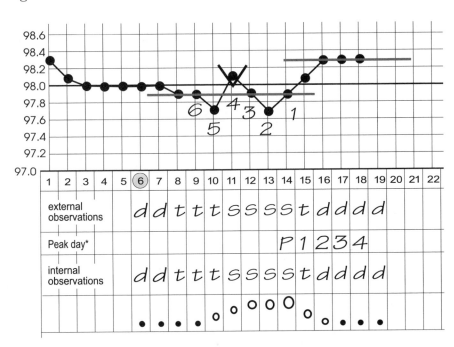

Figure 6.1 A Shaved Low Temperature Level

By looking at the pattern, you can see that the temperatures starting with Day 15 form an obvious upward thermal shift. But when you start to apply the rules, you find that you cannot get any Phase III rule to fit, including the ones in Chapter 12. The standard rule says that you are to set the Low Temperature Level by the highest normal temperature among the pre-shift six. That's Day 11 which is 98.1° F. If you set the LTL at 98.1, by the time you get to Peak Day + 4, the thermal shift is only 2/10 of 1° F. above the LTL. However, you need a cross-checking shift of 4/10 of 1° F. What should you do?

That's why CCL has developed the "shaving" principle.

The basic principle

The basic principle is this: When the interpretation of an **otherwise obvious shift** in temperature levels is held up by **one or two** valid temperatures among the pre-shift six, these higher temperatures may be "shaved" down slightly so that you can apply one of the standard rules.

The basic principle is an effort to apply the common sense of experience to this situation.

The rules for shaving

1. Shave only when there is an obvious thermal shift above the rest of the pre-shift six temperatures.

2. Shave **only one or two** higher temperatures.

3. If there are **two** higher temperatures, shave them down *either* to the **next highest level** among the rest of the pre-shift six *or* to the **arithmetic average** of the pre-shift six, *whichever is higher.* That means that you never set the shaved LTL lower than the arithmetic average of the pre-shift six when you have two out-of-line temperatures.

4. If there is only **one** higher temperature, shave it to the **next highest level**. Don't bother with the arithmetic average test you use with two temperatures.

In Figure 6.1, shave the temperature on Day 11 down to the next highest level, 97.9°. Count Day 15 as part of the overall rising temperature pattern, especially since it is past Peak Day. Draw in a pencil line at 97.9° from Day 7 up through Day 15, and you have just drawn your shaved LTL.

● **To determine the arithmetic average:**

Add all six of the pre-shift six temperatures; divide by six; the answer is the arithmetic average. Round up when the answer ends in .05 to .09; for example, 97.75° = 97.8°. Round down when the answer ends in .01 to .04; for example, 97.74° = 97.7°.

Look at Figure 6.2. Do the temperatures on Days 14-16 constitute a full thermal shift? They do if the LTL can be set at 97.5°.

You can calculate the arithmetic average in two ways: 1) add all the temps and then divide by six; 2) check the temperatures above and below a certain level as in the following example.

In Figure 6.2, select 97.5° as an estimated Low Temperature Level. The temperature on Day 9 is 2/10 above 97.5°, Day 12 is 1/10 above, so they total 3/10ths above the estimated LTL. Day 10 is 1/10 below 97.5° and Day 13 is 2/10 below, so those total 3/10 below the estimated LTL. The temps above and below the estimated LTL balance each other and confirm 97.5° as the arithmetic average as well as the "next highest level" for shaving the temperatures on Days 9 and 12. This is much easier to *do* than to understand from reading.

Use a pencil to draw the LTL at 97.5° and the HTL at 97.9°.

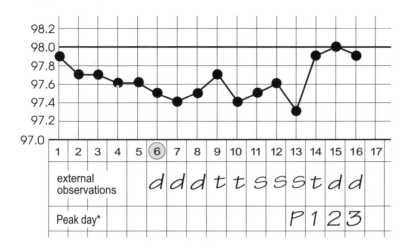

Figure 6.2 Determining the Arithmetic Average

If there are **three** temperatures that are causing the problem, you cannot shave them down to the level of the lower three temperatures. Instead, determine the arithmetic average as described on the previous page. This is called **averaging**. Be sure to check your addition and division; then apply common sense. For example, in Figure 6.3 below, there are three temperatures at 97.7° and three at 97.3°. Just looking at the pattern and applying some common sense, you can see that the average is 97.5°. If you arrived at something else, check your work again. With a pencil, draw the LTL at 97.5° and the HTL at 97.9°.

Ordinarily, we discourage averaging because it is open to mathematical mistakes.

Averaging

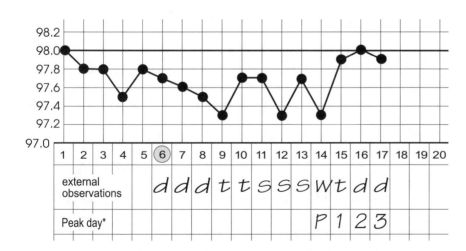

Figure 6.3 Averaging with Three Higher Temperatures

Which Phase III rules?

Can you use shaving with all the Phase III rules? Since we have not yet described the various rules, this is getting ahead of ourselves. However, the rules will refer to the shaving principles, so we placed this chapter right after the chapter on the interpretation of temperature patterns. Here it will be handy for review.

You can use the shaving principles as follows:

Rule C: okay. See Chapter 10.

Rule B: okay. See Chapter 12.

Rule K: okay with *special requirements.*

- With a three day full thermal shift, you need three days of drying-up.
- With a four day thermal shift, you need only two days of drying-up. See Chapter 12.

Rule R: restricted to shaving one temperature only 1/10 of 1° F. See Chapter 12.

Temperature-only: okay. See Chapter 26.

When to use

As indicated above, you use "Shaving" when you see an obvious thermal shift but you can't apply any of the rules on a particular day because of one or two out-of-line temperatures among the pre-shift six.

Important: Never shave or average unless it's really necessary to get a rule to fit—*on a particular day*—in an otherwise obvious situation.

On the other hand, don't be afraid to shave when the situation is obvious except for one or two higher temperatures. For example, check Figure 6.1 again. Imagine that the husband is leaving town for a week on the morning of Day 19. Without shaving, "waiting another day" for the temperature to go up a bit more would mean truly unnecessary waiting for another week.

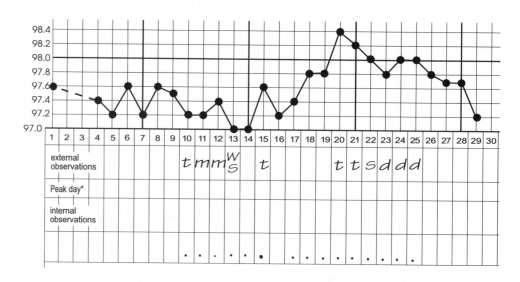

Figure 6.4 Shaving with a Temperature-only Rule

● *On a particular day.* In Figure 6.4, the absence of mucus recordings at the crucial time makes it impossible to apply a sympto-thermal rule, so we turn to the Temperature-only rule explained in Chapter 26. It requires a four-day thermal shift with the last three days at the full HTL. Without shaving, you have to set the base at 97.6°. On Day 21, you tell yourselves, "Tomorrow."

However, to illustrate the point, suppose husband is leaving town early tomorrow morning. What if you ask, "Is there good reason to think we are in Phase III on Day 21?" The answer is "Yes, with shaving." Simply shave the temperature on Day 15 to the next highest level, 97.4°, and you have a shaved LTL of 97.4°. Now you can apply the four-day Temperature-only rule on Day 21.

Workbook exercises

Charts 8, 11, 13, 15 and 22.

All of the charts listed here refer to rules that are explained in Chapters 10-12. Thus, you may want to postpone these Workbook exercises until you have learned the material in those chapters.

Chart 8 provides a good example of when you can shave to get one of the rules to fit. Note that waiting another day and then another still didn't provide a "fit" until Day 23 because of the higher temperatures on Cycle Days 13 and 15. Yet it is obvious that by Day 19 there is a four day thermal shift pattern.

Chart 11 provides a good example of shaving with Rule K. In this case there are *both* three days of full thermal shift and three days of drying-up. (To apply a shaved Rule K with only two days of drying-up, you need four days of thermal shift. This was mentioned above in "Which Phase III rules?" and is explained more thoroughly in Chapter 12.)

Chart 13 provides an example of the temptation to shave where it's not necessary and where, in fact, it doesn't advance the start of Phase III anyway. More examples are in workbook charts 17, 18 and 21.

Chart 15 provides an example of averaging the pre-shift six temperatures.

Chart 22 provides an example of both shaving and averaging.

Self-Test Questions: Chapter 6

(These questions also cover material from previous lessons on the temperature sign.)

1. The first question you ask about the temperature pattern is, "Are there _____ temperatures above the _____ _____ _____?"

2. The second question you ask is, "Are the elevated temperatures _____ above the _____ _____ _____ to satisfy the requirements for a particular rule?"

3. The minimum number of days of drying-up required by any STM rule is _____ days. The only CCL rule that uses this minimum is _____.

4. Every Sympto-Thermal rule for Phase III requires at least _____ days of thermal shift.

5. If you shave temperatures among the pre-shift six and you have three days of thermal shift, you need a minimum of _____ days of drying-up as a cross-check.

6. If it's necessary in order to get one of the Phase III rules to fit, you can shave a maximum of _____ temperatures down to the _____ _____ _____ _____ among the rest of the pre-shift six.

7. True_____ False_____   Shaving can be used with all the CCL Phase III rules.

8. True_____ False_____   If there are three temperatures in the pre-shift six that are higher that the other three, you can shave all three down to the highest of the other three.

9. True_____ False_____   The arithmetic average of the pre-shift six is calculated by adding all six temperatures and dividing by six.

10. True_____ False_____   When you shave two temperatures, you can set the shaved LTL lower than the arithmetic average of the pre-shift six.

11. True_____False_____   If you have five temperatures at 97.6° and shave one temperature of 97.8° to 97.6°, you have a correctly shaved LTL of 97.6°.

Are you doing good charting? Please review once again the end of Chapter 4, "Preparing Your Charts for Review."

Answers to self-test
1. three. . . previous six temperatures 2. enough . . . Low Temperature Level 3. two . . . Rule K 4. three 5. three 6. two. . . next highest temperature level 7. True, but with certain restrictions for Rules K and R. 8. False. If there are three out-of-line temperatures among the pre-shift six, averaging is a possibility. 9. True 10. False 11. True. You don't need to do an arithmetic average check when you shave only one temperature; and even if you did in this case, you could correctly round down from 97.63° to 97.6°.

7

How to Interpret Your Mucus Pattern

In Chapter 3 you learned how to make the external observation for mucus. In this chapter, you will learn how to interpret your mucus pattern in terms of fertility and infertility. You might want to review quickly Chapter 3 on the mucus sign and Chapter 4 on charting before getting into this chapter.

Basic principles

The basic principles for using the mucus sign are these:

1. The presence of cervical mucus before Peak Day is a positive sign that you are fertile.

2. The disappearance of mucus after Peak Day is a negative sign which indicates that you are becoming infertile.

3. You enter Phase III on the evening of the fourth day of mucus dry-up after Peak Day provided it is cross-checked by three days of any standard thermal shift pattern (full, strong or overall).

Development of a typical mucus pattern

Right after menstruation you will typically have several days of dryness—no menstruation and no mucus.

Then your mucus discharge will start as a tacky or sticky substance.

The water content in your cervical mucus increases and the mucus becomes more clear and stretchy; frequently it looks and stretches like raw egg white. The increased water content of the cervical mucus frequently gives you sensations of wetness at the outer lips of the vagina and feelings of lubrication and slipperiness when you wipe after urination.

Then the mucus dries up and generally disappears. It often returns just before menstruation. See page 72.

About 10 to 14 days after the beginning of the dry-up, you will start your next period.

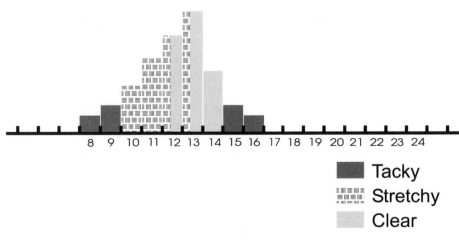

Figure 7.1 A Typical Mucus Pattern

Charting and interpreting the mucus pattern

In Chapter 8 you will learn about making an internal observation for the cervical mucus right at its source, the mouth of the cervix. The primary purpose of the internal observation is to cross-check the external observations. Some women find cervical mucus at the cervical os a day or more before they notice mucus at the vulva, and that gives them the earliest indication that they are in the fertile time. However, some women do not make the internal observation, so here we focus on the external observations.

The dry days right after menstruation are generally infertile. However, there are still a few "dry day pregnancies." We don't know if such pregnancies are the result of faulty observations, or if the woman was truly dry when coitus occurred, or if there was a nearly miraculous sperm survival. The point is, because ovulation is coming, the dry days after menstruation are not quite as infertile as the dry days after ovulation, especially as they get closer to ovulation.

● What is a dry day?

1. If you have *definite feelings of dryness* on the outer lips of the vagina (the labia), and if you see no mucus on your underwear or on the tissue paper after wiping, that's definitely a dry day. Chart it with a **D** in the space for external observations.

2. If you have *no feelings of dryness or wetness* at the vulva—just nothing either way—and if you find nothing on your underwear or on the tissue paper after wiping, that's also a dry day. Chart it with an **N** for "nothing."

3. The next situation is ambiguous. If you observe 1) a bit of shininess on the tissue paper but 2) you cannot lift any mucus from the tissue paper for finger testing and 3) there is no sensation of lubrication when wiping or feelings of wetness at other times, you should make the internal observation as a cross-check. See Chapter 8 for how and when to make the internal observation.

If you do **not** do the internal exam, consider such a day as indicating the beginning of the mucus discharge; chart it with an **M**.

If you do the internal observation and find no mucus at the os, you can consider such a day as still infertile. Chart the internal observation as **D** for dry or **N** for nothing, and chart the external observation also with an **N**.

If you find mucus at the cervical os, you are in the fertile time; record the mucus you observe as **T** or **S**. Chart the external observation as **M**.

4. If you find what you think is seminal residue from marital relations the night before, chart that as **SR**. An SR day is not a dry day because it might be a combination of SR and the beginning of cervical mucus.

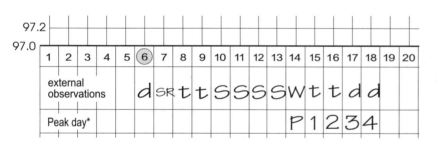

Example 1   Charting a Typical Mucus Pattern

● When does Phase II start?

The beginning of the mucus discharge, even the less-fertile type, marks a positive start of Phase II. This means that the tacky, sticky mucus which generally starts the mucus flow is a sign that you are now in the fertile time of your cycle when you can expect marital relations to cause pregnancy. We call the tacky, sticky mucus "less-fertile," but that's only in comparison to the "more-fertile" types that follow. In normal cycles, "less-fertile" mucus is an early sign that you are now fertile. Chart tacky or sticky mucus with a "**T**." If you notice something but it's not even tacky yet, chart it with an **M**. (The "M" is the symbol of last resort; you use it when you know there's some "less-fertile" mucus present but you can't be more specific. Never use "M" for a more-fertile type of mucus.)

Note well: as your mucus pattern starts, you may notice mucus only on

Note well: as your mucus pattern starts, you may notice mucus only on part of the day. Such a day is still a mucus day and shows that Phase II has started.

part of the day. Such a day is still a mucus day and shows that Phase II has started.

These types of mucus are the "more-fertile" types: produces feelings of lubrication or wetness; stretches more than one-half inch; like raw egg white; clear or cloudy. These are very good days for trying to become pregnant. Chart the days of the "more-fertile" mucus with the appropriate symbols: **C** for clear or **CL** for cloudy; **S** for stretchy; **SL** for feelings of slipperiness or lubrication; **W** for feelings of wetness. We repeat: **W** refers only to sensations of wetness at the vulva; it does *not* refer to what you will always notice in the vagina if you make the internal observation. Likewise, **SL** refers only to vaginal or vulval sensations; it does *not* refer to the slipperiness of mucus between your fingers.

● What is Peak Day?

Peak day is the last day of the more-fertile mucus before the drying-up process starts, even if the more-fertile mucus was present only for part of that day. (A definition of Peak Day is printed on every CCL Daily Observation Chart in the lower left-hand corner of the Notes section.) Peak day is not necessarily the day of peak or greatest fertility. It is certainly not always the day of ovulation. It is not always the day of the greatest quantity of mucus. In fact, you will frequently notice the greatest **quantity** one or two days before the true Peak Day as we illustrate in Figures 7.1 and 7.2. Peak Day is simply the **last day** on which you notice any of the more-fertile types of mucus before the mucus starts to dry up.

● **How do you know which day is Peak Day?** You know Peak Day only by hindsight. You will notice a distinct change from the "more-fertile" mucus to either a "less-fertile" type or complete dryness. Typically you will notice one or two days of merely tacky mucus and then complete dryness. **After one or two days of distinctive change, label as Peak Day the last day on which you noticed the more-fertile mucus.**

Toward the end of your more-fertile mucus days, you may notice both "more-fertile" and "less-fertile" mucus on the same day. Count that day as a "more-fertile" mucus day. It is not yet a part of the drying-up process.

*Note: While the **quality** of cervical mucus is **more** important, the quantity is still important, and certainly a large quantity of mucus cannot be ignored as a sign of continuing fertility.*

● What is a patch of mucus?

A patch of mucus is the length of a mucus episode from its start through its Peak Day. We also call it a "mucus patch." The start will frequently be a day of the less-fertile mucus.

A typical mucus patch lasts five to seven days—sometimes shorter and sometimes longer.

In Figure 7.2, the 7-day mucus patch started with the Tacky mucus on Day 8 and concluded with the W on Day 14. Peak Day was Day 14. The drying-up process started with the Tacky mucus on Day 15.

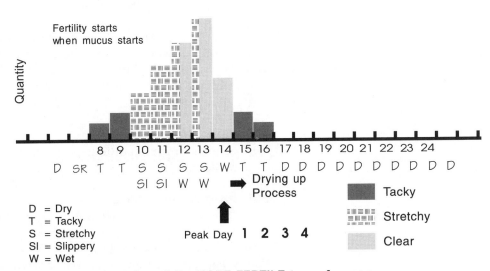

Peak Day = Last day of the MORE FERTILE type of mucus

Figure 7.2   Evaluation of a Typical Mucus Pattern

● When does Phase III start?

The Phase III rule that places most emphasis on the drying-up pattern is called Rule B: "Phase III starts on the evening of Peak Day plus 4 days of drying-up, cross-checked by at least three days of *overall* thermal shift." (See Rule B in Chapter 12.)

Note to beginners. In your first two cycles, wait until you have three days of strong or full thermal shift to cross-check four days of drying-up of the mucus. You should also add one day to your Phase III interpretation in your first two cycles. That means that in your first two cycles your Phase III interpretation will always have at least four days of thermal shift and five days of drying-up. More on this in Chapter 10.

In certain cases, you need only two or three days of mucus drying-up to cross-check full and strong thermal shifts. You will learn these advanced rules in Chapter 12.

● Can you pinpoint ovulation day?

No. You cannot pinpoint the exact day of ovulation either with the mucus sign or with the temperature sign. However, once you have several charted cycles, using those signs together you can get a very good idea which group of three days most likely contained the day of ovulation.

According to published research, ovulation can occur before or after Peak Day in different cycles. Specifically, ovulation sometimes, though rarely, occurs as early as three days before Peak Day (1.5%) and as late as three days after Peak Day (1.5%). Ovulation occurs more frequently on Peak Day (37%) than on any other single day, but it occurs more often on the combination of Peak Day - 1 (20%) and P - 2 (18.5%). It also occurs on P + 1 (14%) and P + 2 (6%). In this sample of 65 cycles, one (1.5%) had no Peak Day.[1]

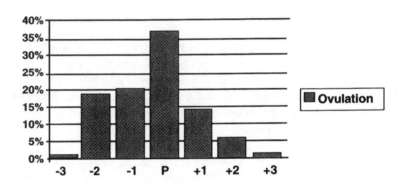

Figure 7.3
Estimated Day of Ovulation in Relationship to Peak Day

The data in Figure 7.3 are estimates based on hormone analyses from a small group of women. The only conclusion you can draw is that Peak Day **cannot** pinpoint Ovulation Day. However, Peak Day still provides an excellent marker, a place to count from, especially when used in conjunction with the temperature sign.

● Irregular mucus patterns

Several unusual mucus patterns are explained in Chapter 27, "Irregular mucus patterns."

● Premenstrual mucus

It is common to have one to three days of mucus, sometimes even the more fertile type, just before menstruation. This is caused by reduced levels of progesterone at the end of the cycle, and therefore it does not indicate fertility. You can ignore this mucus if you had an upward thermal shift around Peak Day in this cycle about 10-12 days previously.

● What is the mucus-only system?

The mucus-only system uses only the mucus sign to determine the fertile and infertile times of the cycle. In Chapter 26, "Mucus-only; Temperature-only," we explain both the mucus-only and the temperature-only systems. We also tell why we continue to prefer the cross-checking Sympto-Thermal Method. We are convinced that you should *learn* each of the common signs of fertility and infertility and how they can cross-check each other, but once you have learned them, it is your choice. You can use the signs in a cross-checking system, or you can use a mucus-only or a temperature-only system. There's more than one way to practice natural family planning, but that does not mean that all the ways are equally easy or effective.

Workbook exercises

Now it's time to apply what you have learned. Turn to the Workbook section. Review Chart 1 to make sure you understand the answer given for Peak Day and where the P-1-2-3-4 is to be recorded. Then chart the Peak Day and the four days of drying-up on all the workbook charts except these: 5, 8, 9, 10, 16, 17, 18 and 20. (Those charts deal with special mucus patterns and situations that will be covered later.) A special note on Chart 14: the wife used **M** to record *any* mucus, so the important thing to watch for here is whatever change in quality she noted. Check all your answers in the Chart Analysis section of the Practical Applications Workbook.

One last point. As you work on the workbook charts, you will be seeing some unusual patterns as well as the more common ones, and this may be confusing. So remember that each of these charts was selected to illustrate a point, and you may never see some of these things in your own charts. On the other hand, it's much better to be prepared ahead of time for the unusual situation than to think you are some sort of oddball if it happens.

Self-Test Questions: Chapter 7

1. In charting mucus, the two letters or symbols used for the less-fertile mucus are _____ and _____.

2. Chart seminal residue as _____.

3. **W** refers to feelings of _____ but only for the _____ observation.

4. True____ False____   The days of the less-fertile mucus before ovulation are infertile.

5. True____ False____   "Peak Day" is always the day you have the most mucus.

6. "Peak day" is the _____ day of the _____ fertile type mucus before the drying-up process begins.

7. Look at the CCL Daily Observation Chart (also Figure 4.1 in this manual). Where on the chart do you find the above definition of Peak Day"?

_____

8. True____ False____   Peak Day usually coincides with the day of greatest quantity of mucus.

9. If you notice both *less*-fertile and *more*-fertile types of mucus on the same day, you must regard it as a day of _____ _____ mucus.

10. In the pre-ovulation (post-menstrual) part of the cycle, the beginning of the mucus indicates the start of the _____ time.

11. According to the basic interpretation of the mucus sign, postovulation infertility (Phase III) starts on the evening of the _____ day of drying-up past the Peak Day.

12. In the Sympto-Thermal Method, the drying-up of the mucus must be cross-checked by at least _____ days of upward thermal shift temperatures.

13. True_____   False_____   After menstruation, you can regard the first day of the mucus patch as infertile if there's only a small amount of the less-fertile type mucus.

14. True_____   False_____   In regular cycles if you have "dry days" between "mucus days" in the early part of the cycle, you can regard the "dry days" as infertile.

15. True_____   False_____   You need at least two days of drying-up to be able to label your Peak Day and apply any of the STM rules.

Please review again the chart review directions, "Preparing your charts for review," at the end of Chapter 4.

Answers to self-test
1. **M** and **T**   2. **SR**   3. wetness. . . external   4. False   5. False   6. last. . . more   7. in the lower left hand corner of the "Notes" section   8. False   9. more-fertile   10. fertile   11. fourth   12. three   13. False   14. False; once the mucus has started, you're in Phase II even if you should have an occasional dry day.   15. True

References
(1) Thomas W. Hilgers, Guy E. Abraham, and Denis Cavanagh, "Natural Family Planning: I. The peak symptom and estimated time of ovulation," *Obstetrics and Gynecology* 52:5 (November 1978) 575-582; Table 3, 579.

8

Internal Observations and Ovulation Pain

In this chapter you will learn about three signs in your fertility cycle—cervical mucus right at the os, physical changes in the cervix, and a sensation called "ovulation pain." These signs are not absolutely essential for your practice of the Sympto-Thermal Method, but you may find them quite helpful. For example, most couples can practice the STM very successfully with just the external mucus observations and the temperature sign. Some women, however, find it much easier to interpret the mucus if they obtain it at its source—the cervical os.

We have two reasons for teaching these signs—practical and psychological. The practical reason: some women have difficulty with the external mucus sign and find more help from the internal observations of the cervical mucus and the cervix. The psychological reason: you cannot choose something unless you know about it. We are giving you the freedom to choose among several morally acceptable options within the overall field of Natural Family Planning. You can read more about our teaching philosophy on the last page of the "Introduction" of this manual.

The internal mucus observation

The purpose of the internal mucus observation is to obtain mucus at its source, the cervical os. Experience has shown that you might notice mucus at the cervical os earlier than you would notice it at the labia—usually one day earlier but sometimes up to three days. On the other hand, you may notice your mucus at both places the same day.

The advantage of this observation is this: you will get the earliest possible indication at the cervical os that the mucus has begun to flow from the cervix. This can be helpful if you are relying upon the mucus sign to indicate the beginning of Phase II.

To make this observation, you insert your index and middle fingers into your vagina to the cervix. You open your fingers and place them on either side of the cervix, about a half inch up. **Gently** draw your fingers toward the tip of the cervix until your fingers are together. Keep them together and withdraw them. Now separate them and look for the mucus. If mucus is present, you

How to make the internal observation for mucus

will see it between your fingertips as you separate them. If it breaks right away or stretches up to a half inch before breaking, you call it Tacky. If it tends to cling and stretches more than a half inch, call it Stretchy.

We emphasize "gently." You are not trying to squeeze any mucus from inside the cervix; you are only collecting what has already come out of the cervical os.

Important: Internal vaginal "wetness" is there all the time, so don't confuse it with the feelings of wetness on the labia. Be sure to read the sidebar in the margin.

Also important: Wash your hands with soap and water before making the internal observations. If you have long fingernails, either trim them, or don't make this observation, or be extremely careful.

Important: *You will always notice "wetness" in the vagina. Such inside wetness is there all the time, so don't confuse it with the feelings of wetness on the labia. That is, "the feeling of wetness" as a sign of fertility refers only to your* **external** *observations—the feeling on the lips of the vagina.*

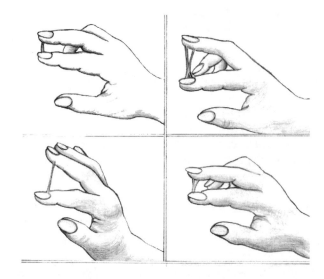

Figure 8.1 Cervical Mucus: Internal Observation

When to start?

Start the internal observation as soon as your period has stopped or by Cycle Day 6 at the latest, even if a bit of spotting should still continue.

When and how frequently?

Once a day is the obvious minimum; twice a day is the maximum.

During Phase I: If you are *not* making the external observations, then make the internal observation twice a day—1) about midday and 2) before bedtime. If you *are* making regular external observations, one internal observation before you go to bed should be sufficient. Making only one internal observation at the end of the day cannot possibly interfere with the quality of your external observations during the day. In some cases, more frequent internal observations may remove too much of the mucus needed for accurate external observations.

During Phase II: If you are having abundant external mucus, you don't need to make the internal observation until near the end of your typical mucus patch. Then start making it at the end of the day to help determine the last day of your more-fertile mucus; make it twice a day if you are not making the external observations.

During Phase III with the Sympto-Thermal Method, there is no need to keep making the internal mucus observation. However, if you are using a mucus-only system, keep making the internal observation as usual at the end of the day or before relations. The reason for that is explained in the "double mucus patch" section in Chapter 27, "Irregular mucus patterns."

● Observation details

When you make the external tissue observation and the internal observation at the same time, make the external observation first.

When you are learning either observation, write down in some detail what you notice. After you become more experienced, you can reduce the detail and use just our basic symbols.

The reason for making the internal observation only once or twice a day when you are making external observations is this: you want to let the internal mucus accumulate enough so that you can notice it at the labia. *Frequent* internal observations may interfere with good external mucus signs.

● Internal mucus symbols

Use **D** or **N** to indicate "no mucus found." Remember, it is never truly dry in the vagina.

The symbols for external mucus are on page 46.

As you separate your two fingers, more-fertile mucus tends to cling and to stretch more than a half-inch. Tacky mucus tends to break soon after you separate your fingers. Use **S** for the more-fertile mucus; use **inches** for the length of stretchy, more-fertile mucus. Use **T** for the less-fertile types of mucus. Use **M** only if you are confused—you find something that certainly is not a more-fertile type but Tacky doesn't seem like a good description either.

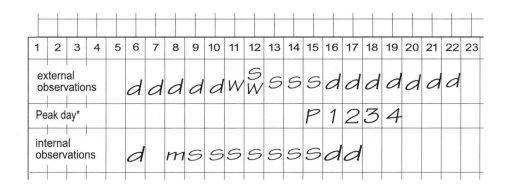

Figure 8.2   Mucus Charting

Mucus charting

In the real life example above, menstruation lasted for five days. No mucus was noticed externally or internally on Cycle Days 6 and 7. On Day 8, some mucus was noticed at the cervical os; this was recorded in the row for internal observations. External feelings of dryness continued up through Day 10. The internal exam indicated the start of the mucus flow three days before mucus was noticed externally. A three-day early warning may be a bit unusual, but the above pattern is an actual case (including the absence of an internal recording on day 7). As noted before, when "D" is recorded for the internal observation, it means "no mucus found."

In Figure 8.2, the last day of the more-fertile mucus—Peak Day—was the same for both internal and external observations. If they are not the same, we recommend being conservative; that means using whichever Peak Day comes last—the external or the internal—as your base for counting the drying-up days.

How to practice the internal observation

Here's how you can practice the two-finger internal observation of your cervical mucus. Assuming you are right-handed, put your left thumb and forefinger together so the tips are even. Now take your right forefinger and middle finger and place them about half way up the fingernails of your left thumb and forefinger. *Gently* draw your right fingers toward the tips of your left thumb and forefinger until your right fingers are together.

That little exercise will give you a fairly good idea of the size of the cervix and how to collect the mucus at the cervical os. Remember, you are not trying to squeeze any mucus out of the cervix; you are just collecting what has already come out of the os.

The cervix

The cervix is the part of the uterus that opens into the vagina. It is firm and cylindrical and about one inch thick. Think of the uterus as a small pear with the small end down and the stem removed. The opening of the cervix—the cervical os (mouth)—feels something like the indentation of the pear where the stem was removed.

What does the cervix do?

Three physical changes occur in the cervix before ovulation, and after ovulation those changes reverse themselves.

During the infertile phases of your cycle, your cervix remains firm, closed, and relatively easy to reach with your longest finger.

As ovulation approaches, the following changes occur as indicated in Figure 8.3.

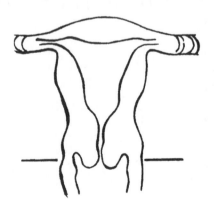 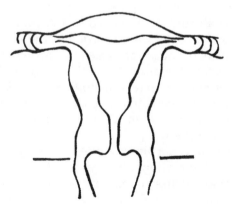 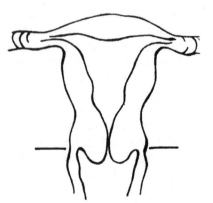

Figure 8.3 Changes in the Cervix

1. The cervical os opens slightly.

2. The tip of the cervix becomes softer; it gets rubbery and its softness is like the walls of the vagina or your facial lips.

3. The cervix rises and is more difficult to reach. Some women may not be able to reach the cervix during Phase II (too high) but find it again after ovulation.

In addition, the cervical mucus makes the cervix feel more slippery.

These signs appear gradually in your fertility cycle; it will probably take you at least two or three cycles of experience to interpret these changes with confidence, perhaps as many as six cycles.

After ovulation, the cervix soon changes back to the way it was before ovulation. These changes occur faster than those before ovulation.

1. The os closes, frequently more tightly than before it started its pre-ovulation opening.

2. The whole cervix becomes firmer; the tip becomes firm like the tip of your nose.

3. The cervix moves lower and is easier to reach; sometimes it is lower than before its pre-ovulation rise.

Also, the absence of cervical mucus makes the cervix feel less slippery compared to the time of the most-fertile mucus.

● **Why does the cervix have those changes?**

The pre-ovulation opening of the cervical os and the rising of the cervix aid sperm migration. We don't know of any function of the softness. The tight closing of the os after ovulation combines with the thickening of the mucus in the cervical canal to prevent the migration of sperm and other organisms into the uterus.

Making the cervix observation is not essential to the practice of the Sympto-Thermal Method, but many married women find it helpful to observe these changes.

How can I observe the cervix changes?

The easiest way to observe the cervix changes is this: Sit on an open toilet. Insert your middle finger through the vagina to touch the cervix. If you cannot reach it during Phase I and Phase III, try pressing down and in on your abdomen with your other hand. This can make the cervix lower and easier to reach.

Note well: If you have to push on your abdomen during Phase I to reach the cervix, then be sure to push every day so you will have the same basis for comparison. If you can reach your cervix without pushing on your abdomen during Phase I but can't reach it during Phase II, don't bother with the pushing. The fact that it has risen so high is a good positive sign that you are in the fertile time.

A second way of making this observation is this: stand with one foot on a stool or low chair, insert your finger, etc.

Another note: if your doctor has told you that you have a "tipped uterus," don't worry. Experience has proved that is no obstacle to making the cervix exam. After all, how did the doctor make that discovery?

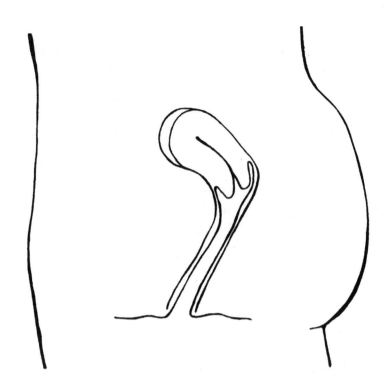

Figure 8.4   Side View of Vagina, Cervix and Uterus

● Finding your cervix

You may find it difficult to find your cervix at first; many women share that difficulty. We have two suggestions.

1. Make your first efforts to find the cervix during Phase III because your cervix may be the easiest to reach in that part of your cycle.

2. Consider asking your husband for help as many other women have done. Once he finds it, he can describe its location and what it feels like so you can find it. Your husband may find this quite arousing, and that's another reason why Phase III would be the best time for such initial help.

Once you have found the tip of your cervix the first time, you should not have any problem finding it afterwards.

When should I observe the cervix?

Make your cervix exam once or twice a day when you make your internal mucus observation.

Start to make your cervix observation beginning on Cycle Day 6; if you have a period that is less than five days, start your cervix exam on the first day after your period stops.

Don't make your cervix exam early in the morning or right after you've taken a good nap. The cervix tends to be consistently higher in the morning. This is probably because the muscles that support the uterus contract a bit during the night as you sleep and then stretch a bit after you have been up and around for a while. We're assuming that the same sort of thing might happen after a long nap.

An experienced user notes: *I have personally found that my cervix is lower before bedtime even if it's been high all day. So I don't check late at night.*

Don't make the cervix observation right after a bowel movement because that may cause the cervical os to open a bit or change its position.

Don't make the cervix observation more than twice a day. You don't want to disturb your external mucus observations.

Should I make the cervix exam every day in Phase II? Normally yes, once a day. The exception would be if you have been having difficulty in becoming pregnant. If that applies to you, once you are in Phase II, don't make any internal exams—either cervix or mucus. It's just possible that in some cases of low fertility, it may be better not to have any possible disturbance of the mucus in the vagina and around the cervix.

If you can't reach the cervix during Phase II, don't worry about it. That's a positive sign you are in the fertile time. When it starts to come down into reaching distance, you should be able to observe the changes near the end of Phase II and the beginning of Phase III.

It's not necessary but it can be helpful to make your cervix exam once a day during Phase III or every two to three days. This gives you the best standard for measuring the changes—opening, rising, and softness.

How do I chart the cervix sign? Use **F** and **S** for Firm and Soft; use **L** and **H** for Low and High; use a dot and an expanding circle to indicate closed and open. Better yet, use the dot and circle to indicate the closed-open sign and also the low-high sign by its position on the chart.

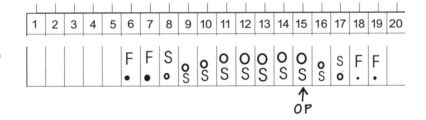

OP = ovulation pain

Figure 8.5   Cervix Charting

In the above example "F" and "S" were used for Firm and Soft. The dot showed "closed," and the gradually opening circles indicated the relative opening of the cervical os. Notice that it closed much more quickly than it opened; this is typical. The location of the circles on the chart showed the rising and then the descent of the cervix. In this case, the first day of closing was Cycle Day 16; that finding can be used in conjunction with the other Sympto-Thermal signs even though some softness continued.

● **Before ovulation**

When your cervix remains low, firm and closed after menstruation, that's a good sign you are still infertile; it provides a great cross-check on the absence of mucus. As soon as your cervix starts to change, that's an indication that your fertile time is starting.

Normally, your cervix changes and your mucus discharge will start on the same day. However, if any of your cervix changes start before your mucus discharge starts, you are getting an extra early sign that Phase II is starting. We have seen a very few charts where the wife charted the opening of the cervix a day or two before she noticed the mucus discharge. They had marital relations on those "dry but open" days and became pregnant.

Here is a "last dry day" pregnancy chart. . . As you can see, I was internally dry on the last day of intercourse for Phase I. However, we did see the cervical sign (opening, softening) on day 10. We basically ignored it (we *knew* we were taking a chance and were willing to accept it) because of the emphasis placed on mucus and dry days. I am certain that day 11 was "dry." . . . This pregnancy is greeted joyfully; we had been discussing for months having another baby, and I feel God just chose for us. Please use my chart as needed. — S.F.

● After ovulation

Here's the Sympto-Thermal rule for the cervix:

"Phase III begins on the evening of the 4th day of closing cross-checked by at least 3 days of overall thermal shift."

In that rule, "closing" stands for any and all of the changes. If you make the observation twice a day and the cervix is open in early afternoon but distinctly closing by bedtime, you can call that your first day of closing.

In other words, once the cervix starts to lower, to close and to become firm, you start counting on the first day of any of those changes. You count four days of changes just as you counted four days of drying-up past the Peak Day with the mucus sign. You cross-check the cervix signs with the temperature sign by having at least three days of a standard thermal shift.

Cervix-only?

The cervical opening is extremely reliable. I have always been amazed how good women are at detecting the changes. But I agree that the cervix observations should be cross-checked as indicated here.

— Konald A. Prem, M.D.

Should I rely solely on my cervix observations and not cross-check them with the other signs? We do not recommend such a procedure because no one has published any research on such a system. It might work just as well or better than a mucus-only system, but we simply don't know at this point in the history of NFP. Our recommendation is that you should cross-check your cervix signs with the mucus sign for the end of Phase I and with the temperature sign for the start of Phase III. For Phase I, that means that if you noticed a mucus discharge before you noticed the cervix changes, you would give priority to the mucus and consider yourself in Phase II (and vice versa). For Phase III, that means that if you do not get a cross-check from a rising temperature pattern, you would not consider yourself to be in Phase III.

If you cannot obtain a thermometer, you should cross-check 4 days of cervix closing with 4 days of mucus dry-up.

If you don't have a thermometer and don't get any help from the mucus sign, then delay the practical start of Phase III until the evening of the 5th day of closing.

The value of experience

Experience with the cervix sign can be a real asset to the mother doing extended nursing and the woman approaching menopause. During those times you might find that the cervix gives you a more clear sign of pre-ovulation infertility than you are getting from the mucus sign.

Because of its possible long range value in those situations, we encourage women not to become discouraged if they have difficulty at first with the cervix sign. It will take many women two to six cycles of daily observations to develop confidence.

You may find that the three physical changes in the cervix don't all work together for you. For example, if you have not had any babies, your cervical os may not open much at all. Or, you may not notice changes in firmness and softness. The change from low to high may not coincide perfectly with the change from firm to soft. Two things need to be said about such situations.

1. First, be glad if you find even one of the three changes really helpful and coinciding well with the mucus and temperature signs.

2. Second, if you don't find any of the cervix changes helpful after six cycles of trying, just don't bother with the effort to observe the physical changes in the cervix.

What if I don't notice all the changes?

In my experience, many women do not like the idea of doing the internal exams. They don't like the idea of inserting one finger for the cervix exam and two fingers for the internal mucus exam. Later, some of these women question their external observations, wondering if they have mucus or not. They try these internal exams and discover how helpful they can be. I empathize with these women because I was one of them. I found these internal exams to be very helpful. They are optional; however, I recommend them because so many other women have also found them helpful.

A note from Sheila K.

Ovulation Pain

Finally, something very brief.

Somewhere around the time of ovulation, you may experience a sensation in the area of one of your ovaries. In the medical literature, this feeling is called "Mittelschmerz," a German word meaning "pain in the middle." Strictly speaking, it refers to the middle of the average cycle.

Some women notice it; others don't. Sometimes it lasts a few hours; in other cycles it may last for two or three days. For some women, the feeling is so slight they can't call it "pain," but some women occasionally experience considerable discomfort, even to the point of doubling over with pain.

What is "ovulation pain"?

The cause of ovulation pain is debated. We are aware of three different explanations.

1. A congestion of mucus in the Fallopian tubes might cause minor swelling and resulting pain. This would coincide with the secretion of cervical mucus, so it would be slightly before and at the time of ovulation. This explanation fits best with the charting of Mittelschmerz for two or three consecutive days before Peak Day and the beginning of the upward thermal shift.

2. A vigorous pulsing of the Fallopian tubes at the time of ovulation and just afterwards may cause this pain. The pulsing of your esophagus, the tube that leads food from your mouth to your stomach, is called peristalsis. It is that same sort of pulsing motion that helps the ovum move through the Fallopian tube toward the uterus.

What causes ovulation pain?

3. A small amount of blood may be released at ovulation; the abdominal lining is sensitive to internal bleeding, and the reaction is pain. Where does the blood come from? The ovarian follicle has to rupture in order to release the ovum; a small surface blood vessel may be broken by the rupture and a slight bleeding may occur.

What does "ovulation pain" tell me?

This sensation or pain does not tell you enough so that you could use it as a primary indicator of when you are fertile and infertile. It might even occur during your sleep so you wouldn't notice it at all. Or you might confuse it with minor intestinal pains or cramps.

However, you can use it as a good secondary sign in conjunction with the other fertility signs. For example, if you experience Mittelschmerz during your mucus patch, it might be a sign you are very close to ovulation.

There's another benefit to knowing about Mittelschmerz. If you experience this as a pain in conjunction with other signs of fertility, you will have a reasonably good idea that it is just Mittelschmerz and not a symptom of some other problem. Being in touch with your natural fertility has its advantages!

A patient of Dr. Konald A. Prem experienced severe abdominal pain. Since Dr. Prem was on vacation, she saw another physician who was not as well acquainted with fertility awareness and Mittelschmerz. The other physician was mystified and admitted the woman to the hospital for exploratory surgery. Dr. Prem returned from vacation, got the message about the patient, visited her in the hospital, found out where she was in her cycle, diagnosed it as severe Mittelschmerz, and saved the woman the unnecessary surgery.

Charting "ovulation pain"

To chart ovulation pain or Mittelschmerz, write an **OP** in the open space just below the boxes for cervix and mucus recordings. If you notice Mittelschmerz for more than one day, record it for each day. Note the "OP" under Cycle Day 15 in Figure 8.5.

Other signs of fertility

Some women may experience other signs that are sometimes associated with fertility. Dr. Konald A. Prem notes that these signs include "increased libido, abdominal bloating, ovulation pain (mittelschmerz), vulvar swelling and slight bloody staining. These usually occur simultaneously with mucorrhea just prior to the temperature rise."[4] Others have mentioned breast swelling after Peak Day and the start of the upward temperature shift.

If you notice these or any other particular signs, note them on your chart. If they occur regularly, they may help your fertility awareness.

Chapter 8: Self-Test Questions

1. The internal observation obtains mucus at its direct _____, the cervical os.

2. True____ False____ The purpose of the internal observation is to detect the mucus as soon as it starts to flow.

3. Some women find mucus at the cervical os as many as _____ days before they notice it at the labia.

4. It takes (how many) _____ fingers to make the internal observation for mucus.

5. During Phase I, how often should you make the internal observation?
   _____

6. During Phase I, when should you make the internal observation?
   _____

7. Too frequent internal observations may _____ the external observations by not giving the mucus enough time to accumulate and flow through the vagina.

8. True____ False____ If you notice wetness in the vagina when you are making an internal observation, you should record a "W" on your chart.

9. True____ False____ When you find no mucus at the os, you should record a "D" or an "N" on your chart.

10. List the three changes that typically occur in the cervix as ovulation approaches: The cervix _____, _____, and _____.

11. True____ False____ Every woman will always be able to notice all three physical changes in the cervix.

12. The _____ finger is used to make the cervix observation.

13. When you make the external and the internal observations at the same bathroom visit, which observation should you make first? _____
    Why?
    _____

14. What is the maximum number of times per day for making the internal observations of the cervix and the cervical mucus? _____

15. It takes some women (how many) _____ to _____ cycles of experience to become familiar and confident with their internal observations.

16. True____ False____ One explanation for Mittelschmerz or ovulation pain is a pre-ovulation congestion of mucus in the Fallopian tube.

Answers to self-test
1. source   2. True   3. three   4. two   5. Once or twice daily   6. a) evening or b) midday and evening   7. obscure
8. False   9. True   10. rises, the os opens, and the tip softens.   11. False   12. middle. You could also use your index finger, but your longest finger works best.   13. external. . . making the internal exam first may obscure the external observation.   14. Two   15. two to six   16. True

References

(1) J.F. Kippley, "The cervix symptom of fertility: a comparative study," *The CCL News* 7:2 (November-December 1980) 2 ff. Also in *International Review of Natural Family Planning* VI:3 (Fall 1982) 272-277.

(2) S.F., Letter and chart (September-October 1993) to CCL, received 8 November 1993.

(3) Edward F. Keefe, "Self-observation of the cervix to distinguish days of possible fertility," *Bulletin of the Sloane Hospital for Women,* VIII:4 (December 1962) 129-136. Dr. Keefe, obstetrician-gynecologist and the medical pioneer of the cervix signs, suggests that a woman who examines her cervix through three cycles should be able to recognize the changing signs.

(4) Konald A. Prem, M.D., "Temperature Method in the Practice of Rhythm," *Child and Family,* Fall, 1968, 313.

9

Basic Fertility Data

Fertility refers to being physically able to conceive babies. We refer to this as "procreation" instead of "reproduction." The word "procreation" reminds us that parents are co-creators along with God in bringing new human persons into existence. Animals reproduce animals; human persons procreate human persons destined for never ending life with God.

This chapter explains both male and female fertility. Male fertility is constant; female fertility occurs in cycles, and basic female hormones control that cycle. That's why we explain the role of hormones in the female fertility cycle.

In one sense, you don't need to study this chapter. You can practice natural family planning without reading this chapter. You can observe your mucus and cervix and temperature changes without knowing what causes them. However, most people like to know the "behind the scenes" story. They want to understand how and why NFP works. If you are among them, read on.

The Man's Part

The husband's part in co-creating human babies is relatively simple compared to that of his wife. His basic sources of fertility are his two testicles. These are contained in a sac called the scrotum, and they make sperm on a regular basis, sometimes hundreds of millions each day. They also produce the male hormone testosterone which causes the various male bodily characteristics. The prostate gland (located beneath his bladder) and two seminal vesicles (one on either side of his bladder) produce a fluid that combines with sperm, and the combination is called semen.

When a husband is sexually excited, his penis stiffens so he can insert it into his wife's vagina. When he is sufficiently stimulated, an ejaculation occurs which expels his semen into his wife's vagina. Millions of sperm may be deposited in any act of sexual intercourse: 200 to 500 million is considered normal. It takes only one of those sperm to join with his wife's egg (ovum) to co-create a new baby.

Sperm are extremely small; they can be seen only with a microscope. Each sperm looks like a tadpole with a head-like body and a tail. The tail thrashes around and enables the sperm to swim upward in his wife's procreative channels to meet the egg. (The procreative channels are explained in "The Woman's Part.") If an egg is present, the wife is fertile, and one of the sperm may unite with it. If the sperm and egg unite, a new human life begins. This process is called conception or fertilization.

Sperm life

If an egg is not available, conception cannot occur even though sperm are present in the procreative channels. Instead, the sperm die within a short time. How long do sperm live after ejaculation? It depends on conditions in the wife's procreative channels, especially her vagina and cervix. If there is no cervical mucus in the vagina, sperm life is very short—usually from a half hour to six hours. Twenty-four hours would be maximum. If cervical mucus is flowing, it's a different story. When cervical mucus is present, in most cases sperm live from one to three days (72 hours). However, in a few cases of very favorable conditions, sperm can live up to five days. Can sperm ever live longer than five days? In very rare cases, it is possible for sperm to live six days or more, but pregnancies caused by such extended sperm life are extremely rare, perhaps about like the chances of winning a huge lottery. You could call such a pregnancy a "small miracle" because it appears that God goes out of his way to bring such a life into being.

Male maturity

A man reaches biological sexual maturity during his teens, sometimes starting even earlier. The growth of hair in the armpits, on the face, in the area around and above his penis, changes in his voice, and sometimes a growth spurt indicate this new biological power.

Physiological sexual maturity is automatic. However, in contrast to his biological sex, a young man's inner sexual maturity is by no means automatic. There is no guarantee he will make progress in true sexual maturity. In fact, he will have to struggle to make progress in chastity; if he does not, he may go backwards. At age 20 he may be more immature than he was at age 12, because at age 20 he might be sinning seriously by sexually exploiting others. Such sins are no small matter. Fornication is the grave matter of mortal sin; it is a sin by which man and woman—whether young or old—exclude themselves from the kingdom of God (Galatians 5:19-21). To put it more bluntly, having sex outside marriage is one way in which people put themselves on the wide and easy path that leads to destruction and the loss of heaven for all eternity (Matthew 7:13). Actions *do* speak louder than words, and God has revealed that by such actions a person is saying "No" to God and to God's revelation about the demands of love.

Much more needs to be said about pre-marital chastity. However, here we simply want to make the point that a young man typically has a struggle of many years to place his biological power at the service of authentic love. And the struggle continues as a married man.

Once a young man's biological sexual power has developed, he is fertile all the time; that means he is capable of fathering a child at any time. By contrast, a woman is fertile only a few days each month.

The Woman's Part

Here we are addressing particularly the wife, but husbands should read this too. As a wife, your part in procreating babies is much more complex than your husband's. While he has a relatively simple system and continuous fertility, you have a more complicated procreative system that gives you a rhythmic cycle of fertility and infertility. You undergo certain hormonal changes each cycle that affect you both physically and emotionally. The practice of natural family planning makes more sense when you understand these changes.

First we will describe your six body parts or organs that are important in your role of procreation. Then we'll show how your menstrual-fertility cycle works. In all of this, we assume that you have normal organs and fertility.

Your sexual organs

1. The ovaries

Ovum is the Latin name for egg, and **ovary** is the name of the organ that has all your eggs—call it your personal egg basket. You have two ovaries, one on each side of your uterus. Each ovary is about the size of an almond. Within each ovary, each ovum has its own container called a **follicle**. Once you have reached a certain level of biological sexual maturity, one of these follicles ripens and ejects an ovum approximately every month except during pregnancy and for a variable time after childbirth. (See Chapters 23-25.)

Actually, a group of follicles start to develop, and one becomes the dominant follicle. As the dominant follicle develops, it secretes the first basic female hormone—**estrogen**. This hormone causes some effects that are very important for your menstrual-fertility cycle. We explain these effects below in the section titled "The Hormonal Cycle."

● **Ovulation**. When you **ovulate**, the dominant ovarian follicle releases the ovum from the follicle and the ovary.

You cannot pinpoint the exact day of ovulation through your mucus and temperature signs. However, in combination they give you a very good idea of the two or three most likely days of ovulation. (Ovulation can be seen through ultrasound images, but that is obviously a very expensive and impractical procedure.) "Pinpointing" ovulation is entirely unnecessary. What you need to know are two things: 1) the outer limits of the fertile time when you are seeking to avoid pregnancy and 2) the most fertile days of the overall fertile time when you are trying to conceive a baby. Your mucus and temperature signs give you that information.

● **Egg life.** After ovulation, your egg lives from 8 to 24 hours. During this time your egg may join with your husband's sperm to begin a new human life. If conception does not occur within 8 to 24 hours, the egg cell begins to disintegrate and can no longer be fertilized.

A second ovulation can occur within 24 hours. That's how fraternal twins are conceived. That means that you can actually *conceive* only on one or two consecutive days per cycle, but don't forget that sperm life is much longer.

After ovulation, the follicle that released the egg has a new role to play and gets a new name—the **corpus luteum** (Latin for the yellow body). Its function is to send out the second basic female hormone—**progesterone**, and it secretes this hormone for about two weeks. Progesterone does several important things related to fertility, and we explain these later in the section on "The Hormonal Cycle."

● **Luteal phase**. The luteal phase of your menstrual cycle is the time between ovulation and the next menstruation; this part of your cycle is under the influence of the corpus luteum which is secreting progesterone. That's a mouthful, and that's why it is called the luteal phase. You can roughly measure the luteal phase in two ways: 1) starting with the first day of elevated temperatures up through the last day before your next period; 2) starting with Peak Day + 1 up through the last day before your next period.

2. The Fallopian tubes

You started life in the Fallopian tube of your mother.

Next to each ovary is the Fallopian tube that connects to the uterus. The free end of the Fallopian tube ends in a loose fringe called the **fimbriae**. These are sticky and move around the ovary to pick up the ovum that is being released. Conception or fertilization takes place in one of the Fallopian tubes when a sperm cell comes through the tube and unites with the ovum. To make that personal, that means that you and your spouse each started life in your respective mother's Fallopian tube.

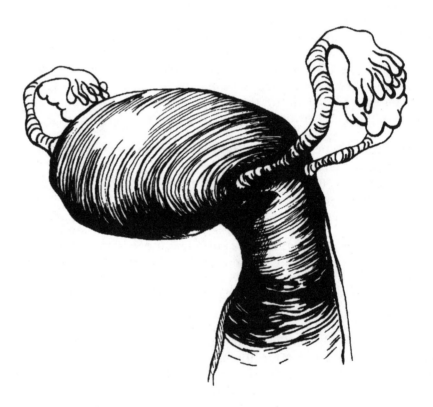

Figure 9.1. A Woman's Procreative Organs

3. The uterus

This organ is sometimes called the womb, and it's where the baby develops. When you are not pregnant, your uterus is the size of a small pear tipped upside down. During pregnancy, it stretches many times that size to accommodate the growing baby. When you are having menstrual cycles, a lining called the **endometrium** builds up inside the uterus in the early part of each cycle. The purpose of this lining is to provide a place for the newly conceived life to implant itself and to give it nourishment. If you conceive a baby, the lining of your uterus remains intact during your pregnancy. (However, a few women continue to have a few periodic bleedings even after they're pregnant.)

If conception does not occur, about two weeks after ovulation this lining disintegrates and passes out of your body in the process called **menstruation**. This is sometimes called a monthly bleeding, but it is not bleeding in the same sense as from a cut. Medical people call it "menses" because it occurs roughly once a month and the Latin word for month is "mensis."

4. The cervix

"Cervix" is the Latin word for "neck." Here it refers to the lower end of the uterus. It's about one inch long and protrudes into the vagina. The opening at the lower end of the cervix is called the cervical **os**. In the inner lining of your cervix are glands or crypts that produce cervical mucus. This is very important for your fertility, and we describe the mucus cycle in "The Hormonal Cycle."

The cervix and the os undergo certain physical changes that we will also describe in "The Hormonal Cycle." During childbirth, the cervix opens wide to allow the baby to pass from the uterus into and through the vagina.

5. The vagina

The vagina is the female sexual organ that receives the male penis and serves as the birth canal. As mentioned before, sperm deposited in the vagina swim up through the cervix if it is open; then they progress through the uterus and into the Fallopian tubes where conception takes place.

6. The breasts

The breasts or mammary glands are also part of your overall procreative physiology even though they are not directly involved in the process of uniting sperm and ovum. During ecological breastfeeding, a baby's suckling suppresses ovulation through a complicated hormonal process. How frequently the baby nurses is the most important factor in determining how long ovulation is suppressed. More on that in Chapters 24 and 25.

The menstrual cycle

Once a girl reaches a certain stage of biological sexual maturity, she begins to have menstrual cycles and periods. "Period" refers to the days of menstruation; "cycle" refers to the time from the first day of one menstruation through the last day before the next menstruation. Some girls menstruate as early as age nine, and a few as late as seventeen; most girls are having menstrual cycles by age 14. You probably will continue to have cycles until you are about 50, but many women stop earlier and others go longer.

A girl's first period is called **menarche** ("men-ar-kee" which comes from the Greek words for "beginning month"). Her cycles at first will tend to be quite irregular. After a few years she will get closer to the adult woman's 28-day average cycle. Sometimes this doesn't happen until she is in her early twenties.

Menopause occurs when your ovaries stop ovulating and when you stop having cycles and periods. **Premenopause** is the transition time from regular fertile cycles to menopause. Medical people call this process the "climacteric"; ordinary folks sometimes call this transition process "*going through* the change in life." More about premenopause in Chapter 33.

● Cycle lengths

On the average, most women start a period about every 28 days. However, this is an average and it may not apply to you. You may regularly have cycles of 25 or 26 days, or you may consistently have cycles of 35 to 40 days.

● Cycle variation

The range from your shortest cycle to your longest cycle is your cycle variation. Almost every woman has some shorter and some longer cycles. For example, if you think you have regular 28 day cycles, once you start keeping accurate records, you will most likely find that occasionally you have cycles ranging from 26 days to 30 days. Generally your cycle variation will be your average cycle plus or minus at least two days each way. We consider a cycle variation of seven days to be normal.

If your cycle variation is eight to 20 days, you have *moderately* irregular cycles. We're talking here about cycles that consistently are 8 to 20 days shorter or longer than each other. We're not talking about someone who almost always has cycles of 28-30 days and then experiences a severe emotional stress that delays ovulation so much that she has a 40 day cycle.

If your cycle variation is 21 days or more, we call that *very* irregular. Both sickness and psychological stress can delay ovulation. Inadequate nutrition, being significantly overweight or underweight, and having too little body fat, as in the case of some female athletes, can also affect the cycle. Some kinds of cycle irregularity can be modified or eliminated; see Chapter 31, "Cycle Irregularities."

● **Regularity of the luteal phase.** Remember, the luteal phase is the time of the cycle between ovulation and the start of your next period. This is the most consistent part of your cycle. For most women in most cycles, the luteal phase is 12 to 14 days. However, some women consistently have shorter or longer luteal phases. The main point is this: the length of your luteal phase will rarely be more than two days shorter or longer than your average luteal phase.

If you have any significant cycle variation, it occurs between menstruation and ovulation as indicated in Figures 9.2 and 9.3.

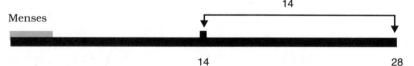

Ovulation on Day 14 plus a 14 day luteal phase.

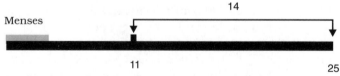

Ovulation on Day 11 plus a 14 day luteal phase.

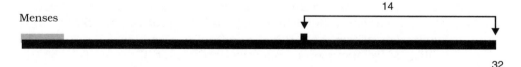

Ovulation on Day 18 plus a 14 day luteal phase.

Figure 9.2 The Regularity of the Luteal Phase

● Cycling

This refers to having one cycle after another. Figure 9.3 shows a typical menstrual cycle. If you are not pregnant or doing ecological breastfeeding, you will have recurring cycles. After you complete one menstrual period, the inner lining (endometrium) of your uterus begins to build up again. Then you ovulate. If you do not conceive in that cycle, your endometrium is discharged about two weeks later. That causes your menstrual bleeding, and a new cycle is under way again.

Your menstrual cycle is also your fertility cycle. That's why we frequently call it the menstrual-fertility cycle. During each cycle you have three phases related to fertility:
Phase I: pre-ovulation infertility
Phase II: the fertile time
Phase III: postovulation infertility.

The fertility cycle

● Phase I

Phase I is the time of **pre-ovulation infertility**, and it begins on the first day of menstruation. The first few days of heavy flow are highly infertile, but once the flow begins to decrease, it is possible to conceive.

In Phase I, you are not quite as infertile as you are in Phase III. That's because after Phase I, you enter the fertile time, Phase II. There is a slight possibility that you could make a mistake and think you were still in Phase I when you were actually in Phase II; there is a very slight possibility that sperm with super extended life might live from Phase I up to the time of ovulation in Phase II.

Chapter 11 gives several "End of Phase I" rules; some are more conservative than others.

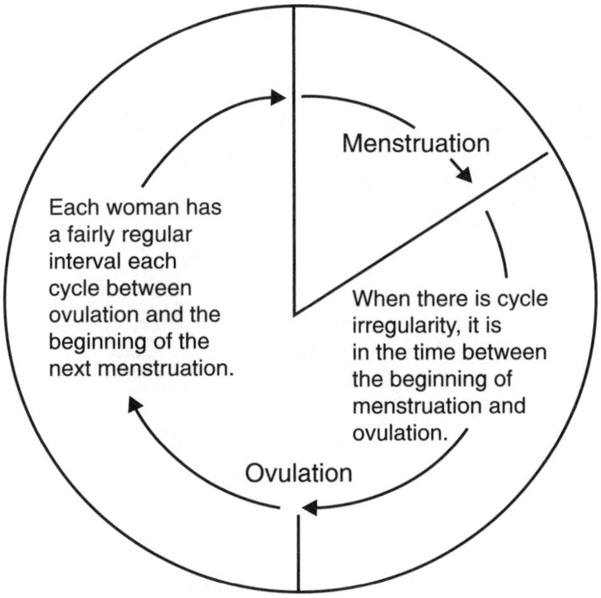

Figure 9.3 The Menstrual Cycle

● Phase II

Phase II is the **fertile time of the cycle** when marital relations can result in pregnancy. If sperm live three to five days and fertilization of the egg can happen only on two days, then there are only five to seven days per cycle on which marital relations can result in pregnancy.[1] However, in practicing NFP to avoid pregnancy, we normally add days before ovulation to take into account the possibility of long sperm life or an extra-early ovulation.

A *positive* sign that Phase II has started is the appearance of cervical mucus, as you learned in Chapters 3 and 7.

A *positive* sign that Phase II has ended is the upward thermal shift of at least three days, as you learned in Chapters 2 and 5. A *negative* sign that Phase II has ended is the disappearance of the cervical mucus for several days. In the Sympto-Thermal Method, we cross-check the positive and the negative signs.

Within the fertile time, some days are more fertile than others. Couples seeking pregnancy should know the *most* fertile days in the overall fertile time, and sometimes they need some other helpful hints. Chapter 21—"If You Don't Succeed at First"—provides extra help.

● Phase III

Phase III is the **infertile time after ovulation**, and it starts several days after ovulation. With the Sympto-Thermal Method, you identify the start of Phase III by cross-checking three or four days of elevated temperatures with two to four days of the drying-up and disappearance of the cervical mucus. More on this in Chapters 10 and 12.

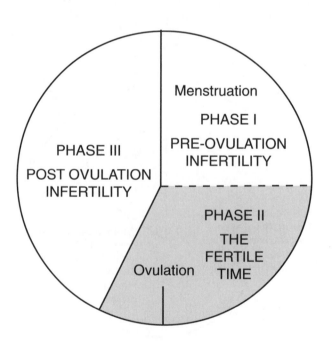

Figure 9.4 The Fertility Cycle

Your hormonal cycle is what causes your menstrual-fertility cycle. A hormone is a chemical substance, made by one of your body's endocrine glands, that affects some other bodily function or organ. You have a number of different hormones; here we are concerned only with the primary ones that affect your menstrual-fertility cycle.

Let us start with the time of menstruation. Shortly after your period starts, your **pituitary gland** (located at the base of your brain) secretes a hormone called **FSH**—follicle stimulating hormone. FSH stimulates the development of an ovarian follicle and the ovum it contains. That ovarian follicle, and probably others too, then secretes the first basic female hormone, **estrogen**. The estrogen causes three effects that are important for your fertility:

1. The inner lining of your uterus (the endometrium) builds up;

2. The glands or crypts lining the inside of the cervix secrete a mucus discharge;

3. The cervical os opens slightly, and the cervix rises a bit and becomes softer.

You can't see or feel what's going on in your uterus, but you can see and feel the cervical mucus, and with the internal observations you can feel the changes in the cervix.

The increasing level of estrogen usually causes your cervical mucus discharge to become more abundant and like raw egg white—clear and stretchy. Your cervix rises higher as your estrogen level increases.

High estrogen levels may also slightly depress your waking temperatures. That's why we use the six temperatures just before the upward shift begins: those half dozen temperatures are the ones most influenced by pre-ovulation estrogen.

About a day before ovulation, your estrogen level reaches its high point; your pituitary gland senses this and secretes another hormone—**LH** or luteinizing hormone—in a big surge. The LH surge stimulates your ovarian follicle to release its egg—the process called ovulation.

After ovulation your estrogen level falls sharply; then it recovers slightly and continues until menstruation at a level that is lower than its preovulation level.

Figure 9.5 (on the next page) illustrates the relationships we have been discussing—the hormones, the menstrual cycle, the ovarian follicle and corpus luteum, and the signs of fertility and infertility, that is, changes in cervical mucus, cervix, and temperature levels.

The follicle that released the egg now gets a new look and a new job. It turns yellow, and therefore is called the yellow body, but all the scientific literature uses the Latin for yellow body—**corpus luteum**. The job of the corpus luteum is to secrete the second basic female hormone—**progesterone**. The higher level of progesterone has five effects that are important for your fertility cycle.

1. Progesterone maintains the inner lining of your uterus at a thick level with a rich blood supply.

2. It suppresses subsequent ovulation in that cycle.

3. Your resting body temperature rises.

4. Your cervical mucus thickens and forms a plug in the cervical canal.

5. Your cervix becomes lower, the tip becomes firm again, and the cervical os closes.

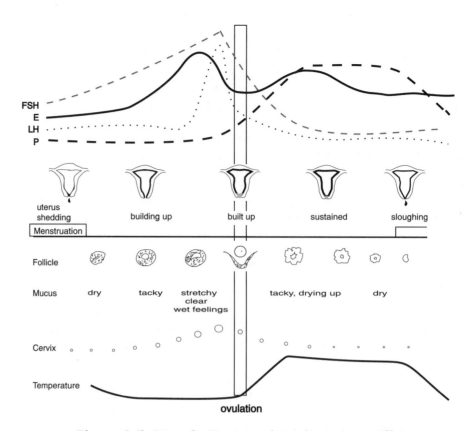

Figure 9.5 Female Hormonal Cycle and Its Effects

As mentioned previously, the corpus luteum continues to secrete progesterone for approximately two weeks. During this time, the progesterone is telling your pituitary gland not to send out FSH; that's how it suppresses additional ovulations in that cycle. When your corpus luteum stops functioning, the level of progesterone in your body drops sharply, and the thick inner lining of your uterus is shed in the bloody discharge called menstruation. The lower level of progesterone no longer inhibits your pituitary gland, so it starts the ovulation process again by secreting FSH. To repeat, the time of the cycle under the influence of the corpus luteum is called the luteal phase.

Check those five effects once again. You cannot see or feel the first two effects of higher progesterone levels, but you can measure or feel or see the last three effects. You can use two or three of them in a cross-checking way to determine the start of Phase III.

The above explanation is simplified but still valid. A more complex explanation would have to include the hypothalamic-pituitary relationship, the luteal phase levels of estrogen and FSH, threshold levels of pre-ovulatory estrogen, and the relationship between the ovaries. That sort of detail is appropriate for a course in physiology, but it is excessive and unnecessary in a manual of this sort. For greater detail, see *A Healthcare Provider's Reference to Natural Family Planning*, a 12-page CCL pamphlet.

Becoming pregnant

The process of becoming pregnant begins when you and your spouse have marital relations at the fertile time. At ejaculation your husband deposits up to 500 million sperm in your vagina. Your cervical mucus nourishes the sperm and provides a river, so to speak, in which they can swim upstream. The sperm swim rapidly (at about 1/8 inch per minute) up through the open cervical os. Some of the sperm continue immediately through the uterus and into the Fallopian tubes. Other sperm stay in the cervical crypts which produce the cervical mucus. Then they move out gradually over the next one to three days and complete their journey into the Fallopian tubes. It is this time-delay mechanism that enables sperm to be present when you ovulate two or three days after relations.

After ovulation, the ovum starts its journey through one of your Fallopian tubes, and soon the ovum meets the sperm. Over a thousand of your husband's sperm may surround your ovum, each one trying to pierce its outer wall. Finally, one sperm penetrates the wall of the ovum which immediately undergoes a change to prevent any others from doing so. His sperm proceeds to unite with the nucleus of your ovum in the process called fertilization or conception, and a new human life has been co-created. All of us began our lives this way. We all started life in our mother's fallopian tubes, and that's where all of our hereditary characteristics were determined. (Fertilization and conception are two words for the same event. We use the terms interchangeably.)

The human person has a primary instinct for survival and it starts working very early in life. Very soon after implantation, your newly conceived little child's placenta begins to make and secrete a hormone called **HCG** (human chorionic gonadotropin.) HCG tells your corpus luteum to keep on secreting its progesterone. Remember, your corpus luteum usually functions only for two weeks, and you menstruate when it stops. Because of your baby's HCG, your corpus luteum keeps working for several months until your baby's placenta takes over the production of progesterone and other hormones for the rest of your pregnancy. In that way the lining of your uterus is maintained and you don't have a period.

Approximately a week after you conceived your new baby's life, he implants in the rich and thick lining of your uterus. After two more weeks, he is taking on familiar physical features and his heart has begun to beat. By six weeks after conception, your baby's brain waves can be measured; by eight weeks after fertilization, your baby has all the organs he will have at birth. If your baby is a girl, when she is born, she will have all the eggs she will ever have.

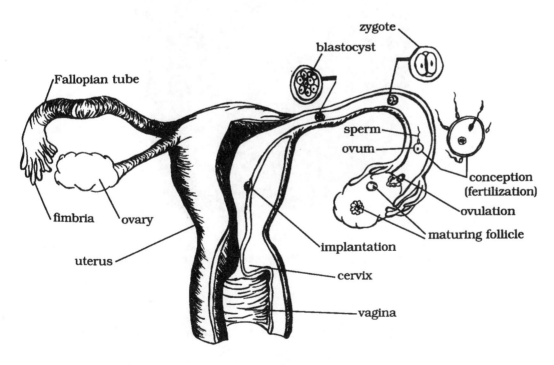

Figure 9.6 The Process of Becoming Pregnant

Female maturity

Like male fertility, physiological sexual maturity proceeds automatically for the young woman. Also like male maturity, true sexual maturity takes years for most women to develop.

There is no question: men and women are different, but each can sexually exploit the other. One difference is this: many young and not-so-young women seem to have no idea how their immodest dress affects men, both young and not-so-young. They dress in such a way as to make their breasts and pubic areas prime objects of visual attention, and then they wonder why men sometimes look at women as sex objects. Or maybe many of them know precisely what they are doing and how to appeal to the weakness of men in this way. And, of course, dressing modestly applies also to men and young men, especially in an age when the active pursuit of homosexuality is so prevalent. What we said in the section on "Male maturity" about the moral implications of illicit sex applies equally to men and to women, young and not-so-young.

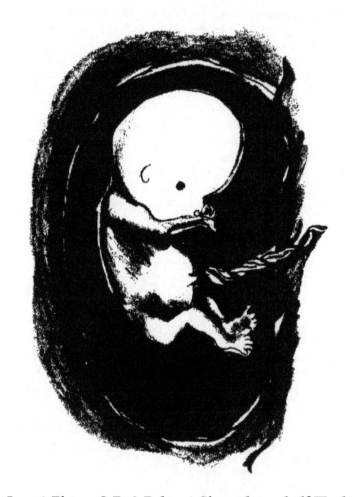

Insert Figure 9.7 A Baby at Six and one-half Weeks

Additional reading

"A Healthcare Provider's Reference to Natural Family Planning"

Self-Test Questions: Chapter 9

1. True_____   False_____   A normally fertile man is fertile all the time, but a normally fertile woman is fertile only some of the time.

2. How many sperm does the normally fertile husband deposit in his wife's vagina at each act of marital relations? _____

3. The hormone that causes the mucus discharge is _____.

4. The hormone that causes your temperature to rise after ovulation is called
   _____.

5. The uterus is another name for the _____.

6. True_____   False_____   A woman has all the eggs (or ova) she will ever have when she is born.

7. A new human person is created at the time of _____.

8. True_____   False_____   You can pinpoint the day of ovulation with the mucus and temperature signs.

9. The time of the cycle between ovulation and the start of the next period is called the
   _____.

10. The most regular part of the cycle is the _____ phase.

11. Identify the phases of the cycle in terms of fertility:
    Phase I: _____
    Phase II: _____
    Phase III: _____

12. High levels of estrogen may slightly _____ a woman's waking temperatures.

Answers to self-test
1. True 2. 200 to 500 million 3. estrogen 4. progesterone 5. womb 6. True 7. conception or fertilization 8. False
9. luteal phase 10. luteal 11. Phase I = pre-ovulation infertility; Phase II = the fertile time; Phase III = postovulation
infertility 12. depress

References

(1) Allen J. Wilcox, M.D., Ph.D., Clarice R. Weinberg, Ph.D., and Donna D. Baird, Ph.D., "Timing of Sexual Intercourse in Relation to Ovulation," *New England Journal of Medicine* 333:23 (December 7, 1995) 1517-1521. Concluded that "nearly all pregnancies can be attributed to intercourse during a six-day period ending on the day of ovulation" (1517).

10

NFP Rules: Beginners

This chapter contains the rules we recommend for beginners.

By way of review, we divide the fertility cycle into three phases:
Phase I is the time of pre-ovulation infertility.
Phase II is the fertile time.
Phase III is the time of postovulation infertility.

Phase I

Count the first day of menstruation* as the first day of Phase I in the vast majority of cycles. Two exceptions are listed immediately below.

● **Two rare exceptions**

1. **Early temperature drop at end of cycle.** What if your waking temperature drops from your thermal shift pattern to or below your Low Temperature Level (in that cycle) *shortly before* your period starts? Such a drop may reflect a sharply reduced level of progesterone, the hormone that inhibits ovulation. If that's so, the hormone cycle that leads up to ovulation is free to get started once again. In this case, the more conservative practice is to count the first day of temperatures at or below your LTL as Day 1 of your new cycle.

2. **Irregular shedding.** The second case is just the opposite of the first and is called irregular shedding. In this case, your temperature remains high during the first few days of spotting or light menstruation, and then it drops. If you have that experience, count as Day 1 the first day of descending temperatures or the first day of heavy flow, whichever comes first. If you have irregular shedding as a consistent pattern, you would do well to read *Fertility, Cycles and Nutrition*,[1] especially chapters six and seven; this problem is often helped by specific nutritional changes.

You may wonder, "What difference does it make?" You will learn why it makes a difference in the next chapter, "Phase I with more experience." For right now, we'll just say what may be obvious: with some rules, the end of Phase I depends on what day you use as Day 1 of the cycle. Probably 99% of the time that's the first day of menstruation.

First day of Phase I

* You know that a bleeding episode is a true menstruation when there was an upward thermal shift in temperatures in the cycle just ended. To learn about a bleeding episode that is not a true menstruation, see Chapter 30, "Breakthrough Bleeding."

● **11:59 p.m.**

An end-of-Phase-I rule in Chapter 11 will tell you the last day of Phase I. More precisely, Phase I ends at 11:59 p.m. on that day.

● **With no experience**

The basic Phase I rule for beginners is this:

Abstain during Phase I for your first one to three cycles.

The reason for that rule is this: you need to get some experience with observing the onset of your cervical mucus without any confusion from seminal residue. If you are a chaste engaged woman, your pre-marriage cycles will fulfill this rule.

If you are coming off the Pill or other hormonal birth control, use the rules in Chapter 29.

● **With a little experience**

If you are married and find you can discern well the onset of mucus in your first cycle, then you don't have to abstain "to get experience" in cycle two. If you get the experience you need by abstaining in Phase I for two cycles, there is no need to abstain "to get experience" in cycle three.

● **After two cycles of experience**

With just two or three cycles of experience, how do you determine the end of Phase I? It depends upon your cycle pattern. Please note: do not count cycles on the Pill in determining your past cycle pattern.

The basic principle is this: the first six days of the cycle are very infertile **IF** you have medium to long cycles—26 days or more with normal luteal phases.

1. If you recall that all of your last 12 cycles have been 26 days long or longer, you can consider Phase I to end on Cycle Day 6, provided you are still dry. See "Clinical Experience Rules" in Chapter 11.

2. Do not extend Phase I beyond Day 6 in your first six cycles.

3. If you have cycles shorter than 26 days, see Chapter 11 for Clinical Experience rules for short cycles.

4. If you have no idea how long your past cycles have been, be conservative. Either abstain during Phase I for your first six cycles, or use a more conservative End-of-Phase-I cutoff such as Day 3, Day 4, or Day 5. More about these in Chapter 11.

● **Early mucus.** Note well: if you notice mucus on Days 4, 5 or 6, consider yourselves in Phase II. Mucus and cervix changes are current experience, and they always take priority over rules based on past history.

● **Shorter periods.** If you have a period that is much shorter than usual, be suspicious. Sometimes that's a tip-off you are going to ovulate much earlier than usual. Be especially watchful for any signs of early mucus or cervix changes, and give them priority if they occur.

Phase II

Avoiding pregnancy

If you are using NFP to avoid or postpone pregnancy, abstain from sexual intercourse and genital contact during Phase II. Why the caution about genital contact? When the mucus is flowing, accidental ejaculation outside the vagina may put semen in contact with the mucus, and the rest is the story of how life begins. Even the small amount of lubrication fluid that comes from the penis of the aroused spouse may transmit sperm through genital contact. The possibility may be small, but it exists.

You will most likely find that lovemaking has a very special meaning when you and your spouse are hoping to conceive a baby, that is, to express your love for each other in a new person. Still, if you are beginners at NFP, we offer a word of advice.

● Beginners

Abstain during the fertile time for the first one to three cycles even if you want to become pregnant as soon as possible.

The reason for that advice is this: you should learn to observe your mucus sign and perhaps your cervix changes before you become pregnant. In that way, you will know what you are looking for when you want to detect the return of fertility after childbirth.

● Experienced couples

Statistically speaking, there is a 25% chance that couples of normal fertility will conceive from a single act of marital relations during the fertile time. (The statistical probability rises with more frequent intercourse.) Other couples will take longer to become pregnant. Some couples will discover that they have an infertility problem. Part IV of this book has six chapters dealing with achieving pregnancy and related subjects, and you will do well to read those chapters before you seek pregnancy.

● Newlyweds

We have a special message for newlyweds. Do not assume that you will achieve pregnancy as soon as you plan to do so. Some very disappointed couples have asked us to emphasize more and more that you may be at the high point of your fertility when you marry. In a very rare case reported to us, a couple conceived on their honeymoon and were never able to conceive after that despite a great desire for more children.

Therefore, we emphasize here as we do elsewhere in this manual: you need a sufficiently serious reason to avoid pregnancy. If you don't have a really good reason to postpone pregnancy, your honeymoon is a wonderful time to start your family. In God's plan, marriage is for family.

Phase III

The basic rule for beginners is this: Use Rule C plus one day for your first one to three cycles.

The "C" of Rule C stands for the most Cautious and Conservative approach. It's a good rule for beginners, but most experienced couples use the other rules described in Chapter 12.

You can use any of the other rules in Chapter 12 in your first three cycles **if** your NFP instructor verifies your interpretation.

● Adding one day

A beginner couple should add one day to their Phase III interpretation for the first one to three cycles. The reason for this has nothing to do with your fertility right now as compared to three cycles from now. However, your **experience** and **understanding** will be much greater after one, two or three cycles than it is right now. Adding the extra day helps to guard against any misinterpretation of the mucus or temperature signs.

Start of Phase III by Rule C

Start of Phase III by Rule C

This is the most conservative rule. It requires **both** three consecutive days of full thermal shift **and** four days of drying-up. The **C** stands for **C**autious and **C**onservative.

**According to Rule C,
Phase III begins on the evening of
1) the 3rd day (or more) of full thermal shift
2) cross-checked by 4 (or more) days of drying-up—whichever comes last.**

Another way of saying the same thing:

With Rule C, Phase III begins on the evening of
1) the 4th day (or more) of drying-up
2) cross-checked by 3 or more days of full thermal shift, whichever comes last.

Clarifications

Phase III starts in the **evening** of the day indicated by the Phase III rule. "Evening" means 6:00 p.m. and later.

A **full thermal shift**: on three **consecutive** days, you have valid waking temperatures that are at least 4/10 of 1° F. above the Low Temperature Level (LTL).

(Other thermal shift patterns are used in Chapter 12, "NFP Rules: Phase III.")

The cervix sign is not included in the rules because it is not essential, and it gets too wordy and complicated to include it. However, note two things:

1. You can get added confidence when you have three or four days of cervix closing to cross-check the mucus drying-up requirements.

2. Once you get experienced with the cervix sign, you can use it as a substitute for the cervical mucus if you aren't getting any help from the mucus sign. That would apply to both the beginning of Phase II and the beginning of Phase III.

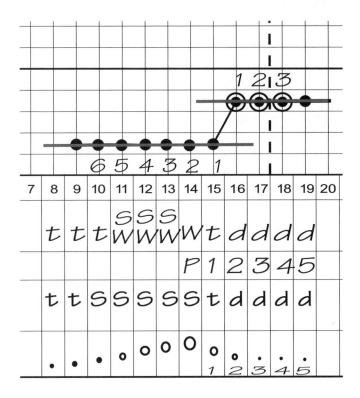

Figure 10.1   Example of Rule C + One Day

Figure 10.1 illustrates Rule C for beginners. (We have numbered the circled temperatures that make the full thermal shift.) In this example, the normal Rule C yields Day 18 as the start of Phase III; adding the extra day for beginners yields Day 19. Note that with Rule C plus one day, you will have four days of thermal shift and five days of drying-up. If the temperature dips a bit on the fourth day, that's okay.

For other examples of Rule C temperature and mucus patterns, see Rule C examples 17-20 in Chapter 12.

Q. What if my temperatures don't form a *full* thermal shift pattern?

A. In Chapter 12, we describe two other rules (B and R) that work with weaker temperature patterns. If you have to use them in your first two or three cycles, do not consider yourselves to be in Phase III until the evening of Peak Day + 5 cross-checked by at least four days of strong or overall thermal shift.

Q. What if I cannot identify a Peak Day in my first few cycles?

A. If you cannot identify a Peak Day in a cycle, use the Temperature-Only Rule in Chapter 26.

105

Self-Test Questions: Chapter 10

1. (Review) The luteal phase is the _____ time of the cycle.

2. The dominant hormone during the luteal phase is _____.

3. To count the length of the luteal phase by temperatures, you start with the _____ of thermal shift up through the last day before your period starts.

4. True____   False____   The luteal phase is usually 12 to 14 days long.

5. LTL stands for _____ _____ _____ .

6. HTL stands for _____ _____ _____.

7. A full thermal shift means that on three _____ days the temperatures are all at least _____/10ths of 1° F. above the Low Temperature Level.

8. True____   False____   Rule C requires three days of full thermal shift cross-checked by four days of drying-up of the mucus.

9. When you add one day for beginners, your Rule C interpretation will always have, after Peak Day, _____ days of drying-up and _____ days of thermal shift of which _____ form a full thermal shift.

10. True____   False____   In describing a thermal shift, "consecutive" means that all three temperatures must be on consecutive days.

11. If the end of Phase I is on day 6, what is the cutoff time?
    a) just before midnight of Day 5   b) 12:00 noon on Day 6
    c) 6:00 p.m. on Day 6   d) just before midnight (11:59 p.m.) on Day 6.

12. If Phase III starts on Day 17, the Phase III startup time is:
    a) 12:01 a.m. on Day 17   b) 6:00 a.m. on Day 17
    c) 6:00 p.m. on Day 17   d) 12:01 a.m. on Day 18

13. Phase I normally starts on
    a) the first day of menstruation
    b) the last day of menstruation
    c) Cycle Day 6.

14. The Couple to Couple League recommends that beginners should use Rule _____ for the start of Phase III.

15. CCL advises beginners to abstain during Phase I for how many cycles: _____

Answers to self-test

1. postovulation 2. progesterone 3. first day 4. True 5. Low Temperature Level 6. High Temperature Level 7. consecutive. . . four 8. True 9. five . . . four . . . three 10. True 11. d) just before midnight (11:59 p.m.) of Day 6 12. c) 6:00 p.m. on Day 17 13. a) the first day of menstruation 14. C plus one day 15. one to three

References

(1) Shannon. See "Resources."

11

NFP Rules: Phase I

In this chapter you will learn four different ways of determining the end of Phase I. Which rule is best for you? That's one of those things you and your spouse will want to work out together. What we can tell you is this: the most liberal rule is the Last Dry Day rule; it probably also has a higher unplanned pregnancy rate—which is still very low. All the other rules are subordinate to the presence of early mucus.

If you find it confusing to have more than one option, we apologize. However, remember that most of the Phase I rules require some experience to use correctly. When you have that experience, the meaning of the different rules will be clear. Also, review the Phase I section of Chapter 10, and then look ahead to "The first few cycles" section of Chapter 15.

First day of Phase I

Normally count the first day of menstruation as the first day of Phase I. For two possible exceptions, see the beginning of Chapter 10.

Knowing your shortest cycle

Some End-of-Phase-I rules are based on your shortest cycle. How do you know the length of your shortest cycle? You keep records. Diary or calendar records of menstruation can be used to calculate cycle lengths for using with the Clinical Experience and 21/20 Day rules. You need charted temperature records to apply the Doering rule. You need at least six cycles for fairly good accuracy; you are better off with 12 or more. Beyond two years is ancient history, so keep your running record based on your last 24 to 30 cycles.

*Note: The Clinical Experience Rules and the 21 Day Rule assume normal luteal phases. Therefore, cycles with 8 days (or less) of rising or elevated temperatures can be ignored for determining your shortest cycle.

● **The value of experience.** On the basis of 4,593 cycles, Dr. John Marshall concluded that you need at least six cycles for predicting the lengths of future cycles. In his study, he found that with six cycles, 82 percent of the next three cycles fell within the same range; if there were 12 cycles, 90 percent of the next three cycles fell within the already recorded range. However, if there were only three cycles, only 64 percent of the next three cycles fell within that range.[1]

1. Clinical Experience Rules

This set of rules is based on the wide experience that **the first six days of the cycle** are highly infertile for most women. The Clinical Experience Rules never go beyond Day 6.

Total abstinence

> **Total Abstinence**
>
> Total abstinence during Phase I is the most conservative option.

● **When to use.** We recommend this for beginners for their first cycle and perhaps their first three cycles so the wife can gain experience with the onset of mucus without any interference from seminal residue. We also suggest this or the Day 3 or Day 4 rules for couples who have extremely serious reasons to avoid pregnancy. With NFP, there are very few true surprise pregnancies, but most of them come from intercourse late in Phase I. (More on this in Chapter 13.)

● **Effectiveness.** Rather obviously, abstinence during Phase I yields a Phase I surprise pregnancy rate of zero.

Day 3 Rule

> **Day 3 Rule**
>
> End Phase I on Cycle Day 3 if you have had cycles of 21 days or less in your last 12 cycles, or if you are in premenopause.

● **When to use.** This is a good rule to use during menstruation in premenopause and when you have a history of very short cycles. Once you have post-menstrual dryness, you may be able to use the Last Dry Day rule.

● **Effectiveness.** Treating the first three days of heavy flow as still in Phase III and starting abstinence on Day 4 will yield a surprise pregnancy rate close to zero.

Basis for estimate: The heavy menstrual flow is hostile to sperm life and migration. One member of the CCL Medical Advisory Board has reported one pregnancy attributable to relations on Cycle Day 3, based on 40 years of experience. CCL Headquarters has no record of any Cycle Day 3 pregnancies from 1971 through 1995.

Note well: you must be sure the bleeding is a true menstruation and *not* breakthrough bleeding. You can know this only if you keep good temperature records and know that a sustained thermal shift has preceded the bleeding episode. More about this in Chapter 30.

Day 4 Rule

    End Phase I on Cycle Day 4 if you have had a cycle of 22 days in your last 12 cycles.

● **When to use.** If you have had a cycle of **22 days** in the last 12 cycles, don't extend Phase I beyond Day 4 during any bleeding or spotting. Once you have post-menstrual dryness, you may be able to apply the Last Dry Day Rule.

● **Effectiveness.** We estimate that having relations only through Cycle Day 4 yields a surprise pregnancy rate not over 1 per 1,000 woman-years.

    Basis for estimate: There are no scientifically controlled studies we can quote. CCL Central has record of only five Cycle Day 4 pregnancies in 22 years of experience (up through 1993).

Day 5 Rule

    End Phase I on Cycle Day 5 if your shortest cycle in the last year was 23 to 25 days.

● **When to use.** If your shortest cycle in the last year was **23 to 25 days**, use a Day 5 cutoff. If you should notice mucus on or before Day 5, consider yourselves to be in the fertile time.

● **Effectiveness.** We estimate that having marital relations up through Cycle Day 5 will have a surprise pregnancy rate of no more than 1 per 200 woman-years (1/2 of 1%) provided the "when to use" rules are followed; that is, you have had no cycles shorter than 23 days in the last year and you have no cervical mucus on Day 5.

    Basis for estimate: There are no scientifically controlled studies we can quote. However, CCL Central has record of only 13 Cycle Day 5 pregnancies in 22 years of experience (1971-1993), and the Day 5 rule simply has to have fewer pregnancies than the Day 6 rule that Doctor Roetzer has researched.

Day 6 Rule

    End Phase I on Cycle Day 6 if your shortest cycle in the last year has been 26 days or longer.

● **When to use.** If your shortest cycle in the last year has been **26 days or longer**, you can use a Day 6 cutoff for Phase I, provided you have no mucus on Day 6.

    Most couples can use a Day 6 rule even when first learning the Sympto-Thermal Method because most women have cycles that are 26 days or longer.

● **Effectiveness.** We estimate that having marital relations up through Cycle Day 6 will have a surprise pregnancy rate not over 1 per 100 woman-years (1%) provided the "when to use" rules are followed; that is, no cycles shorter than 26 days and no mucus on Day 6.

Basis for estimate: Dr. Josef Roetzer has reported a surprise pregnancy rate of only 0.2 per 100 woman-years among couples having relations up through Cycle Day 6. Please note: that is 2/10 per 100 woman-years, or 1 per 500 woman-years. CCL Central has record of 27 Day 6 pregnancies among 88,000 couples taught in 22 years.

Most Day 6 pregnancies have occurred in cases where the woman had previous cycles shorter than 26 days. That's why the rules for Days 4 and 5 were developed.

To repeat:

If you have had short cycles of **25 days or less** during the last 12 cycles, use the rules for Days 3, 4 and 5.

Beyond Day 6

Fertility returns with increasing frequency starting with Cycle Day 7. To go beyond Day 6, you must have enough experience to apply one of the other End of Phase I rules.

2. Previous History Rules

We have two rules based on your own cycle patterns. The 21 Day Rule is based on a wide variety of American, Australian, and European experience. The Doering rule comes from Dr. Gerd K. Doering of Germany. The 21 Day Rule is the simplest to apply; the Doering Rule is more tailored to your specific cycle pattern.

The 21/20 Day Rule

The 21 Day Rule determines the end of Phase I by subtracting 21 from your shortest cycle. It can become a 20 Day Rule with more experience. The difference is this: you can apply the 21 Day Rule after **six** cycles of experience; you can apply the 20 Day Rule after **twelve** cycles of experience. If you wish, you can continue with the more conservative 21 Day Rule; the choice is yours.

> ### The 21 Day Rule
>
> Shortest cycle minus 21 = last day of Phase I, if dry.
>
> ### The 20 Day Rule
>
> Shortest cycle (of last 12 to 24 cycles) minus 20 = last day of Phase I, if dry.

● **"If dry"**

"If dry" means that your mucus flow has not yet started on or before the day indicated as the end of Phase I by this rule. In other words, the 21 and 20 Day Rules are **subordinate to the presence of early mucus.** Mucus is current data and takes precedence over a rule based on your past history.

● **Experience needed.** You need six cycles of experience to apply the 21 Day Rule; you need twelve cycles of experience to apply the 20 Day Rule. (See "Knowing your shortest cycle" at the beginning of this chapter.)

● **Application.** Keep good records. At the end of each cycle, update the "Cycle Variation" section in the upper right hand corner of the CCL chart.

After six cycles you can apply the 21 Day Rule as in these examples:

Shortest cycle	Minus 21	= Last Day of Phase I
31	-21	10
29	-21	8
27	-21	6

After twelve cycles you can apply the 20 Day Rule as follows:

Shortest of last 12-24 cycles	Minus 20	= Last Day of Phase I
31	-20	11
29	-20	9
27	-20	7

However, if you have mucus on or before the day indicated by these rules, you are already in Phase II. So if your 21 or 20 Day Rule indicates Day 8 as the end of Phase I but you notice mucus on Day 8, you are in Phase II on Day 8.

● **Basis of the 21/20 Day Rule.** The practical basis is that it has been working well for years (see effectiveness). The theoretical basis is this: ovulation can occur up to 16 days (rarely more) before the next menstruation; sperm can live up to 5 days (rarely longer). The 21 Day Rule uses the 16 and 5 day figures; experience shows that the 20 Day Rule also works very well.

● **When to use.** Use the 21 or 20 Day Rules when you want a rule that is usually more conservative than the Last Dry Day Rule — or you simply want to set a definite Phase I cutoff. Generally the 21/20 Day Rule will set an end to Phase I a day or more before your mucus starts. However, see sidebar limitation.

● **Effectiveness.** We estimate that the correct application of the 21 and 20 Day Rules will yield a surprise pregnancy rate of not more than 1 per 100 women years (1%).

Basis for estimate: The Los Angeles study found zero unplanned pregnancies among couples who correctly used the 21 Day Rule.[2] CCL Central has record of only 11 surprise pregnancies with the 21 Day Rule among 88,000 couples taught in our first 22 years of experience. Based on experience, the international practice has settled quite consistently on a 20 Day Rule with the mucus cross-check.[3]

● *Limitation.*

Do not use the 21 or 20 Day Rules if you have luteal phases of more than 16 days as measured by temperatures. If you regularly have more than 16 days of rising and elevated temperatures, use the Doering rule (see next page).

The Doering Rule

> **The Doering Rule**
>
> Earliest day of thermal shift minus 7 = Last day of Phase I, if dry.

● **Explanation.** *"Earliest day of thermal shift"* means the first day of upward sustained thermal shift in your last 6 to 12 cycles. Keep good temperature records. Check your past charts to find the first day of upward thermal shift. Then subtract 7. The remainder is the End of Phase I by this rule.

"If dry" means that you still have no mucus on that day. What we said about the 21/20 Day Rule being subordinate to the presence of early mucus applies here too.

● **An exception.** There is one exception to the normal "mucus-dry" requirement with the Doering rule. Dr. Doering achieved high effectiveness with this temperature-only rule without regard to the presence of mucus. Therefore, you can apply the Doering rule in the presence of the *less-fertile* mucus if you meet two requirements:

1) You have a history of long cycles with all-the-time less-fertile mucus from menstruation up to the beginning of the more-fertile mucus;

2) You consistently have at least five days of the more-fertile mucus from its start through Peak Day. Better yet, six or more days.

For example: a woman's shortest cycle is 35 days and she has six days of less-fertile mucus before having six days of the more-fertile mucus. However, **never** apply the Doering rule in the presence of the *more-fertile* mucus.

● **Examples.** If the first day of upward thermal shift in your previous 12 cycles was Day 15, the Doering Rule would yield Day 8 as the End of Phase I in your current cycle provided you still had no mucus. Remember: you have to recalculate if you have an earlier start of elevated temperatures. Some more examples:

First day of thermal shift	Minus 7	Last Day of Phase I
12	-7	5
16	-7	9
18	-7	11

● **Basis of the Doering Rule.** This is part of the temperature-only system used with great success by Dr. G. K. Doering. It has two advantages over the 21/20 Day Rule: it is more closely tied to the time of ovulation, and variations in the luteal phase do not affect it.

● **Experience needed.** You should have at least six cycles of charted temperatures to use the Doering Rule, and 12 is better. (See "Knowing your shortest cycle" at the beginning of this chapter.) If you want to apply it in the presence of all-the-time less-fertile mucus, you certainly need to apply it in theory to your previous cycles to see how it works out, and it would be better to have at least 12 cycles of experience. For example, how close does the Doering Rule put your calculated end-of-Phase-I to Peak Day in those cycles? Then assume a five day sperm life and ovulation on Peak Day or Peak Day minus 1.

We can only say so much in a manual; you do have to use some common sense.

● **When to use.** When you want a rule that is more conservative than the Last Dry Day Rule, you can use the Doering Rule as a substitute for the 21 or 20 Day Rules. It is particularly useful if you have a pattern of consistently short cycles due to short luteal phases. A *short luteal phase* would be less than 10 days of temperatures elevated at least 1/10 of 1° F. above the LTL.

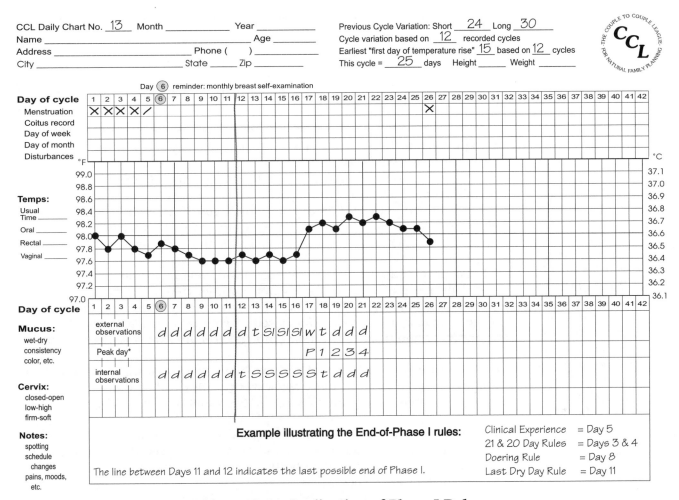

Figure 11.1 Application of Phase I Rules

● **Effectiveness.** We estimate that the proper use of the Doering Rule will yield a surprise pregnancy rate of not over 1 per 100 woman-years.

Basis for estimate: Dr. Doering's temperature-only study indicates a Phase I surprise pregnancy rate of 0.32 per 100 woman-years (about 1/3 of 1% or 1 per 300 woman-years).[4] CCL has not widely taught this rule, and CCL Headquarters has not kept this classification; therefore we have no record of Phase I pregnancies attributed to this rule.

3. The Mucus-related Rules

This section contains the Last Dry Day Rule. It also contains some other rules that are related to the mucus signs and apply to Phase I in general.

The Last Dry Day Rule

> **The Last Dry Day Rule**
>
> Consider yourselves in Phase I up through the last dry day before your cervical mucus starts to flow.
>
> Be sure to follow the "General Phase I Rules" in the next section of this chapter.

● **Limitation**

Your mucus patches in your previous six cycles should be at least five days from the beginning up through Peak Day. Otherwise, you might be having relations very close to ovulation. If your shortest mucus patch in your last six cycles has been six or seven days, you can use the Last Dry Day Rule with even greater confidence.

● **Explanation.** Begin to observe and chart dry days right after your period or by Day 6 at the latest.

Your last dry day is the last possible day of Phase I. The first appearance of cervical mucus is a positive sign you are in Phase II, the fertile time.

A "mucus-dry day" is one on which you observe no cervical mucus either externally or internally. "Observe" includes both feeling and seeing. "Mucus" includes both the less-fertile types and the more-fertile types.

● **Basis.** If you have no cervical mucus in your vagina, sperm life is very short and is measured in terms of a few hours rather than a few days.

Obviously, you know the *last* dry day only by hindsight. You have to make your judgment about *today* based on your observations *today*. Dry days up to the beginning of your cervical mucus discharge are considered infertile.

● **When to use.** Use the Last Dry Day Rule when you want to extend Phase I beyond the limits of the more conservative rules and you have a history of average to long-length mucus patches. See Limitation in sidebar.

● **Experience needed.** You should have at least six cycles of experience in observing and recording your mucus signs. In your last three cycles, you should have been able to identify the beginning of your mucus flow either at the vulva or at the cervical os.

● **Effectiveness.** We estimate that the proper use of the Last Dry Day Rule will yield a surprise pregnancy rate between 3 and 7 per 100 woman-years (97% to 93%).

Basis of estimate: A five nation study of the Ovulation Method yielded a "perfect use" surprise pregnancy rate of 3.1 per 100 woman-years (3.1 %).[5] Later, the authors of that analysis raised their estimate to 3.4% (a probability of 3.4 per 100 woman-years).[6] CCL Central has record of 83 Last Dry Day pregnancies (in 22 years) among couples who said they were following the rules.

While this number (83) is still small in terms of the couples CCL has taught, it compares with 45 from the Clinical Experience Rules, 11 from the 21 Day Rule, and 80 among couples who were not following some of the standard Phase I rules. The women in the five nation study had fairly regular cycles. More research needs to be done on the effectiveness of the Last Dry Day Rule. For the present, we are not sure that the 96.6% level of effectiveness of the Last Dry Day rule can be maintained among couples in all situations. Therefore we have doubled the estimate stemming from that study.

● **Cervix cross-check.** If you make the internal mucus observation, check the cervix, too. If it starts to open, to rise, or to become softer *before* you notice cervical mucus, consider it a sign that you are already in Phase II.

General Phase I Rules

The following rules are related to the observation of your mucus sign, but you need to follow them even if you are not relying on the Last Dry Day Rule. All the other rules are subordinate to the presence of early mucus, so you need to make regular mucus observations.

1. Frequency of observation. Start your charting right after your period or by Day 6 at the latest even if you are still spotting. Make your external observations every time you urinate. Make your internal observations 1) at the end of the day or 2) midday and at the end of the day.

2. Internal observation. We repeat what we wrote in Chapter 8: some women observe the mucus at the cervical os one to three days before they notice it at the vulva. For most of them it's just a one-day "early warning" that Phase II has started. That's why we recommend the internal observation as the best way to find your mucus as soon as it starts.

3. Dry days only. Consider only dry days to be infertile. This is the most basic Phase I rule. Once mucus starts, you are in Phase II.

If you have relations when the mucus is present, do not be surprised when you become pregnant if you are a couple with normal fertility. That includes the days of the "less-fertile" mucus at the beginning of your mucus patch. "Less-fertile" is definitely **not** "infertile."

● **Therefore, when mucus starts, abstain** if you are postponing pregnancy. The main point is this: once your mucus starts, you are in the fertile time even if you should have an occasional dry day.

4. Not in the morning. Do not have marital relations in the morning during Phase I. Why? You want to make sure it's a "dry day," and you know that only by making several observations during the day. Your mucus may have begun to flow while you were asleep but not be noticeable when you wake, especially with the external observation.

Q. My husband leaves for work in the afternoon. Does that mean no Phase I intercourse for us on those days?

A. If you have been up and around for at least five hours and have made several external observations, having relations in the afternoon does not violate this rule. Be sure to make your daily internal observation before getting into bed. If you find mucus, you should tell your husband that the fertile time has started. The same holds true for your evening observation.

5. Not on consecutive days. Do not have marital relations on consecutive days in Phase I. Why? If you have sexual intercourse on Saturday night, you will most likely notice seminal residue on Sunday. But is it just seminal residue or is it maybe seminal residue in the morning and cervical mucus in the afternoon? You simply don't know. One thing is certain: it's not really a "dry day." You should abstain because the most basic Phase I rule is "Dry days only." Be sure to chart **SR** whenever you observe seminal residue.

Example:

Your mucus starts on Day 8 but then you don't notice any mucus on Day 9 or Day 10. You wonder if you are still in Phase II on Days 9 and 10. Yes, you are. The mucus on Day 8 told you that your ovulation process has started. For whatever reason, sometimes the mucus flow starts and stops a bit at first, but once it starts, you are in Phase II.

Q. What if we have relations at night and I am completely dry all the next day. Does the "not on consecutive days" rule still apply?

A. Our standard advice is this: if your seminal residue completely drains during the night and you are truly mucus-dry all day, then you can treat it as a regular "dry day."

On the other hand, we have seen a handful of surprise pregnancies from extended sperm life in cases where the couples had relations on consecutive dry days. We wonder if the first act of intercourse might change the envi-ronment of the vagina (make it less acidic) to make it more favorable to sperm life and longevity. There is no medical evidence to support or disprove this specula-tion, but it is possible that there is more to the "not on consecutive days" rule than we have previously thought.

General questions about Phase I

● Is menstruation infertile?

If you are having a true menstruation, you can regard the first three days of heavy flow as an extension of Phase III.

Remember, you need an upward thermal shift in the cycle that ended just before the start of your period to tell you that you are having a true menstruation and not breakthrough bleeding. (See Chapter 30.) If you are not taking temperatures, you should follow the mucus-only rule of abstaining during any and every bleeding episode even if you think it is menstruation. (Chapter 26 has the mucus-only and temperature-only rules.)

Beyond Day 3, apply the general Phase I rules during the rest of menstruation. You cannot apply the Last Dry Day Rule until your menstrual flow has completely stopped, but you can apply the other rules. So start to make your mucus observations as soon as your heavy flow is over.

● Are all the "General Phase I rules" equally important?

It depends. The basic "dry days only" rule is the most important. However, common sense tells you that if the first six days of the cycle are highly infertile for almost everyone with medium to long cycles, the "not in the morning" and "not on consecutive days" rules don't mean much for most couples for the first six days of the cycle. But if you have cycles shorter than 26 days, then they are important. *After Day 6, all the "general Phase I rules" are very important for everybody.*

● If I notice SR in the morning, should I make observations all day?

Definitely yes. The mucus flow may start that day, perhaps in the afternoon. Make and record your regular observations.

● What if I have tacky mucus days right after menstruation?

Tacky mucus days right after menstruation tell you that your mucus flow has started. You have a positive sign you are in Phase II.

● What if I have post-menstrual days that are neither dry nor wet?

If you never have positive feelings of dryness but regularly detect mucus days, "just nothing" is "dry" for you. That's why you want to get a few cycles of experience before relying on the Last Dry Day Rule.

If you regularly have positive feelings of post-menstrual dryness, but also have "nothing" days before your definite mucus days, the situation is a bit ambiguous. Our recommendation: check the cervical os. If you have no feelings of lubrication while wiping, no mucus on the tissue paper, and nothing at the cervical os, that's a dry day.

If you do not make the internal observation, the combination of no feelings of lubrication while wiping and no mucus on the tissue paper still tells you that you have no external mucus and are still infertile.

● What if I have all-the-time mucus from menstruation until after ovulation?

See Chapter 27, "Irregular mucus patterns."

● What if I have very long cycles and more than one patch of mucus?

The easy answer is this: check your nutrition, your exercise, your weight to height ratio, and your body-fat to weight ratio. Clearing up irregularities in those areas is good for your health and sometimes completely clears up an irregular cycle pattern.

What's a "very long cycle?" Here we enter the area of judgment. We call cycles of 43 days and longer "very long cycles." That is admittedly arbitrary, but such cycles are more than two weeks longer than the classical average of 28 days.

Once you have at least six cycles of experience, you can make some informed judgments based on your own cycle pattern.

All of this applies only if you have a history of very long cycles. If this is the first time for something like this, be sure to check the "Double mucus patch" pattern explained in Chapter 27, "Irregular mucus patterns."

● If your patches have only the "less-fertile" mucus: abstain during the entire mucus patch.

● If you always have a mucus patch of at least five days of the *more-fertile* mucus before your Peak Day that is associated with ovulation, then you can be reasonably certain that the *dry days between* patches of less-fertile mucus are infertile.

● We suggest waiting until the evening of the second dry day *after a patch of less-fertile mucus* before you consider yourselves back into Phase I infertility. If your temperature starts to rise during the dry days, wait until you can apply a standard Sympto-Thermal Phase III rule.

Apply the "End of Phase I" rules to all the charts in the "Practical Applications Workbook" right after Chapter 15.

More than one rule can usually be applied in each chart. Be sure to check the number of previous cycles of experience to see if there is enough experience to apply the 21 or 20 Day Rules, the Doering Rule, and the Last Dry Day Rule. Remember also to check the shortest cycle; you need that data to apply the Clinical Experience rules as well as the 21 and 20 Day Rules.

● **Notations.** If a rule cannot be applied, write N/A for Not Applicable. On the graph, draw a solid line between the last possible day of Phase I and the next day. For example, if Day 8 is the last possible day of Phase I, start your Phase I/II line *between* the boxes for days 8 and 9 at the top of the graph; extend the line downward, and finish between the bottom boxes for days 8 and 9. Then you will have a very graphic picture of the end of Phase I and the start of Phase II.

Workbook exercises

Self-Test Questions: Chapter 11

1. For the general population, the chances of pregnancy from relations on Cycle Day 5 are about one in every _____ woman-years.

2. To apply that statistic to yourself, your shortest cycle in the last year should be at least _____ days long.

3. For the general population, the possibility of pregnancy from relations on Cycle Day 6 is not over 1 per _____ woman-years.

4. For the Day 6 statistic to apply to you, your shortest cycle in the last year should have been at least _____ days long.

5. If you have had very short cycles—21 days or less—in the last year, you should use a Day _____ cutoff during your first six cycles.

6. Imagine that your shortest cycle has been 27 days but you notice a less-fertile mucus today on Day 6. You should regard yourself on Day 6 as:
   a) still in Phase I   b) now in Phase II.

7. Imagine that your mucus discharge hasn't started before Day 9 in your last six cycles. You should start making your mucus observations in this cycle:
   a) right after your days of heavy flow   b) not until Day 8.

8. The 21 and 20 Day Rules are based upon your _____ cycle in the last year.

9. You need at least _____ cycles of experience to apply the 21 Day Rule; _____ for the 20 Day Rule.

10. If the 21/20 Day Rule indicates Day 7 as the end of Phase I and you notice mucus on Day 7, is Day 7 in Phase I or Phase II? Phase _____.

11. True____   False____   The 21/20 Day Rule applies to any cycle pattern, even those with luteal phases of 17 days and more (as measured by days of sustained elevated temperatures).

12. The most "liberal" of the End of Phase I rules is usually the _____.

13. True____   False____   The Doering Rule for the End of Phase I is based on the earliest start of the thermal shift in the last 6-24 cycles.

14. If your "first day of thermal shift" in the last year was Day 15, the Doering Rule would yield Day _____ as the end of Phase I, provided you were still _____.

15. The purpose of the internal test for mucus at the cervical os is to detect the mucus _____ you might notice it at the vulva.

16. The internal observation for mucus at the cervical os requires:
   a) one finger   b) two fingers

17. If you have mucus on Day 8 but then are mucus-dry on Day 9, where are you on Cycle Day 9?   a) Phase I   b) Phase II.

18. True_____ False_____   During Phase I it doesn't make any difference whether you have relations in the morning or the evening.

19. True_____ False_____   The purpose of the not-on-consecutive-days rule is to eliminate confusion between mucus and seminal residue.

20. True_____ False_____   A dry day is known by the sum total of observations made periodically throughout the day.

21. True_____ False_____   The beginning of the mucus—whether it's the less-fertile type or the more-fertile type—is a positive sign that you're in Phase II.

22. True_____ False_____   If there's only a small amount of mucus during the early part of the mucus patch, you can ignore it as a sign of fertility.

23. According to CCL, for you to rely upon the Last Dry Day Rule, the mucus patches in your previous six to twelve cycles should be at least _____ days long, counting from the first day of mucus through Peak Day.

24. In your "Practical Applications Workbook," turn to Chart 20 (mucus helping the temperature interpretation). Note that the "earliest first day of temperature rise" is Day 17. Assume that "Martha Doe" 1) consistently had several days of internal tacky mucus while still dry externally and 2) always had a mucus patch that ended with at least five days of more-fertile mucus (seven days in this cycle). The End-of-Phase-I rule used by Dr. G. K. Doering would yield Day _____ as the last day of Phase I.

25. Work all of Chart 13 (artificially shortened luteal phase). Suppose Day 15 is the earliest first day of thermal shift and that there are 12 charted cycles. In this scenario, the CCL version of the Doering Rule yields Day _____ as the end of Phase I for *future* cycles.

26. In Chart 13, assume 10 cycles of experience and that true mucus (not just SR) was noticed on Day 8. If the mucus patch and the relationship between Peak Day and the thermal shift are typical for this woman, give two reasons why she could have confidence in the Last Dry Day Rule.
    a) _____
    b) _____

Answers to self-test
1. 200 2. 23 3. 100 4. 26 5. three 6. b) now in Phase II 7. a) right after your days of heavy flow 8. shortest 9. six...12 10. Two 11. False; not over 16 days of luteal phase 12. Last Dry Day Rule 13. True 14. eight . . . mucus-dry 15. before 16. b) two fingers 17. b) Phase II 18. False 19. True 20. True 21. True 22. False 23. five 24. ten 25. eight 26. a) There are six days from the start of mucus through Peak Day b) The temperature did not go up until Peak Day + 2.

References

(1) John Marshall, *The Infertile Period*, (Baltimore: Helicon Press, 1969) 86.

(2) Maclyn E. Wade, Phyllis McCarthy, et. al., "A randomized prospective study of the use-effectiveness of two methods of natural family planning," *American Journal of Obstetrics and Gynecology* 141:4 (15 October 1981) 374.

(3) P. Frank and E. Raith, Natürliche Familienplanung-Physiologische Grundlagen, Methodenvergleich, Wirksamkeit—Eine Einführung für Ärzte und Berater—mit einem Geleitwort von G.K. Döring (Berlin: Springer-Verlog, 1985) 62.

(4) G.K. Doring, "The reliability of temperature records as a method of contraception," (Über die zuverlassigkeit der temperaturmethode zur empfangnisverhutung) *Deutsche medizinische wochenschrift* 92:23 (9 June 1967) 1055-1061. Abstracted in 1968 *Yearbook of Obstetrics and Gynecology*, 354.

(5) James Trussell and Laurence Grummer-Strawn, "Contraceptive failure of the ovulation method of periodic abstinence," *Family Planning Perspectives* 22:2 (March/April 1990) 65.

(6) James Trussell and Laurence Grummer-Strawn, "Further analysis of contraceptive failure of the ovulation method," *American Journal of Obstetrics and Gynecology* 165:6 part 2, (December, 1991) 2054.

12

NFP Rules: Phase III

This chapter contains four different sympto-thermal cross-checking rules for determining the beginning of Phase III, the time of postovulation infertility. Mucus-only and temperature-only rules are in Chapter 26; a special rule for coming off the Pill is in Chapter 29.

There is only one purpose in having more than one rule—to provide you with the earliest start of Phase III based on current knowledge and experience. As you will see from the *Workbook* examples and most likely from your own experience, the rising temperature pattern and the disappearance of cervical mucus work together in different ways. The different rules are tailored to meet different real-life situations.

Different thermal shift patterns

You will notice that the temperatures rise in different patterns. Sometimes they jump a full 4/10 of 1° F. from one day to the next and stay there. In other cycles they go up gradually. Sometimes they even zigzag and form a rising sawtooth pattern.

The standard CCL rules recognize three different thermal shift patterns.

● **Full thermal shift.** On three consecutive days, valid temperatures are at least 4/10 of 1° F. above the Low Temperature Level (LTL).

(Rules C and K use this pattern.)

Note that in Example 2, only the last three temperatures make up the full thermal shift. Why? Only the last three are at or above the 4/10 level.

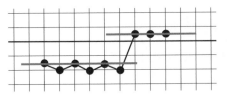

Example 1

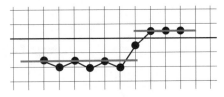

Example 2

Full Thermal Shift Patterns

What if the elevated temperatures do not form a *full* thermal shift? In these cases, we recognize two other patterns—the *strong* thermal shift and the *overall* thermal shift.

● **Strong thermal shift.** On three consecutive days, valid or undisturbed temperatures form this pattern:

1. The first two are at least **2/10** of 1° F. above the Low Temperature Level;

2. The **last** temperature is at or above the High Temperature Level (HTL), that is, 4/10 of 1° F. above the LTL.

(Rule R always uses this pattern; Rule B uses it sometimes.)

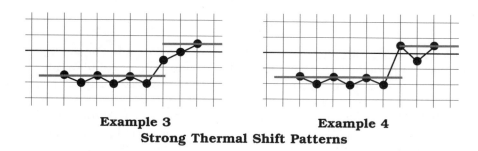

Example 3   **Example 4**
Strong Thermal Shift Patterns

● **Overall thermal shift.** At least three valid temperatures form this pattern:

1. Each one is at least 1/10 of 1° F. above the Low Temperature Level;

2. They are in a rising or elevated pattern;

3. At least one of them has reached the normal HTL of 4/10 of 1° F. above the Low Temperature Level.

(Rule B uses this pattern.)

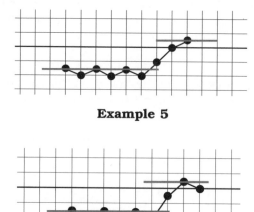

Example 5

Example 6

Overall Thermal Shift Patterns

What if your last temperature falls to within 1/10 of 1° F. of your LTL as in Example 7 below?

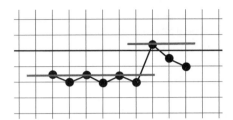

Example 7 Falling Temperature Pattern

Such a pattern would be extremely rare. It would not fulfill the requirements of an overall thermal shift because it is a falling pattern, not rising or elevated. Such a pattern would raise questions such as, "Was the high temperature really an undisturbed temperature?" "Was the LTL properly set?" "Why are the temperatures dropping? Is the corpus luteum functioning properly?" If you should have such a falling pattern, keep taking your temperatures and do not consider yourselves in Phase III until you have a stronger temperature pattern. More on this in "Rule B" below and in "Post-shift return to low temperatures" in Chapter 28.

Rules K, R and B are based on this principle:

The stronger your temperature pattern, the fewer days of mucus drying-up you need as a cross-check.

The basic principle

That principle can also be stated in reverse:
The weaker your temperature pattern, the more days of drying-up you need as a cross-check.

Note: Every sympto-thermal rule requires at least three days of upward thermal shift—full, strong, or overall.

We describe rules K, R, and B in the order of strongest to weakest temperature patterns. Then we describe again the more conservative Rule C and ways of making all the rules even more conservative.

● **Experience needed.** To apply any STM rule, you need to be able to correctly identify your Peak Day. One or two cycles of experience are usually sufficient.

Start of Phase III by Rule K

> ### Start of Phase III by Rule K
>
> According to **Rule K,**
> **Phase III begins on the evening of**
> **1) the 3rd day (or more) of full thermal shift**
> **2) simultaneously cross-checked by 2 (or 3) days of drying-up past the Peak Day.**
>
> The full thermal shift **must be maintained** during the days of drying-up. The last two days of the full thermal shift must be dry or drying-up days.

Basis for Rule K

Rule K is based on the work of Drs. Doering and Vincent.[1,2] They used a temperature-only three-day *full* thermal shift pattern without *any* cross-check from the mucus drying-up and found excellent results. CCL adds a minimum cross-check of two days of drying-up past the peak day. In former editions Rule K, which stands for Kippley, was called Rule A.[3]

● **Rule K with shaving.** In Chapter 6, you learned about "Shaving irregular temperatures" among the pre-shift six. When you have to do that, the temperature pattern is weakened a bit, at least in theory. The practical consequence for Rule K is this: when you have to shave one or two temperatures among the pre-shift six to get Rule K to fit, you need a stronger combination of thermal shift and mucus drying-up.

1. If you have only two days of drying-up, you need four days of thermal shift with the last three at the High Temperature Level.

2. If you have three days of drying-up, you need only the standard three days at the High Temperature Level.

When to use Rule K

Sometimes the temperature pattern is very strong and is ahead of the mucus dry-up as in Example 8. Rule K can sometimes give you a valid start to Phase III one day earlier than Rule R or two days earlier than Rule C.

In Example 8, Rule K takes advantage of the temperature-only research and requires only two days of drying-up to cross-check three days of full thermal shift, thus yielding Day 15 as the start of Phase III. In Example 8 and in Chart 7 of the Practical Applications Workbook, Rule K provides a start to Phase III two days earlier than Rule C.

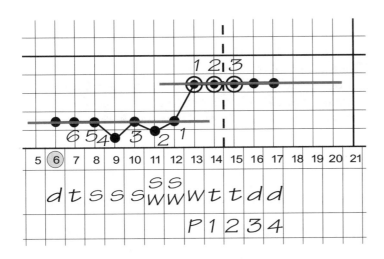

Example 8 Rule K
Strongest Temperature Pattern; Minimum Two-day Dry-up Required

In Example 9 we had to shave the temperatures on Days 8 and 10. Shaving with Rule K calls for either three days of drying-up or four days of thermal shift with the last three at the High Temperature Level. Both of those requirements are met by Day 16, so in Example 9, Rule K yields Day 16 as the start of Phase III.

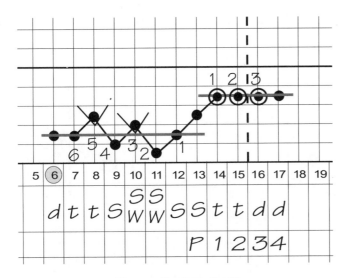

Example 9 Rule K
Shaved LTL Needs Stronger Combination

We estimate the effectiveness of Rule K to be at the 99% level based on the temperature-only work of Doering and Vincent; that is, that surprise pregnancies will be less than 1 per 100 woman-years. In 22 years (1971-1993) CCL Headquarters had record of only four pregnancies resulting from the correct use of Rule K.

Effectiveness of Rule K

NFP Rules: Phase III — 12

Start of Phase III by Rule R

Start of Phase III by Rule R

According to **Rule R,**
Phase III begins on the evening of
1) The 3rd day of drying-up past Peak Day
2) Cross-checked by 3 consecutive days of strong thermal shift past the Peak Day.

Another way of saying the same thing:

Phase III begins on the evening of
1) the 3rd consecutive day of strong thermal shift past Peak Day
2) cross-checked by 3 days of drying-up past Peak Day.

Basis of Rule R

This rule is based on the research of Dr. Josef Roetzer; the "R" stands for his name. There are two things to note:

1. The rising temperatures have to be in a **strong** thermal shift pattern. To repeat, that means that the first two temperatures have to be at least 2/10 of 1° F. above the LTL, and the last temperature has to be at or above the High Temperature Level, that is, 4/10 above the LTL. The three temperatures must be on consecutive days—no missing or disturbed temperatures.

2. All the rising temperatures must be **after** Peak Day. Don't count temperatures that are rising on or before Peak Day.

In Example 10 below, Rule R yields Day 17 as the start of Phase III.

Rule R is always a 3 + 3 rule.

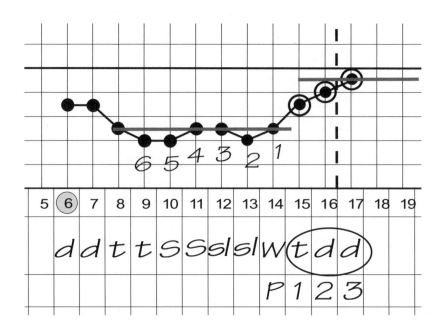

Example 10 Rule R (3 + 3)

Use Rule R only when you are on Peak Day plus 3 and have 3 days of strong thermal shift ending on that day. Rule R is a **3 + 3** pattern.

In other words, when you are on Peak Day plus 3, check your temperature pattern. If Peak Day + 3 is also the 3rd day of strong thermal shift, use Rule R. (Once you reach P + 4, you use either the Rule B or Rule C labels.)

When to use Rule R

*On the other hand, if you have a **full** thermal shift on Peak Day + 3, call it Rule K; if you are on Peak Day + **4** with a strong thermal shift, use Rule B.*

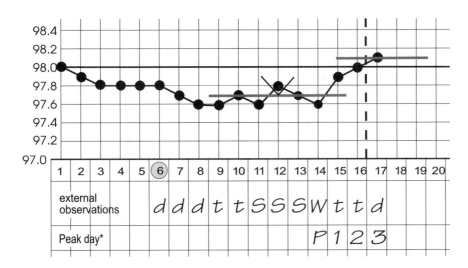

Example 11   Shaving with Rule R

● **Limitation with shaving.** When using Rule R, shave only **one** temperature 1/10 of 1° F.[4] (For normal rules on shaving, see page 64.)

As you can see in Example 11, shaving the temperature on Day 12 still respected the basic principle of three days of rising or well elevated temperatures cross-checking three days of drying-up past the Peak Day. In Example 11, Rule R yields Day 17 as the start of Phase III.

We estimate the effectiveness of Rule R to be at the 99% level based on the work of Dr. Josef Roetzer; that is, surprise pregnancies will be less than 1 per 100 woman-years. In the first 10 years CCL used this rule (1984-1993), we observed only one surprise pregnancy attributable specifically to Rule R.

Effectiveness of Rule R

Start of Phase III by Rule B

Basis of Rule B

This rule starts with the mucus-only rule of Peak Day + 4 and adds a three day temperature cross-check. The "B" stands for Billings—the Australian physicians, John and Lyn Billings, who did so much to popularize the mucus-only approach they called the Ovulation Method. However, the Billings strenuously object to teaching the temperature sign along with the mucus sign. The "Billings Method" is strictly a mucus-only method. For a memory device, you can call Rule B "Billings plus Temperatures for Phase III."

When to use Rule B

Use Rule B when you get to **Peak Day plus 4** and have a temperature cross-check that meets the requirements of either an overall thermal shift or a strong thermal shift. Rule B always needs **at least 3 days** of a cross-checking thermal shift.

Rule B is particularly useful when your temperature pattern is weak and when your mucus dry-up pattern is very clear and helpful.

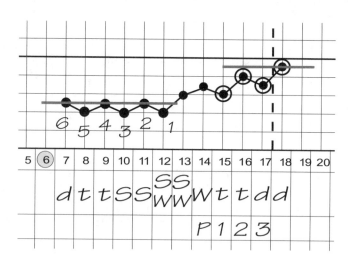

Example 12 Rule B with Overall Thermal Shift

In Example 12, start with Peak Day + 4 which is Day 18. Is it cross-checked by at least 3 days of overall thermal shift? Yes; in fact, by Day 18 there are four days of usable overall thermal shift. Rule B yields Day 18 as the start of Phase III.

Notice that the overall thermal shift actually started on Day 13. However, for Rule B, count only those temperatures that are *past* Peak Day. In Examples 12-14, the **circled temperatures** are the ones that you can use with Rule B.

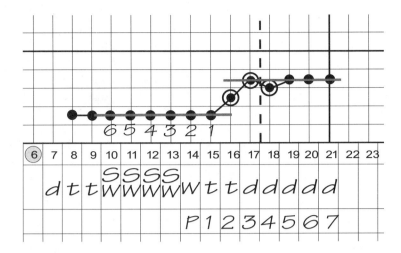

Example 13

In Example 13, start with Peak Day + 4 which is Day 18. Is it cross-checked by at least 3 days of overall thermal shift? Yes. Rule B yields Day 18 as the start of Phase III.

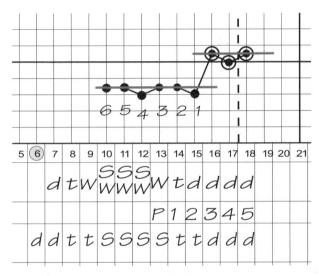

Example 14

In Example 14, note how the drying-up starts two days before the thermal shift starts. As usual, start with Peak Day + 4 which is Day 17. Is Peak Day + 4 on Day 17 cross-checked by at least 3 days of thermal shift? No. You have to wait for a third day of thermal shift. Rule B yields Day 18—Peak Day + 5—as the start of Phase III.

Q. What if my temperature pattern is falling?

A. An overall thermal shift has a rising or elevated temperature pattern.

If your last temperature falls to 2/10 of 1° F. above the LTL, that's okay for an overall thermal shift, but keep taking your temperatures to make sure they stay in a thermal shift pattern (see Example 15).

If your last temperature falls to only 1/10 of 1° F. above the LTL, you are probably in Phase III, but for greater certainty wait another day. If the temperature rises slightly that next day, consider yourselves in Phase III (see Example 16).

If your temperature pattern drops to or below the LTL, you may need to restart your thermal shift count. See "Post-shift dip,""Mid-shift dip," and "Post-shift return to low temperatures" in Chapter 28.

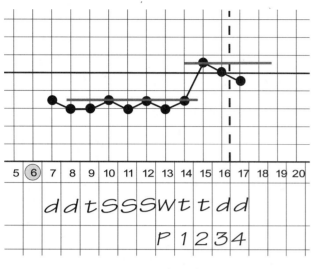

Example 15

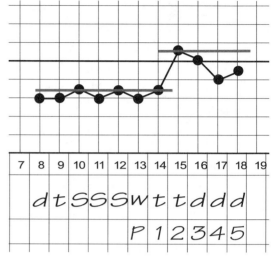

Example 16

Experience needed

Rule B puts primary emphasis on the mucus dry-up. Therefore you need to be able to distinguish Peak Day correctly and with confidence. Two or three cycles of experience will be sufficient for most women. What if you are not confident with your ability to determine Peak Day but would like to apply Rule B because of your temperature patterns? Just add an extra one or two days to your Phase III rule until you become more confident.

Effectiveness of Rule B

We estimate that the effectiveness of Rule B is at the 99% level; that is, the proper application of Rule B will yield not more than one surprise pregnancy per 100 woman-years of use. In 22 years, CCL Headquarters has record of only 12 surprise pregnancies attributable to the correct use of Rule B.

● **Basis.** We are not aware of any study that has specifically measured the effectiveness of Rule B. In fact, we are not aware of any study that has studied the effectiveness of just the Peak-plus-four rule; the mucus-only studies combine both the Last Dry Day Rule for the end of Phase I and the Peak-plus-four Rule for the start of Phase III.

We reason this way: Our records of 22 years (1971-1993) show 137 apparently correct-use surprise pregnancies (or method pregnancies). Of those, only 22 percent (n=30) were Phase III pregnancies. The most recent analysis of the World Health Organization study of the mucus-only method stated a 3.4 percent probability of pregnancy in the first year of correct and consistent use,[5] and that includes both Phase I and Phase III pregnancies.

We apply our experience to the WHO results. Twenty-two percent (22%) of the 3.4 rate is 0.75, that is, less than 1 per 100 woman-years, and that is without the benefit of any temperature cross-check. Cross-check the Peak-plus-four Rule with the tremendous value of three days of thermal shift, and we have no reason to think that the surprise pregnancy rate of Rule B is more than 1 per 100 woman-years of use. That is, the numbers convince us that Rule B has a 99% level of effectiveness.

Note these things about Rule B and how some of them differ from Rule R.

1. Rule B starts with **Peak Day plus 4**; (Rule R uses Peak + 3).

2. Rule B can use an **overall thermal shift**; (Rule R uses only a strong thermal shift). To repeat, in an overall thermal shift, all the temperatures have to be at least 1/10 of 1° F. above the LTL and in a rising or elevated pattern. (In the strong thermal shift, all the temps are at least 2/10 of 1° F. above the LTL.)

3. With Rule B, at least one temperature has to reach the High Temperature Level, but it doesn't have to be the last temperature as with Rule R.

4. With both rules, you count the elevated temperatures only after Peak Day.

● **A "fine point" about Rule B temperatures.** The definition of the "overall thermal shift" used in Rule B does not contain the word "consecutive." With the other Phase III rules, if you *miss* a temperature or have a *disturbed* temperature during the thermal shift, you must re-start your thermal shift count. With Rule B, however, the emphasis is on the drying-up count that gets you four days away from Peak Day.

Therefore, you do not need to restart your temperature count during the Peak-plus-four drying-up count under two conditions:

a) if you forget to take your temperature **one** morning, or

b) if you have **one** disturbed temperature.

In those cases, just ignore that day's temperature and continue your count on the next day.

Note: 1. If you have a *valid* temperature that drops to or below the LTL during the Peak-plus-four count, the standard requirement still holds: you may need to restart your temperature count (see "Mid-shift dip" in Chapter 28).

2. If you have more than one missed or disturbed temperature during the four days of drying-up after Peak Day, you cannot apply Rule B until Peak Day + 5 or later.

Start of Phase III by Rule C

This is the most conservative rule. It requires **both** three consecutive days of full thermal shift **and** four days of drying-up. The C stands for **C**autious and **C**onservative.

According to Rule C,
Phase III begins on the evening of
1) the 3rd day (or more) of full thermal shift
2) cross-checked by 4 (or more) days of drying-up
—whichever comes last.

Another way of saying the same thing:

With Rule C, Phase III begins on the evening of
1) the 4th day (or more) of drying-up
2) cross-checked by 3 or more days of full thermal shift, whichever comes last.

● Perfect coinciding

When the 4th day of drying-up and the 3rd day of full thermal shift occur on the same day, we call it "Perfect coinciding." Example 17 illustrates "Perfect Coinciding." (See also Figure 10.1 in Chapter 10.) Examples 18 and 19 show situations where you have to wait for the cross-check.

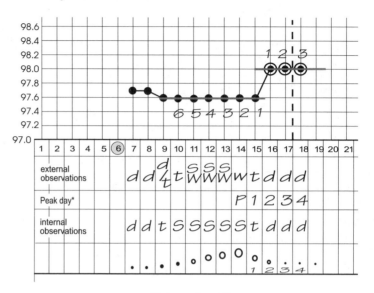

Example 17
Rule C Perfect Coinciding

● Waiting for the other sign

Sometimes you will experience a Perfect Coinciding Rule C. At other times you might have to wait for one of the signs to catch up. That's why we have the words "or more" in the statement of Rule C.

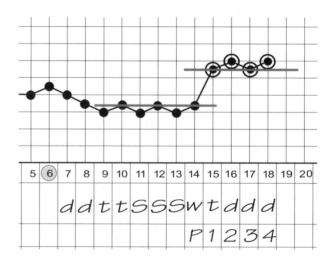

Example 18
Rule C Waiting for 4 Days of Drying-up

For example, you might have 3 days of full thermal shift but only 3 days of drying-up. Rule C calls for 4 days of drying-up. You would need to wait another day. The net result would be 4 days of full thermal shift as well as 4 days of drying-up.

It works the other way, too. You might have four days of drying-up past Peak Day but only two consecutive days of full thermal shift. You would need to wait for another day of full thermal shift temperatures for a Rule C interpretation. Look at the circled temperatures in Example 19.

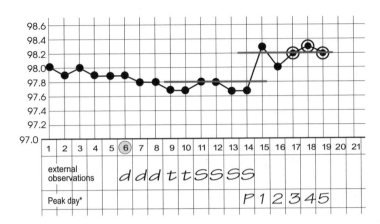

Example 19
Rule C Waiting for 3 Consecutive Days of Full Thermal Shift

Notice that in Example 19 (where Rule C = Day 19) there are four elevated temperatures by Peak Day + 4; however, one of those temperatures is below the High Temperature Level (HTL). Rule C calls for three days of full thermal shift, and a full thermal shift needs three temperatures that are at the High Temperature Level on consecutive days.

That may sound like nit-picking, but we think it's necessary to be clear about what constitutes a full thermal shift and what the requirements are for the most conservative Phase III rule. It illustrates why we have the other rules. (In Example 19, Rule R yields Day 17 as the start of Phase III.)

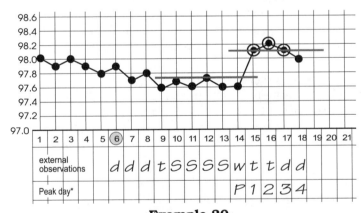

Example 20
Rule C Early Full Thermal Shift

On the other hand, sometimes a full thermal shift is established by the first three consecutive temperatures and the fourth temperature drops by 1/10 or 2/10 of 1° F. as in Example 20 where Rule C yields Day 18. That pattern also fulfills the requirements for Rule C when there are four days of drying-up. (In Example 20, Rule K yields Day 17 as the start of Phase III.)

However, if the temperature dropped 3/10 or more, the situation would become ambiguous; such a pattern would not fulfill the requirements for Rule C. See "Declining temperature pattern" in Chapter 28.

Rule C is frequently far too conservative except for beginners and couples who have the most serious reasons to avoid pregnancy. Even then, most couples who need the highest possible effectiveness would be just as well off simply by using one of the other rules and adding a day. See "Phase III" below.

Effectiveness of Rule C

We estimate that the surprise pregnancy rate with the correct use of Rule C is under 1 per 100 woman years. The Los Angeles study (described in Chapter 13, "More about effectiveness") used Rule C and found zero pregnancies among the couples who followed the rules. However, the study was relatively small, and even Rule C will have an occasional unplanned pregnancy. The analysis of our first 22 years of experience yielded only 14 unplanned pregnancies among couples who said they were using Rule C correctly. There are two possible explanations for the fact that our records of 22 years showed more unplanned pregnancies with Rule C than with any other rule. First, it's possible that many more couples have been using Rule C; second, it's possible that some couples forgot to record coitus at a fertile time. Indeed, in some cases it was difficult to believe that they had correctly recorded coitus, but for purposes of tabulation we have taken their word. If the records are complete and accurate, there have been some "small miracles."

The Most Conservative Approach

If you have the most serious reasons to avoid pregnancy, it is still possible to practice natural family planning. In fact, if you have serious health reasons to avoid pregnancy, then you have all the more reasons to practice NFP and to avoid the health risks of tubal ligation and chemical birth control (the Pill, Norplant, Depo-Provera). You have all the more reason to avoid the lower effectiveness rates of the barrier methods of birth control. At the same time, you may want to increase the effectiveness from a low 99% to a high 99%, that is, from 1 per 100 woman-years closer to 1 per 1000 woman-years or 1 in 10,000 woman-years.

If you are having long and/or irregular cycles, be sure to study Chapter 31. The practical recommendations in that chapter CAN make a difference in your cycle patterns; they CAN make the practice of NFP easier for you even though you have a most serious reason to avoid pregnancy.

Phase I

If you have the most serious reasons to avoid pregnancy, we recommend not using Phase I since most unplanned pregnancies come from relations in late Phase I.

If you choose to use Phase I, use it conservatively. We would not recommend using the Last Dry Day rule because in many cases it is more liberal than the other rules and allows Phase I to get closer to ovulation.

Phase III

You can increase the effectiveness of every Phase III rule simply by adding one or two days more of abstinence. However, there are only three absolutely 100% forms of birth control: 100% abstinence, male castration (removal of both testicles), and female castration (removal of both ovaries).

● **Four day thermal shift.** We do not have any effectiveness studies to indicate the effectiveness of waiting until the evening of the 4th day of thermal shift, but we do have two observations. Dr. Konald A. Prem has told us that in his clinical practice he never saw a couple who became pregnant when they waited until the morning of the 4th day of well-elevated temperatures. Dr. Rudolph Vollman has stated that pregnancies simply are not observed when couples wait for the fourth day of well-elevated temperatures.

While adding one or two days will raise the effectiveness of every Phase III rule, many couples with the most serious reasons to avoid pregnancy will focus on using Rule C, mostly for psychological reasons.

For other conservative recommendations, see page 381.

For a four day thermal shift pattern with Rule C, you do not need all four temperatures at the High Temperature Level. The first temperature can be only 1/10 to 3/10 of 1° F. above the Low Temperature Level. Preferably, the last three should be at the High Temperature Level, but see also Example 20. And, despite Dr. Prem's experience, the more conservative approach is to wait until the evening of the 4th day of thermal shift.

Because of the absence of studies, we cannot quote them; we can only speculate. Our estimate is that adding that fourth day raises the effectiveness of each Phase III rule by a factor of at least 10: from 1 (or less) per 100 woman-years to 1 (or less) per 1,000 woman-years.

● **Five day thermal shift.** Everything that was said about the four day thermal shift applies here as well. The last three days should be at the High Temperature Level for Rule C (but see also Example 20) and well elevated for the other rules. There is no reported research on couples who wait this long. Our estimate is that waiting for a fifth day of well elevated temperatures raises the effectiveness by another ten times—up to 1 pregnancy per 10,000 woman years. Quite frankly, if 10,000 couples were *trying* to become pregnant and waited until the evening of the fifth day of well elevated temperatures, we doubt that any of them would be successful in achieving pregnancy.

Confidence in God

At some point we think you have to put the matter in the hands of the Lord and trust that if He works a small miracle to co-create a new human life, He knows what He is doing and will help you to get through the pregnancy and to be good parents.

When the available research shows an unplanned pregnancy rate of less than one per 100 woman-years and when you abstain for one or two days beyond that, we think you have done all that is reasonable apart from total abstinence. At that point, we think it's time to place the matter in the providential hands of the Lord.

General Questions about Phase III

● **Which rule is best for us?**

Your own cycle pattern best determines which rule is best for you. The rule you use may vary from cycle to cycle.

If you have three days of full thermal shift and only two days of drying-up, there's no need to wait for Peak Day plus four. On the other hand, if you have a thermal shift that's difficult to interpret, wait until Peak Day plus four. If you have a three day *overall* thermal shift by P + 4, there's no need to wait for three days of *full* thermal shift.

● Does Phase III start in the morning or evening?

With every rule Phase III starts in the *evening,* that is, after 6:00 p.m.

● What is the relative effectiveness of the different rules?

We have no reason to believe that the effectiveness of any of the CCL Phase III rules is less than 99% (that is, more than 1 surprise pregnancy per 100 woman-years of use).

Note well: The effectiveness of all the rules depends on three things:
1. Accurate mucus observations in Phase I and Phase II
2. Valid temperature recordings
3. Abstinence from genital contact during Phase II.

Use common sense. If your first day of thermal shift is a disturbed temperature because of sickness, late waking, etc., don't count it. If you are not sure about the first day of drying-up, wait until you are sure the change has occurred.

● Will correct use of the rules give us 100% effectiveness?

No. According to our records, there is even an occasional Rule C surprise pregnancy. Quite frankly, when we see something like that, we have to wonder if the couple forgot to record an act of intercourse or genital contact, but we take their word for it. As long as the husband has his testicles and the woman has her ovaries, there is the possibility, however remote, that relations can lead to pregnancy, and that is true of every form of birth control.

As we have already noted, we think you can reduce the risk of all the Phase III rules to the level of 1 in 1,000 woman-years by adding one day, and you probably can reduce the risk to 1 in 10,000 woman-years by adding two days.

For normal living, the rules are excellent as they stand; if you had a life-or-death reason to avoid pregnancy, you would probably add at least one day as a regular practice. We realize that good medical practice has practically eliminated the life-or-death reason for the mother, but in China the life of a second or third baby is at risk of being killed by coerced abortion.

● What if my thermal shift is less than normal?

That means, what if you have an obvious thermal shift pattern but it doesn't reach the normal level of 4/10 of 1° F. above the Low Temperature Level. First, review Chapter 6, "Shaving irregular temperatures." Second, read Chapter 28, "Irregular temperature patterns."

● What about the mucus-only or temperature-only systems?

If you think you want to use a mucus-only or temperature-only system, study Chapter 26, "Mucus-only; temperature-only." We prefer the confidence of cross-checking signs, but the choice is yours.

Workbook exercises

Complete the following charts in the "Practical Applications Workbook":

Chart 2, applying Rule K
Chart 3, applying Rule R
Chart 4, applying Rule B
Chart 6, applying Rule C
Chart 7, applying Rule K
Chart 11, applying Rule K with shaving
Chart 12, applying Rule R with shaving as an alternative interpretation
Chart 14, noting the need for valid temperatures.

Self-Test Questions: Chapter 12

1. True____   False____   Rule K requires that the two days of drying-up occur on the last two days of the full thermal shift.

    Look at this unlikely situation we have constructed to illustrate some points: There are five days of thermal shift; the first three days are at the full thermal shift level, but the last two are only 3/10 of 1° F. above the LTL. Peak Day occurred on the second day of full thermal shift. Thus, the fifth day of overall thermal shift is P + 3.

2. Can you apply Rule K in this case? Yes____ No____
   Why? _____

3. Can you apply Rule R in this case? Yes____ No____
   Why? _____

4. Add one day of drying-up with a temperature still 3/10 of 1° F. above the LTL. What rule can you now apply? _____

5. Rule K requires at least 3 days of a _____ thermal shift.

6. Rule B requires at least 3 days of an _____ thermal shift.

7. Rule R requires three days of a _____ thermal shift.

8. Turn to Chart 12 ("short luteal phase cycle") in your "Practical Applications Workbook." What do you think of the physician's advice given in Chart 12? _____

   _____

9. One difference between a strong thermal shift and a overall thermal shift is that in a strong thermal shift all the temperatures have to be at least ____/10 of 1° F. above the LTL while the overall thermal shift will count temperatures that are only ____/10 of 1° F. above the LTL.

10. Another difference between the strong thermal shift and the overall thermal shift is that in a strong thermal shift the last temperature must be at least ____/10 of 1° F. above the LTL.

Answers to self-test

1. True 2. No. To apply Rule K, the <u>full</u> thermal shift must be kept up during the required days of drying-up. 3. No. To apply Rule R, the last day of the thermal shift must be a full 4/10 of 1° F. above the LTL. In this example, on P + 3, none of the standard rules can be applied. However, based on general experience with a four-day thermal shift of such strength, we think the woman was in Phase III by the night of P + 2. On P + 3, the only explanation we could give would be that she was in Phase III, based on the general infertility of such a well elevated five-day temperature pattern cross-checked by three days of drying-up. 4. Rule B. Also Rule C (see Example 20 on page 133). 5. full 6. overall 7. strong 8. The physician's advice reflects a makeshift form of calendar rhythm. If it were followed, it would most likely result in pregnancy very quickly. He was saying that Day 21 was the start of Phase III. That day is Peak + 1, frequently the day of ovulation and a very fertile day. 9. strong = two-tenths. . . overall = one-tenth 10. four-tenths

References

(1) G.K. Doering, 1967.

(2) B. Vincent et al., *Methode thermique a et Contraception: Approaches medicale et psychosociologique* (Paris: Masson, 1967) 52-73.

(3) The "K" stands for Kippley. With Dr. Konald A. Prem, John Kippley reasoned that there was no reason to ignore the excellent results of the temperature-only research; they added the two days of drying-up as insurance against being misled by invalid temperatures. For over 20 years we called this Rule A; we have changed the name for consistency: the labels of the other rules are related to names of researchers or the descriptive word (as C for cautious). The "A" didn't stand for anything.

(4) Dr. Josef Roetzer does not use the shaving principle. However, he allows the first temperature of the thermal shift to be only 1/10 of 1°F. above the LTL. Requiring all the strong thermal shift temperatures to be 2/10 of 1°F. above the LTL and shaving by 1/10 of 1°F. only one temperature among the pre-shift six yields similar but not identical results.

(5) James Trussell, Ph.D., and Laurence Grummer-Strawn, Ph.D., "Further analysis of contraceptive failure of the ovulation method," *Am J Obstet Gynecol* 165:6 part 2 (December 1991) 2054.

13

More about Effectiveness

by Thomas W. McGovern, M.D.

Natural family planning: Safe, healthy, and **effective**. How effective? To this simple question there is a not-so-simple answer: It depends — mostly on you. No knowledgeable scientist would deny that for couples who follow the rules, natural family planning can be highly effective for avoiding pregnancy. The notion put forth by some that NFP is not effective is simply false. Unfortunately, there are still some in the scientific community who are not well-informed.

In a paper printed in the highly-regarded *British Medical Journal*, Dr. R.E.J. Ryder addressed doctors and other scientists who need to become better informed.

> It might be argued that natural family planning — being cheap, effective, without side effects, and potentially particularly effective and acceptable in areas of poverty — may be the family planning method of choice for the Third World. The case for and against this may be argued and debated, but whatever the standpoint there is no doubt that it would be more efficient for the ongoing world debate on overpopulation, resources, environment, poverty, and health to be conducted against a background of truth rather than fallacy. *It is therefore important that the misconception that Catholicism is synonymous with ineffective birth control is laid to rest*[1] (emphasis added).

The reality is that NFP can be used at the 99% level of effectiveness by married couples who understand the method and *always* follow the rules.

When you read, "99% level of effectiveness," that's shorthand for "a surprise pregnancy rate (called 'unintended pregnancy rate' in most medical literature) of 1 per 100 woman-years." As you can see, that is technical language. **This chapter is not required reading for learning the art and science of NFP, and that's why most of this chapter is in smaller print.** However, reading the effectiveness data about NFP will give you an added level of confidence in its practice. Understanding this information will also enable you to explain NFP's effectiveness to those who need to become better informed.

Measuring Effectiveness

In general, *effectiveness* is stated in terms of 100% minus the surprise pregnancy rate. A *surprise pregnancy rate* is measured in terms of the number of couples out of 100 using a method for one year who become pregnant. Therefore, a surprise pregnancy rate of 20% or 0.20 means that 20 couples out of 100 would conceive during one year of using that method of birth control. That in turn would yield an effectiveness rate of 80%. While using the term "99% effective" is attractive, it is an oversimplification of what statistically is meant by an "effectiveness rate." In every population, some couples will not become pregnant no matter what method of birth control they use or do not use (the infertility rate of the population). Therefore, if there is only 1 birth per 100 couples using a particular method for 1 year, it does not necessarily follow that the 99 who did not conceive did not do so only because of the method of birth control used. Therefore, it is most accurate to speak in terms of the *surprise pregnancy rate*, even though the oversimplified *effectiveness rate* does state the practical outcome (in terms of couples not becoming pregnant).

Unfortunately, the measurement of effectiveness is not that simple. Patient variables, statistical methods, clinical study criteria, and many other factors enter the determination of a level of effectiveness. Sixteen such factors are listed a few pages later ("Factors influencing actual-use effectiveness"). The result is that apples are being compared with oranges, a fact that does not come through in popular magazine articles about methods of birth control.

Warning! The following discussion is technical. If you bear with it, though, you will gain enough background to be wary when reading any report on the surprise pregnancy rate of any form of birth control. You will also understand the data on which the effectiveness of the sympto-thermal method of NFP is based.

Pearl Index

The first and still most common method used to determine effectiveness is known as the Pearl Index. This is determined using the following formula:[2]

$$Pearl\ Index = \frac{Number\ of\ surprise\ pregnancies}{Number\ of\ months'\ exposure} \times 1200$$

The figure "1200" represents the number of months in which 100 women could conceive during one year. It assumes that each woman had one cycle per month, an average cycle length of 30.4 days. Some studies use the figure "1300" and divide by the number of *cycles* of exposure, assuming that each woman has cycles which average 28 days—a total of 13 cycles per year.

$$Pearl\ Index = \frac{Number\ of\ surprise\ pregnancies}{Number\ of\ cycles'\ exposure} \times 1300$$

The Pearl Index, developed by Raymond Pearl in the 1930s, is popular because it is simple. Only three pieces of information are needed to determine a Pearl Index: the months (or cycles) of exposure contributed, the number of surprise pregnancies, and the reason for leaving the study (pregnancy or other reason).[3] Because of its simplicity, a great deal of information is not communicated.

The Pearl Index assumes a constant risk of pregnancy over time. This is not a valid assumption because early study drop-outs tend to be couples more likely to get pregnant. Also, couples of lower fertility are likely to remain in the study longer. There is also a factor of 'learning by doing'; the longer a couple is in a study, the better they get at using the method.[3-5] Therefore, the longer the study, the lower the Pearl Index will be. This has caused great differences in reported rates among studies of oral contraceptives in which length of duration varied from 12 to 110 months.[2] The Pearl Index also provides insufficient information on factors other than accidental pregnancy which may influence effectiveness rate calculations. Such factors include dissatisfaction with the method, trying to achieve pregnancy, medical side effects, and being lost to follow-up.

For these reasons, two prominent birth control statisticians said in 1966 that the Pearl Index should be abandoned:[3,6]

> "[The Pearl Index] does not serve as an estimator of any quantity of interest, and comparisons between groups may be impossible to interpret....The superiority of life table methods or other estimators that do not assume a constant hazard rate seems clear."[6]

Life Table Calculations

The life table method requires much more work and data gathering when performing an effectiveness study. As the old saying goes, though, "You get what you pay for." This method generates more detailed information that can be used to compare studies. A life table calculates a separate effectiveness rate for each month of the study. It then reports the chance of conceiving during a specified time period, usually 12 months. The life table rates eliminate time-related biases; they go beyond unplanned pregnancy and provide information on other factors that influence continuation.[2] Life table methods are far superior to the Pearl Index approach, yet the Pearl Index continues to be the most frequently reported effectiveness rate in the scientific literature for all methods of birth control.

Furthermore, there are two main types of life tables. The multiple-decrement life table reports 'net' effectiveness rates which are useful for comparing competing reasons for couples dropping out of a study. These rates cannot be used to accurately compare one study to another. The single-decrement life table reports 'gross' effectiveness rates which can be used to accurately compare one study to another.[4,5,7,8,9] (It is not necessary to understand what a 'net' or 'gross' rate is; that is beyond the scope of this chapter.) Sadly, very few data of this nature are available. What is known is reported later in this chapter.

Types of effectiveness rates

To complicate matters further, but to help you better understand the data you may read, there are three types of surprise pregnancy rates which can be reported.[4,5,7,8,9] This cogent system was developed by James Trussell, Ph.D., and colleagues:

Actual-use surprise pregnancy rate: the surprise pregnancy rate which includes all pregnancies in a study and all months (or cycles) of exposure.

Perfect-use surprise pregnancy rate (also known as "Method-related surprise pregnancy rate"): the surprise pregnancy rate which includes only those pregnancies occurring during months (or cycles) when the method was followed according to all the rules. This rate uses only the exposure for cycles in which the rules were followed perfectly.

Imperfect-use surprise pregnancy rate: the surprise pregnancy rate which includes only those pregnancies occurring during months (or cycles) when at least one of the rules of the method was not followed. This rate uses only the exposure for cycles in which at least one of the rules was not followed.

Many studies calculate a **"User-related"** surprise pregnancy rate. The Actual-use rate will typically be higher than the User-related rate because only pregnancies occurring when rules were not followed are included in the numerator of the calculation for User-related rates; all pregnancies are used in the numerator for Actual-use rates. The denominator (all months of exposure) is the same for both calculations.

The main cause for variation in "actual-use" rates among studies of NFP involves the frequent disparity between the stated intention of the user couple and their practice (that is, having intercourse in the fertile time).[10] Many studies exclude all pregnancies that couples reported saying they tried to achieve. However, some scientists view with suspicion, and rightly so, such decisions when made only a few minutes before the act of intercourse. Therefore, most studies require that a "planned pregnancy" be announced at least one cycle before a couple tries to achieve it. Because of this common problem, the rates most important to know are the "perfect-use rates" which a couple can reliably achieve by consistently following the rules.

Even "perfect-use rates" are subject to variation. It is possible to construct a method with rules so onerous that almost no one would follow them. For example, a system could require observation at every bathroom visit even during Phase III and special abstinence rules in Phase III if a single middle-of-the-night mucus observation is missed. If they did not follow those rules during a time they thought was Phase III, the couple would be labeled as engaging in "pregnancy achieving behavior." Such a system would predictably have a very high "perfect-use rate" among the few "perfect-users." Then, because it would transfer so many cycles from an "imperfect-use" category into a "pregnancy seeking" category, such a system could report an erroneously high effectiveness rate for cycles in which there was normal Phase II abstinence.

While those three definitions are simple enough, they have not been followed in the majority of studies on effectiveness of birth control methods.[4] A major error is that the reported perfect-use rates include only the number of method-related pregnancies in the numerator but retain *all* the cycles of exposure (including cycles in which rules were broken) in the denominator. This artificially lowers the perfect-use rate as the following example shows.

A hypothetical study

100 woman-years of exposure
80 woman-years of perfect-use
20 woman-years of imperfect-use
20 pregnancies
2 perfect-use related (all the rules were followed)
18 imperfect-use related (at least one rule was broken)

Actual-use surprise pregnancy rate = 20/100 = 0.20 or 20% (Correct)

Perfect-use surprise pregnancy rate = 2/80 = 0.025 or 2.5% (Correct)

Perfect-use surprise pregnancy rate = 2/100 = 0.02 or 2% (Incorrect. This incorporates all months of imperfect-use in the denominator, thus artificially lowering the rate from 2.5% to 2%. This is how the perfect-use, or method-related, surprise pregnancy rate is most commonly miscalculated in reported studies.[4])

Imperfect-use surprise pregnancy rate = 18/20 = 0.90 or 90% (Correct)

User-related surprise pregnancy rate = 18/100 = 18% (Incorrect. This term has been reported in various studies of NFP. You can see that it uses the numerator of the Imperfect-use rate calculation and the denominator of the Actual-use rate calculation. This improper calculation and the term 'User-related' rate should be abolished from the family planning literature. It calculates a value of no importance.)

Only one NFP study in the medical literature has reported all three of these rates for life-table calculations. An international study of the ovulation method of NFP revealed the following surprise pregnancy rates for the first 12 months of use:[4,5,8]

Actual-use -	20.4%
Perfect-use -	3.1%
Imperfect-use -	86.4%

Do not be surprised that the "imperfect-use" rate approaches the rate of conceiving when using no method of birth control. This merely points out that the ovulation method (mucus-only), or any other NFP method, is unforgiving of risk-taking (not following the rules). The actual-use rate is closer to the perfect-use rate than the "imperfect-use" rate because all the rules were followed in nearly 90% of cycles.[5]

There are no studies reporting the life-table effectiveness of the male condom during perfect use.[11] However, studies have reported both the first year 'actual-use' and 'perfect-use' surprise pregnancy rates for the diaphragm (13-17% and 4-8%), sponge (17% and 11-12%), cervical cap (18% and 10-13%), and first six-month use of the female condom (12% and 2.6%) among U.S. women.[9,11] These studies do not report 'imperfect-use' rates, but being barrier methods, they could also be expected to have very high surprise pregnancy rates from "imperfect use," i.e., having Phase II coitus without the devices.

Pearl Index vs. Life Table Rates

The Pearl Index tends to be higher than life table rates over short periods of time, but lower over longer time periods. However, one cannot predict for an individual study how the Pearl Index would compare to the Life Table Rate since so many factors are involved. It is commonly believed that the highest possible Pearl Index is 100 — all women conceive in the first year of use. If you refer to the Pearl Index calculation, however, you will see that if all the women conceive within the first month, they will each contribute only one cycle of one month of exposure. That would yield the highest possible Pearl Index of 1200 (for months) or 1300 (for cycles).

Life Table Rates (single-decrement type) are comparable between studies; the Pearl Indices are not. Life table rates give detailed information about why couples drop out of studies; the Pearl Indices do not. The Pearl Index only approximates the Life Table Rate if 1) the incidence of pregnancy is low, 2) very few couples drop out of the study, and 3) the rates are compared for equal periods of time.[3] Because these assumptions cannot often be made, it would be best for the entire family planning community to present life table rates in all reported studies.[3,6,7]

Factors influencing measurement of effectiveness

Even though single-decrement life table surprise pregnancy rates may be reported, there are yet other variables between studies that may decrease the similarities between studies. A statistically-ideal study has been proposed which would include a random sample of couples with no refusals allowed, be randomized, double-blind, and prospective with all volunteers followed until the end of the study or until pregnancy occurs.[7] As the authors admit, this is impossible, but the further a study deviates from this ideal design, the less trustworthy are its data.

The four most important factors for determining method effectiveness include[12]

1) quality of the design, execution, and analysis of the study[13]
2) consistent and correct use of a method
3) frequency of intercourse
4) underlying fertility of couples (older vs. younger, previous pregnancies vs. no previous pregnancies)

Other factors influencing study effectiveness include, listed in no particular order:[1,4,5,7,8]

5) women using hormonal birth control before entering the study
6) women breast-feeding before or during the study
7) per cent of cycles in which no intercourse occurred
8) motivation level of the couple to avoid pregnancy
9) tendency of couples to choose methods they think will be effective for them
10) actual participation in a clinical trial vs. a retrospective reporting of data
11) checking for conceptions three months after the study ended to assure that all surprise pregnancies were counted
12) fraction of couples entering study who cannot be accounted for at the end of the study (The 12-month Pearl Index rose from 9.4 to 14.4 when the couples lost-to-follow-up were accounted for in a study of Calendar Rhythm)
13) country or culture where study was performed
14) method of teaching (home study, woman-to-woman, couple-to-couple)
15) effectiveness of teaching
16) (for NFP methods) which set of rules was used.

The topic of couple motivation deserves further mention, especially because some studies distinguish between *limiters* and *spacers*.

Limiters are couples who are using a particular method of family planning to keep their family at its present size. Right now they are telling themselves, "We do not intend to have any more children."

Spacers are couples who are using a particular method to postpone pregnancy. They are telling themselves, "We definitely want to have more children, but right now we want some more spacing."

These designations have nothing to do with any evaluation of their motives. Many couples who were spacers in their twenties and thirties become limiters when they get into their mid-forties. It should be obvious that spacers might change their minds more easily during the course of a study or "take chances." Generally speaking, the more spacers in any given study, the higher the actual-use surprise pregnancy rate will be.

Certainly by now you feel confused and wonder why you have read this far. Fret not! The main purpose of the preceding section is to show you that the effectiveness rates you read in articles about birth control have not been determined by an exact science and that more variability in determining accurate rates exists than you ever imagined. You may soon realize that by selective quoting of studies or manipulation of variables in a study, someone can report results that will show that virtually any method of birth control is better than any other. In other words, the next time you read an article about birth control in a popular magazine — and even in some professional journals — read it "with a grain of salt."

Effectiveness of various methods of birth regulation

First, the big picture. Worldwide, the average woman has the potential to bear 11-13 children during her fertile years if she and her husband never practice any form of birth control. A woman of normal *high* fertility can bear up to 20 children if she marries young and never breastfeeds. In most developing countries all the methods of *systematic* natural family planning and unnatural birth control (including withdrawal) together do not lower this number as much as breastfeeding alone does (Figure 13.1 on page 145).[13,14] The data in Figure 13.1 are calculated from Thapa et al.[13] from figures for 29 developing countries. If developed countries were included, all forms of birth control are found to lower the fertility rate more than breastfeeding.[15]

Ultra-effective

A review article of the effectiveness of all methods of birth control classified those methods with a first year perfect-use surprise pregnancy rate of less than or equal to one surprise pregnancy per 100 woman-years as "ultra-effective" forms of reversible birth regulation.[2] The authors include one form of NFP, intercourse only during Phase III, but some recent studies of the Sympto-Thermal Method of NFP (Phase I and Phase III) suggest this level of effectiveness and will be reported later in this chapter.

Respectably effective

Methods with a first year perfect-use surprise pregnancy rate of 2-6% were rated as "Respectably effective."[2] This includes various sympto-thermal methods and mucus-only methods. The authors made a key point about all methods of birth control:

> "Small numerical differences in method failure rates during perfect use are not as important as personal user preferences, because successful [birth control] is strongly dependent on correct and consistent use at every act of intercourse and on tolerance to side effects that may occur."[2]

In other words, you will achieve greater effectiveness by choosing a method of NFP that best suits you as a couple. An extreme example of this was demonstrated in an actual-use study of the Calendar Rhythm method of NFP and oral contraceptives in the Philippines.[15] After one year of use, there were actual-use surprise pregnancy rates of 28% for oral contraceptives and 36% for the rhythm method. However, for the third year of the study, Calendar Rhythm users had an 18% actual-use surprise pregnancy rate compared to a 23% rate for oral contraceptive users. While this reflects longer use of Calendar Rhythm by successful users, it also demonstrates that Rhythm users who had experienced two years of successful practice were less likely to become pregnant than long-term users of the Pill in that population.

What three methods of birth control are 100% effective? Only those in which a sperm and an egg cannot possibly meet. 1) Total abstinence (sperm and egg made, but no intercourse and therefore no opportunity for fertilization). 2) Male castration—removal of testicles, or orchiectomy (no sperm made; not vasectomy). 3) Female castration—removal of ovaries, or oophorectomy (no eggs made; not tubal ligation). All other methods of birth control have surprise pregnancies associated with their perfect use.

100% effectiveness

The rate of pregnancy ranges between 78 and 94% per year for couples who do nothing to try to prevent conception.[7] In one study of the Hutterite religious group where no form of birth control was used, 89% of women conceived within the first year of marriage. This works out to a life table rate of 0.89 or a Pearl Index of 254.[4]

No method

The rate of pregnancy varies based on previous use of hormonal birth control such as the Pill, whether or not a woman has had a prior pregnancy, and the prevalence of sexually transmitted diseases.[3,4,7,16,17] The pregnancy rate subtracted from 100% is the infertility rate. This is defined as the percentage of women who try to conceive (or do nothing to avoid conception) but do not conceive during a 12 month period.[16] The infertility rate remained at 13-14% in the United States between 1965 and 1982.[16] By 1995, the U.S. infertility rate had risen to 18.5 percent.

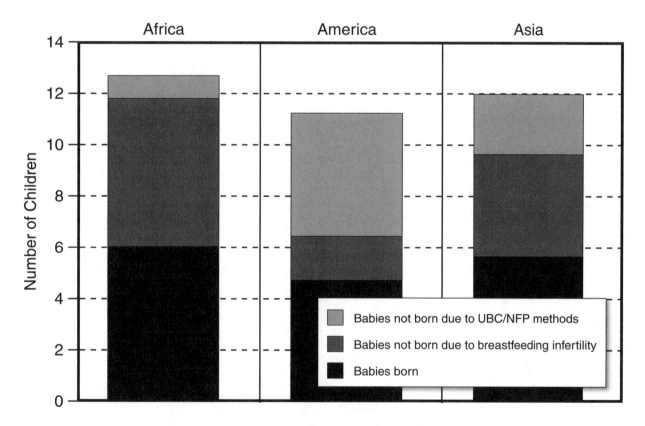

Figure 13.1 The Effect of Breastfeeding on Fertility
(UBC = Unnatural forms of birth control)

This graph illustrates that breastfeeding reduces the fertility rate in Africa by about half, in the Americas by roughly 30%, and in Asia by about 43%.

More on Effectiveness — 13

Effectiveness of unnatural methods of birth control

The vast majority of data on the effectiveness of unnatural methods of birth control come from tables updated periodically by Dr. Robert A. Hatcher and colleagues. The most recent data available are shown in Table 13.1.[12] The next most recent table was published in December of 1992 by other authors based on data from the Alan Guttmacher Institute, an affiliate of Planned Parenthood.[18]

Table 13.1 Surprise Pregnancy Rate in first year of use

Method	Hatcher[12]		Guttmacher[18]	
	Perfect Use	Typical (Actual) Use	Low*	High*
No method (for comparison only)	85%	85%	85%	85%
Spermicide alone	6%	21%	21.6%	25.6%
Withdrawal	4%	19%	14.7%	27.8%
Cervical cap + spermicide (parous women)	26%	36%	12%	38.9%
Cervical cap + spermicide (nulliparous women)	9%	18%	---	---
Diaphragm + spermicide	6%	18%	12%	38.9%
Male condom	3%	12%	9.8%	18.5%
Female condom	5%	21%	---	---
Oral contraceptives	---	3%		
Combined	0.1%	---	3.8%	8.7%
Progestin only	0.5%	---	3.8%	8.7%
Intrauterine devices	0.1-1.5%	0.1-2.0%	2.5%	4.5%
Injectable progestin	0.3%	0.3%	<1%	<1%
Norplant	0.09%	0.09%	<1%	<1%
Tubal ligation	0.4%	0.4%	---	---
Vasectomy	0.10%	0.15%	---	---

* "Low" and "High" refer to rates among women in the U.S.A. more and less likely than average to use the method correctly and consistently. Not to be confused with "perfect use" and "actual use" rates.

Table 13.1 demonstrates some of the many ways numbers can be presented to show different effectiveness rates for the same method of birth control.

Effectiveness of various methods of NFP

One of the problems in interpreting effectiveness rates for "Periodic Abstinence," as most of the scientific world calls NFP, is that there are so many different forms. When an author lumps together a number of results for various types of NFP, he is averaging apples and oranges. As a result, he compares fruit salads, not the same methods of NFP. As an example, in Table 13.2 look at the surprise pregnancy rates quoted by the above two sources.

Table 13.2 Surprise Pregnancy Rate in first year of use

Method	Hatcher[12]		Guttmacher[18]	
	Perfect Use	Average	Low*	High*
Periodic Abstinence	---	20	13.8	19.2
Calendar rhythm	9	---	---	---
Mucus only	3	---	---	---
Sympto-thermal	2	---	---	---
Phase III only	1	---	---	---

Both references lump together all methods of 'periodic abstinence' as if they were the same. This is because the data were derived from the National Surveys of Family Growth. Therefore, the average of 20 surprise pregnancies per 100 couples per year is not based on published prospective studies, but only based on questionnaire-generated data. The number of users of different NFP methods was too small to allow analysis of separate types of NFP. This is where confusion can occur in any publication regarding effectiveness rates.

Hatcher and his colleagues base the 2% and 1% perfect-use rate by extrapolating from the results of the previously quoted ovulation method study which demonstrated a perfect-use surprise pregnancy rate of 3.1%.[5,8] The ovulation method sometimes allows more days for intercourse than some versions of the sympto-thermal method, and the sympto-thermal method (Phase I and Phase III) allows more days of intercourse than would a Phase-III only method.

Now, in Table 13.3 let us take a look at the results of a variety of NFP studies done throughout the world over the last several decades.

Table 13.3
Surprise Pregnancy Rates of Various Sympto-Thermal Methods of NFP
Published in Peer-Reviewed Medical Journals

Country	Year	Method*	Life Table - Actual (Perfect Use)	Pearl Index Actual (Perfect Use)	Reference
Liberia	1990	STM/OM	4.3	--	19
U.S., France Canada, Colombia, Mauritius	1981	STM	7.2	(0.93)†	20
Zambia	1990	STM/OM	8.9	--	19
United States	1981	STM	11.2 (0.0)	--	21
United States	1981	STM	14.4	--	22
Australia	1978	STM	14.3-16.0	--	12
Colombia	1980	STM	19.1	--	23
Germany	1991	STM	--	2.3	24
United Kingdom	1991	STM	--	2.7	25
Europe	1992	STM	--	2.8	26
Italy	1986	STM	--	3.7	27
United Kingdom	1976	STM	--	23.9	28

* Abbreviations:
STM - sympto-thermal method - used a combination of calculation and/or mucus presence to determine end of phase I and combination of mucus and basal body temperature to determine beginning of phase III.

OM - ovulation method (mucus-only) to determine end of Phase I and beginning of phase III (peak day + 4).

STM/OM - volunteers used either of these methods and the results of the study do not differentiate by method.

† - The denominator for this calculation used all months of exposure. Since all the rules were not followed for all the months, the denominator should be smaller and the value of 0.93 quoted in the study should be higher. Given the low "Actual use" rate of 7.2% (life table), we might assume that the rules were followed in at least 80-90% of the months. This would yield a Pearl "Perfect-use" surprise pregnancy rate of 1.0-1.1.

These data demonstrate several points. First, there is a wide variation among *actual-use* surprise pregnancy rates based on individual study and country. The range of these studies for the sympto-thermal method is 2.3-23.9% with a median of 2.8% by Pearl Index and 4.3-19.1% with a median of 11.2% by Life-Table rate. This range is expected because the proportion of couples not following the rules will vary from study to study. All but one STM study showed a rate lower than the 20% average actual-use surprise pregnancy rate[12] or 19.2% rate[18] quoted in Table 13.2. This may be due to the fact that couples under observation in a study sometimes behave differently than those not being observed.

Few STM studies have calculated perfect-use surprise pregnancy rates. Pearl index perfect-use rates could be determined from two of the above listed studies (0.0 and 0.9).[20,21] This suggests that STM can be 99% effective (99% of couples will not conceive in one year of using the method if they follow all of the rules all of the time.) However, these data are too limited to conclusively prove that. One study published in the *Journal of Obstetrics and Gynecology of India* in 1982 found a Pearl Index of 0.2-0.3 in 12,000-19,000 cycles of experience.[29] These were not rates for the first year of use. Some believe these results are valid based on a high level of motivation among very poor people with large average family sizes who accept one to two episodes of coitus each month as normal. Others doubt that the results presented are accurate and point to the limited information present in the article and the fact that the study was not published in a respected, peer-reviewed journal in the field of family planning. Some of the variation between perfect-use rates seen in studies for one method type is due to the fact that not all STM or OM studies used identical rules.

Known effectiveness rates of the various STM rules

The primary work of the Couple to Couple League is to make reliable NFP available to interested couples. It relies upon the research of others. Here we describe some of the studies that support the system that CCL teaches.

Phase I rules

● The 21-Day Rule

The 21-Day Rule had a perfect-use surprise pregnancy rate of 0.00 in a study of Southern California couples sponsored by the National Institutes of Health from 1976-78. This study included 3,399 woman-months of exposure.[21] An Italian study involving approximately 3000 woman-months of exposure found a perfect-use surprise pregnancy rate of 0.00 using a less stringent 19-day rule (the original Calendar Rhythm rule devised by Dr. Kyusaku Ogino around 1930).[27]

In 22 years (1971-1993), CCL's central office received a few (very few, n = 11) unsolicited perfect-use surprise pregnancies that occurred as a result of following the 21-Day Rule. Therefore, we know with certainty that the 21-Day Rule is not perfect.

● The Clinical Experience Rule

An Austrian study examined this in the 1970s.[30] Among 8,532 cycles of exposure, the surprise pregnancy Pearl Index for intercourse on Day 6 was 0.2 per 100 woman-years. The true rate would doubtless be higher, unless it could be shown that intercourse occurred on Day 6 of each cycle. Estimates for Days 3, 4, and 5 are given in Chapter 11.

● Last Dry Day Rule

A study performed in five countries by the World Health Organization involving 725 couples and 7,514 cycles of experience using a mucus-only method of NFP during a one year period yielded a 3.1% life-table perfect-use pregnancy rate and 86.4% imperfect-use surprise pregnancy rate.[5] The actual-use pregnancy rate was 20.4%; rules were followed in 89% of cycles. According to this study, the highest method surprise pregnancy rate that could be assigned to the Last Dry Day Rule is 3.1% <u>if no surprise pregnancies occurred during early coitus in Phase III (no temperature cross-check was used to determine the end of Phase II).</u> However, it is not known if couples who used the method perfectly used the method *to its limit* (every other evening in Phase I right up to the appearance of mucus) or if they themselves reduced their limits (by using a calendar rule) to decrease the probability of conception.

● CCL Anecdotal Data

Finally, between 1972-1993, CCL Central received 107 unsolicited surprise pregnancy charts that were related to the correct use of the various Phase I methods: 83 for Last Dry Day rule, 13 for Clinical Experience rules and 11 for the 21-Day rule. Thus it appears that although we do not have Pearl or Life-table rates available for these data, we do see that 78% of the Phase I method-surprise pregnancies were due to the Last Dry Day rule. Since we don't know the ratios of individuals using the various Phase I rules among those who sent in unsolicited perfect-use surprise pregnancy charts, we don't know if more couples were using the Last Dry Day Rule and therefore more pregnancies occurred in this larger group of users, or if the Last Dry Day Rule is inherently less effective than the other two rules. We suspect that the latter explanation is correct because the Last Dry Day Rule frequently extends Phase I beyond the limits of the other Phase I rules and closer to ovulation.

Phase III rules

● The Los Angeles study

In 1976-1978 the U.S. Department of Health, Education and Welfare conducted a study in Los Angeles to determine the relative effectiveness of the Sympto-Thermal Method and the Ovulation Method.[21] The couples in the STM group used the 21-Day Rule and Rule C; the couples in the OM group followed the standard mucus-only rules. Among couples who followed the rules of their methods, the investigators found zero unplanned pregnancies in the STM group (for a perfect-use 0% surprise pregnancy rate) and six in the OM group (for a 5.7% perfect-use surprise pregnancy rate).

● Vincent: temperature-only

The couples in this mid-Sixties study did not use the mucus sign to cross-check the temperature sign. In 17,496 cycles of using a temperature-only rule to determine the start of Phase III, there was only one clear perfect-use pregnancy.[31] That yields a Pearl Index of .07. One statistical problem is that couples used either three or four days of thermal shift. Although this 1967 study does not meet today's higher standards, it strongly supports the CCL four-day temperature-only rule and Rule K which calls for three days of full thermal shift cross-checked by at least two days of drying-up past Peak Day.

● Doering: temperature-only

The 1967 study of Dr. G.K. Doering is the only one to report on temperature-only rules for both Phase I and Phase III. Some couples had relations only in Phase III; others used Phase I, too.

● **Phase III** was determined by a three-day temperature-only rule. The 307 couples having relations only in Phase III contributed a total of 11,352 cycles and experienced 8 unplanned pregnancies, yielding a user-effectiveness Pearl Index of 0.8. Of those 8 pregnancies, "one was due to misinterpretation of a temperature rise caused by a cold, five were pure patient errors, i.e., intercourse during the fertile phase, and two had incomplete temperature records."[32]

● **Phase I plus Phase III** was used by 689 couples for 48,214 cycles. They experienced 125 unplanned pregnancies, yielding a user-effectiveness Pearl Index of 3.1. Among those 125 pregnancies, 6 were from relations on the second day of upward thermal shift. Of the rest, "12 [couples] had misinterpreted temperature rises from colds, 13 conceived toward the end of the 'safe' postmenstrual period, 56 were patient errors, and 38 had kept incomplete records. . . Conception never occurred on the third day of hyperthermia [well elevated temperatures]."[32]

What was the **Phase I** surprise pregnancy rate among the couples who followed the Doering rules? Dr. Doering tells us that 13 conceived toward the end of Phase I. If all the 689 couples regularly had relations in Phase I in those 48,214 cycles and conceived by surprise only 13 babies, that would yield a Pearl Index of only .32.

Again, this study does not meet today's higher standards. Rather obviously, the couples were in the study for more than the one-year limit currently required, and it is not clear that all the couples using Phase I regularly used it to the limits of the Doering rule. Nevertheless, it continues to support all the temperature-based Phase III rules, and it is the basis of the Doering Phase I rule now being taught by CCL.

● Roetzer: sympto-thermal

In 1968, Dr. Josef Roetzer reported on a group of 180 women who observed 3,542 cycles and experienced 7 unplanned pregnancies, yielding an actual-use Pearl Index of 2.4.[33] Of these 7, only 2 were from couples who followed the rules, yielding a perfect-use Pearl Index of 0.68. In 1978, Roetzer reported a perfect-use Pearl Index of 0.2 for the use of the first six days of the cycle (1 pregnancy in 8,532 cycles).[30] Combining the cycles of both studies, Dr. Roetzer reported 12 unplanned pregnancies in 17,026 cycles observed by 491 fertile women, for an actual-use Pearl Index of 0.8. Among couples having relations only in Phase III, no pregnancies were observed in either study.

As with almost all studies in the Sixties and Seventies, the couples were in the study for more than one year. However, the combined experience of Dr. Roetzer and CCL leads us to think these numbers are fair representations of what can be achieved with the perfect use of Dr. Roetzer's rules. The extremely low actual-use surprise pregnancy rates in the Doering and Roetzer studies suggest that the Austrians and Germans must be among the world's best rules-keepers. The system used by Dr. Roetzer for Phase I is explained in the Clinical Experience section of Chapter 11; his system provides the basis for Rule R which is explained in Chapter 12.

Source of most surprise pregnancies

Various studies support the CCL experience that most perfect-use surprise pregnancies result from coitus too late in Phase I rather than too early in Phase III. The Doering and Roetzer studies which support Table 13.4 have been discussed previously. In addition to the perfect-use Phase III-only data from Vincent and associates discussed previously, they also used a 20-Day rule for the end of Phase I. The Phase III-only perfect-use Pearl Index was 0.07 vs 2.7 for Phase I and Phase III coitus. The actual-use Pearl Indices were 2.7 and 13.3 respectively.[31]

While the example studies do not show life-table rates, they show User-effectiveness Pearl Indices for each author's study, for equal lengths of time. While the rates have not been correctly determined, the same error (including all months of exposure in the denominator) was made consistently. The main point of the table remains valid: the majority of surprise pregnancies occur due to intercourse during the pre-ovulatory time, not during post-ovulatory intercourse.

Table 13.4   Phase III-Only vs. Phases I and III

	User-Effectiveness Pearl Index		Perfect-Use Pearl Index	
	Phase III-only	Phase I & III	Phase III-only	Phase I & III
Doering[32]	0.8	3.1	0.0	0.32
Roetzer[30,33] '68	0.0	2.4	0.0	0.68
'78	0.0	0.8	0.0	0.2
Vincent[31]	4.4	13.3	0.07	2.7

Most of the surprise pregnancies while using Natural Family Planning methods occur because of intercourse late in Phase I. Most of these are presumably due to use of the Last Dry Day Rule (according to CCL unsolicited data). The Clinical Experience and 21-Day Rules have less than a 1-2% estimated perfect-use surprise pregnancy rate.[21,27,30] Nevertheless, many couples will want to decrease the required time of abstinence by using the most liberal Phase I rule, which is the Last Dry Day Rule and which is still very respectably effective.

Points to Remember

1. The rules taught in this manual (except the Last Dry Day Rule) will enable you to practice 98-99% effective NFP if you follow the rules consistently and correctly.

2. The effectiveness of NFP is backed up by scientific studies. Various methods are considered "respectably effective" (2-6% *perfect-use* surprise pregnancy rate) or "ultra-effective" (1% or less *perfect-use* surprise pregnancy rate).

3. All methods of NFP are unforgiving of not following the rules.[34] Rate of conception approaches that of using no NFP as more risks are taken. If you have relations during the fertile time, you can expect to become pregnant.

4. The Sympto-Thermal Method of NFP is more effective than using one fertility sign alone (mucus or temperature-only).

5. The effectiveness you achieve as a couple depends more on how consistently and correctly you practice the method than on which set of rules you use.

Acknowledgement

The author thanks James Trussell, Ph.D., for his critical review of the manuscript.

References

(1) Ryder REJ. "Natural family planning": effective birth control supported by the Catholic Church. *BMJ* 307:723-6. 1993.

(2) Trussell J, Hatcher RA, Cates W, et al. A guide to interpreting contraceptive efficacy studies. *Obstet Gynecol* 76:558-567. 1990.

(3) Potter RG. Application of life table techniques to measurement of contraceptive effectiveness. *Demography* 3:297-304. 1966.

(4) Trussell J. Methodological pitfalls in the analysis of contraceptive failure. *Statistics in medicine* 10:201-220. 1991.

(5) Trussell J, Grummer-Strawn L. Further analysis of contraceptive failure of the ovulation method. *Am J Obstet Gynecol* 165:2054-2059. 1991.

(6) Sheps MC. Characteristics of a ratio used to estimate failure rates: Occurrences per person year of exposure. *Biometrics* 22:310-321. 1966.

(7) Trussell J, Kost K. Contraceptive failure in the United States: A critical review of the literature. *Studies in family planning*. 18:237-82. 1987.

(8) Trussell J, Grummer-Strawn L. Contraceptive failure of the ovulation method of periodic abstinence. *Fam Plan Perspect* 22:65-75. 1990.

(9) Trussell J, Strickler J, Vaughan B. Contraceptive efficacy of the diaphragm, the sponge and the cervical cap. *Fam Plan Perspect* 25:100-105, 135. 1993.

(10) Discussion and recommendations. *Am J Obstet Gynecol* 165:2068. 1991.

(11) Trussell J, Sturgen K, Strickler J, Dominik R. Comparative contraceptive efficacy of the female condom and other barrier methods. *Fam Plan Perspect* 26:66-72. 1994.

(12) Hatcher RA, Trussell J, Stewart F, et al. *Contraceptive Technology: Sixteenth Revised Edition*. Irvington Publishers, New York. 1994.

(13) Thapa S, Short RV, Potts M. Breast feeding, birth spacing and their effects on child survival. *Nature* 335:679-683. 1988.

(14) Howie PW. Natural regulation of fertility. *Brit Med Bull* 49:182-199. 1993.

(15) Laing JE. Natural family planning in the Philippines. *Stud in fam plan* 15:49-61. 1984.

(16) Gray RH. Epidemiology of infertility. *Curr Opin Obstet Gynecol* 2:154-158. 1990.

(17) Li Y, Wang JL, Qian SZ, Gao ES, Tao JG. Infertility in a rural area of Jiangsu province: an epidemiologic survey. *int J Fertil* 35:347-349. 1990.

(18) Choice of contraceptives. *Med Let* 34:111-114. 1992.

(19) Gray RH, Kambic RT, Lanctot CA, et al. Evaluation of natural family planning programmes in Liberia and Zambia. *J Biosoc Sci* 25:249-258. 1993.

(20) Rice FJ, Lanctot CA, Garcia-Devesa C. Effectiveness of the sympto-thermal method of natural family planning: an international study. *Int J Fertil* 26:222-230. 1981.

(21) Wade ME, McCarthy P, Braunstein GD, et al. A randomized prospective study of the use-effectiveness of two methods of natural family planning. *Am J Obstet Gynecol* 141:368-376. 1981.

(22) Kambic R, Kambic M, Brixius AM, et al. A thirty-month clinical experience in natural family planning. *Am J Pub Health* 71:1255-1257. 1981.

(23) Medina JE, Cifuentes A, Bernathy JR, et al. Comparative evaluation of two methods of natural family planning in Colombia. *Am J Obstet Gynecol* 138:1142-1147. 1980.

(24) Frank-Herrmann P, Freundl G, Baur S, et al. (includes Doring GK). Effectiveness and acceptability of the sympto thermal method of natural family planning in Germany. *Am J Obstet Gynecol* 165:2052-2054. 1991.

(25) Clubb EM, Pyper CM, Knight J. A pilot study on teaching natural family planning (NFP) in general practice. Proceedings of the Conference at Georgetown University, Washington, DC, 1991.

(26) European Natural Family Planning Study Groups. Prospective European multi-center study of natural family planning (1989-1992): interim results. *Adv Contracept* 9:269-283. 1993.

(27) Barbato M, Bertolotti G. Natural methods for fertility control: A prospective study - first part. *Int J Fertil* 48-51. 1988.

(28) Marshall J. Cervical-mucus and basal body-temperature method of regulating births: field trial. *Lancet* 2(7980):282-283. 1976.

(29) Ghosh AK, Saha S, Chatterjee D. Symptothermia vis a vis fertility control. *J Obstet Gynecol India* 32:443-447. 1982.

(30) Roetzer J. Sympto-thermal method - Ten years of change. *Linacre Quarterly* 45:358-374. 1979.

(31) Vincent B, Aymard A, Aymard M, et al. *Methode thermique et contraception: Approches medicale et psycho-sociologique*, Masson et Ciet, Eds. Paris: Masson, 1967, 52-73.

(32) Doering GK. The reliability of temperature records as a method of contraception. *Deutsche med wochenschr* 92:1055-1061. 1967.

(33) Roetzer J. Supplemented BBT and regulation of conception. *Archiv fuer gynaekologie* 206:195-214. 1968.

(34) Trussell J. Natural Family Planning - Effective only if used perfectly. *BMJ* 307:1003. 1993.

14

It's Not 100%

This chapter contains 11 charts to illustrate the chapter title, "It's Not 100%."

It is erroneous and unfair for articles in the popular press to ignore the extremely high effectiveness of natural family planning that we illustrated in the last chapter. The same sort of errors are frequent in birth control brochures that are handed out in many doctors' offices. It is simply unconscionable for U.S. government publications to ignore the Los Angeles study— research funded and supervised by a department of the U.S. federal government (mentioned briefly in Chapters 1 and 13).

It would also be unfair for us to give the impression that couples who use NFP never have any unplanned pregnancies. They do. As we have mentioned before, there are only three 100% methods of birth control: 100% abstinence during the fertile years, removal of both ovaries, and removal of both testicles. Although the Los Angeles study found a 100% effectiveness rate among couples using a conservative version of the Sympto-Thermal Method (21 Day Rule and Rule C), we know from our years of experience that the 100% level of effectiveness cannot be maintained. Occasionally a true surprise pregnancy will occur.

Unplanned pregnancies are of two types: 1) the real surprise and 2) unplanned but no surprise.

1. The true surprise pregnancy occurs when the couple correctly follow the rules and still become pregnant. As indicated in Chapter 13, these are very rare. In the previous chapter Dr. McGovern called these "perfect-use" surprise pregnancies. They are also called "method" surprise pregnancies.

2. The "unplanned but no surprise pregnancy" occurs when spouses do not follow the rules and become pregnant. If you ignore the abstinence rules, you are inviting pregnancy. For example, becoming pregnant from relations on a day of early mucus should certainly be no surprise to anyone who has taken good NFP classes or read this book. In the more technical literature these are called "imperfect-use" pregnancies; they are also called "user" surprise pregnancies.

Fairness and unfairness

Two types of unplanned pregnancies

Method Surprise Pregnancies

We take the word of couples who report surprise pregnancies; we presume they kept accurate records of coitus and remembered any sort of genital contact during the fertile time. Sympto-Thermal Phase I surprise pregnancies are somewhat explainable; Sympto-Thermal Phase III surprise pregnancies are truly baffling. Sometimes both seem to require a small miracle by the Lord. However, that is not true of method-related pregnancies when the method was Calendar Rhythm.

Calendar rhythm

We are starting with Calendar Rhythm because even today some people still think modern NFP is not much different from the Calendar Rhythm of the 1930s and 1940s.

Back in the 1960s, some retired friends told us they had practiced Calendar Rhythm during their entire fertile years with 100% success, having their three children just when they wanted them. There is no question that Calendar Rhythm worked very well when the couple followed the rules **AND** the wife had regular cycles.

However, if she had any of several kinds of cycle irregularity, the rules simply didn't work. For example, the Calendar Rhythm rules assumed a luteal phase of 14 to 16 days. If a woman consistently had luteal phases of only 10 days, she might consistently become pregnant despite following the rules. Or if ovulation was unusually delayed, the couple would still be in Phase II when they thought they were in Phase III.

In other cases where there was a history of long cycles, the Phase III rule was so conservative that it was very discouraging.

Calendar Rhythm Formula

The formula for Calendar Rhythm was very simple:
Shortest Cycle minus 19 = Last Day of Phase I
Longest Cycle minus 10 = First Day of Phase III.

To see for yourself how this formula would work—or not work—apply it to the Workbook charts. For example, in Chart 7 and some others, the Calendar Rhythm Phase I rule would be allowing relations on a day when the mucus had already started. In Chart 9, the Calendar Rhythm Phase III rule would have a couple thinking they were in Phase III when they were clearly still in Phase II but having a delayed ovulation. In Charts 4, 7, and 11, the Calendar Rhythm Phase III rule requires considerably more abstinence than is necessary with modern NFP.

We do not recommend Calendar Rhythm—and never have. However, if you should want to use it, be sure to use the 21 Day Rule for determining the End of Phase I. (See Chapter 10 for details.) Also, be on the alert for any stress situation that might delay ovulation. In such cycles, abstain from the start of Phase II to the start of the next menstruation, hoping that it is a true menstruation and not the breakthrough bleeding described in Chapter 30. The more you understand the possible variations from the "regular" cycle, the more amazing it is that calendar rhythm worked as well as it did for so many couples.

Figure 14.1 shows an apparent "dry day" pregnancy. The external mucus sign and the cervix sign apparently did not give the woman a sufficiently early message that she was in her fertile time. The couple was using the Last Dry Day rule for the End of Phase I. Relations on Day 7, a dry day, apparently resulted in pregnancy. We think it is extremely unlikely that relations on Day 16 caused the pregnancy because of the five days of very strong thermal shift cross-checked by three days of drying up.

Apparent dry day

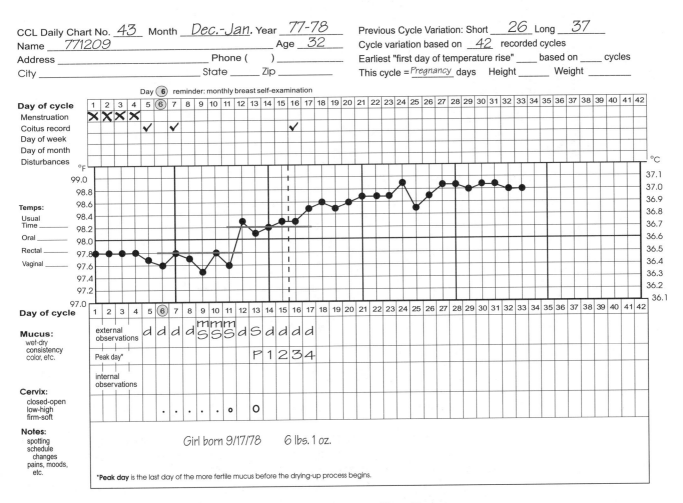

Figure 14.1   Apparent Dry Day Pregnancy

This woman typically had only three or four days of discernible mucus.

From a strictly scientific perspective, we would expect to see more unplanned pregnancies from the use of the Last Dry Day Rule than from the other Phase I rules because the Last Dry Day Rule is the most liberal rule. That is, it generally extends Phase I closer to ovulation. It is still a very good rule, but to reduce the possibility of "dry day" pregnancies, we make two recommendations:

1) In addition to your external observations throughout the day, also make the internal observation. Each night in Phase I, check for mucus directly at the cervical os.

2) Use the Last Dry Day Rule only if you consistently have mucus patches at least five days long from the start of the mucus through Peak Day.

Extended sperm survival?

Figure 14.2 and particularly Figure 14.3 move into the area of the "small miracle" if the couples correctly remembered and recorded their acts of marital relations and any genital contact.

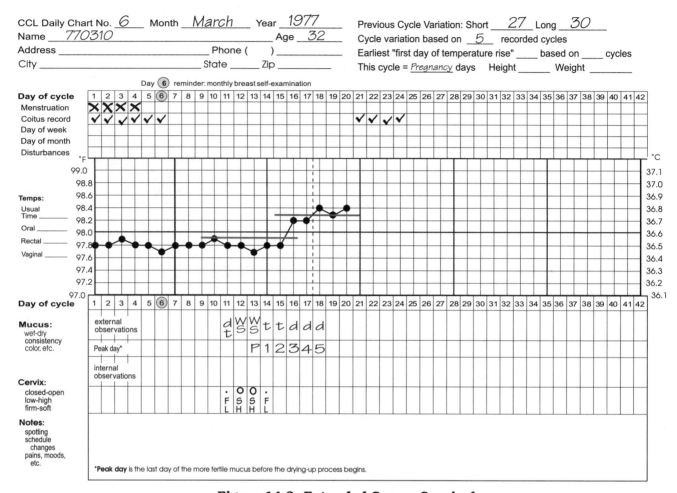

Figure 14.2 Extended Sperm Survival

The couple were not following the not-on-consecutive-days rule, but they abstained after Day 6 until well into Phase III. She should have recorded mucus observations beginning with Day 5.

However, even if she noticed mucus on Day 6, extended sperm survival provides the most plausible explanation for this pregnancy.

Ovulation is estimated to occur—rarely—as early as three days before Peak Day. If that happened here—on Day 10—sperm would have to live only four days, longer than usual but not yet super-long. However, with the temperature rise not starting until the third day **after** Peak Day, we think that ovulation before Day 12 is highly unlikely. Everything considered, we think that this pregnancy most likely required a sperm life of 6 to 8 days, and that happens very rarely. We speculate that it is possible that coitus on consecutive days modified the vaginal environment—made it more alkaline—and thus possibly contributed to extended sperm survival.

This unplanned pregnancy was truly a great-surprise pregnancy. First, Day 6 was the last day of Phase I by both the Clinical Experience Rule and the 21 Day Rule, and no mucus was observed and recorded. Second, it required very extended sperm life. What are the odds of that sort of combination? Who can say? It's not a miracle, but it surely looks as if God gave it his special assistance.

The couple who gave us the chart in Figure 14.3 said that they did not have marital relations or any genital contact for the first 15 days of the cycle. Assuming that to be true, this is an example of a genuine Phase III method surprise pregnancy, an extremely rare occurrence.

A Phase III pregnancy

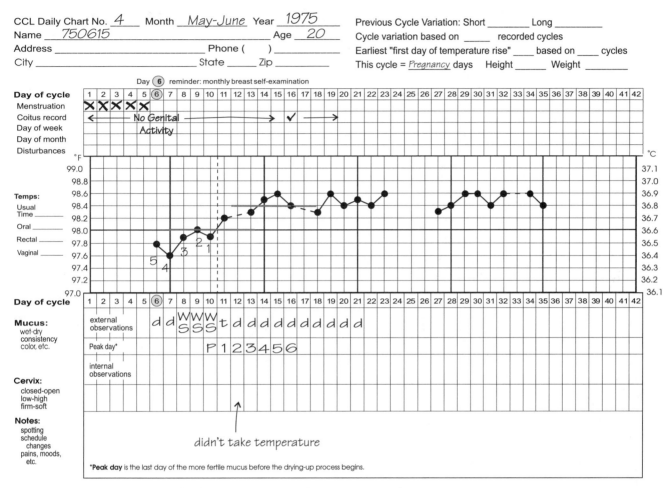

Figure 14.3 A Phase III Surprise Pregnancy

The LTL is set at 98.0° based on the five temperatures on Cycle Days 6 through 10. We consider the temperature on Day 11 to be part of the overall thermal shift pattern, but even if you used the Day 11 reading to set the LTL at 98.2°, you would still have a Rule B interpretation on Day 15.

Ovulation can occur as late as Peak Day plus 3. However, with the elevated temperatures on Days 11 and 13, it's hard to accept that in this case. A second ovulation can occur within 24 hours after the first. That would still require an egg life of 48 hours, and the textbooks say that doesn't happen. In the last analysis, we don't have a good explanation. It's not a miracle in the strict sense, but it is so unexplainable in terms of normal fertility that we call it "a small miracle."

Quite frankly, we really wondered if the couple forgot to record an incident of genital contact during Phase II, but the couple assured us they had no sexual contact until Day 16. Thus, if their memory is correct, all we can say about this pregnancy chart is that it shows that we cannot promise 100%. Once in a while a pregnancy occurs for which we have no explanation—except that God must have really wanted that child to come into being.

User Surprise Pregnancies

Most so-called surprise pregnancies are "imperfect use pregnancies." They result from a lack of motivation or erroneous interpretations; most of them are best labeled "unplanned but no surprise." The comment of the young couple who gave us the chart in Figure 14.11 is typical: "Not planned but it was not a surprise. This is our first! Keep up the great work."

We include these because you can learn much from the experience of other couples.

Obviously in Phase II

The couple who sent us the chart in Figure 14.4 had this to say: "This was not a wanted pregnancy, but it was not unwanted either. . . We just got careless—cut too many corners."

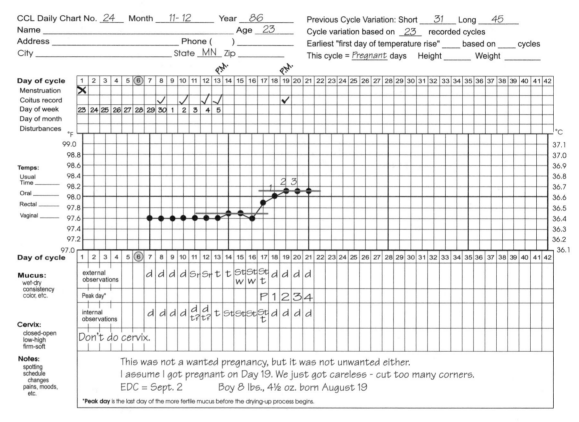

Figure 14.4   Lack of Motivation

What Phase I rules did the couple choose to ignore?

1. They did not abstain once she noticed mucus, and she certainly found mucus on Day 13, probably on Days 11 and 12 also.

2. Judging from her notation of "evening" on Day 13 and the notation of SR on Day 12, they had relations in the morning on Day 12.

3. They also ignored the not-on-consecutive-days rule.

4. The earliest beginning of Phase III was Day 20 by Rule R; coitus on Day 19 was one day too soon by any of the standard rules.

Relations on Days 12 and 13 most likely caused this pregnancy.

This chart does not illustrate any sort of failure. On the contrary, it simply shows that the presence of less-fertile cervical mucus indicates fertility.

The chart in Figure 14.5 dates back to 1961 and speaks for itself. If you have a sufficiently serious reason to use NFP to postpone pregnancy, you have to find ways other than marital relations to say "Goodbye, I love you," and "Hello again, I love you."

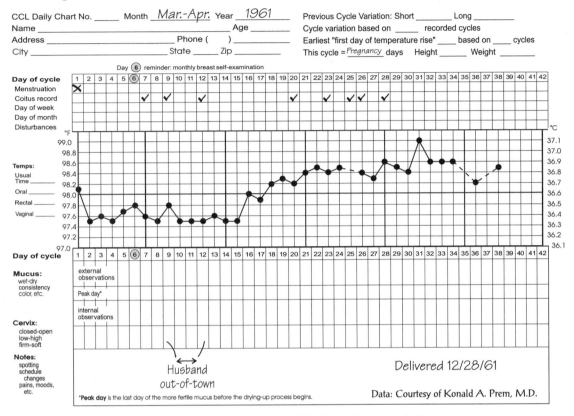

Figure 14.5   Absence, Lack of Motivation, and Pregnancy

The couple learned NFP from Dr. Konald A. Prem. In 1961 he was not promoting the mucus sign as he did later. However, he would have told the couple to consider themselves in Phase II after Day 7.

This chart does not show any sort of failure, but it does point to a challenge in the practice of natural family planning. Yes, a little absence does tend to make the heart grow fonder. Yes, many married couples like to make love on "special occasions" such as departures and homecomings. But no, having marital relations on such occasions is by no means a necessity for a happy marriage.

In such cases, the attitudes of both spouses—and perhaps especially the husband—are very important. If every night that he has gone to bed alone he has *dwelt* on the thought of having relations upon their reunion, he's making problems for himself. If he watches provocative television or movies or lets the sometimes provocative dress of some women get to him, he is simply not making the effort every husband needs to make to grow in chaste, sexual maturity.

Certainly the traveling man is usually going to want to embrace his wife when they are reunited, but such an embrace does not have to include marital relations. The sexually mature couple can express the warmth, tenderness and gentleness of marital love in a physical embrace without feeling compelled to follow their erotic tendencies to their culmination in the marriage act. The next morning they may well have real satisfaction and self-esteem at having expressed their marital love in non-genital ways—more than if they had followed the cultural pattern of equating lovemaking with coitus.

Two possibilities

Sometimes it is difficult to say which act of coitus caused the pregnancy, and that's the case in Figure 14.6. Relations on Day 8 most likely caused this pregnancy, but the coitus on Day 16 cannot be ruled out.

This chart also provides a handy summary of several things that add up to "how not to do it" if you're serious about avoiding pregnancy.

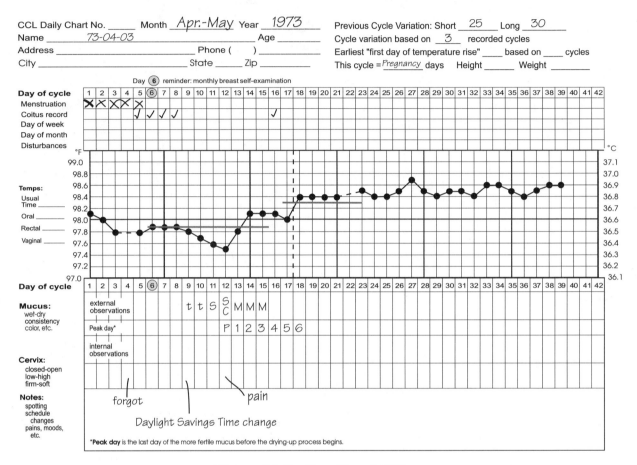

Figure 14.6   Two Possibilities

● Ignoring Phase I rules

Refresh your memory on the standard Phase I rules. Beginners should abstain in Phase I for the first one to three cycles. You need six cycles of experience to go beyond Day 6 and to apply the 21 Day Rule and the Last Dry Day Rule. Not in the morning. Not on consecutive days. Daily observations and recordings.

In Figure 14.6 you see four of those rules being ignored: 1) not making and recording daily mucus observations; 2) ignoring the not-on-consecutive days rule; 3) going beyond Day 6 without enough experience; 4) apparently using the Last Dry Day Rule without enough experience.

● Insufficient mucus observation

You need to make and record mucus observations every day past menstruation until you are in Phase III. In this chart, no observations were recorded on Days 6, 7, and 8. Perhaps the woman thought that any vaginal discharge was only seminal residue and was not the beginning of her mucus patch; that shows the reason for the not-on-consecutive-days rule. That rule is particularly important if you extend Phase I beyond the limits of the 21 Day Rule or Day 6, whichever is earlier.

● Insufficient temperature rise

The couple apparently thought the three day temperature rise on Days 14, 15, and 16 was enough. That's incorrect. All of those temperatures are only 2/10 of 1° F. above the Low Temperature Level of 97.9°. Even the weakest temperature rise (the overall thermal shift) requires that at least one temperature reach the High Temperature Level. That doesn't happen until Day 18, so the earliest Phase III interpretation in this case would be "Rule B = Day 18."

In their three previous cycles, they had thermal shifts of 4/10 to 6/10 of 1° F. The wife knew her temperature was still too low on Day 16, but the couple were no longer serious about avoiding pregnancy.

We might state the obvious: experience helps in the interpretation of difficult patterns. Your LTL and HTL will not change much from one cycle to the next.

● Paying too much attention to insignificant details

The couple talked themselves into regarding Day 16 as possibly the start of Phase III by focusing too much on two details.

1. They gave primary importance to the "pain" on Day 12. Mittleschmerz can occur before ovulation; use it only as a secondary sign to confirm the other signs.

2. They also paid too much attention to the dip on Day 12 and told themselves that on Day 16 they were four days past the dip. For more analysis of that mistake, see Figure 14.10 and "Focusing on a dip."

● Day 8 or Day 16?

No one can say for sure which act of marital relations caused this pregnancy. However, extended sperm life is a more common cause of pregnancy than is extended ovum life. In addition, Day 16 was Peak Day + 4 and was cross-checked by three days of weak thermal shift. Thus, we think it is most likely that relations on Day 8 caused this pregnancy, but Day 16 remains a possibility.

Misinterpreting the mucus sign

There are three ways to misinterpret the mucus sign of fertility. Each of the next three charts illustrates one of these.

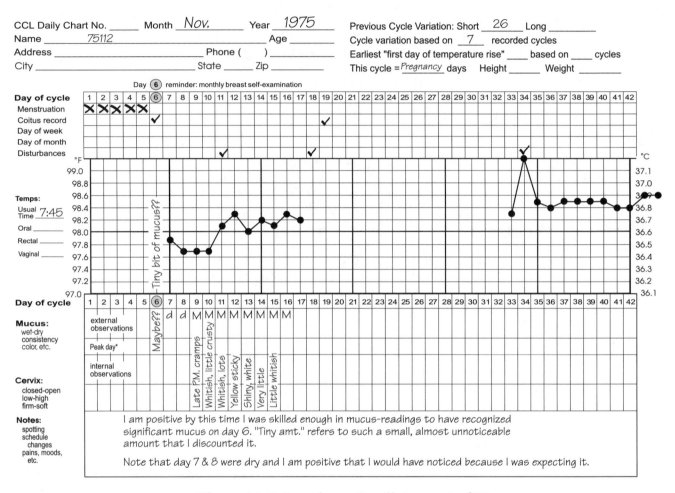

Figure 14.7 Ignoring a Small Amount of Mucus

● Ignoring a small amount

The couple who gave us the chart in Figure 14.7 noticed a small amount of mucus on Day 6, but they decided to ignore it as a sign of fertility. Relations that night resulted in pregnancy.

Day 6 was one day beyond the limits of the 21 Day Rule.

The Clinical Experience Rule yields Day 6—but only if it is still a dry day.

The obvious lesson: even a small amount of mucus indicates the beginning of the fertile time.

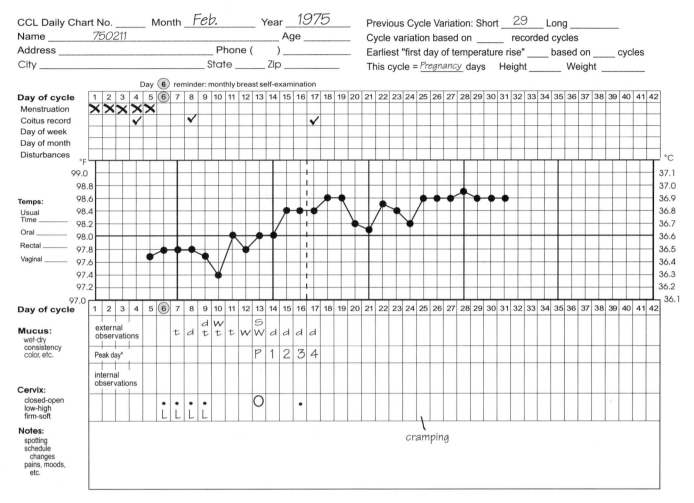

Figure 14.8 Mucus Followed by a Dry Day

● Ignoring the start of Phase II

The standard rule for normal cycles is this: once your mucus starts, you are in Phase II, even if you should have a dry day after a mucus day.

In Figure 14.8, the mucus started on Day 7. Day 8 appeared to be dry. Marital relations on the night of Day 8 resulted in pregnancy.

This chart dates back to 1975, and at that time we were not emphasizing the internal observation. If the woman had been making the internal observation for mucus, it is very possible she would have found it on Day 8.

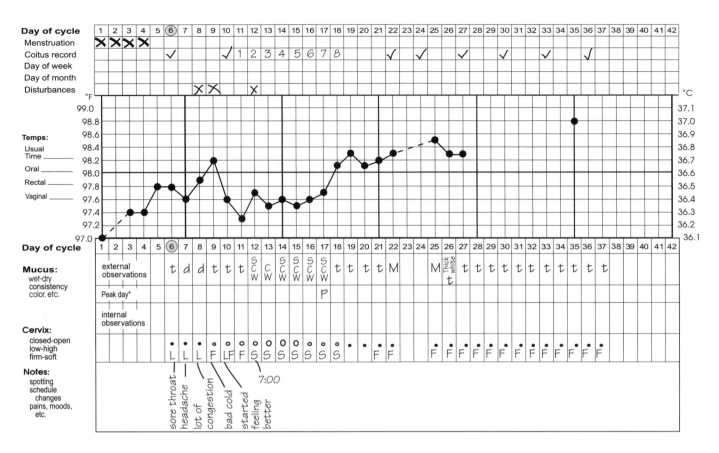

Figure 14.9 Ignoring the Less-fertile Mucus

● Ignoring the less-fertile mucus

The couple who gave us the chart in Figure 14.9 misunderstood our instructions. They thought the *less-fertile* type mucus was *infertile*. Wrong. Every kind of mucus from your cervix can nourish and transport your husband's sperm. The *more-fertile* types do an even better job, but for many couples, the *less-fertile* mucus—even if it's only tacky— does an excellent job of aiding sperm migration and conception.

The lesson is this: before ovulation, you have to regard every kind of mucus as a positive sign that you are in Phase II, the fertile time.

There's another lesson you can learn from this chart. This was only the second cycle of Sympto-Thermal experience for this couple. Do you remember what we recommend for beginners?

1. No relations during Phase I during the first one to three cycles so you can learn to detect the beginning of your mucus without any confusion from seminal residue.

2. Then, use the Clinical Experience rules for the next few cycles, and remember, they never take you beyond Day 6.

● Only a single observation

Here's another way to have an "unplanned" pregnancy that is really no surprise: rely on the Last Dry Day rule and make only one external mucus observation each day. That's completely insufficient.

Actually, no matter what Phase I rule you are using, you need to make your external mucus checks **periodically throughout the day in Phase I**. The most practical way to do this: make an external observation every time you urinate in Phase I. No extra time; no extra bother; just some awareness.

Just as there is more than one way to misinterpret or ignore the mucus sign, so also with the temperature sign.

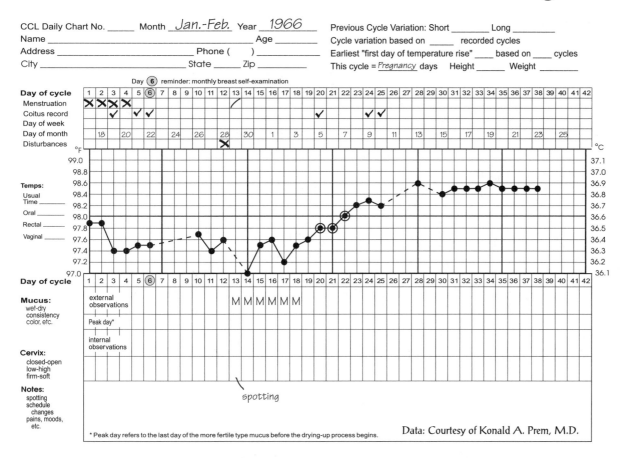

Figure 14.10 Focusing on a Pre-Shift Dip?

● Focusing on a dip

You may wonder how a couple could think they were in Phase III on Day 20. Here's our guess. Years ago, some writers associated a temperature dip with ovulation. Perhaps this couple heard or read something like that. Perhaps they focused on the dip on Day 17 and told themselves it might be associated with ovulation and then counted the next three days as rising temperatures.

In reality, Day 20 is only the FIRST day of thermal shift above the LTL set by the pre-shift six temperatures.

The lesson is this: if you are seeking to avoid pregnancy, ignore any temperature dips. For your upward thermal shift pattern, count only the temperatures that are consecutively above the Low Temperature Level.

Sometimes high levels of estrogen have a temperature depressing effect. Thus a temperature dip near the end of your typical mucus patch might signal a time of optimum fertility, a good time to seek pregnancy. However, it is far too unreliable to be used in any way when you are trying to avoid pregnancy.

This chart dates back to 1966. At that time Dr. Prem was instructing couples to determine the start of Phase III mostly by the temperature sign. Couples were recording mucus, but they were not identifying Peak Day and counting days of drying up. If Day 18 was the true Peak Day, then Rule B would indicate that Phase III started on the evening of Day 22.

● Not waiting for three temperatures

One of the early discoveries about the temperature sign was that pregnancies occur with some regularity from relations on the second day of thermal shift.

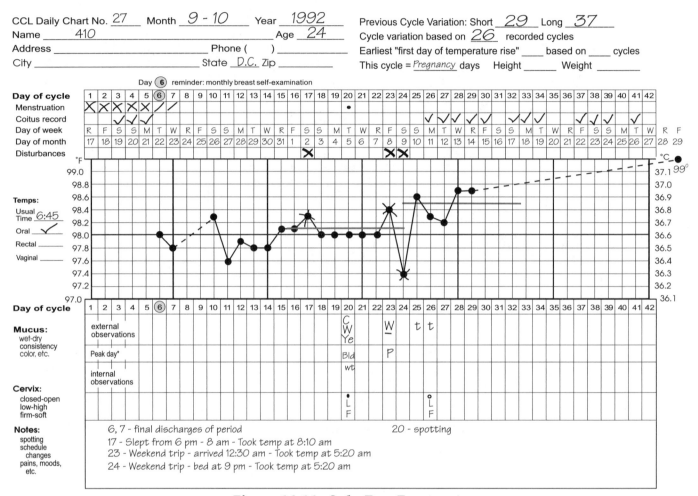

Figure 14.11 Only Two Temperatures

The couple set a shaved LTL at 98.0° and the HTL at 98.4° and wondered if they had misinterpreted the temperature pattern. Well, they didn't need to shave the LTL, but that had nothing to do with the pregnancy. Either way, Day 26 is still only the second day of thermal shift, and **you need three valid elevated temperatures for every Sympto-Thermal rule**. With her questionable Peak Day and no mucus recordings for Day 24, they should have waited at least until Day 28.

Summary Comment

We have shown you a number of "surprise" or unplanned pregnancies because we believe that honesty is the best policy. We cannot promise 100% effectiveness with natural family planning. Occasionally there will be a true method surprise pregnancy as well as the "imperfect use" unplanned pregnancies.

We would like to see a similar honesty from those dealing in Pills, implants, IUDs, sterilization, and the barrier methods. We challenge them to print the surprise pregnancy rates and the medical side effects of those methods in full size print, not in nearly unreadable small print such as this.

We believe that when you consider everything from effectiveness to health to morality, the natural methods of conception regulation described in this book are the best methods of family planning the world has ever known.

A key element for the happy and successful use of natural family planning is attitude, and the same thing is true if you should have an unplanned pregnancy. One of the guiding principles of the Couple to Couple League is that every child—whether asked for or not—is a gift from God and is to be loved and respected for her or his own sake. Each child will bring unexpected joy; each child is the living incarnation of personal spousal love.

As you know, it has become a deadly custom in much of the world to kill unplanned babies. We think this is at least partly the result of absolutizing the idea of the "planned family" and thus closing minds and hearts to the acceptance of the "unplanned" child. The acceptance of abortion did not come on the scene overnight. It grew out of other ideas such as absolute personal freedom, absolute family planning, and a confusion of love with the pleasure of genital intercourse. However, many of us know from personal experience and many others know with a deep-down intuition that love is shown much more in the acceptance of adversity and difficulties for a good cause than by being self-willed. We know intuitively or have learned that pleasure and long-range happiness are not at all the same.

We think it is appropriate to conclude a chapter on surprise pregnancies with a reminder that the value of family planning is only relative. What we need to emphasize is the love we must have for all who enter our lives, whether at conception or as adults, whether we really invited that person or not.

Planning says something about how we think we might respond to an imagined future. Our response to the present is the test of our love.

If you have a pregnancy that is "unplanned" or in any way is a surprise to you, please send the chart and the two preceding charts to CCL in Cincinnati. We have no reason to think that CCL couples are not achieving a 99% level of perfect-use effectiveness. However, records of genuine surprises

---

Not 100%. . .

Still the best. . .

The importance of attitude

The relativity of planning

Informing CCL

It's Not 100% — 14

are extremely important for any further refinement of the method, and records of imperfect-use surprises are important for improving our teaching. You may also want to review your charts with your teachers.

Workbook exercise   Go back to the section on Calendar Rhythm in this chapter. Apply calendar rhythm rules to the workbook charts as suggested and compare with STM interpretations.

Self-test Questions: Chapter 14

Some of these questions refer to material in previous chapters.

1. A "perfect use" surprise pregnancy is another term for a _____ surprise pregnancy.

2. The above term means that the couple used the method _____ and still became pregnant.

3. Limiters are couples who are
   a) anti-baby
   b) using their birth control method to keep their family at its present size and do not now intend to have another baby
   c) both over 35.

4. True_____   False_____   A spacer couple are using their birth control method to postpone the next pregnancy but intend to have another baby.

5. True_____   False_____   Doctors Josef Roetzer and G. K. Doering reported zero unplanned pregnancies from coitus during the time of postovulation infertility designated by their rules.

6. True_____   False_____   Dr. Maclyn Wade reported zero unplanned "method" pregnancies in the STM group of the 1976-1978 HEW Los Angeles study.

7. True_____   False_____   Because several studies have shown a 100% method effectiveness rate for various Phase III rules, we can claim that those rules are 100% effective for everyone.

8. True_____   False_____   Normal ovum life is longer than normal sperm life.

9. True_____   False_____   Sperm life is never longer than 72 hours.

10. True_____   False_____   The raw egg white, stretchy mucus is probably more conducive to sperm migration than the merely tacky mucus.

11. True____ False____   The first day of the less-fertile, tacky mucus indicates in a positive way that the fertile time (Phase II) has started.

12. True____ False____   Physical changes in the cervix can indicate the start of Phase II.

13. True____ False____   Calendar rhythm can work well for couples when the wife is regular in every way—mucus patch, time of ovulation, and luteal phase.

14. True____ False____   Delayed ovulation is a common source of unplanned pregnancies with the calendar rhythm method.

15. According to CCL rules, if you want to use the Last Dry Day Rule, you should consistently have mucus patches that are at least _____ days long from start through Peak Day. Shorter mucus patches may _____ the effectiveness of the Last Dry Day Rule.

Answers to self-test
1. method 2. correctly 3. b) using their birth control method to keep their family at its present size and do not now intend to have another baby 4. True 5. True. See Chapter 13. 6. True. See Chapters 1 and 13. 7. False 8. False 9. False 10. True 11. True 12. True 13. True 14. True 15. five. . . reduce

15

Getting Started & Quick Review

Let's assume you have just finished your first NFP class or the first lesson in the *CCL Home Study Course*, or have just browsed a couple of chapters in this book. Do you want a quick summary of how to get started? Do you want a quick reference to key sections of this manual? If so, you'll find this chapter helpful.

For Beginners

1. For the wife. Figure out where you are in your cycle—how many days it has been since the start of your last period. If it's been 10 days, then begin your recordings on Day 10 of the CCL Daily Observation Chart. (See "Resources" for obtaining charts.) Start making your mucus observations, at least externally, today—after each urination. If you are ready to start the cervix observation, then record those observations too. While you are doing that, you might as well try the internal mucus observation.

2. For the husband. Tonight, shake down the thermometer over the bed. Tomorrow morning, give it to your wife when the alarm goes off. After 5 to 9 minutes, take it back and place it in its holder. When you get up, record the reading on the temperature graph; then store the thermometer someplace out of sight and out of reach of little people's hands. Far back in a top dresser drawer usually is best.

The first steps

1. Keep loving each other regardless of whether or not you are having relations. Times of sexual restraint should be times of care and consideration; they need not be times of restraint from all physical embracing. Keep up your marital courtship and enjoy the honeymoon later on.

2. Keep your attitudes positive and work together as a team. With the proper attitudes, periodic abstinence is good and healthy for the marriage relationship.

3. Develop a prayer life, a personal relationship with God who will give you every grace you need.

4. Keep good records on a daily basis. Incomplete records greatly complicate the process of interpretation.

5. Feel free to seek technical or personal support from your NFP teachers. Enjoy continued support every other month through *CCL Family Foundations*.

Important reminders

If you are coming off the Pill or other hormonal birth control, be sure to review Chapter 29.

Review

It may take two to six cycles to develop confidence in your interpretation of your mucus observations.

● Mucus

Review Chapters 3 and 7.

Make your external mucus observations at each urination. The beginning of your mucus discharge, even the less-fertile type, signals the start of the fertile time. The internal observation sometimes reveals the appearance of mucus a day or more before you notice it externally.

Record your observations at the end of each day. Be sure to mark **D** when you are "dry." Use the symbols at the bottom of the chart for the other recordings. The more-fertile mucus is described in various ways: clear or cloudy, stretchy, like raw egg white, producing sensations of vaginal lubrication or wetness.

Peak Day is simply the last day of the more-fertile mucus. You know it only by hindsight. Label Peak Day after it is followed by 2 to 4 days of drying-up. Rule C plus one day is recommended for beginners. That means beginners should have 4 days of thermal shift and 5 days of drying-up past the Peak Day for the start of Phase III, the time of postovulation infertility.

● Temperature

Review Chapters 2 and 5.

Use a basal thermometer and take your temperatures either orally, rectally or vaginally. Take your temperature for a couple of minutes when you wake up; and be sure to take it at the same waking time each day during Phase II. In case of a variation of 1/2 hour or more, indicate the time on the chart, write an "x" in the disturbance row, and regard it as a disturbed temperature if it is out of line with the other temperatures in the pre-shift six.

Read the thermometer and mark the reading on your chart. Also record any disturbances—such as a cold or a fever—that might have affected your temperature.

To determine the thermal shift, ask yourself two questions:

1. Are there at least 3 temperatures above the previous 6 temperatures?

2. Are those 3 temperatures **enough** above the pre-shift six to fulfill the requirements of one of the Phase III rules?

After you find a group of 3 temperatures above the previous 6 temperatures, the following terms are used. The 6 temperatures immediately before the upward shift begins are called the **pre-shift six**. The undisturbed high temperatures among the pre-shift six set the **Low Temperature Level (LTL)**.

Rule C (which we recommend for beginners in the first two or three cycles) requires—after Peak Day—three consecutive days of **full** thermal shift to cross-check four days of drying-up. Then, in your first two or three cycles, add one day so you have at least five days of drying-up and four days of full thermal shift.

● Cervix

Review "The cervix" section in Chapter 8.

Examine the cervix once or twice a day—evening or afternoon and evening. Use the same position. During the infertile times, the cervix is firm and easier to reach. As ovulation approaches, the cervix becomes softer and more difficult to reach; the mouth of the cervix opens a little, usually enough to accept a finger tip, especially if you have had a baby.

Record the cervix changes by using the symbols given on the chart.

It may take you two to six cycles to develop skill and confidence in your cervix observations.

● Ovulation pain

Review the "Ovulation Pain" section in Chapter 8.

This is a secondary sign, but sometimes you may find it helpful.

● Phase I: Pre-ovulation infertility

Review Chapters 10 and 11.

We recommend that you abstain from all genital contact during Phase I for the first 1 to 3 cycles when you are just starting your NFP observations, even if you want to become pregnant very soon. In this way, you will be able to become familiar with the onset of your mucus flow without any interference from seminal residue or the vaginal mucus from sexual excitement. With this experience, the woman who soon achieves pregnancy will know what she is looking for when fertility returns after childbirth.

When you start having relations in Phase I, first use the rules in Chapter 10. With more experience you can use the rules in Chapter 11. We suggest not having relations in Phase I beyond Day 5 or Day 6 until you have six cycles of keeping NFP records and you are confident about your mucus observations—and perhaps your cervix observations, too. The Day 5 rule assumes short cycles in the 23-25 day range; the Day 6 rule assumes that your short cycles are 26 days and longer.

● Phase II: The fertile time

Study Chapter 20.

If you have had difficulty in achieving pregnancy, also study Chapters 21 and 22.

If you are seeking to avoid or postpone pregnancy, the fertile time calls for creative continence. Read Chapter 17 and learn how to make this time one of growth in your marital relationship.

● Phase III: Postovulation infertility

Review Chapters 10 and 12.

When you are just beginning the Sympto-Thermal Method, we suggest that you add one day to whatever rule you use. In Chapter 10 we suggested starting with Rule C plus one day, and that was repeated above in the section on "Temperature."

If you are having difficulty interpreting your temperature and/or mucus patterns, get in touch with your local CCL teacher or with CCL Headquarters for assistance. After those first two or three cycles, you may be ready to apply all the Phase III rules where applicable. Remember that Phase III begins in the evening of the day indicated by a particular rule.

The first few cycles

Experience is a great help in natural family planning, and we suggest the following steps while you gain that experience. These steps assume you are a married couple. The great advantage of a woman learning NFP observations while in a chaste engagement is that she gains her observation experience before marriage.

● Your first INCOMPLETE cycle

If you start the Sympto-Thermal Method early enough in your cycle to establish a pre-shift six and a thermal shift, you should be able to determine clearly the start of Phase III by one of the rules mentioned below. If you start observations too late to establish a pre-shift six and a subsequent thermal shift, we recommend abstinence during the first incomplete cycle.

● Your first COMPLETE cycle

Begin a new chart with the first day of menstruation. Begin your mucus observation right after menstruation or by Day 6 at the latest. Abstain during Phase I and Phase II during the first cycle.

Use **Rule C** to determine the start of Phase III and add one day as a precaution against misinterpretation due to inexperience.

If the mucus is of little or no help in the first cycle, use the **4-day Temperature-only** rule described in the Temperature-only section of Chapter 26. Add one extra day for beginners.

If you are unsure, contact your teachers. With their help, you may be able to apply one of the other rules (described in Chapter 12) in your first few cycles.

If you are **coming off the Pill** (or other hormonal birth control such as Norplant or Depo-provera), be sure to review the special 5-day Temperature-only rule in Chapter 29. This rule already has the extra day for beginners built into it.

The point is this: if you have a good indication of being in Phase III by one of the above rules, it is not necessary to abstain during Phase III of the first complete cycle.

● Your second and third cycles

We recommend abstinence during Phases I and II during your first two or three complete cycles. As you gain skill in your mucus and/or cervix observations and as you and your spouse gain confidence in the interpretation of your temperatures, you can drop the "extra day for beginners" for your Phase III interpretation. Some couples still may want to use the conservative Rule C to determine the start of Phase III.

● Cycles four through six

If you have not had cycles shorter than 26 days in the last 12 cycles, you can consider yourselves to have a 90% probability of being in Phase I up through Day 6. Depending upon the strength of the temperature shift and the clarity of the drying-up of the mucus, you might start using Rules K, R and B instead of Rule C for the start of Phase III.

● After six cycles

Six cycles of experience should be sufficient for most couples to use either the 21 Day Rule, the Doering Rule, or the Last Dry Day Rule to determine the end of Phase I. Be sure to review the details in Chapter 11.

With Experience

Once you gain sufficient experience, your practice of NFP will most likely fall into a fairly regular pattern. The following examples may help to give you a good idea of what the practice of NFP will be like for experienced couples in various circumstances.

You have two children and are hoping for more but you really like to space your babies two years apart. You had an early return of fertility at seven months postpartum, so you would like to postpone pregnancy for another eight months. Your shortest cycle has been 27 days.

As Mrs. A, you will begin making and recording mucus observations (and probably cervix observations, too) as soon as your period ends or by Day 6 at the latest. You have noted that both the 21 Day Rule and the Clinical Experience rules indicated Day 6 as the end of Phase I. You are confident in your mucus and cervix observations; you always have a mucus patch at least five days long. Therefore, you decide to rely upon the Last Dry Day Rule and/or the opening of the cervix. You have relations beyond Day 6; you follow the standard Phase I rules—dry days only, not in the morning, and not on consecutive days.

As soon as you notice the beginning of a mucus discharge or some changes in the cervix, you tell your husband. You both decide whether to seek pregnancy now or to limit your display of love and affection to non-genital ways. You discuss the matter long before going to bed. If you choose to avoid pregnancy, you avoid genital contact beginning with the first day of the show of cervical mucus (or changes in the cervix).

You notice that in a few days the mucus has become clear and stretchy, and then it begins to thicken and to dry up again. Perhaps you notice a little "ovulation pain" just before or around Peak Day. Then your temperature records show that your waking temperature is rising. You experience several dry or drying-up days that coincide with a sustained higher temperature level. When the sympto-thermal signs indicate the beginning of Phase III, you resume coital relations with confidence that you are in the phase of postovulation infertility. On the chart, you can calculate the start of your next menstrual period based on the usual length of your luteal phase.

Couple B. have more serious reasons for wanting to avoid pregnancy at this time. As Mr. and Mrs. B, you do not want to run the slight risk of not noticing the start of the mucus pattern and therefore you want to be more conservative than Couple A. For at least six months you have been limiting coitus to Phase III. During this six months, your shortest cycle has been 25 days and your longest cycle has been 30 days.

According to the 21 Day Rule, Phase I ends on Day 4 (25-21=4). According to the Clinical Experience rules, Phase I ends on Day 5. You decide which rule to follow.

You continue to record all your sympto-thermal observations, and you use a combination of at least 3 days of thermal shift and 2 to 4 days of drying-up (according to which rule you use—K, R, B, or C) to determine the start of Phase III.

Couple A (minimum Phase I abstinence)

Aside from differences in family size, this will be the typical family planning process for many couples.

Couple B (using the 21 Day Rule or CE Rules)

Couple C (very conservative)

You have what you consider the most serious reasons for avoiding pregnancy. Unless you are very experienced in observing, recording and interpreting the mucus and cervix signs of fertility, you will refrain from genital contact from the beginning of menstruation until the beginning of Phase III. If you decide to have coitus in Phase I, you will follow the more conservative rules and will not have relations beyond Days 5 or 6. The chances of becoming pregnant using conservative rules for the end of Phase I and the beginning of Phase III are very low and are described in the appropriate sections of Chapters 10 and 12. Some couples with the most serious reasons for avoiding pregnancy may decide to have coitus only in Phase III and to abstain in Phases I and II.

Couple D (great cycle irregularity)

Almost no one is perfectly regular, having a built-in 28-day menstrual clock. Most women have a range of three to five days between their shortest and longest cycles. However, when a woman varies from 20 days in one cycle to 45 days in the next cycle, she's highly irregular—and also an exceptional case. A few of these women may occasionally go for three months between menses.

If your cycles are highly irregular, be sure to study Chapter 31.

If you are Couple D and are serious about avoiding pregnancy, you will refrain from genital contact during Phase I and Phase II while you learn how to observe the mucus and cervix signs of fertility.

Once you have six cycles of experience and feel confident in your mucus and cervix observations, you may decide to apply the Clinical Experience rules up through Cycle Day 6. Be watchful for the appearance of cervical mucus during the days of light flow and afterwards; the Day 6 rule assumes that your mucus discharge has not yet started.

After your menstruation has stopped and dry days have been established, you can consider yourselves in Phase I infertility, applying the standard Phase I rules—dry days only, not in the morning, not on consecutive days, and preference for the internal observations.

At the first sign of mucus or the opening or rising of the cervix, you will recognize that Phase II has started and will refrain from genital contact until the beginning of Phase III.

The biggest advantage of the mucus and cervix signs is that they indicate the approach of ovulation right here and now. In a long cycle, sexual abstinence is normally not required for an extended time using these signs. On the other hand, the couple who rely solely on the postovulation thermal shift may have, in a long cycle, a rather long time of abstinence from coital relations.

Although it has been well emphasized in previous chapters, we repeat again that coitus before ovulation carries with it an inherently higher possibility of conception than coitus during postovulation infertility for two reasons: 1) the possibility of not detecting the mucus or cervix signs, and 2) the possibility of unusually extended sperm survival. For the experienced couple, the first possibility may be extremely small, but some couples with severe cycle irregularity may find the previous guidelines for Couple C appropriate for themselves.

Couple N (nursing mother)

This couple are new parents, and Mrs. N is nursing her baby according to the natural plan described in Chapter 24. Thus her menstrual periods and fertility may not return for 6, 12, or even 24 months.

About 6% of all extended-nursing mothers will become pregnant before their first period if they do not practice systematic NFP. Many couples who want only the natural spacing of ecological breastfeeding between babies will ignore all signs of fertility and look forward to the next pregnancy. Others will decide to use the sympto-thermal signs only after the first menstruation. Still others will start making their systematic sympto-thermal observations before the first period.

If Mrs. N wants to detect the return of fertility before her first period, she will begin looking for the pre-ovulation signs of mucus and cervix changes—especially after the baby has reached six months and is eating some solids. She may also begin her temperature recordings. When she detects mucus or cervix changes, they will refrain from genital contact if they need more spacing, and she will certainly start her temperatures if she has not already done so. If this is true pre-ovulation mucus, she will also soon notice a sustained postovulation rise in her temperature pattern. (See Chapter 25 for actual cases.)

Note: *a mother's experience with one baby is no guarantee of the same experience with her next baby. For example, with Baby #1 the mother may not ovulate until after her first postpartum menstruation, but with Baby #2 she might ovulate before her first menstruation.*

Couple P (premenopause)

Mrs. P is approaching menopause. Her cycles are becoming more irregular. For some, this will be a wakeup call. It's a sign that this is probably the last chance to have another baby. For others, a combination of age, fatigue, and the demands of their older children may provide increased motivation to avoid pregnancy at this stage in life. For our purposes, Couple P think they have sufficiently serious reasons not to be seeking pregnancy at this point in life, and they want to adopt a more conservative pattern of interpretation. They decide to end Phase I on Day 3 because of the possibility of a very short cycle. Some couples, however, will consider themselves back in Phase I after menstruation and during the days of no mucus and no cervix indications of fertility. They also begin requiring a four day thermal shift pattern for the start of Phase III. If the temperature drops to or below the LTL just before menstruation, they will count the first day of such low temperatures as Day 1 of the new cycle. Apart from these changes, Couple P will probably follow a pattern very similar to that of Couple D.

Couple S (seeking pregnancy)

Mr. and Mrs. S are looking forward to having a baby, so they review Chapter 20. Mrs. S eats a balanced diet and makes sure she is consuming 400 micrograms of folic acid daily to reduce the possibility of certain birth defects. (Most pre-natal supplements have this amount.) Then they pray for the gift of a child, a healthy pregnancy and a healthy baby. They will probably find a special meaning and pleasure in the marital embrace knowing that they are asking God to bless their love for each other with its expression in a new person.

Mrs. S will continue to consume a good pre-natal dietary supplement in addition to eating properly. After 21 days of elevated temperatures they establish the "due date" and notify her physician.

If they do not achieve pregnancy in the first cycle, they will not be too surprised. In cycle 2, to maximize their mutual fertility, they abstain during Phase I and until the more-fertile mucus starts. They will have marital relations every other day up through Peak Day + 2 or the first day of elevated temperatures, whichever comes first. If they do not achieve pregnancy within three cycles, they should read or re-read Chapters 21 and 22. If she achieves pregnancy but suffers a miscarriage, they will review Chapter 32.

Mrs. S will most likely enjoy good health during pregnancy, but some women encounter problems. Such women, in addition to seeking medical advice, would also do well to obtain *Managing Morning Sickness* and *Fertility, Cycles and Nutrition*, both by Marilyn Shannon (see "Resources").

About four months pregnant, Mrs. S starts to attend childbirth meetings and breastfeeding meetings so she is well prepared and can establish her local support system. It can be an exciting time, one of mutual growth and learning as a married couple.

Conclusion of Part I: Introduction and Basics

Two important parts of the successful practice of natural family planning are proper instruction and adequate understanding. The Couple to Couple League tries hard to ensure proper instruction and adequate understanding through its regular classes, its home study course, and through this manual. If you could compare your understanding of your fertility and natural family planning before you started instruction and after you have finished Part I of this manual, you would probably be amazed at how much you have learned. However, don't stop now. The best and some of the most interesting aspects of NFP are in the rest of the manual.

If you are like most of us, you will experience occasional difficulties when you practice chaste periodic abstinence. If you are like many women, you may also experience occasional difficulty in having marital intercourse. For various reasons, many women feel little or no inclination to marital relations on some occasions when their husbands feel so inclined. Therefore it involves sacrifice and generosity both to give and to abstain.

With the proper attitudes and convictions, however, any such difficulties remain small ones and become stepping stones toward increased marital maturity, mutual self-respect, and true sexual freedom. Therefore, another important part of the successful practice of natural family planning is a combination of mutual motivation, cooperative attitudes, and letting God into your decisions so that you do the right things for the right reasons. That's what Part II of this manual is all about.

There is no question that natural family planning provides an extremely effective method of conception regulation, and it does this without any harmful physical or psychological side effects. In addition it provides its own benefits of developing the whole person and fostering marital maturity. In short, NFP is good for family planning, it is good for character development, and it is good for marriages. With almost everybody concerned about birth control and with almost everybody also concerned about the family and the need for character development and acting on principle, what's the world waiting for?

Please—don't be bashful about sharing with others the gift of NFP.

Part II

Practical Applications Workbook

Practical Applications Workbook

**A workbook for applying
the Sympto-Thermal Rules
used by
The Couple to Couple League**

The 24 charts in this workbook section show how to apply the rules to a number of different cycle patterns. Some of these patterns are common and others are uncommon. Some of the charts are very easy to interpret; others are not so easy. By working your way through these charts, you will gain about two years of vicarious experience, yet it is highly doubtful that you will personally experience the sort of variety you will see in these charts. Our interpretations are in the "Chart Analysis" found at the end of the Workbook section. By completing the charts and reviewing the "Chart Analysis," you will help to prepare yourself for unusual situations.

Before the Fourth Edition of *The Art of Natural Family Planning*, the "Practical Applications Workbook" was a separate publication called *The Practical Applications Booklet*. The current workbook contains many of the 20 charts contained in the previous booklet.

The charts came from CCL couples, many of them in their first cycles of using the Sympto-Thermal Method. The lack of recorded experience and other data sometimes impedes a more thorough analysis, but each chart still teaches us something.

You will notice that a number of the charts are dated in the early 1970s and in the early 1990s. Those are the times when we were putting together the first edition and the current edition of this workbook.

As you review some of the interpretations toward the end of the Workbook, you will see alternative interpretations. The application of principles to concrete situations is an art as well as a science.

Summary of Rules

The following summary is **not complete**. Be sure to review Chapters 10-12.

THE END OF PHASE I can be determined in four ways (see Chapter 11):
1. (p. 108) The *Clinical Experience* rules for the first six days of the cycle;
2. (p. 110) The *21/20 Day Rule*: Shortest previous cycle minus 21 = last day of Phase I. After 12 cycles: Shortest previous cycle minus 20 = last day of Phase I.
3. (p. 112) The *Doering Rule*: Earliest day of sustained thermal shift minus 7 = last day of Phase I.
4. (p. 114) *The Last Dry Day Rule*: The last dry day = the last day of Phase I.

THE START OF PHASE III can be determined in several ways:
- (p. 131) **RULE C** (the most conservative interpretation): Phase III begins on the evening of
   1. the 3rd day (or more) of full thermal shift
   2. cross-checked by 4 or more days of drying-up, whichever comes later.
When the 3rd day of full thermal shift and the 4th day of drying-up are the same day, it is called **perfect coinciding.**
   *Note that a **full** thermal shift consists of three or more consecutive days of temperatures which are at least 4/10 of 1° F. above the Low Temperature Level (LTL).*

   Rules K, R, and B are based on this principle:
   The stronger the temperature pattern, the fewer days of drying-up are required (Rules K and R);

   or

   The weaker the temperature pattern, the more days of drying-up are required (Rule B).

- (p. 124) **RULE K** (more emphasis on the *full* thermal shift): Phase III begins on the evening of
   1. the 3rd day of **full** thermal shift
   2. simultaneously cross-checked by 2 (or 3) days of mucus drying-up past the Peak day.
   *See Rule C above for conditions for a **full** thermal shift.*

- (p. 126) **RULE R** (3 + 3 rule using the *strong* thermal shift): Phase III begins on the evening of
   1. the 3rd day of drying-up past Peak day
   2. cross-checked by 3 consecutive days of **strong** thermal shift past Peak day.
   *Conditions for a **strong** thermal shift:*
      1. Temperatures on three consecutive days are at least 2/10 of 1° F. above the LTL.
      2. The last temperature is at or above the normal HTL of 4/10 of 1° F. above the LTL.

- (p. 128) **RULE B** (more emphasis on the drying-up): Phase III begins on the evening of
   1. the 4th day (or more) of drying-up past Peak day
   2. cross-checked by 3 (or more) days of **overall** (or strong) thermal shift past Peak day.
   *Conditions for an **overall** thermal shift:*
      1. Three or more temperatures are at least 1/10 of 1° F. above the LTL.
      2. They are in an rising or elevated pattern.
      3. At least one of them reaches the normal HTL of 4/10 or 1° F. above the LTL.

- (p. 407) **POST-PILL** (temperature-only rule plus a day for beginners): Phase III begins on the evening of
      1. the 5th day of thermal shift with the last three on consecutive days at or above the High Temperature Level
      2. cross-checked by drying-up or dryness on at least the last day of the thermal shift.
   Be sure to study Chapter 29, "Coming off the Pill."

   Note: **Phase III** starts on the **evening** of the day indicated by a rule.

Abbreviations:
   LTL = Low Temperature Level
   HTL = High Temperature Level

CCL Daily Chart No. _10_ Month _Dec.-Jan._ Year _1974-75_

Name _____ Age _____

Address _____ Phone ( ) _____

City _____ State _____ Zip _____

Previous Cycle Variation: Short _27_ Long _32_

Cycle variation based on _9_ recorded cycles

Earliest "first day of temperature rise" ____ based on ____ cycles

This cycle = _28_ days Height _____ Weight _____

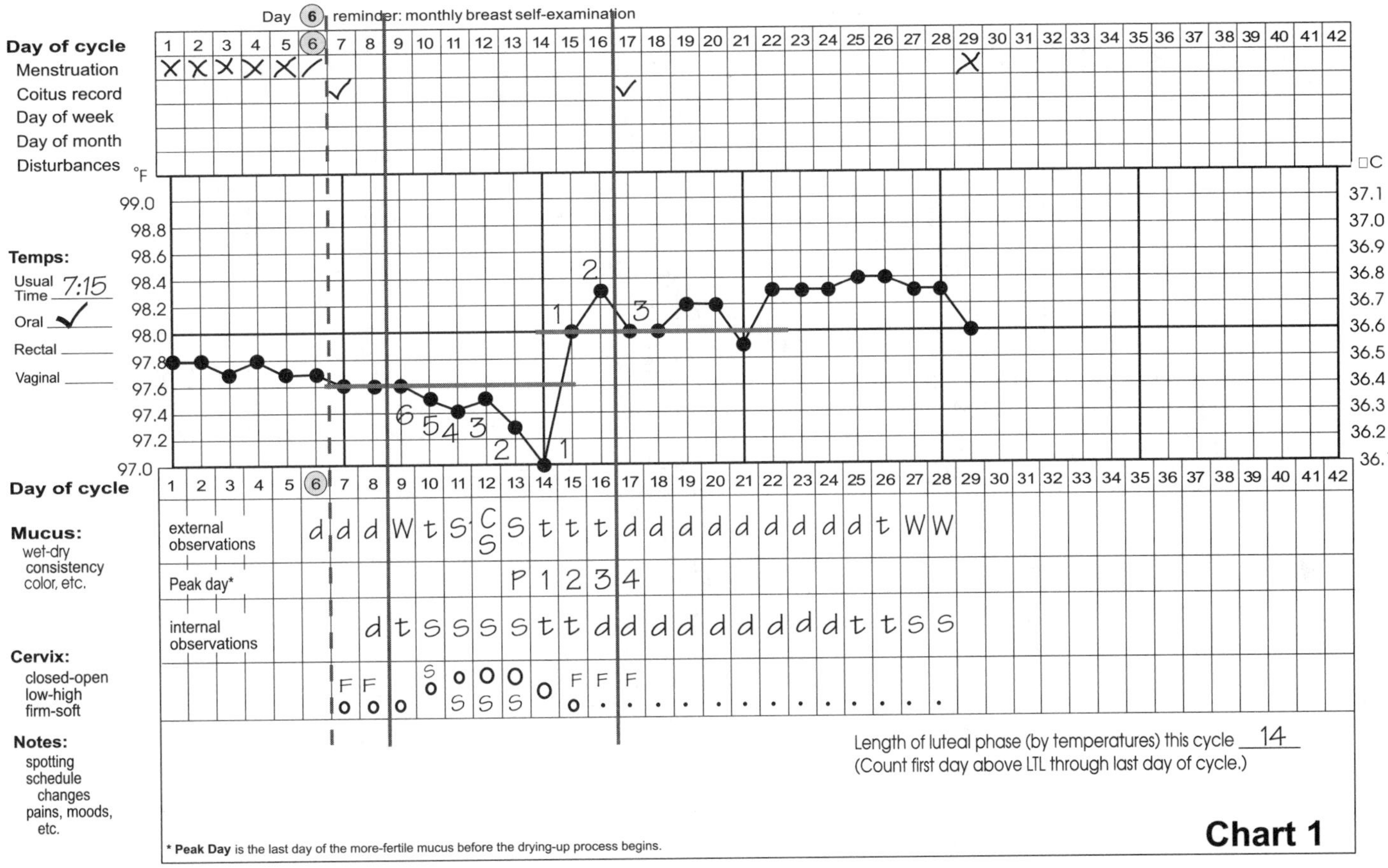

Chart 1

* **Peak Day** is the last day of the more-fertile mucus before the drying-up process begins.

Length of luteal phase (by temperatures) this cycle _14_
(Count first day above LTL through last day of cycle.)

End of Phase I:

Clinical experience _6_ 21/20 day rule _6_ Doering _n/a_ Last dry day _8_

Pre-shift six _9 - 14_ Low Temp Level _97.6_ High Temp Level _98.0_

"Peak" day _13_ First day of cervix closing _14_

Start of Phase III: Rule _PC_ = _17_ Rule C = _17_

NOTES:

Rule C, perfect coinciding; see Chapter 10 and Chapter 12, p. 131.

Name _____ Age 23
Address _____ Phone ( ) _____
City _____ State _____ Zip _____

Previous Cycle Variation: Short 24 Long 32
Cycle variation based on 21 recorded cycles
Earliest "first day of temperature rise" 13 based on 12 cycles
This cycle = 28 days Height 5' 4" Weight 108 lbs.

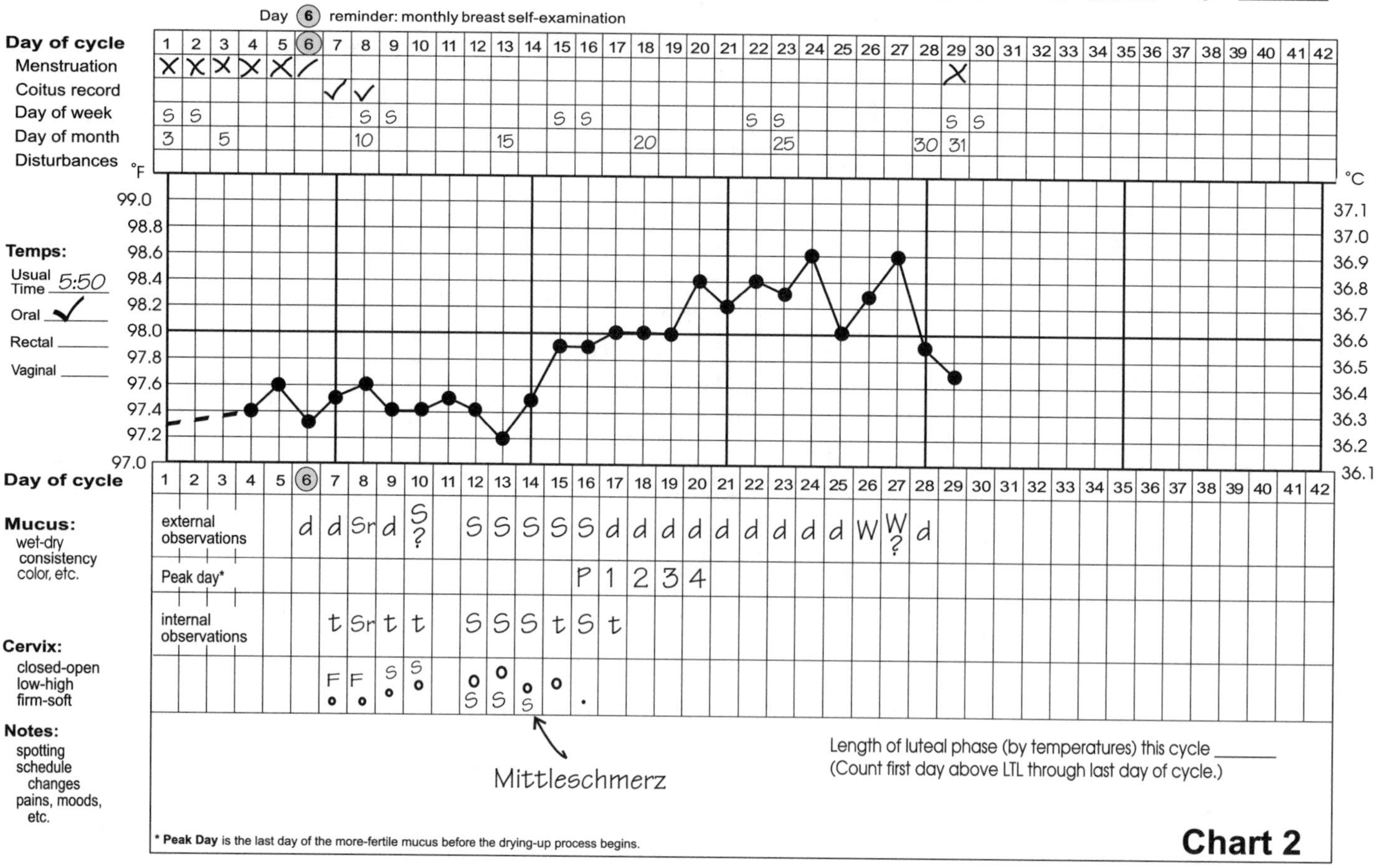

Day ⑥ reminder: monthly breast self-examination

Day of cycle	1	2	3	4	5	⑥	7	8	9	10	11	12	13	14	15	16	17	18	19	20	21	22	23	24	25	26	27	28	29	30	31	32	33	34	35	36	37	38	39	40	41	42
Menstruation	X	X	X	X	X	✓																							X													
Coitus record							✓	✓																																		
Day of week	S	S					S	S						S	S						S	S						S	S													
Day of month	3		5				10						15						20				25					30	31													
Disturbances																																										

Temps:
Usual Time 5:50
Oral ✓
Rectal _____
Vaginal _____

Temperature graph (°F left axis 97.0–99.0, °C right axis 36.1–37.1)

Day of cycle	1	2	3	4	5	⑥	7	8	9	10	11	12	13	14	15	16	17	18	19	20	21	22	23	24	25	26	27	28	29	30	31	32	33	34	35	36	37	38	39	40	41	42

Mucus: wet-dry, consistency, color, etc.

external observations: d d Sr d S? | S S S S S d d d d d d d d d d W W? d (days 7–29)

Peak day*: P 1 2 3 4 (at days 16–20)

Cervix: closed-open, low-high, firm-soft

internal observations: t Sr t t | S S S t S t (days 7–18)

cervix row: F° F° S°S S°S | O°S O°S O°S O° · (days 7–14)

↗ Mittleschmerz

Length of luteal phase (by temperatures) this cycle _____
(Count first day above LTL through last day of cycle.)

Notes: spotting, schedule changes, pains, moods, etc.

* **Peak Day** is the last day of the more-fertile mucus before the drying-up process begins.

Chart 2

End of Phase I:

Clinical experience ____ 21/20 day rule ____ Doering ____ Last dry day ____

Pre-shift six _____ Low Temp Level _____ High Temp Level _____

"Peak" day _____ First day of cervix closing _____

Start of Phase III: Rule ____ = _____ Rule C = _____

NOTES:

A typical Rule K interpretation; see Chapter 12, p. 124.
Phase I rules; see Chapter 11.

CCL Daily Chart No. __1__ Month ___Jan.___ Year __1993__

Name _____ Age __33__

Address _____ Phone ( ) _____

City _____ State _NC_ Zip _____

Day ⑥ reminder: monthly breast self-examination

Day of cycle	1	2	3	4	5	⑥	7	8	9	10	11	12	13	14	15	16	17	18	19	20	21	22	23	24	25	26	27	28	29	30	31	32	33	34	35	36	37	38	39	40	41	42
Menstruation	/	X	X	X	X	/	/																									X										
Coitus record	✓				✓																	✓	✓		✓			✓		✓												
Day of week	S							S	S					S	S					S		S				S	S								S	S						
Day of month	31	1			5					10					15					20					25					30												
Disturbances																																										

Temps:
Usual Time _6:40_
Oral ✓
Rectal ____
Vaginal ____

°F
99.0 — 37.1 °C
98.8 — 37.0
98.6 — 36.9
98.4 — 36.8
98.2 — 36.7
98.0 — 36.6
97.8 — 36.5
97.6 — 36.4
97.4 — 36.3
97.2 — 36.2
97.0 — 36.1

Day of cycle	1	2	3	4	5	⑥	7	8	9	10	11	12	13	14	15	16	17	18	19	20	21	22	23	24	25	26	27	28	29	30	31	32	33	34	35	36	37	38	39	40	41	42

Mucus:
wet-dry
consistency
color, etc.

external observations: d | d | W Sr | W | W | O | S | sl | sl | W | W | W | W | d | d | d | d | d | d | d | d | d | d | d | d | d | d

Peak day*: P | 1 | 2 | 3 | 4

internal observations: F | O | O | O | t | S | S | S | S | t | d | d | d | Sr | Sr | d | d | Sr | d | Sr | d | d
(1" | 1½" | 2" | 2" | 1½")

Cervix:
closed-open
low-high
firm-soft

o | o | O | O | O | O | O | O | O | O | o | o | · | · | · | · | · | · | · | · | · | ·
F | F | F

Notes:
spotting
schedule
changes
pains, moods,
etc.

Length of luteal phase (by temperatures) this cycle _____
(Count first day above LTL through last day of cycle.)

Chart 3

* **Peak Day** is the last day of the more-fertile mucus before the drying-up process begins.

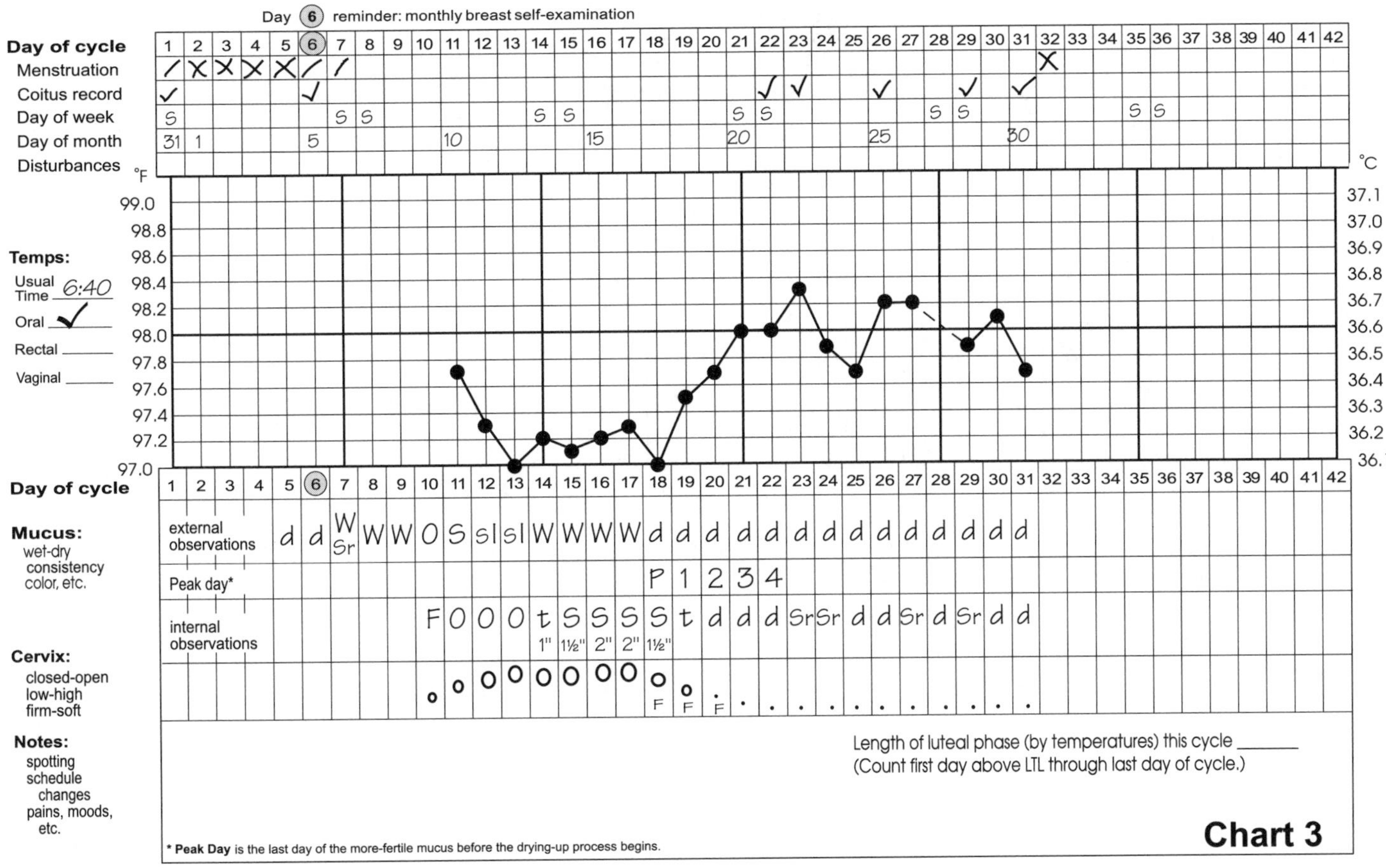

End of Phase I:
    Clinical experience ____ 21/20 day rule ____ Doering ____ Last dry day ____

Pre-shift six _____ Low Temp Level _____ High Temp Level _____

"Peak" day _____ First day of cervix closing _____

Start of Phase III: Rule ____ = _____ Rule C = _____

NOTES:

    A typical Rule R interpretation; see Chapter 12.

CCL Daily Chart No. _91_ Month ___Dec.___ Year ___1993___

Name _____ Age __41__

Address _____ Phone ( ) _____

City _____ State _____ Zip _____

Previous Cycle Variation: Short __24__ Long __31__

Cycle variation based on _90_ recorded cycles

Earliest "first day of temperature rise" __13__ based on __24__ cycles

This cycle = __27__ days   Height _5'5"_ Weight _122 lbs._

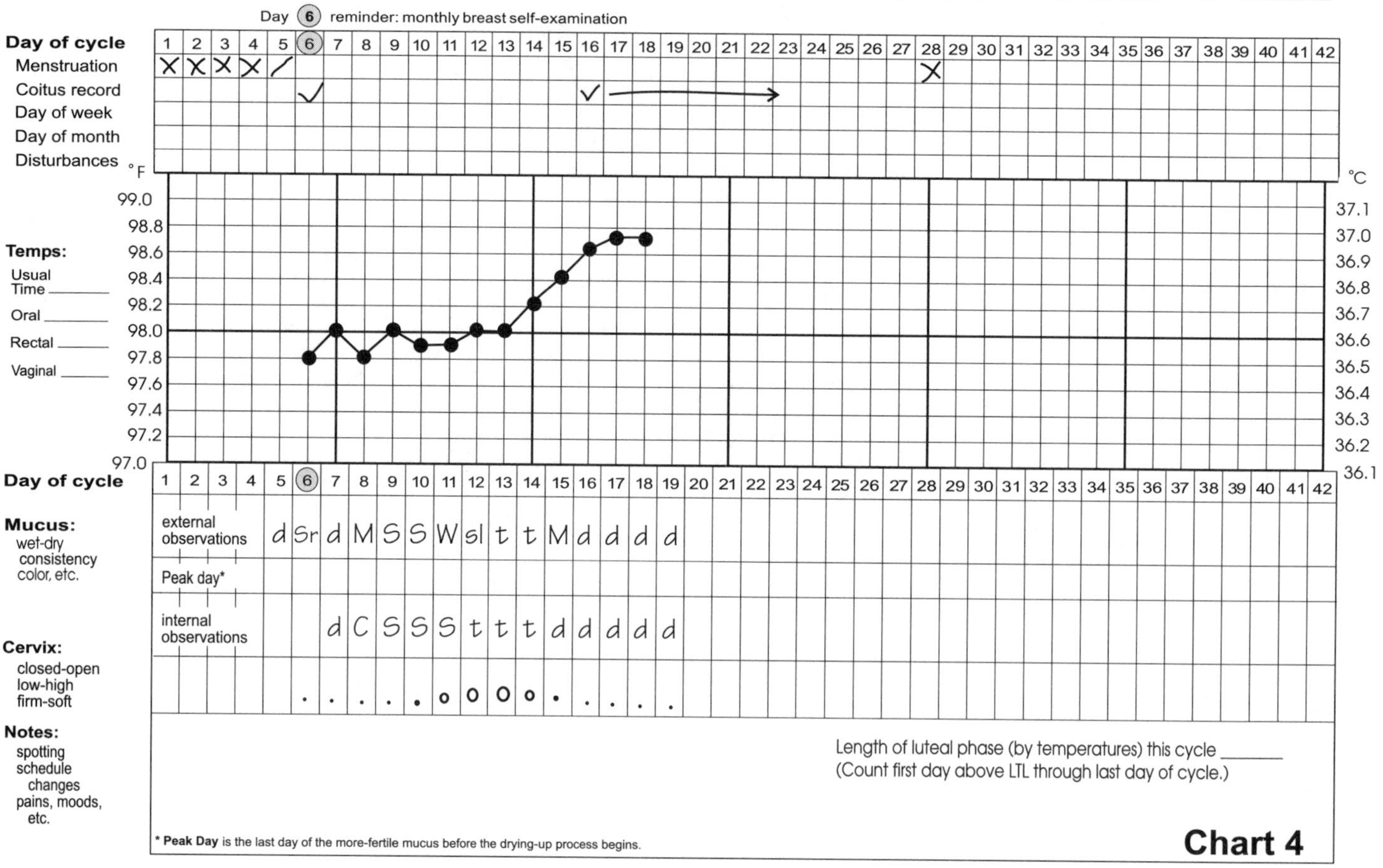

Day ⑥ reminder: monthly breast self-examination

Day of cycle	1	2	3	4	5	⑥	7	8	9	10	11	12	13	14	15	16	17	18	19	20	21	22	23	24	25	26	27	28	29	30	31	32	33	34	35	36	37	38	39	40	41	42
Menstruation	X	X	X	X	/																							X														
Coitus record							✓									✓	→	→	→																							
Day of week																																										
Day of month																																										
Disturbances																																										

Temps:
Usual Time _____
Oral _____
Rectal _____
Vaginal _____

°F / °C temperature grid:
99.0 / 37.1
98.8 / 37.0
98.6 / 36.9
98.4 / 36.8
98.2 / 36.7
98.0 / 36.6
97.8 / 36.5
97.6 / 36.4
97.4 / 36.3
97.2 / 36.2
97.0 / 36.1

Day of cycle	1	2	3	4	5	⑥	7	8	9	10	11	12	13	14	15	16	17	18	19	20	21	22	23	24	25	26	27	28	29	30	31	32	33	34	35	36	37	38	39	40	41	42

Mucus:
wet-dry
consistency
color, etc.

external observations	d	Sr	d	M	S	S	W	sl	t	t	M	d	d	d	d

Peak day*

internal observations	d	C	S	S	S	t	t	t	d	d	d	d	d

Cervix:
closed-open
low-high
firm-soft

	.	.	.	.	.	.	o	o	o	o	.	.	.	.	.

Notes:
spotting
schedule changes
pains, moods, etc.

Length of luteal phase (by temperatures) this cycle _____
(Count first day above LTL through last day of cycle.)

* **Peak Day** is the last day of the more-fertile mucus before the drying-up process begins.

Chart 4

End of Phase I:

   Clinical experience _____ 21/20 day rule _____ Doering _____ Last dry day _____

Pre-shift six _____   Low Temp Level _____   High Temp Level _____

"Peak" day _____   First day of cervix closing _____

Start of Phase III: Rule ____ = _____   Rule C = _____

NOTES:

   A typical Rule B interpretation; see Chapter 12.

CCL Daily Chart No. __1__ Month _Feb.-March_ Year ___1994___   Previous Cycle Variation: Short _____ Long _____
Name _____ Age __26__   Cycle variation based on _____ recorded cycles
Address _____ Phone (____) _____   Earliest "first day of temperature rise" ____ based on ____ cycles
City _____ State _VA_ Zip _____   This cycle = __27__ days Height _5' 6"_ Weight _115 lbs._

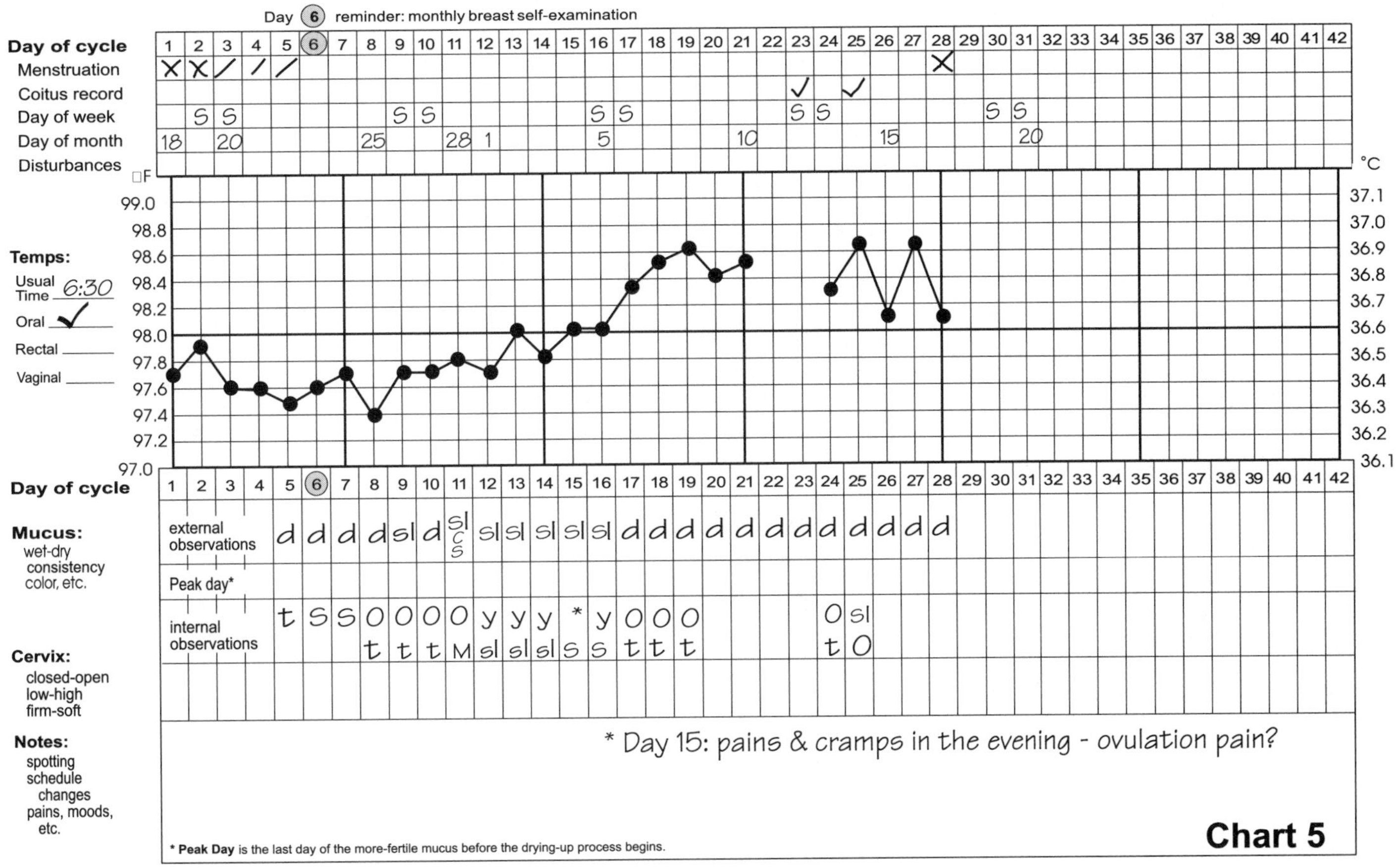

Day ⑥ reminder: monthly breast self-examination

Day of cycle	1	2	3	4	5	⑥	7	8	9	10	11	12	13	14	15	16	17	18	19	20	21	22	23	24	25	26	27	28	29	30	31	32	33	34	35	36	37	38	39	40	41	42
Menstruation	X	X	/	/	/																							X														
Coitus record																							✓		✓																	
Day of week		S	S						S	S						S	S						S	S				S	S													
Day of month	18		20						25			28	1				5					10				15				20												
Disturbances																																										

Temps:
Usual Time _6:30_
Oral ✓
Rectal _____
Vaginal _____

Day of cycle	1	2	3	4	5	⑥	7	8	9	10	11	12	13	14	15	16	17	18	19	20	21	22	23	24	25	26	27	28	29	30	31	32	33	34	35	36	37	38	39	40	41	42

Mucus:
wet-dry
consistency
color, etc.

| external observations | d | d | d | d | d | sl d | d | sl/c/s | sl | sl | sl | sl | sl | d | d | d | d | d | d | d | d | d | d | d | | | | | | | | | | | | | | | | | | |

Peak day*

| internal observations | t | S | S | O/t | O/t | O/t | O/M | y/sl | y/sl | y/sl | */s | y/s | O/t | O/t | O/t | | | O/t | sl/O | | | | | | | | | | | | | | | | | | | | | | | |

Cervix:
closed-open
low-high
firm-soft

Notes:
spotting
schedule
changes
pains, moods,
etc.

* Day 15: pains & cramps in the evening - ovulation pain?

Chart 5

* **Peak Day** is the last day of the more-fertile mucus before the drying-up process begins.

End of Phase I:
    Clinical experience _____ 21/20 day rule _____ Doering _____ Last dry day _____

Pre-shift six _____   Low Temp Level _____   High Temp Level _____

"Peak" day _____   First day of cervix closing _____

Start of Phase III: Rule _____ = _____   Rule C = _____

NOTES:

    Just off the Pill; see Chapter 29.

Practical Applications Workbook

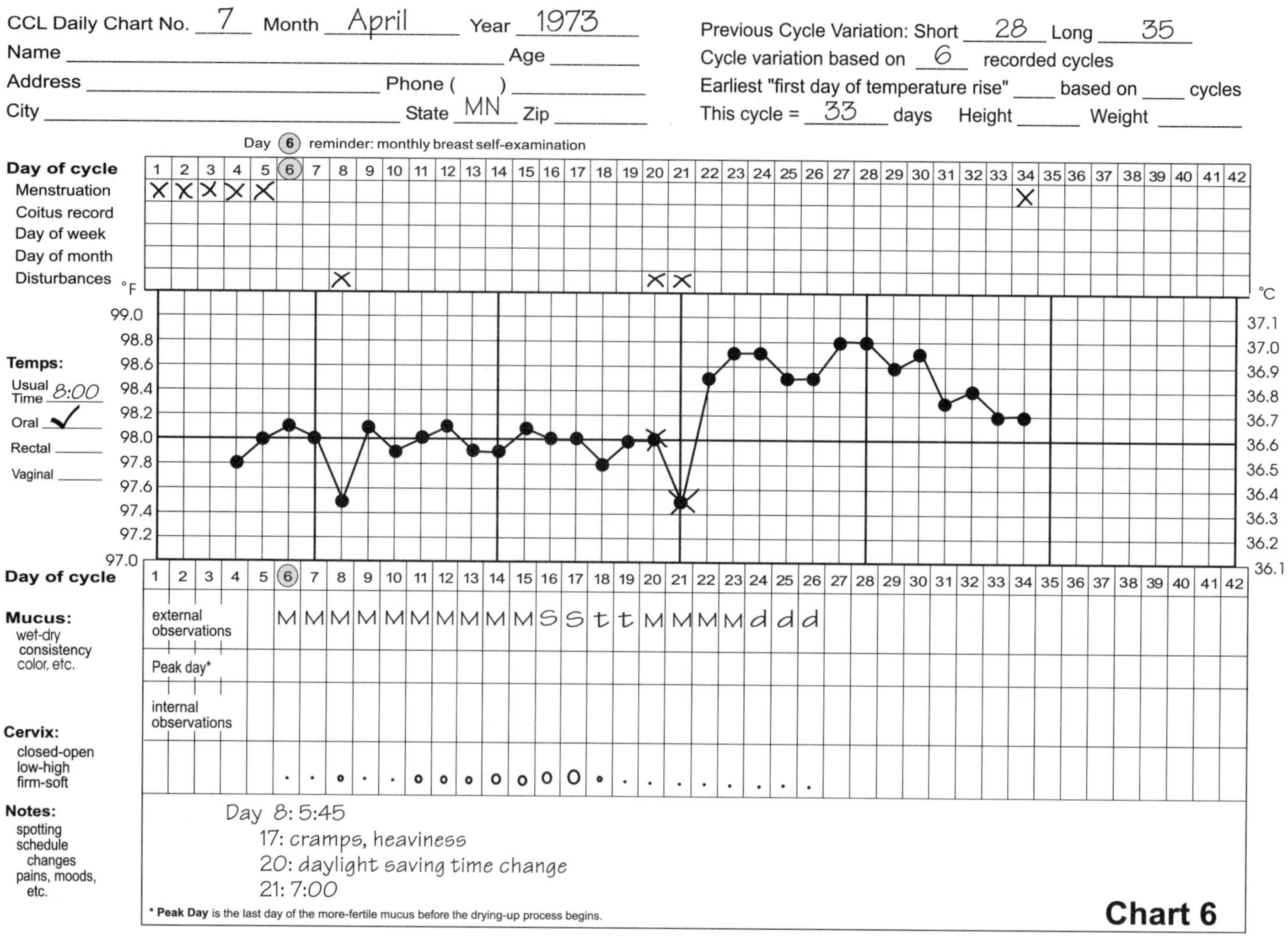

CCL Daily Chart No. __7__ Month __April__ Year __1973__

Name _____ Age _____
Address _____ Phone ( ) _____
City _____ State __MN__ Zip _____

Previous Cycle Variation: Short __28__ Long __35__
Cycle variation based on __6__ recorded cycles
Earliest "first day of temperature rise" ____ based on ____ cycles
This cycle = __33__ days   Height _____ Weight _____

Day ⑥ reminder: monthly breast self-examination

Day of cycle	1	2	3	4	5	⑥	7	8	9	10	11	12	13	14	15	16	17	18	19	20	21	22	23	24	25	26	27	28	29	30	31	32	33	34	35	36	37	38	39	40	41	42
Menstruation	X	X	X	X	X																													X								
Coitus record																																										
Day of week																																										
Day of month																																										
Disturbances								X												X	X																					

Temps:
Usual Time __8:00__
Oral ✓
Rectal ____
Vaginal ____

°F / °C temperature grid (99.0/37.1 down to 97.0/36.1)

Day of cycle	1	2	3	4	5	⑥	7	8	9	10	11	12	13	14	15	16	17	18	19	20	21	22	23	24	25	26	27	28	29	30	31	32	33	34	35	36	37	38	39	40	41	42

Mucus:
wet-dry
consistency
color, etc.

external observations: M M M M M M M M M S S t t M M M M d d d

Peak day*

internal observations

Cervix:
closed-open
low-high
firm-soft

(cervix markings): · · o · · · o o o O o O O o · · · · · · · · ·

Notes:
spotting
schedule changes
pains, moods, etc.

Day 8: 5:45
17: cramps, heaviness
20: daylight saving time change
21: 7:00

* Peak Day is the last day of the more-fertile mucus before the drying-up process begins.

Chart 6

End of Phase I:
    Clinical experience ____   21/20 day rule ____   Doering ____   Last dry day ____

Pre-shift six _____   Low Temp Level _____   High Temp Level _____

"Peak" day _____   First day of cervix closing _____

Start of Phase III: Rule ____ = _____   Rule C = _____

NOTES:

Necessity of temperature cross-check of drying-up process.

CCL Daily Chart No. __22__ Month __Oct.__ Year __1974__

Name _____ Age __34__

Address _____ Phone ( ) _____

City _____ State _____ Zip _____

Previous Cycle Variation: Short __26__ Long __30__
Cycle variation based on _last 12_ recorded cycles
Earliest "first day of temperature rise" _12_ based on _12_ cycles
This cycle = __25__ days   Height _____ Weight _____

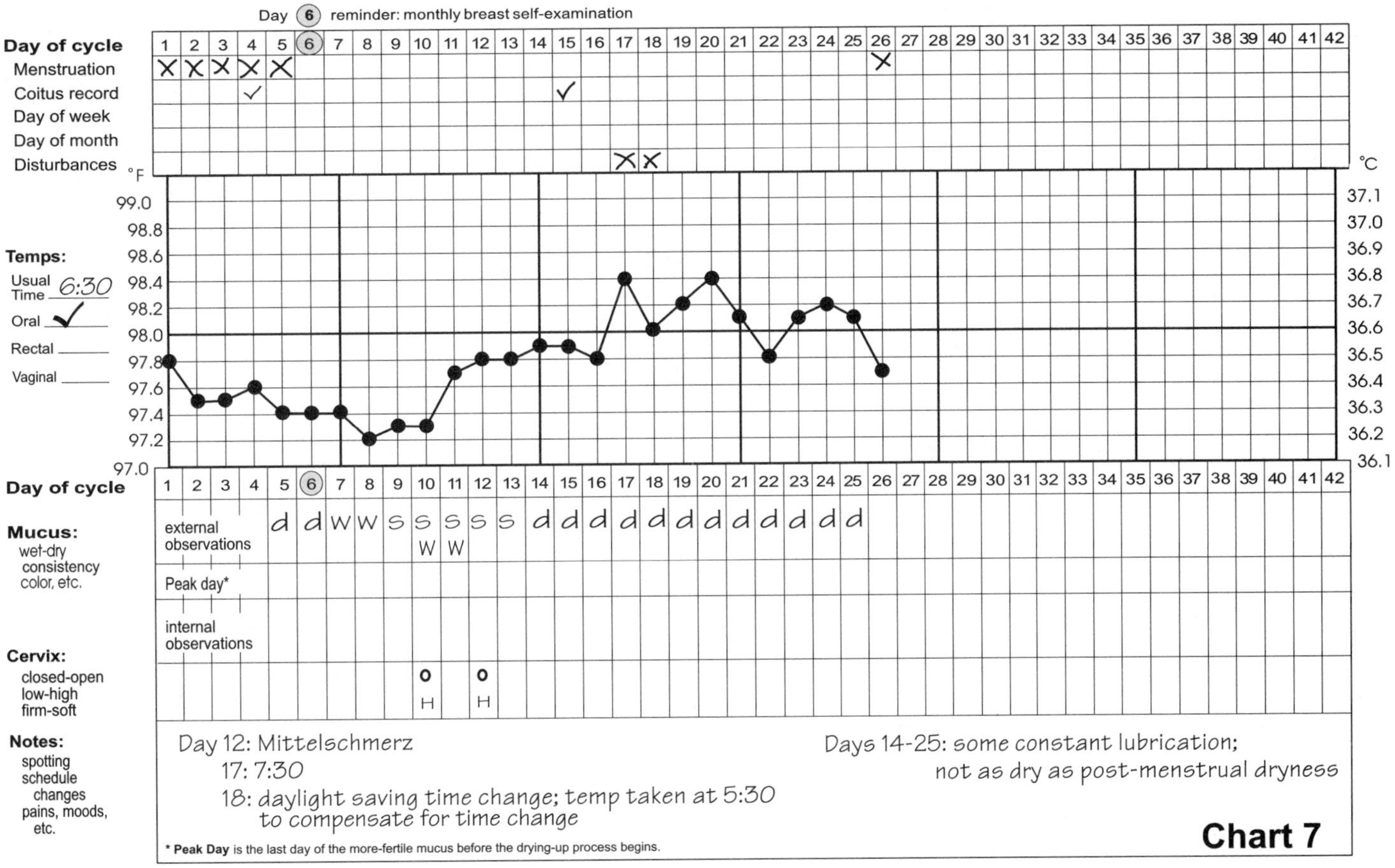

Day ⑥ reminder: monthly breast self-examination

Day of cycle	1	2	3	4	5	⑥	7	8	9	10	11	12	13	14	15	16	17	18	19	20	21	22	23	24	25	26	27	28	29	30	31	32	33	34	35	36	37	38	39	40	41	42
Menstruation	X	X	X	X	X																					X																
Coitus record				✓											✓																											
Day of week																																										
Day of month																																										
Disturbances																X	X																									

Temps:
Usual Time __6:30__
Oral ✓
Rectal _____
Vaginal _____

Day 12: Mittelschmerz
   17: 7:30
   18: daylight saving time change; temp taken at 5:30
      to compensate for time change

Days 14-25: some constant lubrication;
   not as dry as post-menstrual dryness

Chart 7

Mucus: wet-dry consistency color, etc.

Day of cycle	1	2	3	4	5	⑥	7	8	9	10	11	12	13	14	15	16	17	18	19	20	21	22	23	24	25	26
external observations		d	d	W	W	S	S	S	S	S	S		d	d	d	d	d	d	d	d	d	d	d			
(W row)							W	W																		

Peak day*

internal observations

Cervix: closed-open low-high firm-soft

	1	2	3	4	5	⑥	7	8	9	10	11	12
										O	O	
										H	H	

Notes: spotting schedule changes pains, moods, etc.

* **Peak Day** is the last day of the more-fertile mucus before the drying-up process begins.

End of Phase I:

    Clinical experience _____   21/20 day rule _____   Doering _____   Last dry day _____

Pre-shift six _____   Low Temp Level _____   High Temp Level _____

"Peak" day _____   First day of cervix closing _____

Start of Phase III: Rule _____ = _____   Rule C = _____

NOTES:

    Necessity of mucus cross-check of thermal shift.
    For more on daylight saving time changes, see Chapter 5.

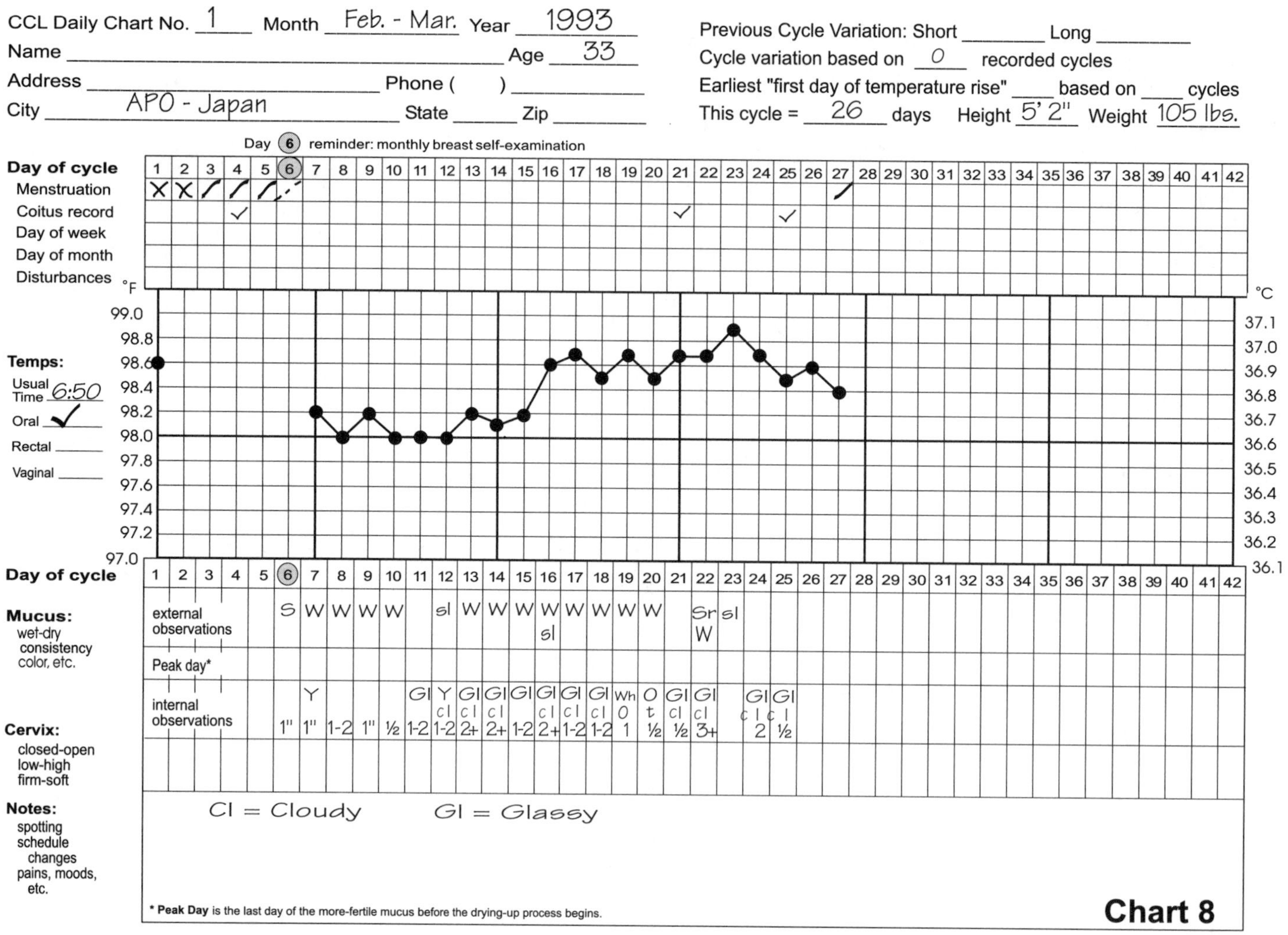

CCL Daily Chart No. __1__ Month __Feb. - Mar.__ Year __1993__

Name _____ Age __33__

Address _____ Phone ( ) _____

City _____APO - Japan_____ State _____ Zip _____

Previous Cycle Variation: Short _____ Long _____
Cycle variation based on __0__ recorded cycles
Earliest "first day of temperature rise" ____ based on ____ cycles
This cycle = __26__ days   Height __5' 2"__   Weight __105 lbs.__

Day ⑥ reminder: monthly breast self-examination

Day of cycle	1	2	3	4	5	⑥	7	8	9	10	11	12	13	14	15	16	17	18	19	20	21	22	23	24	25	26	27	28	29	30	31	32	33	34	35	36	37	38	39	40	41	42
Menstruation	X	X	/	/	/	:																					/															
Coitus record				✓																	✓				✓																	
Day of week																																										
Day of month																																										
Disturbances																																										

Temps:
Usual Time __6:50__
Oral __✓__
Rectal _____
Vaginal _____

°F
99.0   37.1
98.8   37.0
98.6   36.9
98.4   36.8
98.2   36.7
98.0   36.6
97.8   36.5
97.6   36.4
97.4   36.3
97.2   36.2
97.0   36.1
°C

Day of cycle	1	2	3	4	5	⑥	7	8	9	10	11	12	13	14	15	16	17	18	19	20	21	22	23	24	25	26	27	28	29	30	31	32	33	34	35	36	37	38	39	40	41	42

Mucus:
wet-dry
consistency
color, etc.

external observations: S W W W W _ sl W W W W W W W W _ Sr sl
(row 2 under day 13: sl) (day 21: W)

Peak day*

internal observations:
Y Gl Y Gl Gl Gl Gl Gl Gl Wh O Gl Gl   Gl Gl
   cl cl cl   cl cl cl t cl cl   cl cl
1" 1" 1-2 1" ½ 1-2 1-2 2+ 2+ 1-2 2+ 1-2 1-2 1 ½ ½ 3+   2 ½

Cervix:
closed-open
low-high
firm-soft

Notes:
spotting
schedule
changes
pains, moods,
etc.

Cl = Cloudy   Gl = Glassy

* Peak Day is the last day of the more-fertile mucus before the drying-up process begins.

Chart 8

End of Phase I:
    Clinical experience _____ 21/20 day rule _____ Doering _____ Last dry day _____

Pre-shift six _____   Low Temp Level _____ High Temp Level _____

"Peak" day _____   First day of cervix closing _____

Start of Phase III: Rule ____ = _____   Rule C = _____

NOTES:

    Shaving irregular temperatures; see Chapter 6 and Chart 22.
    Temperature-only rule; see Chapter 26.

CCL Daily Chart No. _17_ Month ____April____ Year __1975__

Name _____ Age __34__

Address _____ Phone ( ) _____

City _____ State _____ Zip _____

Previous Cycle Variation: Short __26__ Long __34__

Cycle variation based on __16__ recorded cycles

Earliest "first day of temperature rise" ____ based on ____ cycles

This cycle = __42__ days   Height _____ Weight _____

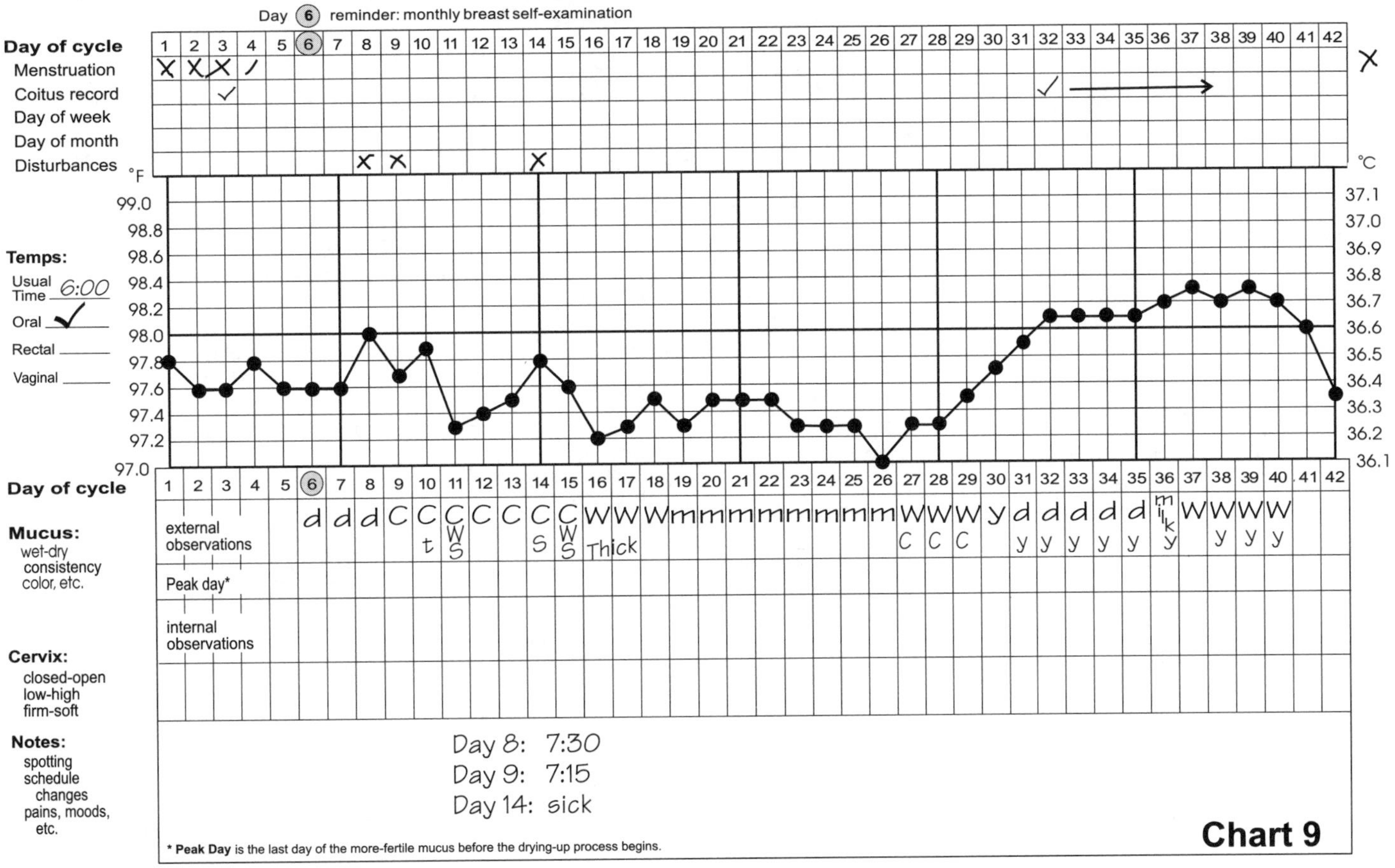

Day of cycle	1	2	3	4	5	⑥	7	8	9	10	11	12	13	14	15	16	17	18	19	20	21	22	23	24	25	26	27	28	29	30	31	32	33	34	35	36	37	38	39	40	41	42	X
Menstruation	X	X	X	/																																							
Coitus record			✓																													✓	→										
Day of week																																											
Day of month																																											
Disturbances									x	x				x																													

Temps:
Usual Time _6:00_
Oral ✓
Rectal ____
Vaginal ____

°F: 99.0 98.8 98.6 98.4 98.2 98.0 97.8 97.6 97.4 97.2 97.0

°C: 37.1 37.0 36.9 36.8 36.7 36.6 36.5 36.4 36.3 36.2 36.1

Day of cycle	1	2	3	4	5	⑥	7	8	9	10	11	12	13	14	15	16	17	18	19	20	21	22	23	24	25	26	27	28	29	30	31	32	33	34	35	36	37	38	39	40	41	42

Mucus:
wet-dry
consistency
color, etc.

external observations: d d d C C C C C C C W W W m m m m m m m m m W W W y d d d d d m:ilk W W W W
(with: t, W S, S, W S, Thick, C C C, y y y y y y y:y, y y y)

Peak day*

internal observations

Cervix:
closed-open
low-high
firm-soft

Notes:
spotting
schedule
changes
pains, moods,
etc.

Day 8: 7:30
Day 9: 7:15
Day 14: sick

* **Peak Day** is the last day of the more-fertile mucus before the drying-up process begins.

Chart 9

End of Phase I:

Clinical experience _____ 21/20 day rule _____ Doering _____ Last dry day _____

Pre-shift six _____ Low Temp Level _____ High Temp Level _____

"Peak" day _____   First day of cervix closing _____

Start of Phase III: Rule ____ = _____   Rule C = _____

NOTES:

"Double peak" mucus pattern. See Charts 17, 21 and Chapter 27.

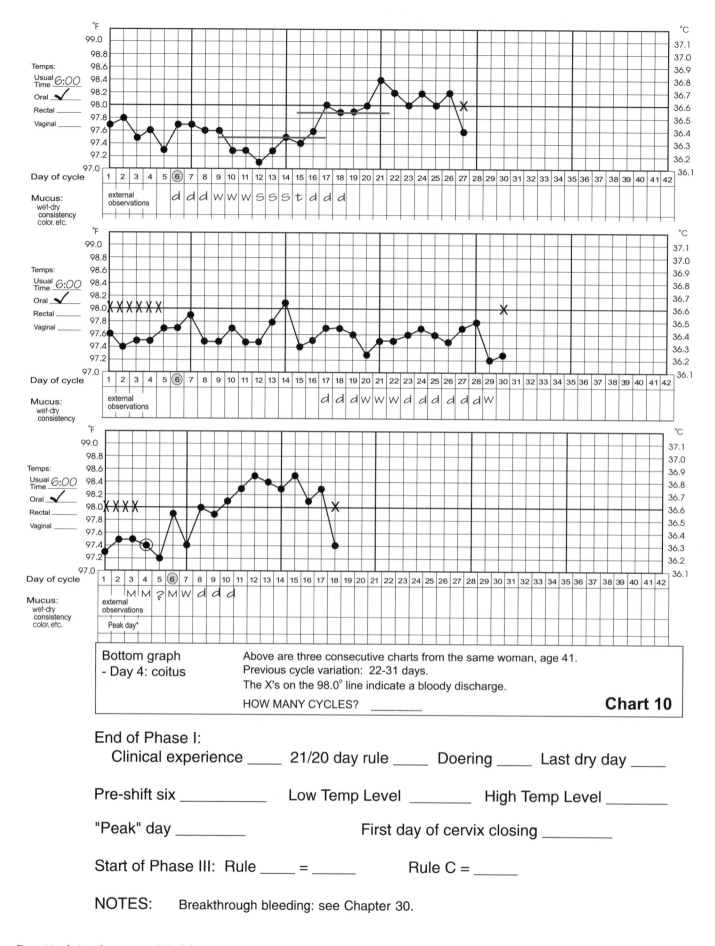

**Bottom graph
- Day 4: coitus**

Above are three consecutive charts from the same woman, age 41.
Previous cycle variation: 22-31 days.
The X's on the 98.0° line indicate a bloody discharge.

HOW MANY CYCLES? _____

Chart 10

End of Phase I:

    Clinical experience _____ 21/20 day rule _____ Doering _____ Last dry day _____

Pre-shift six _____ Low Temp Level _____ High Temp Level _____

"Peak" day _____ First day of cervix closing _____

Start of Phase III: Rule _____ = _____ Rule C = _____

NOTES: Breakthrough bleeding: see Chapter 30.

CCL Daily Chart No. __25__ Month __July-Aug.__ Year __1994__

Name _____ Age __36__

Address _____ Phone ( ) _____

City _____ State __IN__ Zip _____

Previous Cycle Variation: Short __23__ Long __30__

Cycle variation based on __24__ recorded cycles

Earliest "first day of temperature rise" ____ based on ____ cycles

This cycle = __24__ days   Height __5' 3½"__ Weight __126 lbs.__

Day ⑥ reminder: monthly breast self-examination

Day of cycle	1	2	3	4	5	6	7	8	9	10	11	12	13	14	15	16	17	18	19	20	21	22	23	24	25	26	27	28	29	30	31	32	33	34	35	36	37	38	39	40	41	42
Menstruation	X	X	X	X	X																				X																	
Coitus record																	✓					✓																				
Day of week	S	S						S	S					S	S							S	S																			
Day of month	23		25							31	1				5					10					15																	
Disturbances																																										

Day of cycle	1	2	3	4	5	6	7	8	9	10	11	12	13	14	15	16	17	18	19	20	21	22	23	24	25	26	27	28	29	30	31	32	33	34	35	36	37	38	39	40	41	42

Temps:
Usual Time _____
Oral _____
Rectal _____
Vaginal _____

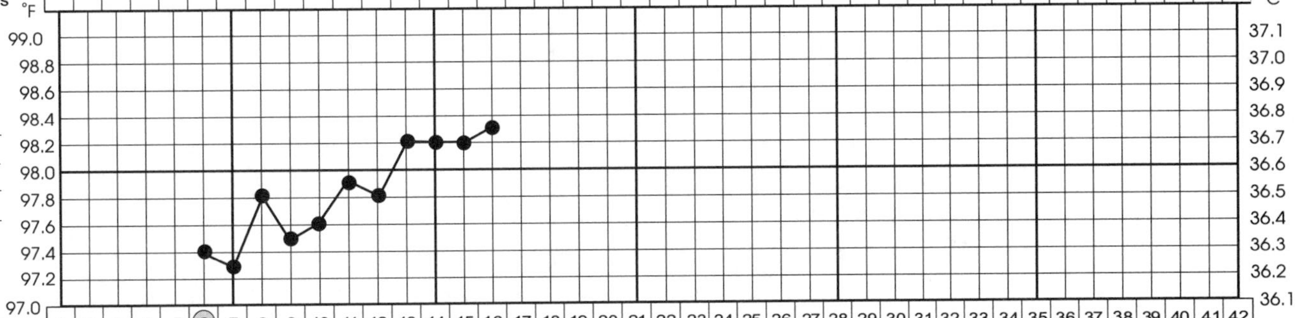

Mucus: wet-dry consistency color, etc.

external observations: d t W sl S d w t t t t t t

Peak day*

internal observations

Cervix: closed-open low-high firm-soft

Notes: spotting schedule changes pains, moods, etc.

* **Peak Day** is the last day of the more-fertile mucus before the drying-up process begins.

Chart 11

End of Phase I:

Clinical experience _____   21/20 day rule _____   Doering _____   Last dry day _____

Pre-shift six _____   Low Temp Level _____   High Temp Level _____

"Peak" day _____   First day of cervix closing _____

Start of Phase III: Rule ____ = _____   Rule C = _____

NOTES:

Shaving with Rule K.
See Chapters 6 and 12.

CCL Daily Chart No. __7__ Month ____July____ Year __1973__

Name _____ Age _____

Address _____ Phone ( ) _____

City _____ State _____ Zip _____

Previous Cycle Variation: Short __28__ Long __40__

Cycle variation based on __6__ recorded cycles

Earliest "first day of temperature rise" ____ based on ____ cycles

This cycle = __29__ days Height _____ Weight _____

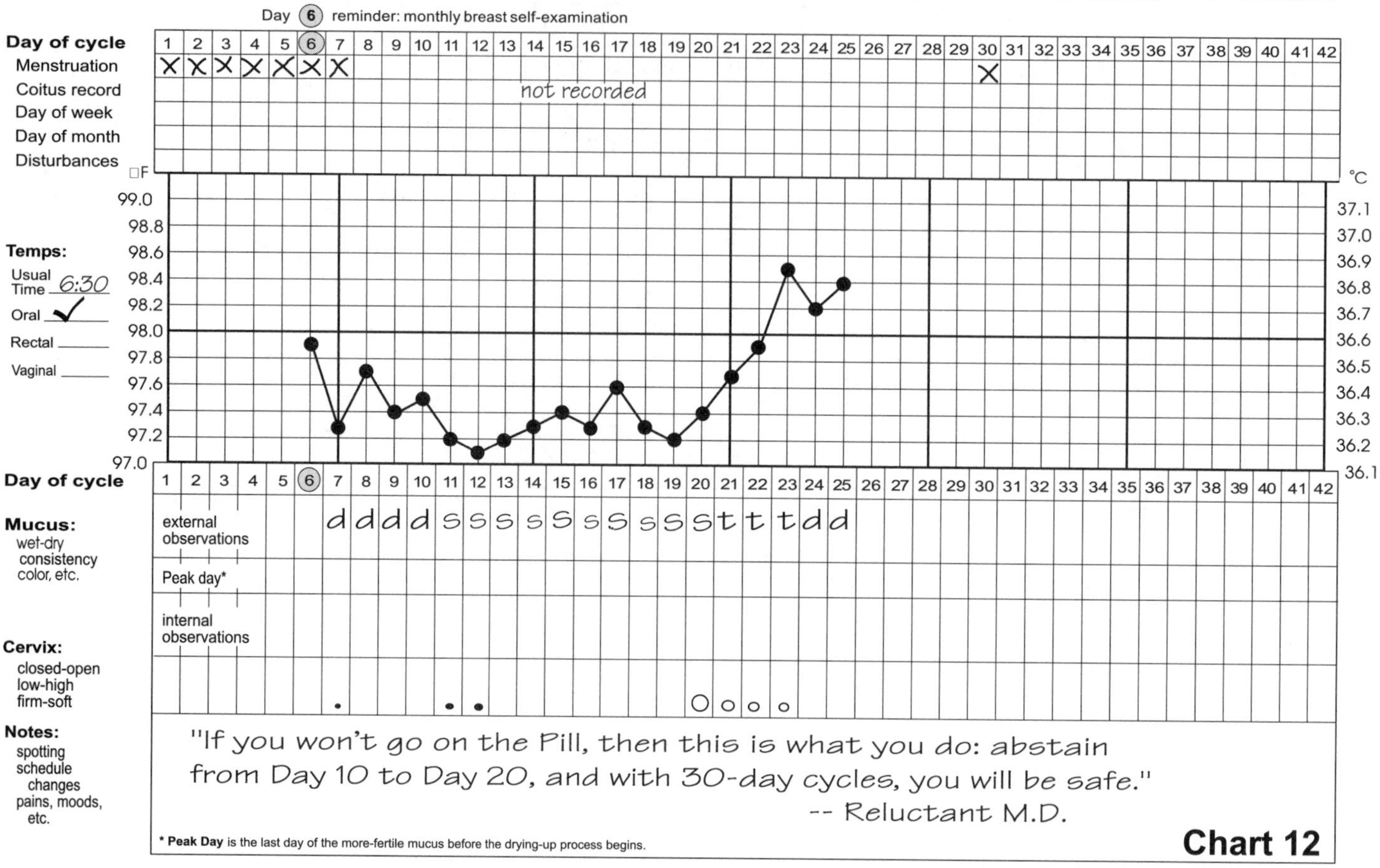

Day ⑥ reminder: monthly breast self-examination

Day of cycle 1–42

Menstruation: X X X X X X X (days 1–7), X (day 30)

Coitus record: *not recorded*

Day of week

Day of month

Disturbances

Temps:
Usual Time __6:30__
Oral ✓
Rectal ____
Vaginal ____

Mucus: wet-dry consistency color, etc.

external observations: d d d d s s s s s S s s s S s S t t t d d

Peak day*

internal observations

Cervix: closed-open, low-high, firm-soft

Notes: spotting, schedule changes, pains, moods, etc.

"If you won't go on the Pill, then this is what you do: abstain from Day 10 to Day 20, and with 30-day cycles, you will be safe."
-- Reluctant M.D.

* **Peak Day** is the last day of the more-fertile mucus before the drying-up process begins.

Chart 12

End of Phase I:

Clinical experience ____   21/20 day rule ____   Doering ____   Last dry day ____

Pre-shift six _____   Low Temp Level _____   High Temp Level _____

"Peak" day _____   First day of cervix closing _____

Start of Phase III: Rule ____ = _____   Rule C = _____

Length of luteal phase (by temps) in this cycle _____

NOTES:

A true short luteal phase cycle; nutrition check needed.
Alternative interpretation: shaving with Rule R.

Shaved LTL _____   Rule R = ____   Rule C = _____

Do you agree with the M.D.? _____

Why or why not? _____

CCL Daily Chart No. __2__   Month __Sept.__   Year __1974__

Name _____ Age __24__

Address _____ Phone ( ) _____

City _____ State __MN__ Zip _____

Previous Cycle Variation: Short __27__ Long __30__

Cycle variation based on memory* recorded cycles

Earliest "first day of temperature rise" ____ based on ____ cycles

This cycle = __21__ days   Height _____ Weight _____

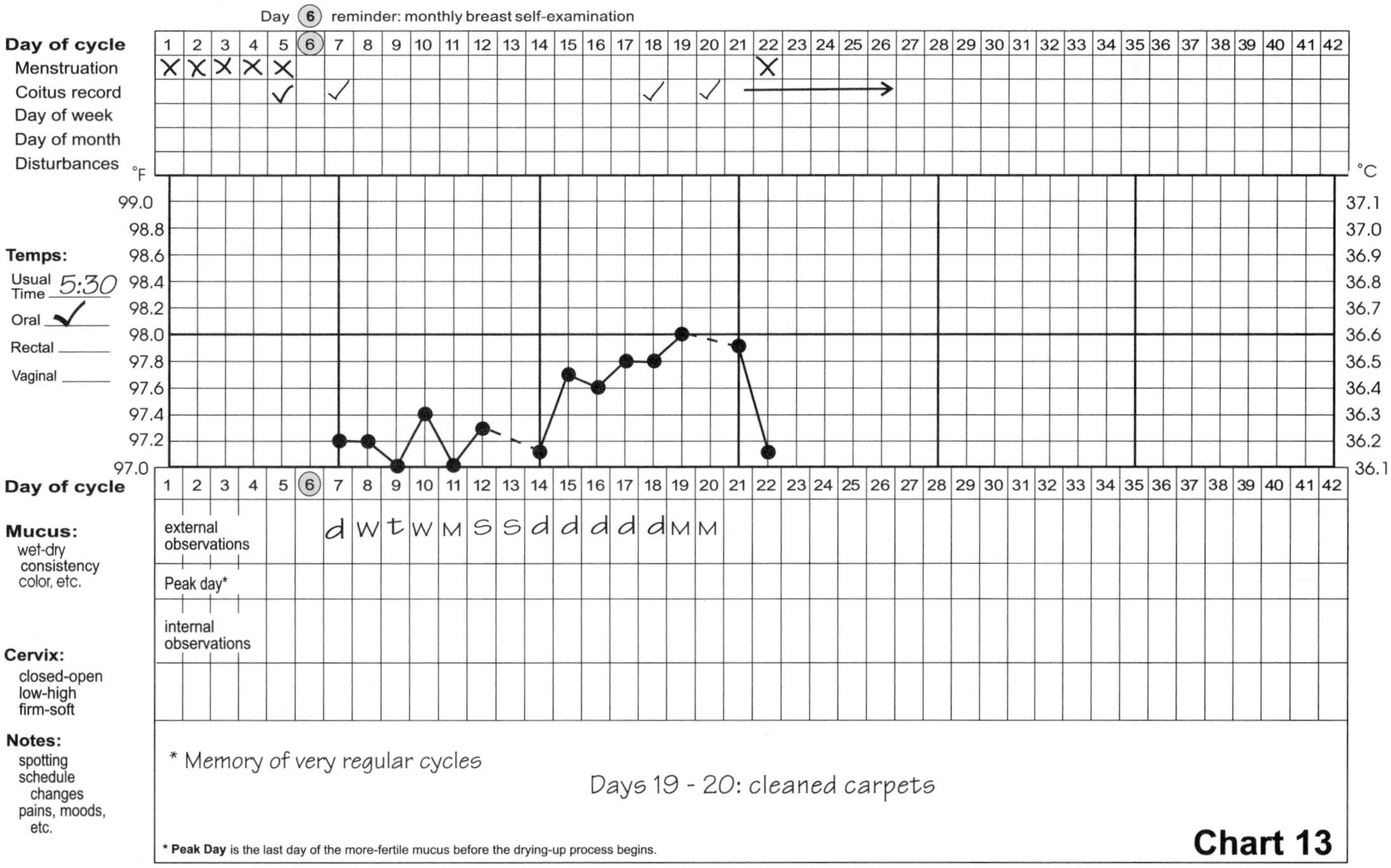

Day ⑥ reminder: monthly breast self-examination

Day of cycle	1	2	3	4	5	⑥	7	8	9	10	11	12	13	14	15	16	17	18	19	20	21	22	23	24	25	26	27	28	29	30	31	32	33	34	35	36	37	38	39	40	41	42
Menstruation	X	X	X	X	X																	X																				
Coitus record						✓		✓									✓		✓	→→→																						
Day of week																																										
Day of month																																										
Disturbances																																										

Temps:

Usual Time _5:30_

Oral _✓_

Rectal ____

Vaginal ____

Day of cycle 1 2 3 4 5 ⑥ 7 8 9 10 11 12 13 14 15 16 17 18 19 20 21 22 23 24 25 26 27 28 29 30 31 32 33 34 35 36 37 38 39 40 41 42

°F temperatures: 99.0 / 98.8 / 98.6 / 98.4 / 98.2 / 98.0 / 97.8 / 97.6 / 97.4 / 97.2 / 97.0
°C: 37.1 / 37.0 / 36.9 / 36.8 / 36.7 / 36.6 / 36.5 / 36.4 / 36.3 / 36.2 / 36.1

Mucus:
wet-dry
consistency
color, etc.

external observations: d w t w M S S d d d d d M M

Peak day*

internal observations

Cervix:
closed-open
low-high
firm-soft

Notes:
spotting
schedule
changes
pains, moods,
etc.

* Memory of very regular cycles

Days 19 - 20: cleaned carpets

Chart 13

* **Peak Day** is the last day of the more-fertile mucus before the drying-up process begins.

End of Phase I:

Clinical experience _____   21/20 day rule _____   Doering _____   Last dry day _____

Pre-shift six _____   Low Temp Level _____   High Temp Level _____

"Peak" day _____   First day of cervix closing _____

Start of Phase III: Rule ____ = _____   Rule C = _____

NOTES:

An artificially shortened luteal phase.

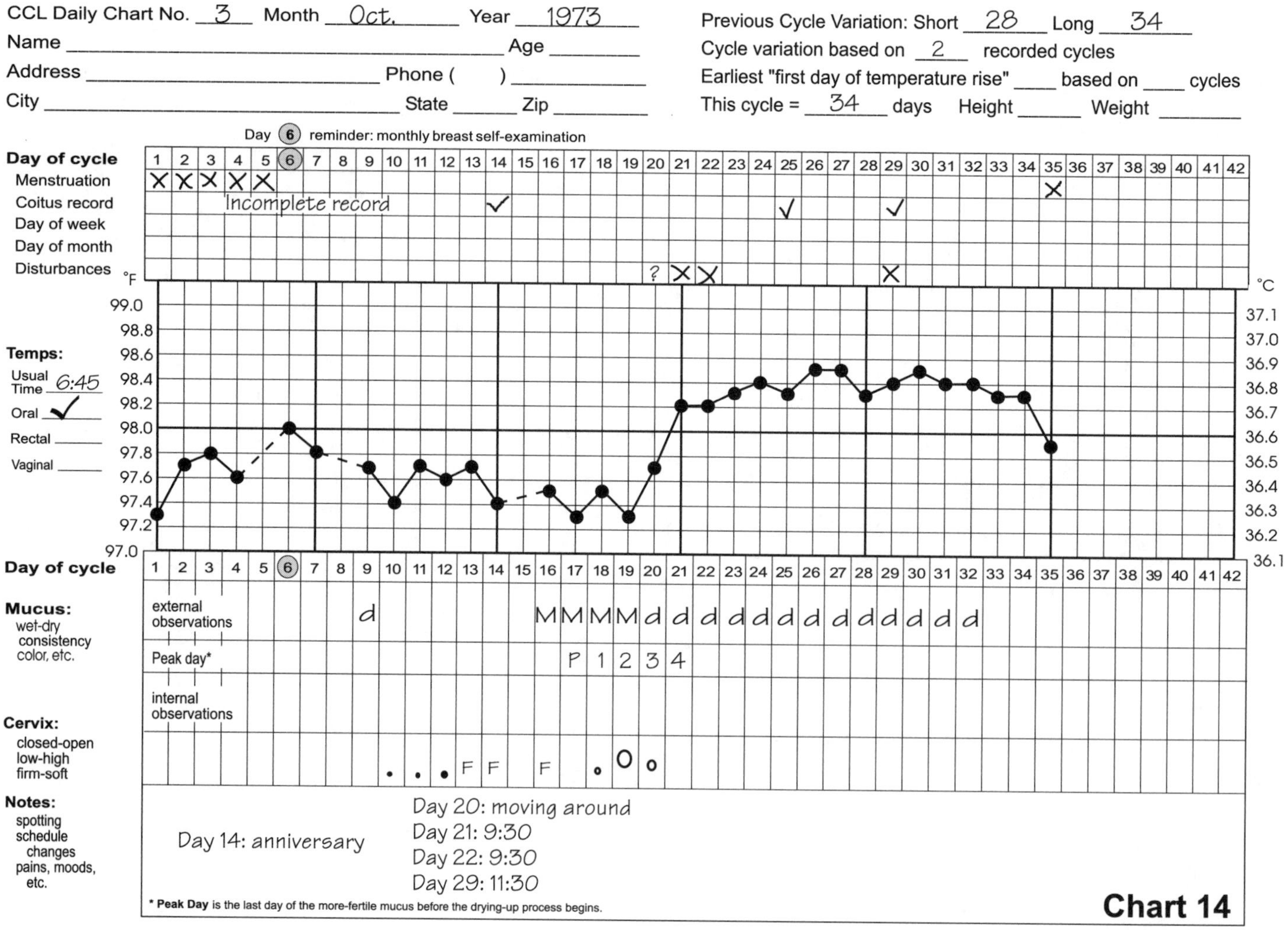

CCL Daily Chart No. __3__ Month __Oct.__ Year __1973__

Name _____ Age _____

Address _____ Phone ( ) _____

City _____ State _____ Zip _____

Previous Cycle Variation: Short __28__ Long __34__

Cycle variation based on __2__ recorded cycles

Earliest "first day of temperature rise" ____ based on ____ cycles

This cycle = __34__ days   Height _____ Weight _____

Day ⑥ reminder: monthly breast self-examination

Day of cycle	1	2	3	4	5	⑥	7	8	9	10	11	12	13	14	15	16	17	18	19	20	21	22	23	24	25	26	27	28	29	30	31	32	33	34	35	36	37	38	39	40	41	42
Menstruation	X	X	X	X	X																														X							
Coitus record				Incomplete record										✓							✓				✓																
Day of week																																										
Day of month																																										
Disturbances														?	X	X												X														

Temps:
Usual Time __6:45__
Oral ✓
Rectal _____
Vaginal _____

Mucus:
wet-dry
consistency
color, etc.

Cervix:
closed-open
low-high
firm-soft

Notes:
spotting
schedule
changes
pains, moods,
etc.

Day of cycle	1	2	3	4	5	⑥	7	8	9	10	11	12	13	14	15	16	17	18	19	20	21	22	23	24	25	26	27	28	29	30	31	32	33	34	35	36	37	38	39	40	41	42
external observations									d						M	M	M	M	d	d	d	d	d	d	d	d	d	d	d	d												
Peak day*																	P	1	2	3	4																					
internal observations																																										
								•	•	•	•	F	F		F			•	O	o																						

Day 14: anniversary

Day 20: moving around
Day 21: 9:30
Day 22: 9:30
Day 29: 11:30

* Peak Day is the last day of the more-fertile mucus before the drying-up process begins.

Chart 14

End of Phase I:

    Clinical experience ____ 21/20 day rule ____ Doering ____ Last dry day ____

Pre-shift six _____   Low Temp Level _____   High Temp Level _____

"Peak" day _____   First day of cervix closing _____

Start of Phase III: Rule ____ = _____   Rule C = _____

NOTES:

    Necessity for valid Peak day and accurate Phase II temperatures.

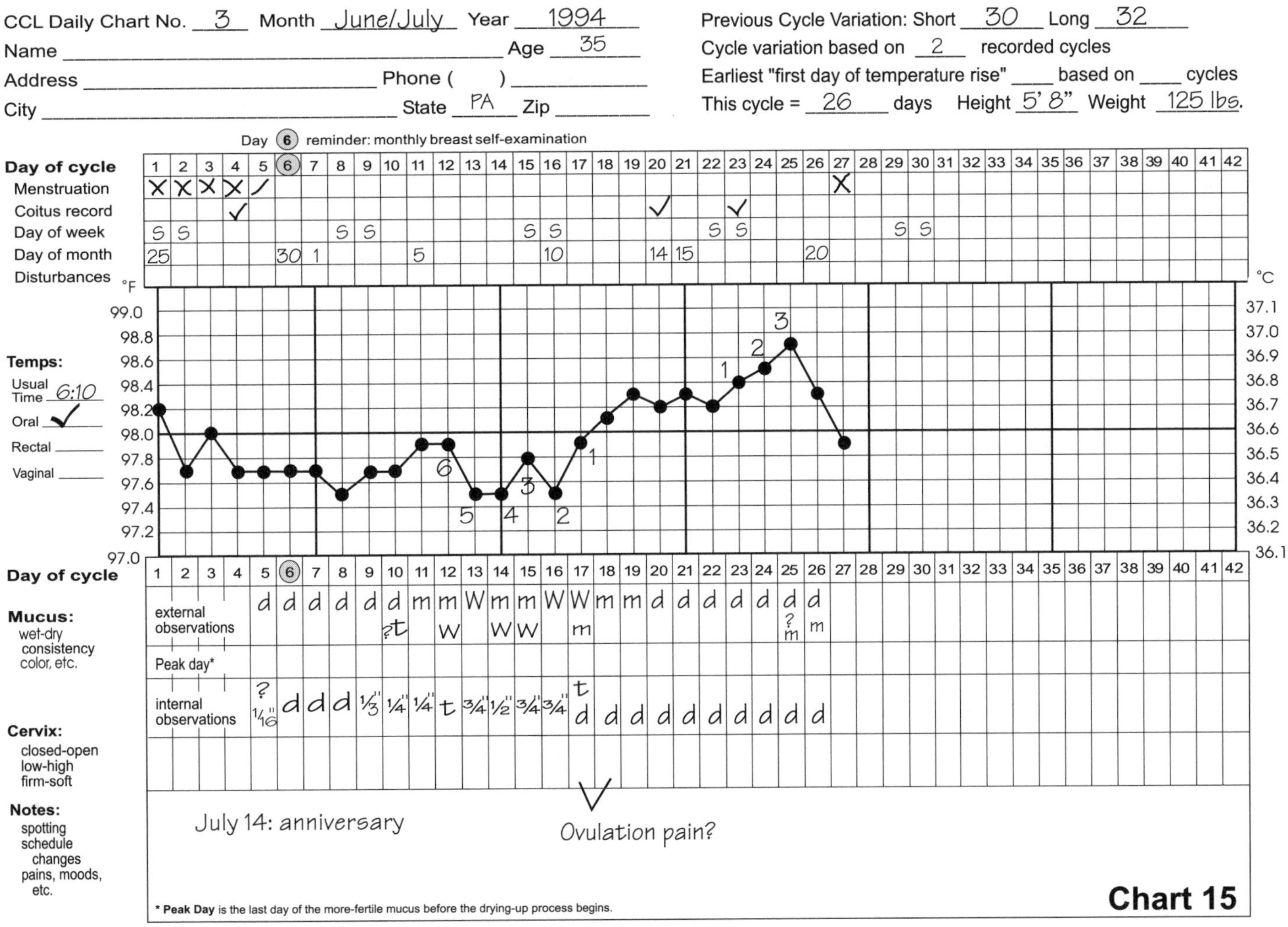

CCL Daily Chart No. __3__ Month _June/July_ Year __1994__

Name _____ Age __35__

Address _____ Phone ( ) _____

City _____ State _PA_ Zip _____

Previous Cycle Variation: Short __30__ Long __32__

Cycle variation based on __2__ recorded cycles

Earliest "first day of temperature rise" ____ based on ____ cycles

This cycle = __26__ days   Height _5' 8"_ Weight _125 lbs._

Day ⑥ reminder: monthly breast self-examination

Day of cycle	1	2	3	4	5	⑥	7	8	9	10	11	12	13	14	15	16	17	18	19	20	21	22	23	24	25	26	27	28	29	30	31	32	33	34	35	36	37	38	39	40	41	42
Menstruation	X	X	X	X	/																						X															
Coitus record					✓															✓			✓																			
Day of week	S	S						S	S					S	S							S	S						S	S												
Day of month	25						30	1				5					10			14	15					20																
Disturbances																																										

Temps:
Usual Time _6:10_
Oral ✓
Rectal _____
Vaginal _____

(Temperature chart °F / °C with plotted points; mucus notations "6", "5", "4", "2", "3", "1" marked along the low temperatures. Peak-related numbers "1", "2", "3" marked along the rising temperatures.)

Day of cycle	1	2	3	4	5	⑥	7	8	9	10	11	12	13	14	15	16	17	18	19	20	21	22	23	24	25	26	27	28	29	30	31	32	33	34	35	36	37	38	39	40	41	42

Mucus:
wet-dry
consistency
color, etc.

external observations: d d d d d d m m W m m W W m m d d d d d d d d
(with: ?t under 10; W under 12; W W under 14-15; m under 16; ?m under 26)

Peak day*

internal observations: ? 1/16 d d d 1/3 1/4 1/4 t 3/4 1/2 3/4 3/4 t d d d d d d d d d d

Cervix:
closed-open
low-high
firm-soft

Notes:
spotting
schedule
changes
pains, moods,
etc.

July 14: anniversary   Ovulation pain?

* **Peak Day** is the last day of the more-fertile mucus before the drying-up process begins.

Chart 15

End of Phase I:
   Clinical experience ____ 21/20 day rule ____ Doering ____ Last dry day ____

Pre-shift six _____   Low Temp Level _____   High Temp Level _____

"Peak" day _____   First day of cervix closing _____

Start of Phase III: Rule ____ = _____   Rule C = _____

NOTES:

   Averaging the pre-shift six.
   Nutrition check: double-check exercise and nutrition habits.

CCL Daily Chart No. __23__ Month __Mar.-Apr.__ Year __1992__

Name _____ Age __26__

Address _____ Phone ( ) _____

City _____ State __TX__ Zip _____

Previous Cycle Variation: Short __26__ Long __51__

Cycle variation based on __22__ recorded cycles

Earliest "first day of temperature rise" ____ based on ____ cycles

This cycle = __32__ days   Height __5' 6"__   Weight __ha ha, nice try!__

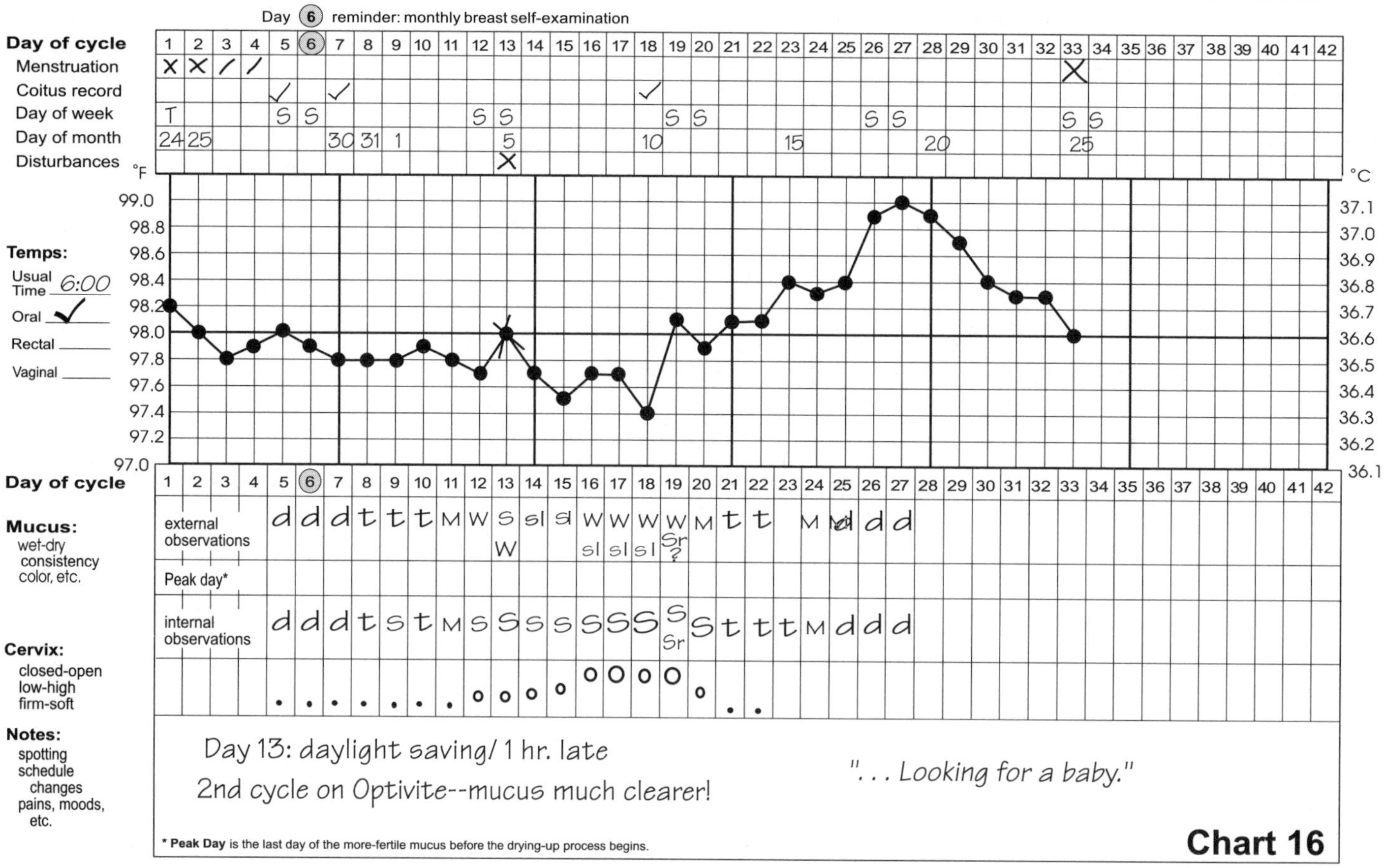

Day ⑥ reminder: monthly breast self-examination

Day of cycle	1	2	3	4	5	6	7	8	9	10	11	12	13	14	15	16	17	18	19	20	21	22	23	24	25	26	27	28	29	30	31	32	33	34	35	36	37	38	39	40	41	42
Menstruation	X	X	/	/																													X									
Coitus record					✓		✓											✓																								
Day of week	T				S	S						S	S					S	S					S	S							S	S									
Day of month	24	25						30	31	1			5					10					15					20					25									
Disturbances													X																													

Temps:
Usual Time __6:00__
Oral ✓
Rectal ____
Vaginal ____

Day of cycle	1	2	3	4	5	6	7	8	9	10	11	12	13	14	15	16	17	18	19	20	21	22	23	24	25	26	27	28	29	30	31	32	33	34	35	36	37	38	39	40	41	42

Mucus:
wet-dry
consistency
color, etc.

external observations: d d d t t t M W S sl sl W W W W M t t M d d d
(W below day 13; sl below 15,16,17; Sr? below 19)

Peak day*

Cervix:
closed-open
low-high
firm-soft

internal observations: d d d t s t M S S S s S S S S/Sr S t t t M d d d

(cervix dots: • • • • • • • o o o o o o o o o • •)

Notes:
spotting
schedule
changes
pains, moods,
etc.

Day 13: daylight saving/ 1 hr. late

2nd cycle on Optivite--mucus much clearer!

"... Looking for a baby."

Chart 16

* Peak Day is the last day of the more-fertile mucus before the drying-up process begins.

End of Phase I:

  Clinical experience ____   21/20 day rule ____   Doering ____   Last dry day ____

Pre-shift six _____   Low Temp Level _____   High Temp Level _____

"Peak" day _____   First day of cervix closing _____

Start of Phase III: Rule ____ = _____   Rule C = _____

NOTES:

  Can Phase III start on Day 22? See analysis for this chart.

CCL Daily Chart No. __14__ Month ___March___ Year ___1978___

Name _____ Age __24__

Address _____ Phone ( ) _____

City _____ State _____ Zip _____

Previous Cycle Variation: Short __30__ Long __52__

Cycle variation based on __13__ recorded cycles

Earliest "first day of temperature rise" ____ based on ____ cycles

This cycle = __38__ days Height _____ Weight _____

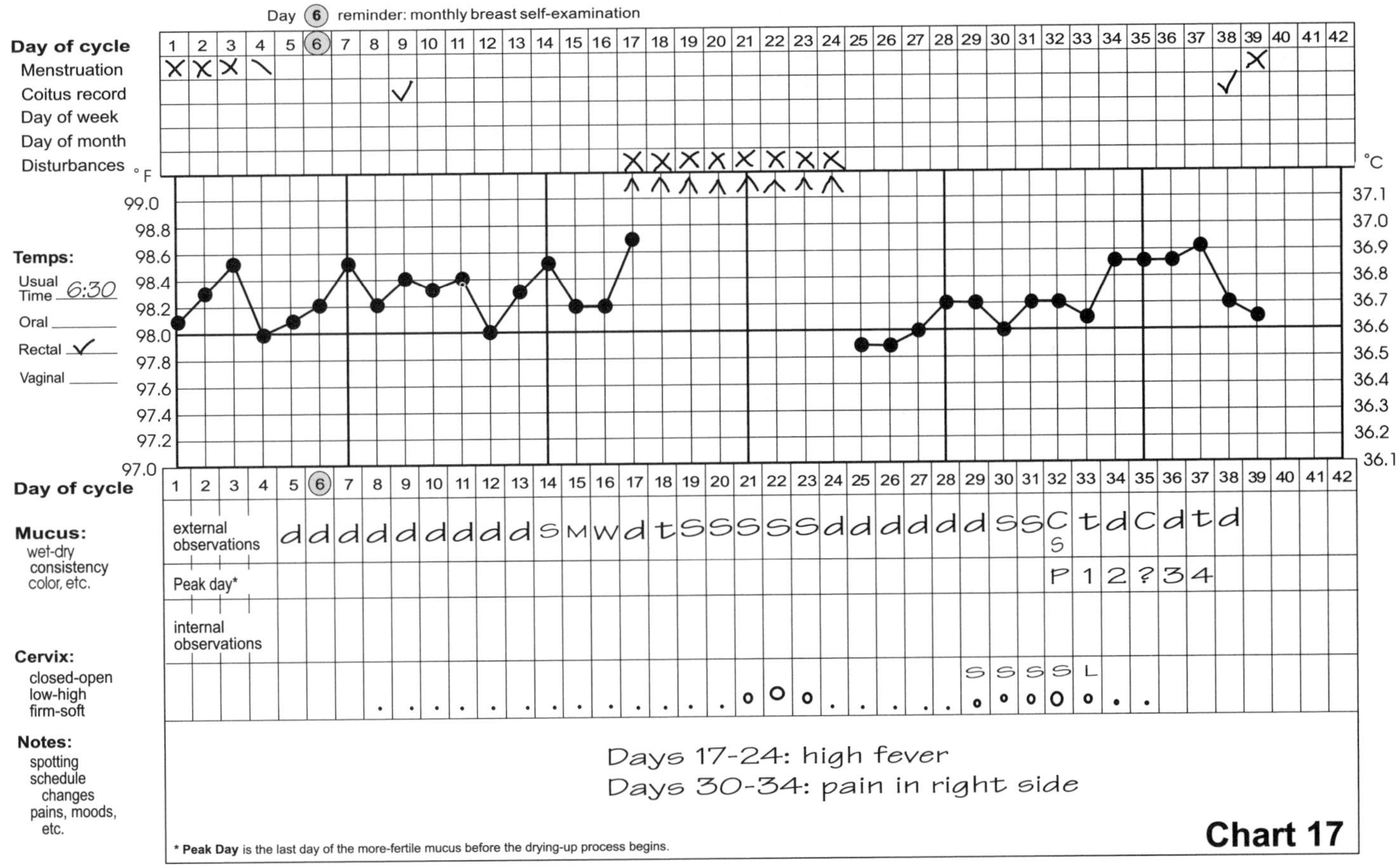

Day ⑥ reminder: monthly breast self-examination

Day of cycle	1	2	3	4	5	⑥	7	8	9	10	11	12	13	14	15	16	17	18	19	20	21	22	23	24	25	26	27	28	29	30	31	32	33	34	35	36	37	38	39	40	41	42
Menstruation	X	X	X	＼																																			X			
Coitus record									✓																													✓				
Day of week																																										
Day of month																																										
Disturbances																	X	X	X	X	X	X	X	X																		

Days 17-24: high fever
Days 30-34: pain in right side

Temps:
Usual Time __6:30__
Oral _____
Rectal ✓
Vaginal _____

°F: 99.0 / 98.8 / 98.6 / 98.4 / 98.2 / 98.0 / 97.8 / 97.6 / 97.4 / 97.2 / 97.0

°C: 37.1 / 37.0 / 36.9 / 36.8 / 36.7 / 36.6 / 36.5 / 36.4 / 36.3 / 36.2 / 36.1

Day of cycle	1	2	3	4	5	⑥	7	8	9	10	11	12	13	14	15	16	17	18	19	20	21	22	23	24	25	26	27	28	29	30	31	32	33	34	35	36	37	38	39	40	41	42
Mucus: external observations	d	d	d	d	d	d	d	d	d	d	s	M	W	d	t	S	S	S	S	S	S	d	d	d	d	d	d	d	S	S	C s	t	d	C	d	t	d					
Peak day*																																P	1	2	?	3	4					
internal observations																																										

Cervix:
closed-open
low-high
firm-soft

| | | | | | | | | | | | | | | | | | | | | | | o | O | o | | | | | | S | S | S | S | L | | | | | | | | |
| | | | | . | . | . | . | . | . | . | . | . | . | . | . | . | . | . | . | . | o | O | o | . | . | . | . | . | o | o | o | O | o | . | . | | | | | | |

Notes:
spotting
schedule
changes
pains, moods,
etc.

* Peak Day is the last day of the more-fertile mucus before the drying-up process begins.

Chart 17

End of Phase I:

Clinical experience ____ 21/20 day rule ____ Doering ____ Last dry day ____

Pre-shift six _____ Low Temp Level _____ High Temp Level _____

"Peak" day _____ First day of cervix closing _____

Start of Phase III: Rule ____ = _____ Rule C = _____

NOTES:

The split dry-up; sickness and delayed ovulation;
see Chapter 27, Figures 27.1 and 27.3.

CCL Daily Chart No. __9__ Month _____Feb._____ Year __1973___

Name _____ Age _____

Address _____ Phone ( ) _____

City _____ State _____ Zip _____

Previous Cycle Variation: Short __31__ Long __37__

Cycle variation based on __8__ recorded cycles

Earliest "first day of temperature rise" ____ based on ____ cycles

This cycle = __27__ days   Height _____ Weight _____

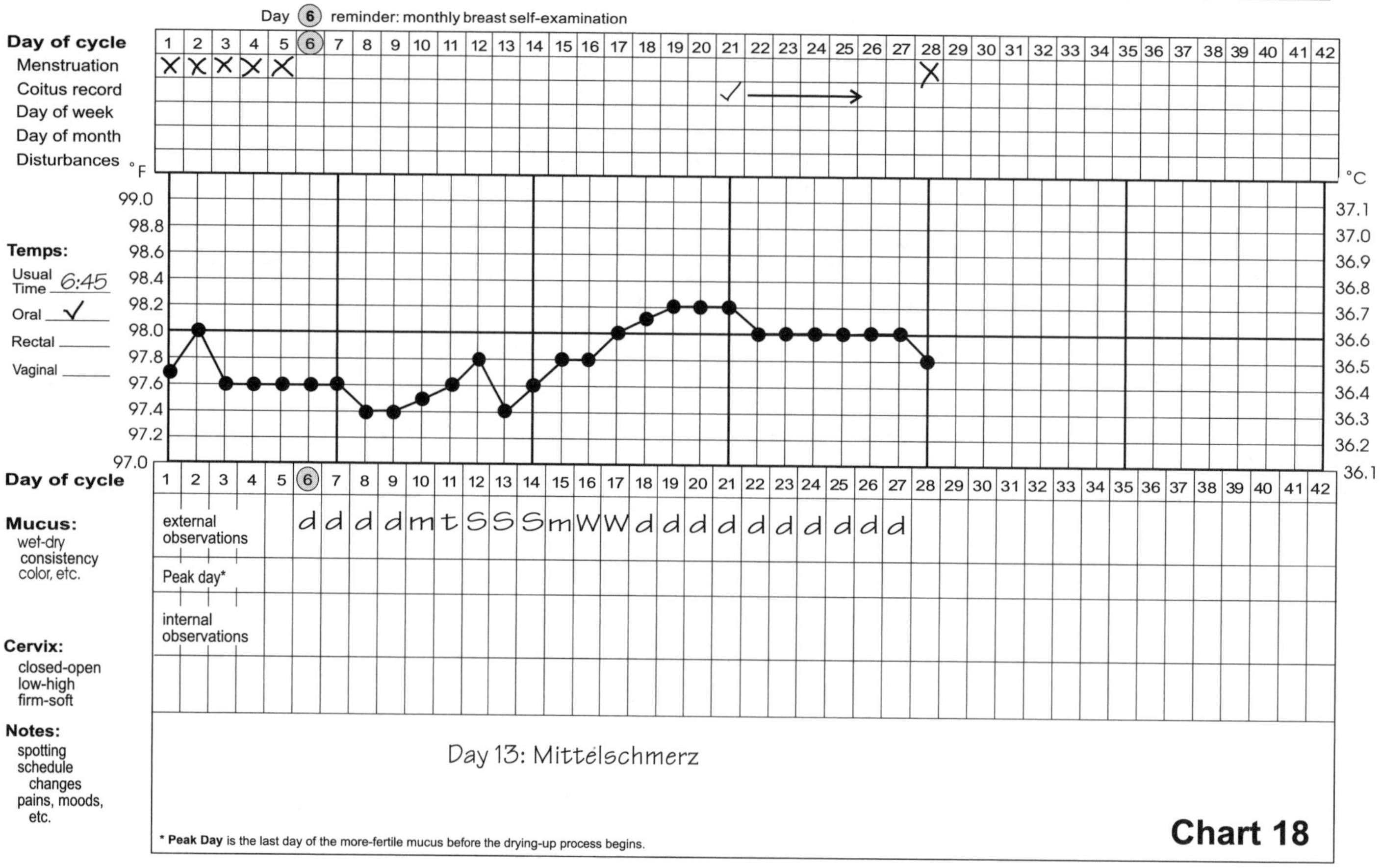

Day ⑥ reminder: monthly breast self-examination

Day of cycle	1	2	3	4	5	⑥	7	8	9	10	11	12	13	14	15	16	17	18	19	20	21	22	23	24	25	26	27	28	29	30	31	32	33	34	35	36	37	38	39	40	41	42
Menstruation	X	X	X	X	X																							X														
Coitus record																					✓	→																				
Day of week																																										
Day of month																																										
Disturbances																																										

Temps:
Usual Time _6:45_
Oral ✓
Rectal ____
Vaginal ____

°F																																											°C
99.0																																											37.1
98.8																																											37.0
98.6																																											36.9
98.4																																											36.8
98.2																																											36.7
98.0																																											36.6
97.8																																											36.5
97.6																																											36.4
97.4																																											36.3
97.2																																											36.2
97.0																																											36.1

Day of cycle	1	2	3	4	5	⑥	7	8	9	10	11	12	13	14	15	16	17	18	19	20	21	22	23	24	25	26	27	28	29	30	31	32	33	34	35	36	37	38	39	40	41	42

Mucus:
wet-dry
consistency
color, etc.

external observations: d d d d m t S S S m W W d d d d d d d d d d

Peak day*

internal observations

Cervix:
closed-open
low-high
firm-soft

Notes:
spotting
schedule
changes
pains, moods,
etc.

Day 13: Mittelschmerz

Chart 18

* **Peak Day** is the last day of the more-fertile mucus before the drying-up process begins.

End of Phase I:

 Clinical experience _____ 21/20 day rule _____ Doering _____ Last dry day _____

Pre-shift six _____   Low Temp Level _____   High Temp Level _____

"Peak" day _____   First day of cervix closing _____

Start of Phase III: Rule ____ = _____   Rule C = _____

NOTES:

 The "split peak" mucus pattern; see Chapter 27, Figure 27.2.

CCL Daily Chart No. __5__ Month __March__ Year __1973__

Name _____ Age __40__

Address _____ Phone ( ) _____

City _____ State _____ Zip _____

Previous Cycle Variation: Short __27__ Long __37__

Cycle variation based on __4__ recorded cycles

Earliest "first day of temperature rise" ____ based on ____ cycles

This cycle = __33__ days Height _____ Weight _____

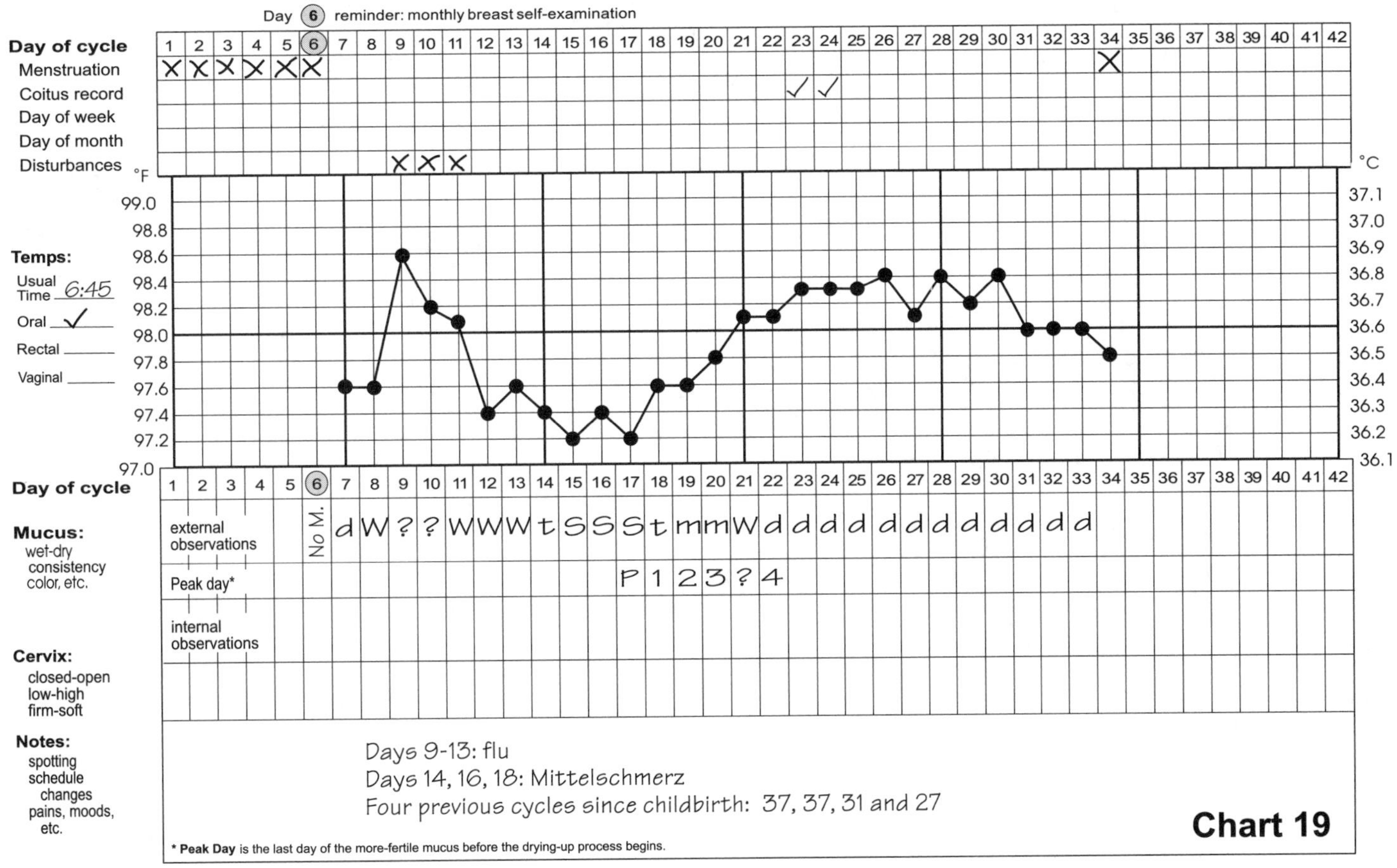

Day ⑥ reminder: monthly breast self-examination

Day of cycle	1	2	3	4	5	⑥	7	8	9	10	11	12	13	14	15	16	17	18	19	20	21	22	23	24	25	26	27	28	29	30	31	32	33	34	35	36	37	38	39	40	41	42
Menstruation	X	X	X	X	X	X																												X								
Coitus record																						✓	✓																			
Day of week																																										
Day of month																																										
Disturbances									X	X	X																															

Temps: Usual Time __6:45__ Oral ✓ Rectal ____ Vaginal ____

Temperature readings (°F):
- Day 7: 97.6
- Day 8: 97.6
- Day 9: 98.6
- Day 10: 98.2
- Day 11: 98.1
- Day 12: 97.4
- Day 13: 97.6
- Day 14: 97.4
- Day 15: 97.2
- Day 16: 97.4
- Day 17: 97.2
- Day 18: 97.6
- Day 19: 97.6
- Day 20: 97.8
- Day 21: 98.1
- Day 22: 98.2
- Day 23: 98.3
- Day 24: 98.3
- Day 25: 98.3
- Day 26: 98.45
- Day 27: 98.15
- Day 28: 98.45
- Day 29: 98.2
- Day 30: 98.45
- Day 31: 98.05
- Day 32: 98.05
- Day 33: 98.05
- Day 34: 97.85

Day of cycle	1	2	3	4	5	⑥	7	8	9	10	11	12	13	14	15	16	17	18	19	20	21	22	23	24	25	26	27	28	29	30	31	32	33	34	35	36	37	38	39	40	41	42
Mucus: external observations						No M.	d	W	?	?	W	W	W	t	S	S	S	t	m	m	W	d	d	d	d	d	d	d	d	d	d	d	d									
Peak day*																	P	1	2	3	?	4																				
internal observations																																										

Cervix: closed-open, low-high, firm-soft

Notes: spotting schedule changes pains, moods, etc.

Days 9-13: flu
Days 14, 16, 18: Mittelschmerz
Four previous cycles since childbirth: 37, 37, 31 and 27

Chart 19

* Peak Day is the last day of the more-fertile mucus before the drying-up process begins.

End of Phase I:
    Clinical experience ____ 21/20 day rule ____ Doering ____ Last dry day ____

Pre-shift six _____ Low Temp Level _____ High Temp Level _____

"Peak" day _____ First day of cervix closing _____

Start of Phase III: Rule ____ = _____ Rule C = _____

NOTES:

Temperatures helping the mucus interpretation; a split dry-up.

CCL Daily Chart No. __14__ Month __July-Aug.__ Year ____1994____

Name _____ Age _____

Address _____ Phone ( ) _____

City _____ State _VA_ Zip _____

Previous Cycle Variation: Short __27__ Long __35__

Cycle variation based on __13__ recorded cycles

Earliest "first day of temperature rise" __17__ based on __12__ cycles

This cycle = __28__ days   Height _5' 4"_ Weight _125 lbs._

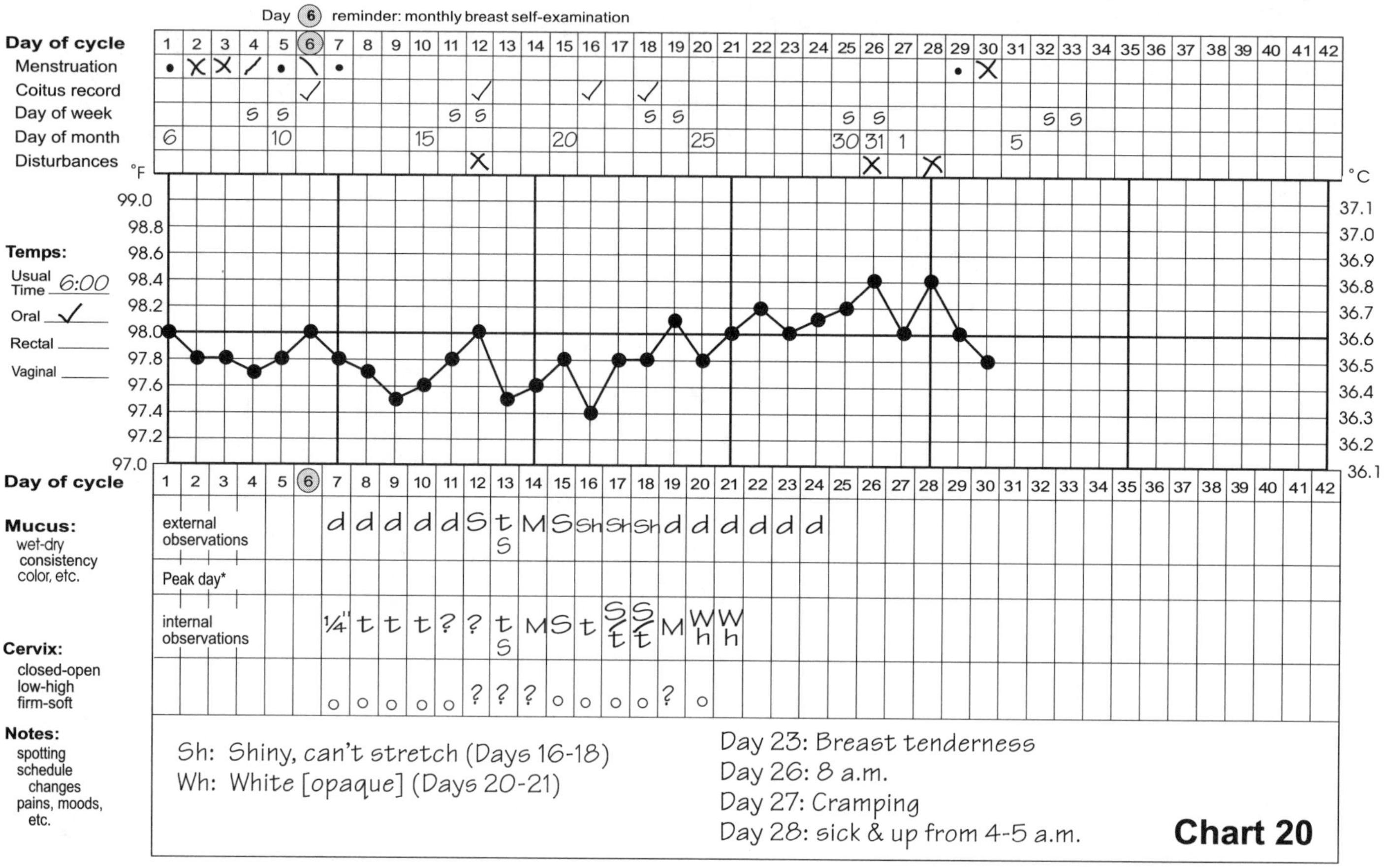

Day ⑥ reminder: monthly breast self-examination

Day of cycle	1	2	3	4	5	⑥	7	8	9	10	11	12	13	14	15	16	17	18	19	20	21	22	23	24	25	26	27	28	29	30	31	32	33	34	35	36	37	38	39	40	41	42
Menstruation	•	X	X	/	•	◡	•																						•	X												
Coitus record					✓							✓			✓		✓																								
Day of week			S	S								S	S				S	S					S	S					S	S												
Day of month	6				10					15					20					25					30	31	1			5												
Disturbances												X													X		X															

Temps:
Usual Time _6:00_
Oral ✓
Rectal ____
Vaginal ____

Day of cycle	1	2	3	4	5	⑥	7	8	9	10	11	12	13	14	15	16	17	18	19	20	21	22	23	24	25	26	27	28	29	30	31	32	33	34	35	36	37	38	39	40	41	42

Mucus:
wet-dry
consistency
color, etc.

Cervix:
closed-open
low-high
firm-soft

Notes:
spotting
schedule
changes
pains, moods,
etc.

external observations	d	d	d	d	d	S t/S	t	M	S	Sh	Sh	Sh	d	d	d	d	d	d
Peak day*																		
internal observations	¼"	t	t	t	?	?	t/S	M	S	t	S t	S t	M	W h	W h			
	o	o	o	o	o	?	?	?	o	o	o	o	?	o				

Sh: Shiny, can't stretch (Days 16-18)
Wh: White [opaque] (Days 20-21)

Day 23: Breast tenderness
Day 26: 8 a.m.
Day 27: Cramping
Day 28: sick & up from 4-5 a.m.

Chart 20

End of Phase I:
    Clinical experience _____ 21/20 day rule _____ Doering _____ Last dry day _____

Pre-shift six _____   Low Temp Level _____ High Temp Level _____

"Peak" day _____   First day of cervix closing _____

Start of Phase III: Rule _____ = _____   Rule C = _____

NOTES:

    Mucus helping the temperature interpretation.
    Seeking pregnancy.

Name _____ Age 30

Address _____ Phone ( ) _____

City _____ State MD Zip _____

Previous Cycle Variation: Short 28 Long 42 (prior to pregnancy)

Cycle variation based on 0 recorded cycles

Earliest "first day of temperature rise" ____ based on ____ cycles

This cycle = 39 days   Height 5' 6"   Weight 109 lbs.

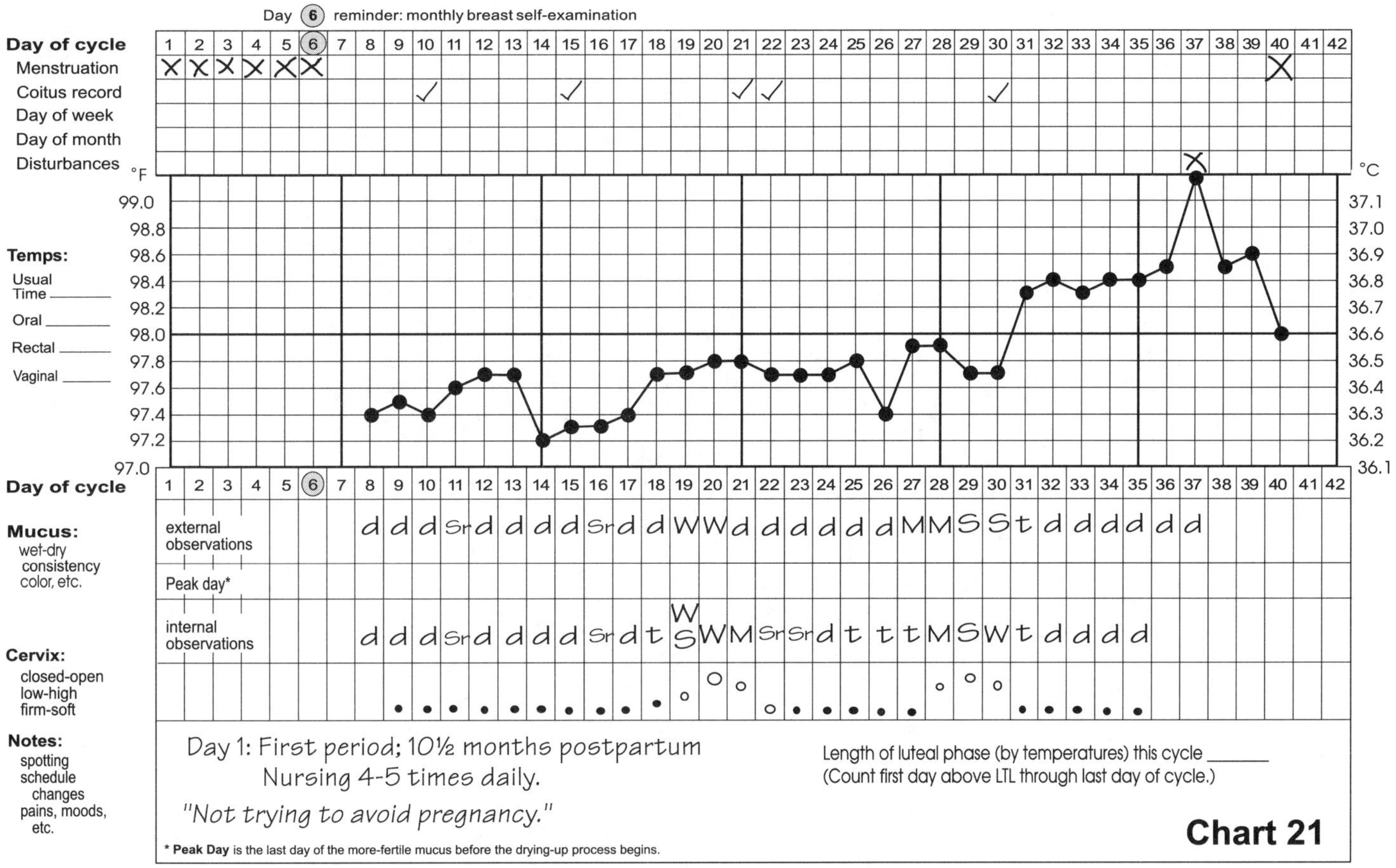

Day ⑥ reminder: monthly breast self-examination

Day of cycle | 1 2 3 4 5 ⑥ 7 8 9 10 11 12 13 14 15 16 17 18 19 20 21 22 23 24 25 26 27 28 29 30 31 32 33 34 35 36 37 38 39 40 41 42

Menstruation: X X X X X X ... X (day 40)

Coitus record: ✓ (10) ✓ (15) ✓ (21) ✓ (22) ✓ (29)

Day of week

Day of month

Disturbances: X (day 37)

Temps:
Usual Time _____
Oral _____
Rectal _____
Vaginal _____

°F scale: 99.0, 98.8, 98.6, 98.4, 98.2, 98.0, 97.8, 97.6, 97.4, 97.2, 97.0
°C scale: 37.1, 37.0, 36.9, 36.8, 36.7, 36.6, 36.5, 36.4, 36.3, 36.2, 36.1

Day of cycle | 1 2 3 4 5 ⑥ 7 8 9 10 11 12 13 14 15 16 17 18 19 20 21 22 23 24 25 26 27 28 29 30 31 32 33 34 35 36 37 38 39 40 41 42

Mucus:
wet-dry
consistency
color, etc.

external observations: d d d Sr d d d d Sr d d W W d d d d d d M M S S t d d d d d d

Peak day*

internal observations: d d d Sr d d d d Sr d t W/S W M Sr Sr d t t t M S W t d d d

Cervix:
closed-open
low-high
firm-soft

(cervix dots/circles row)

Notes:
spotting
schedule
changes
pains, moods,
etc.

Day 1: First period; 10½ months postpartum
Nursing 4-5 times daily.

"Not trying to avoid pregnancy."

Length of luteal phase (by temperatures) this cycle _____
(Count first day above LTL through last day of cycle.)

* Peak Day is the last day of the more-fertile mucus before the drying-up process begins.

Chart 21

End of Phase I:

Clinical experience ____   21/20 day rule ____   Doering ____   Last dry day ____

Pre-shift six _____   Low Temp Level _____   High Temp Level _____

"Peak" day _____   First day of cervix closing _____

Start of Phase III: Rule ____ = _____   Rule C = _____

NOTES:

Return of fertility while breastfeeding;
Phase II coitus and non-pregnancy: see chart analysis.

CCL Daily Chart No. __14__ Month __Oct.__ Year __1973__

Name _____ Age __22__

Address _____ Phone ( ) _____

City _____ State _____ Zip _____

Previous Cycle Variation: Short __26__ Long __33__

Cycle variation based on __13__ recorded cycles

Earliest "first day of temperature rise" ____ based on ____ cycles

This cycle = __27__ days   Height _____ Weight _____

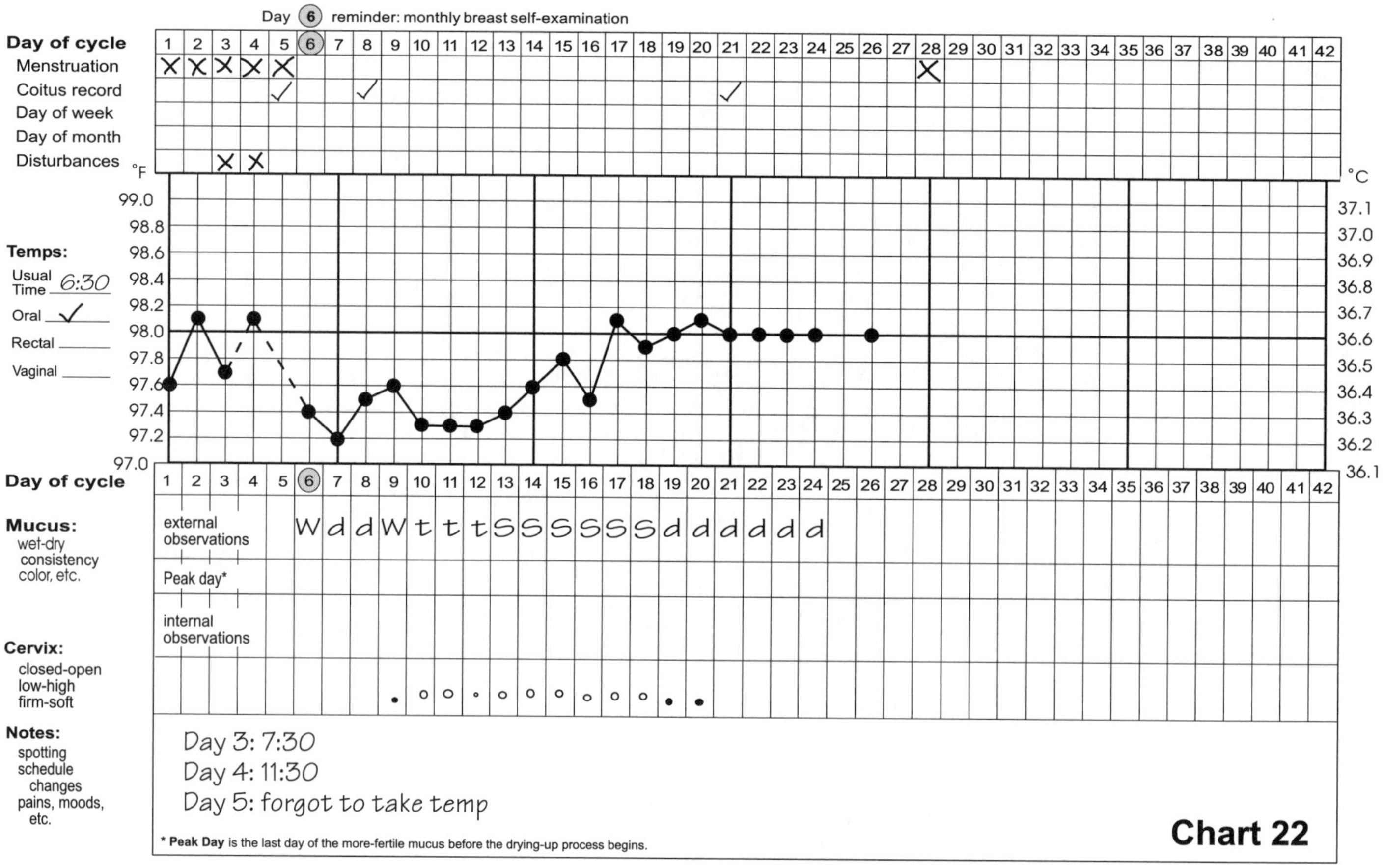

Day ⑥ reminder: monthly breast self-examination

Day of cycle	1	2	3	4	5	⑥	7	8	9	10	11	12	13	14	15	16	17	18	19	20	21	22	23	24	25	26	27	28	29	30	31	32	33	34	35	36	37	38	39	40	41	42
Menstruation	X	X	X	X	X																							X														
Coitus record						✓		✓													✓																					
Day of week																																										
Day of month																																										
Disturbances			X	X																																						

Temps:
Usual Time __6:30__
Oral ✓
Rectal ____
Vaginal ____

Day of cycle	1	2	3	4	5	⑥	7	8	9	10	11	12	13	14	15	16	17	18	19	20	21	22	23	24	25	26	27	28	29	30	31	32	33	34	35	36	37	38	39	40	41	42

Mucus:
wet-dry
consistency
color, etc.

external observations: W d d W t t t S S S S S S S d d d d d d d

Peak day*

internal observations:
• o o • o o o o o o o • •

Cervix:
closed-open
low-high
firm-soft

Notes:
spotting
schedule changes
pains, moods, etc.

Day 3: 7:30
Day 4: 11:30
Day 5: forgot to take temp

* Peak Day is the last day of the more-fertile mucus before the drying-up process begins.

Chart 22

End of Phase I:
  Clinical experience ____   21/20 day rule ____   Doering ____   Last dry day ____

Pre-shift six _____   Low Temp Level _____   High Temp Level _____

"Peak" day _____   First day of cervix closing _____

Start of Phase III: Rule ____ = _____   Rule C = _____

NOTES:

  Shaving and averaging irregular temperatures; see Chart 8 and Chapter 6.

CCL Daily Chart No. 7 Month Oct. Year 1978

Name ______ Age 41

Address ______ Phone ( ) ______

City ______ State ______ Zip ______

Previous Cycle Variation: Short 26 Long 30

Cycle variation based on 6 recorded cycles

Earliest "first day of temperature rise" ____ based on ____ cycles

This cycle = 28 days Height ______ Weight ______

Day (6) reminder: monthly breast self-examination

Day of cycle	1	2	3	4	5	6	7	8	9	10	11	12	13	14	15	16	17	18	19	20	21	22	23	24	25	26	27	28	29	30	31	32	33	34	35	36	37	38	39	40	41	42
Menstruation	X	X	X	X	X																								X													
Coitus record																																										
Day of week																																										
Day of month																																										
Disturbances																																										

Temps: Usual Time 6:30 Oral ✓ Rectal ______ Vaginal ______

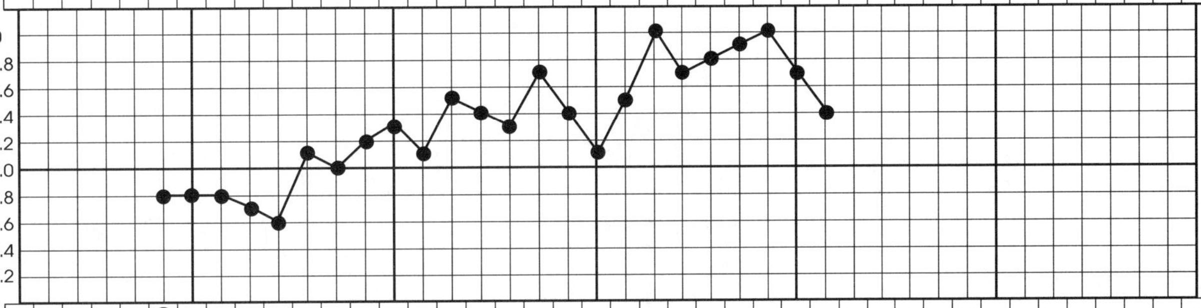

Day of cycle	1	2	3	4	5	6	7	8	9	10	11	12	13	14	15	16	17	18	19	20	21	22	23	24	25	26	27	28	29	30	31	32	33	34	35	36	37	38	39	40	41	42
Mucus: wet-dry, consistency, color, etc. — external observations						d	d	d	d	d		S EW	S EW	W	EW t	EW t	t	t	t	t																						
Peak day*																P	1	2	3	4																						
internal observations																																										
Cervix: closed-open, low-high, firm-soft																																										

Notes: spotting, schedule changes, pains, moods, etc.

EW = mucus like raw egg white

* **Peak Day** is the last day of the more-fertile mucus before the drying-up process begins.

Chart 23

End of Phase I:

Clinical experience ____ 21/20 day rule ____ Doering ____ Last dry day ____

Pre-shift six ______ Low Temp Level ______ High Temp Level ______

"Peak" day ______ First day of cervix closing ______

Start of Phase III: Rule ____ = ____ Rule C = ____

NOTES:

Mucus assisting the temperature interpretation.

CCL Daily Chart No. _32_ Month ___March___ Year _____

Name _____ Age _____

Address _____ Phone ( ) _____

City _____ State _____ Zip _____

Previous Cycle Variation: Short __25__ Long __31__

Cycle variation based on __31__ recorded cycles

Earliest "first day of temperature rise" ____ based on ____ cycles

This cycle = __28__ days Height _____ Weight _____

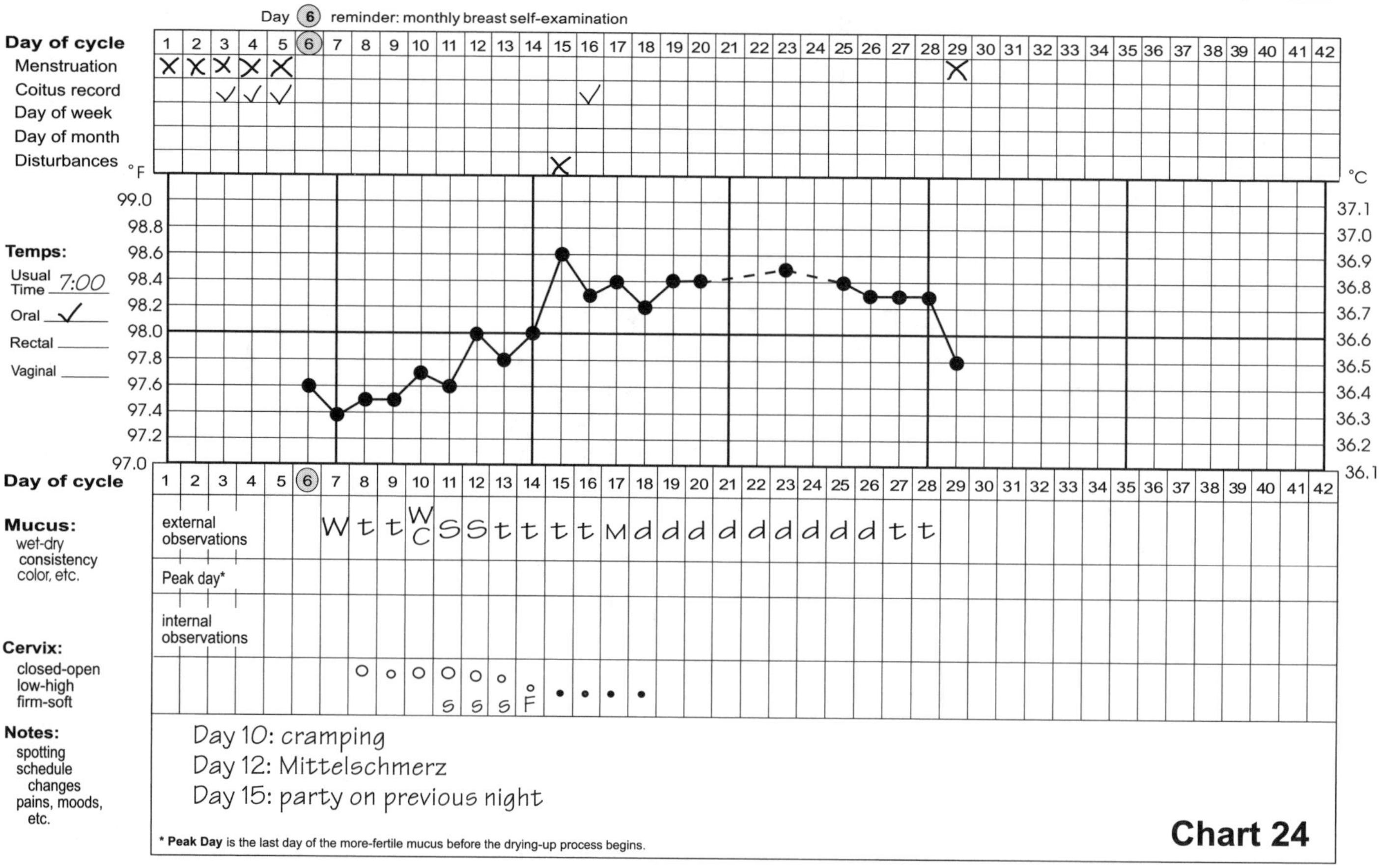

Day ⑥ reminder: monthly breast self-examination

Day of cycle	1	2	3	4	5	⑥	7	8	9	10	11	12	13	14	15	16	17	18	19	20	21	22	23	24	25	26	27	28	29	30	31	32	33	34	35	36	37	38	39	40	41	42
Menstruation	X	X	X	X	X																								X													
Coitus record			✓	✓	✓										✓																											
Day of week																																										
Day of month																																										
Disturbances															X																											

Temps:
Usual Time _7:00_
Oral ✓
Rectal ____
Vaginal ____

°F / °C temperature grid (Chart 24):
99.0 / 37.1
98.8 / 37.0
98.6 / 36.9
98.4 / 36.8
98.2 / 36.7
98.0 / 36.6
97.8 / 36.5
97.6 / 36.4
97.4 / 36.3
97.2 / 36.2
97.0 / 36.1

Day of cycle	1	2	3	4	5	⑥	7	8	9	10	11	12	13	14	15	16	17	18	19	20	21	22	23	24	25	26	27	28	29	30	31	32	33	34	35	36	37	38	39	40	41	42

Mucus: wet-dry consistency color, etc.

external observations: W t t W/C S S t t t t M d d d d d d d d d t t

Peak day*

internal observations

Cervix: closed-open low-high firm-soft

internal observations row: O (d7) o (d8) O (d9) O/S (d10) O/S (d11) o/S (d12) °F/S (d13) • (d14) • (d15) • (d16) • (d17)

Notes: spotting schedule changes pains, moods, etc.

Day 10: cramping
Day 12: Mittelschmerz
Day 15: party on previous night

* Peak Day is the last day of the more-fertile mucus before the drying-up process begins.

Chart 24

End of Phase I:

Clinical experience ____ 21/20 day rule ____ Doering ____ Last dry day ____

Pre-shift six _____ Low Temp Level _____ High Temp Level _____

"Peak" day _____ First day of cervix closing _____

Start of Phase III: Rule ____ = _____ Rule C = _____

NOTES:

A good situation for Rule B.

Chart Analysis

Chart 1. Perfect Coinciding

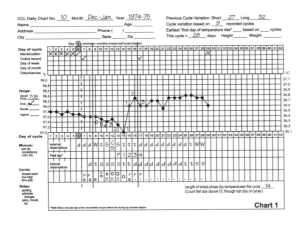

End of Phase I: Clinical Experience: = 6   21/20 day rule = 6
Doering = n/a   Last dry day = 8
Pre-shift six: 9-14   LTL: 97.6°   HTL: 98.0°
Peak day: 13   First day of cervix closing: 14
Start of Phase III: Rule C = 17, Perfect Coinciding in this case

End of Phase I. This cycle shows five days of mucus starting with the first day (Day 9) through Peak day. A five-day mucus patch is the **minimum** we recommend to rely on the Last Dry Day Rule beyond the limits of the 21 Day Rule. That is, if you usually experience less than five days of mucus between its first appearance and Peak day inclusive, the Last Dry Day Rule may not give you sufficient notice of fertility. Another way of saying the same thing: the possibility of a so-called "dry-day" pregnancy is reduced if the mucus appears at least four days before Peak day (Peak day minus 4). If there are less than four days of mucus before Peak day, you will probably have a better indication of the end of Phase I by one of the other rules.

Start of Phase III. Chart 1 illustrates the perfect coinciding of all the signs to indicate the beginning of Phase III. The third day of thermal shift, the fourth day of drying-up, and the fourth day of cervix closing all coincide on Day 17. Postovulation infertility begins on the evening of that day.

Chart 2. A typical Rule K interpretation

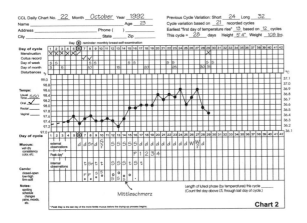

End of Phase I: Clinical Experience = 5   21/20 day rule = 4
Doering = 6   Last dry day = 6
Pre-shift six: 9-14   LTL: 97.5°   HTL: 97.9°
Peak day: 16   First day of cervix closing: 16
Start of Phase III: Rule K = 18   Rule C = 20

End of Phase I. The woman noticed internal mucus on Day 7. Therefore Day 6 was the last dry day. The Doering rule starts with the first day of thermal shift in the last 12 cycles, here recorded as Day 13. Then you subtract 7, which yields Day 6.

The 20 Day version of the 21/20 Day Rule can be applied when there are more than 12 cycles of experience. Here it yields Day 4. That interpretation policy is followed in the *Workbook* analyses; you, of course, are free to use the more conservative 21 Day Rule.

The couple continued to have intercourse on Days 7 and 8, knowing they were in Phase II. That's "taking chances." For a couple of normal fertility, such "taking chances" will normally result in pregnancy in a few cycles. This cycle was 28 days, but her short cycle was 24 days, meaning that ovulation most likely occurs earlier in some cycles than it did in this cycle.

The couple compounded their "chance-taking" by having relations on consecutive days. Though some women think they can distinguish between mucus and seminal residue, they cannot determine if the beginning of a mucus discharge is starting *at the same time* that she notices the seminal residue. Furthermore, there is some reason to suspect that relations on consecutive days may change the vaginal environment and extend the life of sperm from the second coitus.

Start of Phase III. The upward thermal shift precedes the mucus dry-up. Still, Rule K needs at least two days of drying-up to cross-check three or more days of full thermal shift. You can apply Rule K on Day 18 because there are four days of full thermal shift and two days of drying-up. Rule C yields Day 20, and that appears to be excessively conservative except in the case of an ultra-serious reason to avoid pregnancy.

Chart 3. A typical Rule R interpretation

End of Phase I: Clinical Experience = 6? 21/20 day rule = n/a
Doering = n/a   Last dry day = n/a
Pre-shift six: 13-18   LTL: 97.3°   HTL: 97.7°
Peak day: 18   First day of cervix closing: 18
Start of Phase III: Rule R = 21   Rule C = 22

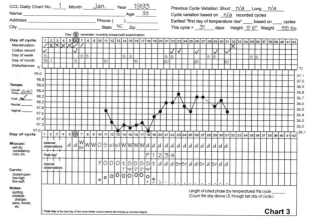

End of Phase I. The chart records a woman's first cycle of charting. Because of her lack of experience, all the Phase I rules that require some charting and fertility awareness experience are not applicable. However, if a woman knows from her past experience that her last 12 normal cycles (no Pill cycles) have been at least 26 days long, the couple can use the Clinical Experience rule that ends Phase I on Day 6. Nevertheless, CCL's general recommendation remains that couples do best to abstain in Phase I during their first cycle so the wife can experience the start of the mucus without any confusion from seminal residue.

Start of Phase III. There are three days of strong thermal shift which cross-check three days of drying-up past Peak day. Therefore Rule R yields Day 21 as the start of Phase III. Rule C requires three days of full thermal shift cross-checked by four days of drying-up. Day 22 meets those requirements.

In general. The woman who completed this chart lived in a state in which CCL had very few teachers, so she took the *CCL Home Study Course.* In her very first cycle she was successful in observing external mucus changes, internal mucus, and changes in the cervix, as well as taking her temperatures. We certainly recommend starting the temperature taking by Day 6 at the latest, and there was a little confusion about recording the internal mucus. Apart from that, the chart demonstrates good self-instruction.

Chart 4. A typical Rule B interpretation

End of Phase I: Clinical Experience = 5   21/20 day rule = 4
Doering = 6   Last dry day = 7
Pre-shift six: 8-13   LTL: 98.0°   HTL: 98.4°
Peak day: 12   First day of cervix closing: 14
Start of Phase III: Rule B = 16   Rule C = 17

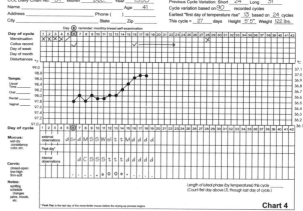

Phase I. The recording of SR (seminal residue) on Day 6 infers that the coitus was in the morning of that day. The standard rule is "not in the mornings" in Phase I, especially beyond the limits of the Clinical Experience rules. The reason for that rule is that mucus may be starting to flow but is not yet noticeable due to the woman's horizontal position all night.

The woman's mucus patch was five days, the minimum recommended for using the Last Dry Day rule.

Phase III. Three days of strong thermal shift cross-check four days of drying-up after Peak day. Rule B yields Day 16 as the start of Phase III. Rule C needs three days of *full* thermal shift to cross-check four or more days of drying-up. Day 17 fulfills those requirements. Rule B can be satisfied with three days of "overall thermal shift." If the temperature on Day 14 had been at 98.1°, Rule B would still yield Day 16.

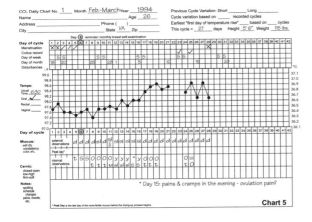

Chart 5. Just off the Pill

End of Phase I: Not applicable in first three cycles off the Pill
Pre-shift six: 11-16   LTL: 98.0°   HTL: 98.4°
Peak day: 16 but n/a   First day of cervix closing: No data
Start of Phase III: Just-off-the-Pill rule = Day 21

Phase I. The Pill companies warn against becoming pregnant for three months after your last Pill. They are afraid of birth defects caused by the Pill and the possibility of litigation and liability. Since most unplanned pregnancies come from coitus in late Phase I, we encourage couples to abstain from marital relations during Phases I and II for the first three cycles off the Pill.

The couple correctly set the LTL at 98.0 using Days 11-16 as the pre-shift six. The temperatures on Days 17-19 are the first three that are consecutively above the previous six.

Phase III. The Just-off-the-Pill rule or Post-Pill rule is primarily a five-day Temperature-only rule (see Chapter 29). It starts with the basic four-day Temperature-only rule explained in Chapter 26. Then it adds one day for beginners. The first two days of upward thermal shift do not have to be a full 4/10 of 1° F. above the LTL, but the last three days must be consecutively at the High Temperature Level. In this case, the last four days are at or above the HTL.

Sometimes the more-fertile mucus continues well into the start of the thermal shift. Normally we like to see at least one day of drying-up or less-fertile mucus to cross-check the thermal shift. In this particular case, the woman had an almost classic mucus patch, especially with the external observations. In other cases, the mucus in the first one or two cycles off the Pill may be continuous or otherwise impossible to interpret with confidence. Therefore, we rely upon the Temperature-only rule until the woman has some experience with a normal mucus pattern. Our **standard recommendation:** Use the Post-Pill rule for the first three cycles off the Pill.

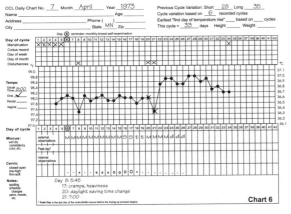

Chart 6. Necessity of temperature cross-check of mucus drying-up

End of Phase I: Clinical Experience = 6   21/20 day rule = n/a
                Doering = n/a   Last dry day = n/a
Pre-shift six: 14-19   LTL: 98.1°   HTL: 98.5°
Peak day: 17   First day of cervix closing: 18
Start of Phase III: Rule C = 24

End of Phase I. Chart 6 shows all-the-time mucus from menstruation until the start of Phase III. Under such circumstances, the Last Dry Day rule is not applicable since there are no Phase I dry days. (For an exception, see p. 386.) Both the 21 Day Rule and the Clinical Experience rules normally presume the absence of any mucus. However, much of the experience with the first six days of the cycle was gained without reference to mucus. Therefore, if this woman HAS A HISTORY of all-the-time mucus with plenty of days of the more-fertile mucus, it is highly probable that the usual very low fertility of Cycle Day 6 would apply in this case, especially since the Clinical Experience Rule of Day 6 is also within the limits of the 21 Day Rule. If the 21 Day rule yielded something before Day 6, the couple might use the 21 Day rule or at least not go beyond Day 5.

Setting the LTL. Ignore the temperatures on Cycle Days 20 and 21 in setting the LTL because they were probably *lower* than if taken at the normal time. It usually takes your body three days to adjust to time changes. Due to spring daylight saving time, the temperature reading on Day 20 was, in effect, taken one hour earlier, and the reading on Day 21 was, in effect, taken about two hours earlier. Therefore, use the temperatures on Days 14-19 to set the LTL.

Start of Phase III. Chart 6 illustrates the sympto-thermal requirement for at least three days of elevated temperatures to cross-check the days of drying-up. Ovulation sometimes, though rarely, occurs as late as Peak day + 3, and that might have happened here, thus explaining the delay in the start of the thermal shift (Day 22) after Peak day (Day 17). The use of the cross-checking signs is the essence of the Sympto-Thermal Method.

Chart 7. Necessity of mucus cross-check of thermal shift

End of Phase I: Clinical Experience = 6   21/20 day rule = 6
                 Doering = 5   Last dry day = 6
Pre-shift six: 5-10   LTL: 97.4°   HTL: 97.8°
Peak day: 13   First day of cervix closing: n/a
Start of Phase III: Rule K = 15   Rule C = 17

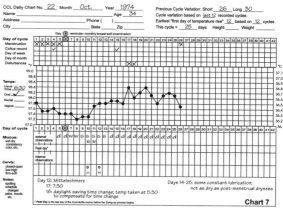

End of Phase I. Three rules indicate Day 6 as the end of Phase I. **Next cycle:** Since *this* is a 25 day cycle, the end of Phase I for *subsequent* cycles will be Day 5 by the 20 Day Rule and Day 5 also by the Clinical Experience rules. The Doering Rule will yield Day 4 in future cycles.

Start of Phase III. The main purpose of this chart is to illustrate a basic sympto-thermal requirement: you need at least two to four days of drying-up (depending upon the rule) to cross-check the elevated temperature pattern. When you have several days of full thermal shift, you have to wait for at least two days of drying-up to apply Rule K.

    This chart complements the previous one. Chart 6 shows the need to wait for at least three days of higher temperatures to cross-check the mucus drying-up; Chart 7 shows the need to wait for a minimum of two days of drying-up to cross-check the thermal shift pattern.

Chart 8. Shaving irregular high temperatures; temperature-only rule

End of Phase I: Clinical Experience = ?   21/20 day rule = n/a
                 Doering = n/a   Last dry day = n/a
Pre-shift six: 10-15   LTL: S-98.1°   HTL: 98.5°
Start of Phase III: Temperature-only = 19

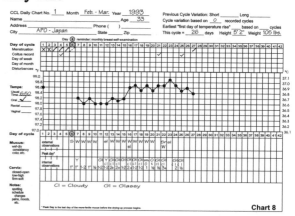

End of Phase I. This chart records the first cycle of NFP charting for the couple, an American military couple serving in Japan and self-instructing themselves with the *CCL Home Study Course.* Although the wife did not record any previous cycle variations, apparently they thought that her cycles were long enough to apply the Clinical Experience rules up through Day 4. The other rules require charting or experience and are not applicable to this cycle.

Start of Phase III. After menstruation, this woman experiences a continuous discharge of the more-fertile mucus for the rest of the cycle. When the mucus sign provides no help to determine the start of Phase III, we use the Temperature-only Rule described in Chapter 26. This rule requires four days of thermal shift with the last three temperatures consecutively at the High Temperature Level. If you set the Low Temperature Level at 98.2, you don't find the requirements for the Temperature-only Rule until Day 23. The experienced eye recognizes that such an interpretation is far too conservative. Therefore we use the shaving principle.

Shaving irregular high temperatures is explained in Chapter 6. In this chart, by Day 19 you see four well elevated temperatures. When you try an LTL of 98.2 and an HTL of 98.6, you see that Temperature-only Rule doesn't fit because the temperature on Day 18 falls below the HTL. In the presence of such an obvious thermal shift, shave the temperature readings on Days 13 and 15 to the next highest level, 98.1. The HTL becomes 98.5, and everything falls into place to apply the Temperature-only Rule on Day 19.

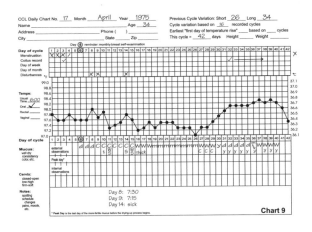

Chart 9

Chart 9. The Double Peak mucus pattern

End of Phase I: Clinical Experience = 6   21/20 day rule = 6
                          Doering = n/a   Last dry day = 8
Pre-shift six: 23-28   LTL: 97.3°   HTL: 97.7°
Peak days: 18 and 29   First day of cervix closing: n/a
Start of Phase III: Rule K = 32   Rule C = 33

End of Phase I. If you have any questions about the Phase I interpretations, check Chapter 11 again. We do not have the data to apply the Doering rule.

Start of Phase III. The main purposes of this chart are 1) to illustrate the "double peak" mucus pattern and 2) to show a non-stretchy mucus patch. The "double peak" pattern is explained in Chapter 27, "Irregular mucus patterns."

1. A mucus patch can come and go without ovulation occurring. The mucus patch from Day 9 through Day 18 gave every indication of fertility, but its Peak day was not cross-checked by a thermal shift. A second patch of the more-fertile mucus occurs on Days 27, 28 and 29. Day 29 is the second Peak day, and this time the drying-up is cross-checked by a full thermal shift to indicate the start of Phase III on Day 32 by Rule K and on Day 33 by Rule C.

2. Sometimes a more-fertile mucus patch produces no stretchy mucus. No problem: the feeling of wetness is a very important indicator of fertility. Note well the short second mucus patch on Days 27-29. No indication of stretchiness is recorded in the second patch, but the woman did experience distinctive feelings of wetness.

The Sympto-Thermal Method provides no indication of being in Phase III before Day 32. However, the rules of the mucus-only method (Ovulation Method or OM) would have indicated Day 22 as the start of Phase III. Couples following that method must continue to be watchful for the reappearance of the more-fertile mucus and abstain again if they notice it. See more on this in Chapter 27.

If a woman using the OM is normally dry in Phase III but experiences a continuation of less-fertile mucus after a Peak day as in this cycle, the couple should continue to abstain.

The mucus that begins on Day 37 also produced feelings of wetness. Some women usually have a few days of wetness just before menstruation. STM users can ignore such mucus if they have had a thermal shift in that cycle, but OM users should treat it as a potential sign of fertility. Such complications and uncertainties lead CCL to recommend the cross-checking Sympto-Thermal Method.

Chart 10. Breakthrough bleeding

This series of graphs shows two cycles. The top graph shows a cycle of 26 days; the middle and bottom graphs show one cycle of 46 days interrupted by breakthrough bleeding that starts on Cycle Day 30. Breakthrough bleeding is explained in Chapter 30.

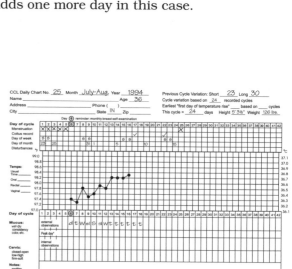

End of Phase I. Top cycle: Assume that the woman has had six cycles of experience. Note that her previous short cycle was 22 days. Clinical Experience = 4   21 day rule = 1   Doering = n/a because of no data   Last dry day = Day 8

Second cycle: The Clinical Experience rules and the 21 Day Rule remain the same. However, we cannot apply the Last Dry Day Rule because the woman did not record mucus observations until Day 17. We cannot assume that "no recording" means "no mucus."

Start of Phase III. Top cycle. The first cycle has a clearly defined thermal shift after Peak day. Therefore: Pre-shift six = 10-15, LTL = 97.5, HTL = 97.9, Peak day = 14, Rule B = 18 as the start of Phase III. The thermal shift leaves no doubt that the bleeding that starts on Day 27 is a menstruation and that Day 27 is really Day 1 of the next cycle.

The second cycle starting with the middle graph has a short mucus patch on Days 20-22 that is **not** followed by a thermal shift. When a bloody discharge starts on Cycle Day 30, it has **not** been preceded by a thermal shift. Therefore, that bleeding **cannot** be considered to be a true menstruation and the start of Phase I. Because the bloody discharge is followed immediately by mucus and a thermal shift, the bloody discharge is called "breakthrough bleeding."

The couple thought the bleeding (bottom graph, Days 1 - 4) was menstruation so they started a new chart and had coitus on what they thought was Cycle Day 4 in the bottom graph, as indicated by the circle around the temperature reading. In reality, "Day 4" of the bottom graph was Cycle Day 33 and a very fertile time. "Day 1" of the bottom graph is Day 30 of the cycle started in the middle graph.

In the bottom graph, the temperature on "Day 6" is a pre-shift spike. (See Chapter 28, "Irregular Temperature Patterns.") Shave it down to 97.5, the next highest level among the pre-shift six of Days "2" through "7," and check out the arithmetic average (= 97.48). Shaved LTL = 97.5; HTL = 97.9. Peak day = "7"; Rule K = "Day 10" (really Cycle Day 39) as the start of Phase III. Rule C adds one more day in this case.

Chart 11. Shaving with Rule K

End of Phase I: Clinical Experience = 5   21/20 day rule = 3
                      Doering = n/a   Last dry day = 6
Pre-shift six: 7-12   LTL: S-97.8°   HTL: 98.2°
Peak day: 12   First day of cervix closing: n/a
Start of Phase III: Rule K = Day 15   Rule C = Day 16

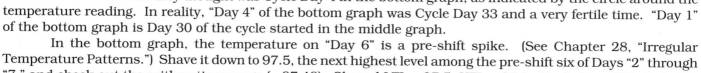

End of Phase I. The application of the rules is self-explanatory. If you consistently have mucus patches of six days from start through Peak day as in this cycle, you can use the Last Dry Day with confidence. Five days is the minimum recommended.

Application of Rule K with shaving. By Day 15, you see three days of elevated temperatures that would be a full thermal shift except for the temperature on Day 11. You can shave and apply Rule K when you have either one of two options: 1) three days of drying-up and three days of full thermal shift (after shaving) or 2) only two days of drying-up cross-checked by four days of higher temperatures with the last three at the High Temperature Level.

The first option applies here. Shave the temperature down to the next highest level, 97.8, and Rule K yields Day 15.

See Chapter 6, "Shaving irregular temperatures" and Rule K in Chapter 12.

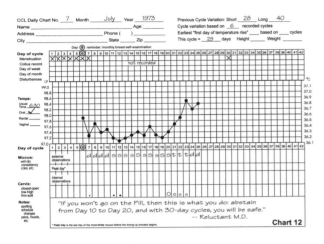

"If you won't go on the Pill, then this is what you do: abstain from Day 10 to Day 20, and with 30-day cycles, you will be safe."
-- Reluctant M.D.

Chart 12

Chart 12. Shaving with Rule R

End of Phase I: Clinical Experience = 6   21/20 day rule = 7
              Doering = n/a   Last dry day = 10
Pre-shift six: 15-20   LTL: 97.6°   HTL: 98.0°
Peak day: 20   First day of cervix closing: insufficient data; perhaps 21
Start of Phase III: Rule B = 24   Rule C = 25
Alternative interpretation: Shaved LTL: 97.5°   Rule R = 23
    Rule C = 24

End of Phase I. Self explanatory.

Shaving with Rule R. Without shaving, Rule B = 24 and Rule C = 25. What if it's Day 23 and husband is leaving the next day for a week's trip? Would intercourse on Day 23 be "taking chances" or can one of the rules yield Day 23?

For shaving with Rule R, we take our tips from Dr. Josef Roetzer who developed the basis for this rule. With Rule R, you can shave one temperature in the pre-shift six group by 1/10 of 1° F. Therefore, shave the temperature on Day 17 by 1/10, and your shaved Low Temperature Level is 97.5°. With this bit of shaving, Rule R clearly yields Day 23 as the start of Phase III.

The physician's advice. This chart dates back to 1973, and some physicians used variations of the calendar rhythm method. This variation was called the 10-10 system, and it was irresponsible advice even in 1973. It would have the couple thinking they were infertile on Day 21. In reality, Day 21, which is Peak day + 1, is a highly fertile day, perhaps the day of ovulation.

Long mucus patch; short luteal phase. The ten-day mucus patch and the nine-day luteal phase (as measured by temps and mucus) *perhaps* indicate a hormonally unbalanced cycle. The woman might be able to shorten the mucus patch and lengthen the luteal phase through better nutrition. CCL publishes *Fertility, Cycles and Nutrition* to help women discover how to improve their nutrition and possibly their cycle patterns. (See "Resources.")

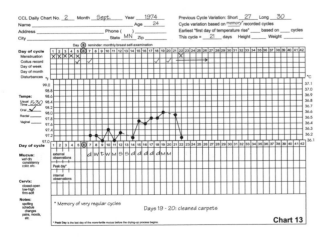

* Memory of very regular cycles

Days 19 - 20: cleaned carpets

Chart 13

Chart 13. Artificially shortened luteal phase

End of Phase I: Clinical Experience = 6? 21/20 day rule = 6?
              Doering = n/a   Last dry day = n/a
Pre-shift six: 8-14   LTL: 97.4°   HTL: 97.8°
Peak day: 13   First day of cervix closing: n/a
Start of Phase III: Rule B = 17   Rule C = 19

End of Phase I. The question mark for the Clinical Experience application means that no record of mucus observations on Day 6 makes the rule somewhat doubtful. You need to begin making and recording observations the day after menstruation stops and by Day 6 at the latest. The question mark for the 21 Day Rule indicates some doubt about the value of a previous cycle history where the only record is memory. On the other hand, many women have an excellent memory of such things. The Doering Rule and the Last Dry Day Rule are not applicable because the woman has only one cycle of experience.

Start of Phase III. Rule B yields Day 17 as the start of Phase III. Coitus on the night of Day 17 would have a risk of pregnancy of less than 1 in 100 woman-years. By waiting for the fourth day of this strong thermal shift, the couple probably reduced the chance of pregnancy to something closer to 1 in 1000 woman-years.

Short luteal phase and short cycle. This cycle was only 21 days long. Does it form the basis for the Clinical Experience and 21 Day rules in future cycles? Not in this case. The luteal phase was artificially shortened by the vigorous and unaccustomed physical exertion on Days 19 and 20. Both the mucus and the temperature signs point to ovulation around Days 13 to 15, just where you would expect it in cycles in her normal range of 27 to 30 days.

    The purpose of the Clinical Experience and 21/20 Day rules is to guard against early ovulation and/or the possibility of not detecting early cervical mucus. Since the cycle was shortened by external circumstances, nothing would be gained by using this cycle as the basis for those rules.

Chart 14. Need for valid Peak day and valid temperatures
End of Phase I: Clinical Experience = 6? 21/20 day rule = n/a
              Doering = n/a   Last dry day = n/a
Pre-shift six: 14-20   LTL: 97.7°   HTL: 98.1°
Peak day: 19   First day of cervix closing: insufficient data;
   may be Day 19
Start of Phase III: Rule C = 25

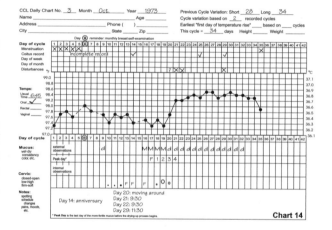

Chart 14

End of Phase I. The first six days of the cycle are very infertile for women with cycles of 26 days and longer. The question mark for the Clinical Experience reflects the lack of a "dry" recording. All the other rules are not applicable because of the lack of experience. Even with experience, she should not apply the Last Dry Day Rule. To use it, you need to record your observations beginning by Day 6 at the latest.

Phase II. Day 14 coitus was most likely in Phase II.

Start of Phase III. Chart 14 illustrates a mistake in the mucus interpretation—labeling Day 17 as Peak day when it was not followed the next day by *a change in the quality* of the mucus. Perhaps the woman made one of the most common mistakes—calling the day of the *most* mucus the Peak day. See Chapter 7, "How to interpret your mucus pattern."

    Chart 14 also shows unusable temperatures at a critical time—right at the end of Phase II. The temperature on Day 20 offers no problem if "moving around" simply meant moving around for the five minutes she was taking her temperature, so we included it among the pre-shift six. However, the temperatures on Days 21 and 22 were taken almost two hours later than usual. That makes them so questionable you cannot use them as part of the thermal shift pattern. The late temperature on Day 29 makes no difference. The point is that you need valid temperatures during Phase II.

    Start the thermal shift count on Day 23. Rule C indicates Day 25 as the start of Phase III. With the information given, no STM rule yields anything earlier. However, if the woman had taken her temperatures on Days 21 and 22 between 6:45 and 7:15, and if they had started an overall thermal shift, Rule B would have yielded Day 23 as the start of Phase III. Furthermore, with a valid temperature on Day 15, a pre-shift six of 14 - 19, an LTL of 97.5, more information about Day 20, and valid temperatures on Days 21 and 22, Rule R might have yielded Day 22 as the start of Phase III.

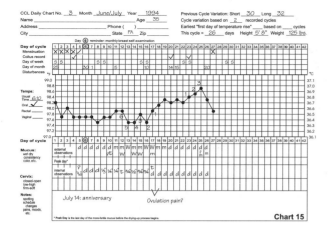

Chart 15

Chart 15. Averaging the pre-shift six

End of Phase I: Clinical Experience = 6   21/20 day rule = n/a
             Doering = n/a   Last dry day = n/a
Pre-shift six: 12-17   LTL: 97.7° avg.   HTL: 98.1°
Peak day: 17   First day of cervix closing: perhaps 17.
Start of Phase III: Rule K = 20   Rule C = 21
             Rule B without shaving = 21

End of Phase I. This woman's first charted cycle was 32 days, the next was 30, and this cycle is 26 days. With that sort of variation, the couple would be well advised not to extend Phase I beyond Day 5 until they have a few more cycles on which to base their cycle variation.

Selecting the pre-shift six. Should the temperature on Day 17 be counted as the last day of the pre-shift six or the first day of the thermal shift? It's not a "rule," but it's a guiding principle that if such temperature is on or before Peak Day, include it in the pre-shift six, unless it is obviously part of the thermal shift pattern. That's why we selected Days 12 - 17 as the pre-shift six.

Averaging the pre-shift six temperatures. By Day 20, you see three elevated temperatures cross-checked by three days of drying-up. However, the temperatures on Days 12 and 17 interfere with a Rule R interpretation. Even shaving those two readings to 97.8 doesn't provide a fit on Day 20. When it is so obvious that there is a good thermal shift cross-checking the drying-up, you can average the pre-shift six, Days 12-17. The result is 97.68 = 97.7   Rule K yields Day 20. Without shaving or averaging, the LTL is 97.9, and Rule B yields Day 21.

Nutrition check. With a slightly delayed ovulation, a somewhat short luteal phase, and only 125 pounds on a 5' 8" frame, there is reason to ask the woman to double-check her exercise and nutrition habits.

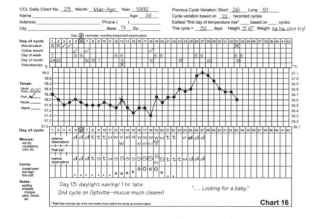

Chart 16

Chart 16. Common sense or rationalizing?

End of Phase I: Clinical Experience = 6   21/20 day rule = 6
             Doering = n/a   Last dry day = 7
Pre-shift six: 12, 14-18   LTL: 97.7°   HTL: 98.1°
Peak day: 20   First day of cervix closing: 20
Start of Phase III: Rule K = 23   Rule C = 24

End of Phase I. This woman has been experiencing a long mucus discharge before ovulation. She noted that this was her second cycle on Optivite, the dietary supplement formulated to assist cycle normality, and that her mucus pattern was much more clear. If she continued to have a very long mucus discharge, the couple might consider relying more upon the opening of the cervix and the appearance of the more-fertile mucus. They would check their last 12 charts to see if those indicators gave them at least six days of warning before Peak day or the first day of thermal shift before deciding to ignore those early days of the less-fertile mucus. However, they should *not* make such a change while making other changes—such as a big change in nutrition—that might change the cycle pattern and cause ovulation to occur earlier.

Phase III. With an LTL of 97.7, there is no question that Rule K yields Day 23 as the start of Phase III. However, consider the temperatures on Days 19-22. When you see such a strong four-day thermal shift cross-checked by the minimum of two days of drying-up, you wonder if there is some way for the rules to fit on Day 22.

There isn't. The average of the pre-shift six is 97.6, which gives a High Temperature Level of 98.0, but that doesn't help; the temperature on Day 20 dips below 98.0 and spoils a normal Rule K interpretation for Day 22.

On the other hand, the experienced person who views this pattern "knows" that Phase III starts on Day 22 if her normal HTL is between 98.0 and 98.2. Four days of thermal shift with three at the full HTL don't "just happen." There are no indications of sickness, late temperatures, or daylight saving changes at that point in the cycle. The "common sense" explanation is that the elevated temperatures are due to increased progesterone which doesn't come in large quantities until after ovulation.

The conclusion: An interpretation that Phase III starts on the evening of Day 22 does not fit the normal rules. However, it is still a reasonable judgment if 98.1 is in her normal HTL range. We base it on the strength of the four-day thermal shift cross-checked by the two days of drying-up internally and three days of drying-up externally. If the temperature on Day 20 had stayed at 98.1, there would be no question that you could validly apply Rule K on Day 22 with the LTL of 97.7. The "common sense" interpretation says that the dip on Day 20 does not invalidate the strength of the four day pattern, especially since the dip is followed by two more days at the full HTL.

Oh yes. The wife has a sense of humor about her weight, and the couple were "looking for a baby," as they put it. Coitus on Day 18 was at the most fertile time of the cycle. This couple had previously had a problem of secondary infertility; they conceived a few months after this cycle.

Please see the note about non-pregnancy at the end of Chart 21.

Chart 17. The split dry-up; sickness and delayed ovulation

End of Phase I: Clinical Experience = 6   21/20 day rule = 10
                  Doering = n/a   Last dry day = 13
Pre-shift six: 28-33   LTL: 98.2°   HTL: 98.6°
Peak days: 23, 32   First days of cervix closing: 23, 33
Start of Phase III: Rule B = 37   Rule C: n/a

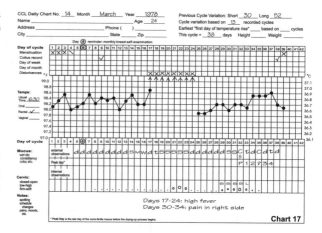

Chart 17

End of Phase I. Self explanatory.

Rectal temperatures. The temperature pattern in this chart is higher throughout the entire cycle compared to most charts in this workbook. That's probably because these are rectal temperatures.

Sickness and delayed ovulation. Sickness is a physical stress that can delay ovulation, and that is apparently what happened in this cycle. As the woman's brain and nervous system reacted to the sickness and shut down the process of ovulation, the level of estrogen dropped, causing the initial drying-up of the mucus and closing of the cervix. The second mucus patch was associated with ovulation as indicated by the progesterone-caused thermal shift immediately afterwards.

Note that in both this cycle and the one illustrated in Chart 9, the second mucus patch was very short. Note also that in Chart 9 there was a 14 day luteal phase (as measured by temperatures) while the cycle in Chart 17 has a very short luteal phase—only five days as measured by temperatures, six from Peak day. We have no sure explanation for this shortness, but we guess that it may have been due to the sickness with its high fever.

The lesson: If you are seeking to postpone pregnancy and experience wifely sickness in Phase I or Phase II, make sure you have a sympto-thermal indication of being in Phase III.

Start of Phase III. The first Peak day occurred on Day 23 and was accompanied by the closing of the cervix, but it was not cross-checked by a thermal shift. The couple wisely considered themselves still in Phase II. The mucus reappeared on Day 30, and a second Peak day occurred on Day 32—which was cross-checked this time by a thermal shift as well as the closing of the cervix.

● **The split dry-up pattern.** Note the more-fertile mucus on Day 35. Do you have to call this another Peak day and restart the drying-up count? With a mucus-only system, you would. In the presence of a good thermal shift, you do not.

Three factors allow us to ignore the mucus on Day 35. 1) The more-fertile mucus appeared for only a single day. 2) The mucus appeared during an obvious and strong thermal shift. 3) In addition, the cervix remained closed. In such a case, label the single day of mucus with a question mark and skip it in counting the four days of drying-up. The requirements for Rule B are met by the evening of Day 37.

We call this the "split dry-up pattern" and explain it in Chapter 27, "Irregular mucus patterns." The mucus on Day 35 was probably caused by a postovulation secondary rise in estrogen. (See Chapter 9, Figure 9.5.)

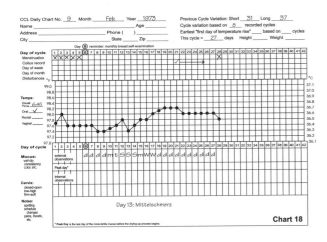

Chart 18. The split peak pattern

End of Phase I: Clinical Exp. = 6   21/20 day rule = 10, but n/a
                      Doering = n/a   Last dry day = 9
Pre-shift six: 11-16   LTL: 97.8°   HTL: 98.2°
Peak days: 14 and 17   First day of cervix closing: n/a
Start of Phase III: Rule R = 20   Rule C = 21

Selecting the pre-shift six. The temperature on Day 17 is obviously part of the thermal shift. Days 15 and 16 are debatable. Since they are before the Peak day and the final Peak day was Day 17, we included Days 15 and 16 in the pre-shift six, following the general principle of trying to keep the last day of the pre-shift six close to Peak day. This guiding principle is not, however, a hard and fast rule.

End of Phase I. Based on the previous short cycle, the 21 Day Rule indicated Day 10 as the end of Phase I. However, you cannot apply that rule if the mucus has already started. Thus Day 9 is the last possible day of Phase I in this cycle. In subsequent cycles, you would use this 27 day cycle to set the 21 Day Rule.

The split peak. The split peak drying-up pattern is explained in Chapter 27; see Figure 27.2. Here we draw your attention to three conditions which make a split peak pattern: 1) you have 1-3 days of drying-up past the first Peak day; 2) your temperature remains low; 3) you have a second mucus patch of one or more days.

Treat the split peak pattern just like a double mucus patch. (The only difference is that double mucus patch requires four or more days of drying-up between the two mucus patches.) Restart the drying-up count after the second Peak day and look for at least three days of temperature cross-check for the start of Phase III.

In this chart, label Day 14 as Peak day, 15 as 1, 16 blank, 17 as the second Peak day, and Days 18-21 as four days of drying-up.

Start of Phase III. Set the LTL at 97.8 and the final Peak day on 17. Rule R yields Day 20, and Rule C yields Day 21 as the start of Phase III.

If her cycle history consistently showed an LTL of not over 97.6, we would not call "wrong" a pre-shift six of 9 - 14, a shaved LTL of 97.6, and a Rule K interpretation yielding Day 19 as the start of Phase III.

Chart 19. Temperatures helping the mucus interpretation: a split dry-up

End of Phase I: Clinical Experience = 6   21/20 day rule = n/a
  Doering = n/a   Last dry day = n/a
Pre-shift six: 14-19   LTL: 97.6°   HTL: 98.0°
Peak day: 17   First day of cervix closing: n/a
Start of Phase III: Rule B = 22   Rule C = 23

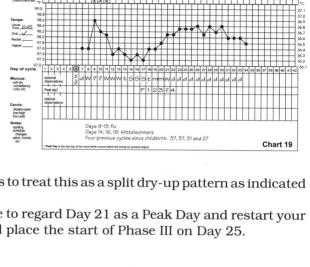
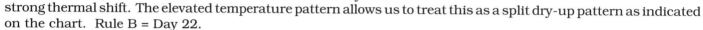

Chart 19

End of Phase I. The indication of "no mucus" on Day 6 allows the application of the Clinical Experience rules up through Day 6. If the woman had six or more recorded cycles, the 21 Day Rule would have yielded Day 6, and the Last Dry Day Rule would have indicated Day 7 as the end of Phase I.

Start of Phase III. The mucus drying-up pattern is confused by the return of wetness on Day 21. However, the next day (22) dryness has returned, and it is the third day of a strong thermal shift. The elevated temperature pattern allows us to treat this as a split dry-up pattern as indicated on the chart. Rule B = Day 22.

If you were using a mucus-only system, you would have to regard Day 21 as a Peak Day and restart your drying-up count. A four-day mucus-only interpretation would place the start of Phase III on Day 25.

Alternate Interpretation:
Pre-shift six: 12-17   LTL: S-97.4°   HTL: 97.8°   Start of Phase III: Rule C = 22
This interpretation (with shaving) follows the guidelines of having the last day of the pre-shift six on or nearly on Peak Day when there's a choice, but it does not advance the start of Phase III. In such cases, we prefer the unshaved interpretation.

Chart 20. Mucus helping the temperature interpretation

End of Phase I: Clinical Exp. = 6   21/20 day rule = 7, n/a (mucus)
  Doering = 10(Mod)   Last dry day = ?
Pre-shift six: 13-18 or 15-20   LTL: S-97.7° or S-97.8°   HTL: 98.1° or 98.2°
Peak day: 18   First day of cervix closing: Insufficient notations
Start of Phase III: Rule B = Day 22 or 23, depending upon LTL. See below.

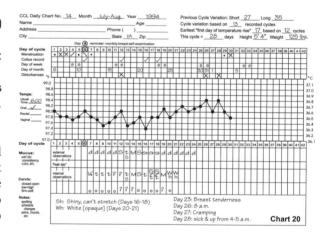
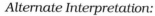

Chart 20

This chart shows that the couple were seeking but did not achieve pregnancy in this cycle. From that perspective it is an easy chart, and they had relations at the appropriate times. However from the perspective of a couple seeking to postpone pregnancy, it is a difficult chart. We will take it step by step.

End of Phase I. The Clinical Experience rule is the only truly clear and unambiguous aspect of this chart, indicating Day 6 as the end of Phase I. The "10(Mod)" for Doering means that a couple can apply the modified Doering rule in the presence of the less-fertile mucus if the wife consistently has all-the-time less-fertile mucus from menses to the start of the more-fertile mucus. You cannot apply the Last Dry Day Rule because there are no true dry days after menstruation. The question mark asks whether what she is observing internally is truly cervical mucus. What she noticed on Day 7 could have been seminal residue. Days 8-10 raise questions that only the woman herself can answer. We would not advise ignoring the less-fertile mucus beyond the limits of the Doering rule.

Phase III. You never see three consecutive temperatures that are above the previous six unshaved temperatures. The question is, "Which temps do you count as the thermal shift?" Look at Peak day. Can you find a series of elevated temperatures beyond Peak day? If you shave Day 19 to the next highest level, you have a shaved LTL of 97.8 and an HTL of 98.2. The temperatures on Days 21-23 provide a sufficient thermal shift so that Rule B yields Day 23 as the start of Phase III. This interpretation is reinforced by the consistently higher level of all the temperatures starting with Day 21.

An alternative interpretation is also based on Peak day. Select the six temperatures ending on Peak day. Average those pre-shift six (Days 13-18), and the result is 97.7. With that as the LTL, the four temperatures on Days 19-22 make a thermal shift to cross-check the four days of drying-up, so Rule B would yield Day 22 in that scenario.

When matters are as difficult as they are in this chart, we would prefer the first interpretation. We think it is better to shave just one temperature than to average all six. The fifth day of drying-up gives added confidence to the first interpretation that Rule B = 23.

Please see the note on non-pregnancy at the end of Chart 21.

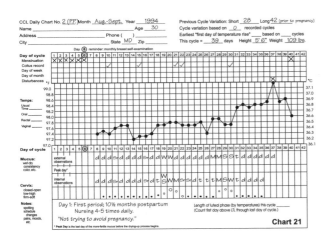

Chart 21. Return of fertility while breastfeeding

End of Phase I: Clinical Experience = 6   21/20 day rule = 7

Doering = n/a   Last dry day = 17

Pre-shift six: 25-30   LTL: 97.9°   HTL: 98.3°

Peak days: 20 and 30   First days of cervix closing: 21 and 31

Start of Phase III: Rule K = 33   Rule C = 34

End of Phase I. When you apply the 21 Day Rule to postpartum cycles, use the shortest cycle in the year before you became pregnant. This couple had sufficient pre-pregnancy experience to use the Last Dry Day Rule.

Phases II and III. It is very tempting to see a thermal shift starting on Day 18, but it lacks two important factors. First, the apparent shift was not preceded by *any* days of mucus; second, there were only four lower temperatures, and the "elevated" temperatures were in the same range as those before the lower four (Days 14-17).

The internal mucus on Day 18 positively indicated the start of Phase II. The <u>first</u> mucus patch and the cervix changes were short. The <u>second</u> mucus patch started with the internal observations on Day 25 and lasted six days; it was followed by a sharp full thermal shift.

Short luteal phase. Nine days of elevated temperatures constitute a short luteal phase. Such short luteal phases are natural and common in the early postpartum cycles among mothers who continue to breastfeed after their first period. What this mother can expect in succeeding cycles is that ovulation will occur earlier and that the luteal phase will gradually lengthen.

Note on Phase II coitus and non-pregnancy. In Charts 16, 20, and 21 you have seen records of couples having intercourse during the fertile time and not becoming pregnant. Such records could lead some couples to imitation, to "taking chances" so we include this reminder: when you have relations at the fertile time, you can normally expect pregnancy. Of course, that assumes you have normal fertility. When you see a chart showing coitus in Phase II and non-pregnancy, you cannot draw any conclusions. The couple might have low mutual fertility. The cycle might be hormonally disturbed. Or it might just be that even among normally fertile couples seeking pregnancy, sometimes it takes a few cycles to achieve pregnancy.

In these charts, the Chart 16 couple had previously had a problem with secondary infertility; judging from the time it took them to conceive they would seem to be a couple of below-average mutual fertility. The unusual patterns in Chart 20 may indicate a cycle that was hormonally disturbed. Chart 21 shows a short luteal phase in a breastfeeding cycle. Such cycles are sub-fertile for many breastfeeding mothers, but many others do achieve pregnancy despite a history of short luteal phases.

The point is this: having marital relations during the fertile time is "pregnancy achieving behavior."

Chart 22. Shaving and averaging

End of Phase I: Clinical Experience = 5   21/20 day rule = 5
Doering = n/a   Last dry day = 8 (assuming Day 6 was SR)

Pre-shift six: 11-16   LTL: S-97.6°   HTL: 98.0°
Peak day: 18   First day of cervix closing: 19
Start of Phase III: Rule K = 21   Rule C = 22
Alternative interpretation: Averaged LTL: 97.5   Rule K = 20

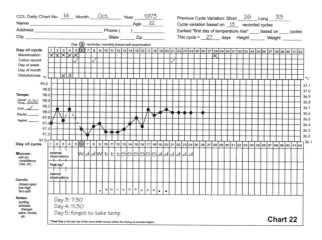

End of Phase I. On the basis of previous cycle history, the Clinical Experience Rule yields Day 6. However, that day must be dry to apply the rule. Whether the "W" is mucus or, more probably, seminal residue, the Phase I rules preclude intercourse on Day 6. If that discharge was truly cervical mucus, then Phase II began on Day 6.

The 21 Day Rule yields Day 5. Can the 20 Day Rule be applied? There are more than 12 cycles, and it would yield Day 6, but it cannot be applied in the presence of mucus or SR that day.

If we assume that the discharge on Day 6 was only seminal residue, the Last Dry Day Rule yielded Day 8. The discharge on Day 9 was probably seminal residue or a combination of SR and the less-fertile mucus that continued on Day 10.

Shaving. The temperature on Day 15 has to be shaved to the next highest level to get any of the Phase III rules to fit. With Rule K, you need three days consecutively at the full thermal shift level, 98.0, so Rule K yields Day 21.

Averaging. The four-day thermal shift on Days 17-20 is so strong that it invites the effort to see if the rules will allow a Day 20 interpretation. Averaging the pre-shift six (11-16) yields an LTL of 97.48 that rounds up to 97.5. When you average or shave and want to apply Rule K with only two days of drying-up, you need four days of thermal shift with the last three at the HTL. Those requirements are met on Day 20.

Chart 23. Unusual discordance of mucus and temperature

End of Phase I: Clinical Experience = 6   21/20 day rule = 5
Doering = n/a   Last dry day = 10
Pre-shift six: 10 - 15   LTL: S-98.1°   HTL: 98.5°
Peak day: 16   First day of cervix closing: n/a
Start of Phase III: Rule B = 20   Rule C = 24

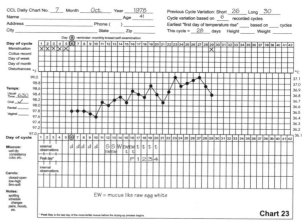

End of Phase I. Self explanatory, but we would recommend using the internal observation of the mucus. With a cycle range of 26 to 30 days, experience suggests that extending Phase I to Day 10 is pushing it unless she is so experienced that she can observe the first sign of mucus at the cervical os.

Start of Phase III. The problem is that the mucus discharge doesn't *start* until an upward thermal shift has started. Such a discordance is weird and hints that the cycle may be hormonally irregular. Normally, the upward thermal shift starts very close to Peak day. So if you look for a thermal shift starting close to Peak day, you see that on Peak day itself the temperatures start into a higher pattern. Counting Days 10-15 as the pre-shift six and shaving Days 13 and 14 to the next highest level, you have a shaved LTL of 98.1. On that basis you find a very strong Rule B on Day 20 with a five day overall thermal shift. Rule C yields Day 24, and that is far too conservative for normal use.

An alternative interpretation might use a pre-shift five of Days 6 - 10 to set the LTL at 97.8; Rule K would yield Day 18 as the start of Phase III. That interpretation respects the general rule of "three above the previous six" but seems unrealistic in the face of the mucus discharge. With the temperatures tending downward and the "weirdness" of the overall pattern, we would advise waiting until Peak + 3. On Day 19 (Peak + 3), the temperature has also strengthened. A Rule K interpretation on Day 19 would be reasonable.

Chart 24. Rule B with disturbed temperature

End of Phase I: Clinical Exp. = 5   21/20 day rule = 5
                  Doering = n/a   Last dry day = 6?
Pre-shift six: 6-11   LTL: 97.7°   HTL: 98.1°
Peak day: 12   First day of cervix closing: 13
Start of Phase III: Rule B = 16   Rule C = 18

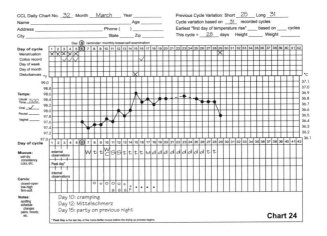

Chart 24

End of Phase I. Coitus on consecutive days may hinder the observation of early mucus. Second, it may assist extended sperm life. That is, the first coitus may change the vaginal environment from acidic to alkaline, thus aiding sperm life, just as cervical mucus does. Those factors are the reasons for the "not-on-consecutive-days" rule in Phase I. This rule is especially important past the limits of the Clinical Experience rule for your cycle pattern. However, the days within the limits of the Clinical Experience rule for your pattern are so infertile that the rule is much less important. Therefore, we do not think the couple in this case were "taking chances."

Start of Phase III. The temperatures on Days 12-14 definitely do not make a full thermal shift as required for Rule K, even if you shave Day 10 to 97.6°. The disturbed and therefore invalid temperature on Day 15 eliminates the possibility of a shaved Rule R. The earliest interpretation is Rule B = 16.

Practical Applications Workbook

Part III:

Does God Care about Birth Control?

You will find that you will soon learn all you need to know about the "technique" of Natural Family Planning. Making your daily observations, charting, and knowing where you are in your cycle will soon become more or less "second nature."

You will also find that no one who is at all informed will really challenge you about the value of the different signs of fertility or infertility. If someone has some sincere questions about the method, you'll be able to answer most of them quite well by the time you're half way through your NFP learning process or have charted for two or three cycles. Articles in the media tend to question or misrepresent the effectiveness of NFP as a method of family planning, but once you study Chapter 13, you will be able to answer such statements.

However, you will find that there are other questions that keep coming up over and over again, and these are concerned with morality and religion. In short, "Does God care what you do about birth control?" We believe He does. Chapter 18 provides the reasons for that belief from the Bible and Tradition; Chapter 19 applies human reason and observation to this issue. However, in Chapter 16 we start this part of the book with a review of the principles for deciding whether God is calling you to achieve or to postpone pregnancy, and Chapter 17 shows how NFP can have a good effect upon your marriage.

You may be tempted to skip over some of these chapters. Please don't. Regardless of your faith or religious preference, if you read the newspapers or watched the news on television during the '80s and '90s, you learned at least one thing about Pope John Paul II: he has vigorously proclaimed the very unpopular teaching of the Catholic Church that it is a serious moral evil to use unnatural methods of birth control. It is probably obvious to you that he is not doing this just because it's his job to promote the teaching of his Church but that he also *really believes* it. Why?

If you are an atheist or agnostic, you should have enough intellectual curiosity to want to know why the leader of the world's largest Christian church keeps himself on such a collision course with contemporary culture. You should also grant these premises: if there is a God, then surely 1) He can reveal how man is called to live and 2) He can keep his truth alive despite the shortcomings of those through whom He chooses to work.

If you are Catholic, Part II will provide you with a short and clear explanation of the teachings of your Church regarding birth control.

If you are Protestant or Jewish or whatever you may be, you may find yourself surprisingly in agreement with Catholic teaching on birth control once you see it in context.

For a fuller picture, read CCL's booklet, *Birth Control and Christian Discipleship*; it's been a real eye-opener for many. For a more extended treatment of the moral, religious, and theological aspects of birth control and the rest of the sexual revolution, read *Sex and the Marriage Covenant* by John F. Kippley. Called "must reading for anyone concerned with marriage, sexuality and the family" by one of its reviewers, *Sex and the Marriage Covenant* is a readable explanation of traditional Christian teaching about sexuality in the context of what couples do when they enter the marriage covenant. See "Resources" near the end of this manual.

We start this part of the manual with a chapter dealing with the moral use of natural family planning. We wish it were shorter, but we thought it best to put you in contact with the original sources.

16

Planning, Providence and Prudence

For many couples, the biggest question about natural family planning is this: "Should we use it to achieve pregnancy or to postpone it." Why?

Many couples come to recognize that marriage is for family, not just for enjoying each other. They recognize the general biblical call to generosity in having children, and they also recognize that God's plan includes a natural spacing of babies. They want to do what is right by God, and they also wonder whether the Lord is calling them to conceive another child right now in their present circumstances. In our experience, the couples who are most concerned about these things are generally practicing Catholics and Evangelical Protestants.

In addition, some wonder if it is being untrusting on their part to do ANY planning, to exercise ANY prudence. They wonder if they should not just put all their trust in the Providence of God and just let the babies come as they may. When couples adopt the position that *they* should not do any planning, we call it "providentialism." When they go further and say that *no one*, and least no one who believes in God, should use NFP for *any* prudential reasons, we call it "extreme providentialism."

In this chapter we are not going to rehash the "extreme providentialism" debate. We make a few references to it in Chapter 18. Suffice it to say that our experience indicates that the proponents of this view accept the Catholic position once they understand it. Therefore, we will attempt to explain Catholic teaching regarding providence and prudence in family planning. For a more complete review, see "The Moral Use of Natural Family Planning" by Prof. Janet E. Smith.[1]

I. Principles

As mentioned above, for many couples the most difficult aspect of NFP is whether to use it to achieve or to avoid pregnancy. That's because there are two complementary principles involved—the call to generosity and the call to Christian prudence. They are not contradictory principles, but sometimes they appear to tug in different directions.

The Call to Generosity

The first general principle is that spouses are called to be generous in the service of life. Marriage is for family. Specifically, if a young couple should attempt to marry with the intention of never having any children, it would not be a true marriage unless they had extremely serious reasons for avoiding pregnancy. This principle is founded on both the Bible and Tradition.

Genesis 1:28

And God blessed them, and God said to them,
"Be fruitful and multiply, and fill the earth and subdue it;
and have dominion over the fish of the sea
and over the birds of the air
and over every living thing that moves upon the earth."

You've probably heard the joke, "Wouldn't it be nice if all the commandments were as easy to keep as the first part of this one." The fact remains, however, that this is the first commandment of the Bible and it has not been deleted or completely fulfilled. Despite the gloomy talk of the anti-population propagandists, all the world's population could fit in the state of Texas with 1361 square feet per person.[2] Except for Ireland, the Western European countries have been experiencing a below-replacement population rate for years. The only factors that keep the U.S. population increasing are immigration and babies born out of wedlock. In Europe and North America, married couples are not having enough children to sustain the population.

Psalms 127 and 128

These verses are regularly quoted in the discussion about the biblical perspective on family planning. If you want to start nit-picking, you will be able to note that these verses reflect a time when a number of strapping sons gave credibility to a father when he met his enemies. That generally is not the case today, but with the breakdown of civility in the West, it may again be the case in the future. Such verses say nothing about the man who has a household of four or five daughters, nor about the couple who are past their youth but certainly not past their mutual fertility. Still, these verses provide a good introduction to the widespread biblical teaching that children are a blessing from the Lord.

Lo, sons are a heritage from the LORD,
the fruit of the womb a reward.
Like arrows in the hand of a warrior
are the sons of one's youth.
Happy is the man who has his quiver full of them!
He shall not be put to shame
when he speaks with his enemies in the gate *(Ps 127: 3-5)*.

Your wife will be like a fruitful vine within your house;
your children will be like olive shoots around your table.
Lo, thus shall the man be blessed who fears the LORD
(Ps 128: 3-4).

It is important to realize that in the first modern papal condemnation of unnatural methods of birth control, there are both a call to generosity in the service of life and the acceptance of the principle of spacing babies through natural family planning. The reasoning of Pope Pius XI concerning generosity emphasizes the supernatural destiny of Man:

> Besides, God wishes men to be born that they may be worshippers of God, that they may know Him and love Him and finally enjoy Him forever in heaven; and this end, since man is raised by God in a marvelous way to the supernatural order, surpasses all that eye has seen, and ear heard, and all that has entered into the heart of man.[3]

God had no need to create the universe. He did so simply to share his goodness with others. By entrusting procreation to couples, He put Himself in the position of needing spouses to cooperate in the procreation of those "others" with whom God wants to share his life and happiness in heaven for all eternity. There is also no question that spouses benefit by being parents and that children benefit from having ample brothers and sisters.

During the 1940s, the temperature sign had been added to the Calendar Rhythm that was developed in the early 1930s. This addition made it much more effective. There was no question that it had attained such efficiency that it could be used with selfish intent and results. Perhaps that is part of the background for the teaching of Pope Pius XII in 1951. It's a long quotation, and the language is not always easy, but it's an important one.

> The mere fact that the couple do not offend the nature of the act and are prepared to accept and bring up the child, which in spite of their precautions came into the world, would not be sufficient in itself to guarantee the rectitude of intention and the unobjectionable morality of the motives themselves.
>
> The reason for this is that marriage obliges to a state of life which, while conferring certain rights, also imposes the fulfillment of a positive work in regard to the married state itself. In such a case, one can apply the general principle that a positive fulfillment may be omitted when serious reasons, independent from the good will of those obliged by it, show that a similar demand cannot reasonably be made of human nature. . .
>
> But upon couples who perform the act peculiar to their state, nature and the Creator impose the function of helping the conservation of the human race. . . The individual and society, the people and the state, the Church itself depend for their existence on the order established by God on fruitful marriage. Therefore, to embrace the married state, continuously to make use of the faculty proper to it and lawful in it alone, and on the other hand, to withdraw always and deliberately with no serious reason from its primary obligation would be a sin against the very meaning of conjugal life.
>
> There are serious motives, such as those often mentioned in the so-called medical, eugenic, economic and social "indications," that can exempt for a long time, perhaps even the whole duration of the marriage, from the positive and obligatory carrying out of the act. From this it follows that observing the non-fertile periods alone can be lawful only under a moral

Pius XI

Pope Pius XI issued Casti Connubii, *"Chaste Marriage," on December 31, 1930, to reaffirm traditional Christian teaching against unnatural forms of birth control.*

Pius XII

Pope Pius XII made this "Address to the Italian Catholic Union of Midwives" on October 29, 1951 to warn against the selfish use of natural family planning.

aspect. Under the conditions mentioned it really is so. But if, according to a rational and just judgment, there are no similar grave reasons of a personal nature or deriving from external circumstances, then the determination to avoid habitually the fecundity of the union while at the same time to continue satisfying their sensuality, can be derived only from a false appreciation of life and from reasons having nothing to do with proper ethical laws.[4]

The main points from this statement are these:

1. Married couples have a positive obligation to procreate and to educate their children.

2. The good of the couple, the Church, and society depend upon married couples fulfilling this obligation.

3. Positive obligations can be reduced or eliminated for sufficiently serious reasons. This applies to the obligation of procreation; the most serious reasons could exempt a couple from this normal duty for their entire fertile years.

4. However, to avoid children always and deliberately without an extremely serious reason would be "a sin against the very meaning of marriage."

5. There are different sorts of reasons that can constitute grave or sufficiently serious reasons for avoiding or postponing pregnancy. (See the next section, "The Call to Christian Prudence," for more on this.)

Vatican II

The Second Vatican Council document titled *Gaudium et Spes* (*The Church in the Modern World*), addressed the issues of marriage, love, and family planning in 1965. The following quotation comes from section 50 titled "The fruitfulness of marriage." (We will quote other portions of Section 50 when we discuss planning and prudence.)

Gaudium et Spes was issued on December 7, 1965.

50.1 Marriage and married love are by nature ordered to the procreation and education of children. Indeed children are the supreme gift of marriage and greatly contribute to the good of the parents themselves. . . Without intending to underestimate the other ends of marriage, it must be said that true married love and the whole structure of family life which results from it is directed to disposing the spouses to cooperate valiantly with the love of the Creator and Savior, who through them will increase and enrich his family from day to day.

50.2 Married couples should regard it as their proper mission to transmit human life and to educate their children; they should realize that they are thereby cooperating with the love of God the Creator and are, in a certain sense, its interpreters. . .

Whenever Christian spouses in a spirit of sacrifice and trust in divine providence carry out their duties of procreation with generous human and Christian responsibility, they glorify the Creator and perfect themselves in Christ. Among the married couples who thus fulfill their God-given mission, special mention should be made of those who after prudent reflection and common decision courageously undertake the proper upbringing of a large number of children.[5]

It has been fashionable in some quarters to give the impression that any call to generosity in the service of life went out with Vatican II. It should be clear that such opinions are definitely not founded on the actual teaching of Vatican II.

In 1968, Pope Paul VI addressed the moral use of natural family planning in two sections of *Humanae Vitae*. In section 10, titled "Responsible Parenthood," he said:

> If we look further to physical, economic, psychological, and social conditions, responsible parenthood is exercised by those who, guided by prudent consideration and generosity, elect to accept many children. Those are also to be considered responsible who, for serious reasons [*seriis causis*] and with due respect for moral precepts, decide not to have another child for either a definite or an indefinite amount of time (Janet E. Smith translation in *Why Humanae Vitae Was Right*).

Paul VI said more about this in section 16, "The Morality of Recourse to the Infertile Period." We do not wish to be nit-picking, but the translation of key words *does* make a difference. For example, in the paragraph above, the NC News Service translation translates *"seriis causis"* as "grave motives." The problem is, that sort of terminology can give the impression that a woman has to have one foot in the grave to justify the use of NFP, and that simply is not true. Therefore in what follows we will give the translation by classics scholar Janet E. Smith; then in brackets we provide the Latin in italics and the NC News translation of the key words in quotation marks.

> Certainly, there may be serious reasons [*justae causae*, "serious motives"] for spacing offspring. . .
> The Church is not inconsistent when it teaches both that it is morally permissible for spouses to have recourse to infertile periods and also that all directly contraceptive practices are morally wrong, even if spouses seem to have good and serious reasons [*argumenta . . . honesta et gravia*, "honest and serious"] for using these.
> It cannot be denied that the spouses in each case have, for defensible reasons [*probabiles rationes*, "plausible reasons"], made a mutual and firm decision to avoid having a child. . .
> . . . when for good reasons [*justae rationes*, "just motives"] offspring are not desired (*H. V.*, n. 16).

More will be said about these texts in the concluding section on "Responsible Parenthood: Prudence in Planning."

Pope John Paul II celebrated Mass on the Washington Mall when he visited the United States in October 1979. The following quotation is from his homily at that Liturgy. Even secular television commentators were impressed by the reasons he gave in his call to married couples to be generous in having children.

> Human life is precious because it is the gift of a God whose love is infinite: and when God gives life, it is for ever. Life is also precious because it is the expression and the fruit of love. This

Humanae Vitae

Humanae Vitae *was issued on July 25, 1968 to respond to questions raised by the Pill.*

John Paul II

In his first visit to the United States, Pope John Paul II made these remarks in his homily on October 7, 1979.

is why life should spring up within the setting of marriage, and why marriage and the parents' love for one another should be marked by generosity in self-giving. The great danger for family life, in the midst of any society whose idols are pleasure, comfort and independence, lies in the fact that people close their hearts and become selfish. The fear of making permanent commitments can change the mutual love of husband and wife into two loves of self—two loves existing side by side, until they end in separation. . .

In order that Christian marriage may favor the total good and development of the married couple, it must be inspired by the Gospel, and thus be open to new life—new life to be given and accepted generously. The couple is also called to create a family atmosphere in which children can be happy, and lead full and worthy human and Christian lives.

To maintain a joyful family requires much from both the parents and the children. Each member of the family has to become, in a special way, the servant of the others and share their burdens (cf. Gal 6:2; Phil 2:2). Each one must show concern, not only for his or her own life, but also for the lives of the other members of the family: their needs, their hopes, their ideals.

Decisions about the number of children and the sacrifices to be made for them must not be taken only with a view to adding to comfort and preserving a peaceful existence. Reflecting upon this matter before God, with the graces drawn from the Sacrament, and guided by the teaching of the Church, parents will remind themselves that it is certainly less serious to deny their children certain comforts or material advantages than to deprive them of the presence of brothers and sisters, who could help them to grow in humanity and to realize the beauty of life at all its ages and in all its variety.

If parents fully realized the demands and the opportunities that this great sacrament brings, they could not fail to join in Mary's hymn to the author of life—to God—who has made them his chosen fellow-workers.[6]

In brief, here John Paul II teaches
1) the preciousness of human life and its eternal destiny
2) the dangers of materialism
3) that children benefit their parents
4) the challenges and demands of love in parenting
5) the great value of siblings to each other.

The Catechism

This teaching is summarized as follows in the *Catechism of the Catholic Church.*

Fecundity is a gift, an *end of marriage,* for conjugal love naturally tends to be fruitful. A child does not come from outside as something added on to the mutual love of the spouses, but springs from the very heart of that mutual giving, as its fruit and fulfillment. So the Church, which "is on the side of life"[a] teaches that "each and every marriage act must remain open to the transmission of life."[b] "This particular doctrine, expounded on numerous occasions by the Magisterium, is based on the inseparable connection, established by God, which man on his own initiative may not break, between the unitive significance and the procreative significance which are both inherent to the marriage act"[c7] (n. 2366).

In summary, the teaching of the Bible and Tradition make it clear: there is no question that NFP needs to be learned and practiced in the context of the Gospel and the call to generosity in the service of life. Couples need sufficiently serious reasons to avoid pregnancy. When they use NFP to avoid pregnancy, they need to ask themselves periodically if those sufficiently serious reasons still exist.

The Call to Christian Prudence

After the above, you may think it strange to continue with this section. However, Christian teaching is frequently "both this and that." Every heresy starts with an emphasis on just one truth and eventually denies a corresponding truth. Just as Catholic teaching insists on both the full divinity **and** the full humanity of Jesus Christ, so it also insists on both the call to generosity **and** the right of parents to exercise Christian prudence.

We start with a sentence from *Casti Connubii* (*On Chaste Marriage*), the 1930 encyclical in which Pope Pius XI vigorously reaffirmed the traditional Christian teaching against all unnatural forms of birth control.

Pius XI

> Nor are those considered as acting against nature who in the married state use their right in the proper manner, although on account of natural reasons either of time or of certain defects, new life cannot be brought forth.[8]

The first meaning of that paragraph is that the teaching against contraception does not exclude marital relations during menopause or by infertile couples. However, we think it also applies to NFP. In the 1920s, scientists had discovered the first of the principles on which natural family planning is based—that ovulation occurs approximately two weeks before the next menstruation. Even though Calendar Rhythm was not yet promoted, we think the Pope must have been informed about the scientific principles. Besides, well before the actual physical principles were known, theologians had discussed the morality of marital relations during the infertile times—if there were such times. Such moral questions reached the appropriate office of the Vatican. As a result, the Vatican gave its approval to the *principle* of NFP in the 19th century. We think that Pope Pius XI combined the already accepted moral principle with the new scientific discoveries. Thus the above statement is the first statement at the papal level approving the use of NFP.

Pius XII

During the postwar period, discussion about the moral use of NFP was renewed. We repeat three sentences from the 1951 address of Pope Pius XII to Italian midwives. They set the stage for all that follows.

> There are serious motives, such as those often mentioned in the so-called medical, eugenic, economic and social "indications," that can exempt for a long time, perhaps even the whole duration of the marriage, from the positive and obligatory carrying out of the act. From this it follows that observing the non-fertile periods alone can be lawful only under a moral aspect. Under the conditions mentioned it really is so.[9]

Vatican II

This quotation starts with a repetition of a sentence quoted previously and continues with what was omitted there.

> 50.2 Married couples should regard it as their proper mission to transmit human life and to educate their children; they should realize that they are thereby cooperating with the love of God the Creator and are, in a certain sense, its interpreters. This involves the fulfillment of their role with a sense of human and Christian responsibility and the formation of correct judgments through docile respect for God and common reflection and effort; it also involves a consideration of their own good and the good of their children already born or yet to come, an ability to read the signs of the times and of their own situation on the material and spiritual level, and, finally, an estimation of the good of the family, of society, and of the Church.
>
> It is the married couple themselves who must in the last analysis arrive at these judgments before God. Married people should realize that in their behavior they may not simply follow their own fancy but must be ruled by conscience—and conscience ought to be conformed to the law of God in the light of the teaching authority of the Church, which is the authentic interpreter of divine law.[10]

Humanae Vitae

We quote here the full paragraph from which we previously quoted part of the first sentence.

> Certainly, there may be serious reasons [*justae causae*] for spacing offspring; these may be based on the physical or psychological condition of the spouses or on external factors. The Church teaches that [in such cases] it is morally permissible [for spouses] to calculate [their fertility by observing the] natural rhythms inherent in the generative faculties and to reserve marital intercourse for infertile times. Thus spouses are able to plan their families without violating the moral teachings set forth above (n. 16).[11]

In December 1990, Pope John Paul II addressed a group of NFP teachers and emphasized that couples are called to discern God's will for them. He also strongly criticized a secular, closed-to-life, use of NFP techniques. In short, he calls for truly Christian prudence.

> Through this sense of responsibility for love and life, God the Creator invites the spouses not to be passive operators, but rather "cooperators or almost interpreters" of His plan (*Gaudium et Spes*, n. 50). In fact, they are called, out of respect for the objective moral order established by God, to an obligatory discernment of the indications of God's will concerning their family. Thus in relationship to physical, economic, psychological and social conditions, responsible parenthood will be able to be expressed "either by the deliberate and generous decision to raise a large family, or by the decision, made for serious moral reasons and with due respect for the moral law, to avoid for the time being, or even for an indeterminate period, another birth" (*Humanae Vitae*, n. 10).[12]

". . .called . . . to an obligatory discernment . . ."

"Called. . . to an obligatory discernment of the indications of God's will concerning their family." That's a strong statement about the need to pray and think about family size.

In this same talk, the Pope went on to stress that morality needs to be taught right along with the techniques of natural family planning. In doing so he neatly balanced what he said above with the call to openness to parenthood. Referring to NFP instruction, he said:

> This intrinsic connection between science and moral virtue constitutes the specific and morally qualifying element for recourse to natural methods. It should be clear that what is of concern here is more than just simple "instruction" divorced from the moral values proper to teaching people about love. In short, it allows people to see that it is not possible to practice natural methods as a "licit" variation of the decision to be closed to life, which would be substantially the same as that which inspires the decision to use contraceptives: only if there is a basic openness to fatherhood and motherhood, understood as collaboration with the Creator, does the use of natural means become an integrating part of the responsibility for love and life.[13]

We also want to quote some additional comments from this talk even though they are not directly related to the subject of planning.

> In applying this scientific knowledge to regulating fertility, technology in no way substitutes for the involvement of the persons and neither does it intervene by manipulating the nature of the relationship, as is the case with contraception in which the unitive meaning of the conjugal act is deliberately separated from its procreative meaning. To the contrary, in practicing natural methods science must always be joined with self-control, since, in using them, virtue—that perfection belonging specifically to the person—is necessarily a factor.
>
> Thus we can say that periodic continence, practiced to regulate procreation in a natural way, *requires a profound understanding of the person and of love.* In truth, that requires mutual listening and dialogue by spouses, attention and sensi-

tivity for the other spouse and constant self-control: all of these are qualities which express real love for the person of the spouse for what he or she is, and not for what one may wish the other to be. The practice of natural methods requires personal growth by the spouses in a joint effort to strengthen their love.[14]

Read those last two sentences again. They help to show how much the Pope truly does understand what married life and love is all about.

Summary

Catholic teaching about the moral use of NFP is clear: there do exist good reasons for postponing pregnancy, and individual couples have to make the decisions about seeking and avoiding pregnancy. No one can do it for them.

On the other hand, there are all sorts of reasons that are frivolous or selfish. They are prudent only in a highly materialistic, money counting, and pleasure seeking sense of "prudence." Couples would find it difficult to defend such reasons before the Lord.

II. Responsible Parenthood: Prudence in Planning

For a couple of normal fertility, it is easy to plan but it may be difficult to be prudent. The reasons for this are easy to see after a bit of thought.

Prudence versus materialism

Most of us are highly influenced by the materialism of Western culture that generally regards babies as liabilities instead of assets. We stand in constant need of the Gospel corrections. The public life of Jesus starts with the temptation to materialism, and Jesus answers, "Not by bread alone does man live but by every word that comes forth from the mouth of God" (Mt 4:4). In the Beatitudes, Jesus teaches, "Blessed are the poor in spirit, for theirs is the kingdom of heaven" (Mt 5:3).

The anti-materialism of Jesus is a major theme in the Gospel of Luke. It is in Luke that we read the parable of the rich man with the two barns who hears from God, "You fool, this very night you will meet your Maker. Those things you have stored up, whose will they be?" (Lk 12:20). In that same chapter, we are told to trust in God's providence and to stop worrying about what to eat and wear (22-31). We are told to lay up our treasures in heaven by giving alms because "where your treasure is, there will your heart be also" (32-34). In Luke 16 we are told bluntly, "You cannot serve God and money" (13), and the last part of Luke 16 relates the extremely sobering account of the rich man who goes to a place of torment and the poor beggar Lazarus who goes to heaven.

Those of us who are influenced by the materialism in which we live need to realize that true prudence is far different from the purely money oriented calculation that passes for prudence in the culture of secular materialism. And how can we even start to compare ordinary middle-class material well-being with that of former ages in history or with that of less developed nations today?

Prudence versus presumption

Some of us have worked very hard to free ourselves from secular materialism, and some of us may need the lesson of Jesus in his second temptation. Here the tempter challenges Him to jump off the top of the temple. Jesus responds, "Thou shalt not tempt the Lord thy God" (Mt 4:7). In other words, "Thou shalt not demand a miracle to counter your own free choice."

The question here is this: when, if ever, is "trusting God" a matter of presumption, not a virtue but a fault at best? Are there some circumstances in which we might be **obliged** to practice NFP to avoid pregnancy?

Yes. Since we live in extreme times, there are extreme examples. What if you lived in a country such as China in the 1980s and 1990s and already had the one or two children "permitted" by government policy? What if you knew that another child in the womb would be forcibly killed by abortion? We think you would be morally obliged to abstain during the fertile times to avoid pregnancy and consequent forced abortion. (To show *your* rejection of such a government policy, try not to buy products made in such countries, and write letters to the ambassadors of such countries.)

Are there less extreme cases in which we might be obliged to practice NFP to avoid pregnancy? Drawing from his experience as a priest and bishop before he became Pope John Paul II, Karol Wojtyla wrote:

Obliged to practice NFP to avoid pregnancy? Obviously, another morally permissible choice would be total abstinence. However, we think that in most cases it is better for the couple to practice periodic rather than total abstinence.

There are, however, circumstances in which this disposition [to be a responsible parent] itself demands renunciation of procreation, and any further increase in the size of the family would be incompatible with parental duty. A man and a woman moved by true concern for the good of their family and a mutual sense of responsibility for the birth, maintenance, and upbringing of their children, will then limit intercourse and abstain from it in periods in which this might result in another pregnancy undesirable in the particular conditions of their married life and family.[15]

Without being materialistic, it is easy to imagine such circumstances. Serious health problems. Dire poverty. Active persecution. And you may be able to think of others.

Sufficiently serious reasons

For most of us, the question will not be, "Are we *obliged* to avoid pregnancy?" For most of us, the recurring question will be, "Are we *justified* in avoiding pregnancy right now?" In other words, not "Must we?" but "May we?"

To put it in the words of *Humanae Vitae,* do we have reasons that are grave or serious, just, worthy and weighty, and defensible? Do these terms mean that we have to have one foot in the health or economic or social grave? Professor Janet E. Smith offers her opinion:

It is my view that the common rendering of some of these phrases, such as "serious reasons" or "grave reasons," may suggest weightier reasons are required than is necessary. I believe the phrase "just reasons" to reflect more precisely what is meant. Trivial reasons will not do, but reasons less than life-threatening conditions will.[16]

After quoting from *Gaudium et Spes* as we have done above, she concludes,

It seems right to say, then, that the Church teaches that in planning their family size, spouses need to be just to all their obligations: those to God, to each other, to the family they already have, and to all their commitments. They need to have defensible reasons, ones that are not selfish but that are directed to a good beyond their own comfort and convenience.[17]

Elsewhere in this book we have used the term "sufficiently serious reasons" to designate such just and defensible reasons for using natural family planning to avoid pregnancy. "Sufficiently serious" means unselfish. "Defensible" means that if you met the Lord tonight, you could honestly tell Him that you thought that He was calling you, through your circumstances, to avoid pregnancy for the present (if that is your current decision). That's why the decision takes mutual discussion and prayer.

● Obligations to our children

We all need to understand that procreation also involves the education of our children. This does not by any means refer only to educating them in reading, writing, and arithmetic. It means primarily bringing them up in the ways of the Lord—religion and character formation. As the Pope indicated in 1979, another sibling may be a big help in character formation.

Some people have great inner resources; others have less. In some areas parents have great confidence that they can delegate much of the education of their children to teachers in schools; in other areas, parents have concluded that they need to educate their children at home.

1. Inner resources. Some parents have great emotional and physical energy and strength; others have less. Some parents are blessed with wonderful health; the health of other parents makes it more difficult to care for a large number of children. Some wives are blessed with husbands who help with the care and education of the children, but the travel and other demands of some husbands' employment leave them all too little time to be as helpful as they would like to be. (Many husbands are leaving such overly-demanding jobs in order to be with their families, but not everyone may have that choice.)

2. Age of children. As your older children move into their teen years, you may find that you need to spend more time with them. (The easy years of child rearing are from 2 to 12. Enjoy those years to the fullest.) On the other hand, sharing in a few of the responsibilities of child care may be the best thing that can happen for many teenagers.

3. "Nature" of your children. Some children are easy-going; others are demanding. Some children are blessed with excellent health; others may have a chronic problem that takes much time and energy on the part of their parents.

4. Education. There is no question that parents are the primary educators of their children. It is one of their greatest privileges and duties. In some geographic areas, parents think they can delegate much of the education of their children to private or public schools. In other geographic areas, the quality of such education leads many parents to conclude that they should educate their children at home. Others make the home-education decision simply because they believe it is best for their children even when the local schools enjoy a good reputation. Regardless of the reasons, home education generally places most of the responsibility upon the full-time homemaking mother. Most such mothers find home education is a real joy, but it is also real work. Some mothers receive great practical help from their husbands; others receive only moral support. We once heard a homeschooling mother of five, the youngest a baby, give her teaching responsibilities as their reason for using NFP for spacing. Five years later, they believed that they could then handle the additional responsibilities, and had their sixth child.

We are not trying to provide a bunch of excuses or rationalizations for parents who just don't like the work involved in rearing children. We are simply saying that at some point, the very real responsibilities you have to your existing children may provide a serious reason for keeping your family at its present size—at least for the present.

● Obligations to others

In some cases, the care of parents, dedication to public service or to apostolic work within the Church and similar commitments will certainly be factors in the exercise of Christian prudence. On the other hand, dedication to commitments outside the family—the primary apostolate—can sometimes be more of an excuse than a valid reason.

● Family size

The Church does not officially promote any size as the ideal. The norm is generosity according to your circumstances, and for most of us that means a size that requires sacrifice on our part as parents. However, individuals have made suggestions about family size. Janet Smith quotes a friend of hers who was quite relieved when they had their third child since he believed that was the critical number for adequate family interaction. Dr. Herbert Ratner has told many audiences that he believes that five children is the minimum for optimum socialization of the children. It seems to be an almost universal experience that it is easier to raise three to five children than it is to raise one or two, or at least that it is more difficult to raise the first two children.

Newlyweds

Many newlyweds plan to delay pregnancy until they are well established financially. They may have a serious need to reflect upon the anti-materialism teachings of Jesus as they are assembled in the Gospel of Luke. Other newlyweds want to start a family right away, but they have no experience of paying for their own basic food, rent and utilities. Because of such great variation, it's hard to give any specific advice, so we will limit ourselves to a few general observations.

1. Too little money can be a source of marital stress, but sometimes this is the stress we need to make us grow.

2. Too much money can be an equal or greater source of stress. Spending money that you didn't have to work hard for can develop bad habits of overspending and create real problems. Proper tithing can help put things in perspective.

3. "Too little money" frequently means "too much debt." That, in turn, frequently means that the newlyweds bought expensive furniture and appliances. Then they're afraid that kids will damage it.

To our young friends we say this: you need only a minimum of furniture to get started. You can get almost everything you need from estate sales, etc. The big exception: invest in a king-size bed so there's room for you and your children, but you don't need either a headboard or a footboard. We've been married over 30 years and have never missed them.

4. Delayed childbearing can create serious problems in your relationship unless you truly do have sufficiently serious reasons for such delays. You and your spouse can look into each other's eyes only for so long. Then you start noticing the pimples—your mutual personality defects. In the natural order of things, a newly married couple soon direct their energies to their children, children who are the physical expressions of their love, their joint projects. Children are a great blessing and joy to their parents in more ways than one.

5. We have never seen "Getting to know each other" listed as a sufficiently serious reason for delaying pregnancy. Isn't the purpose of the engagement period to get to know each other through the exchange of ideas? Too often, the pre-engagement and engagement periods are so social that the couple hardly have time to discuss the important things of life. We suggest that our book, *Marriage Is for Keeps*,[18] can be a valuable tool for raising the important questions—whether the couple are pre-engaged, engaged, or married.

6. Marriage is for family. What Vatican II teaches about children really is true:

> By its very nature the institution of marriage and married love
> is ordered to the procreation and education of the offspring, and
> it is in them that it finds its crowning glory.[19]

Q. Should we discuss our "family plans" with a priest?

R. If you are perplexed whether you have sufficiently serious reasons to postpone pregnancy, you might find it helpful to discuss your situation with a Christ-centered priest or other third party. Such an impartial third party might help you to evaluate your circumstances and your reasoning. Such a person can also help you understand if you are being too strict with yourselves.

It seems to us that the two sides of Catholic teaching about family size—generosity and prudence—are summed up in section 50.2 of *Gaudium et Spes* and by the homily of Pope John Paul II on the Washington Mall.

The Pope himself drew attention to both sides of this teaching in a brief message to pilgrims in July 1994 as the battle about population and birth control was warming up for the full scale confrontation at the United Nations Conference on Population and Development in Cairo.

> Unfortunately, *Catholic thought is often misunderstood* on this point [about "responsible parenthood"], as if the Church supported an ideology of fertility at all costs, urging married couples to procreate indiscriminately and without thought for the future. But one need only study the pronouncements of the Magisterium to know that this is not so (italics in original).
>
> Truly, in begetting life the spouses fulfill one of the highest dimensions of their calling: they are *God's co-workers*. Precisely for this reason they must have an extremely responsible attitude. In deciding whether or not to have a child, they must not be motivated by selfishness or carelessness, but by a prudent, conscious generosity that weighs the possibilities and circumstances, and especially gives priority to the welfare of the unborn child.
>
> Therefore, when there is a reason not to procreate, this choice is permissible and may even be necessary. However, there remains the duty of carrying it out with criteria and methods that respect the total truth of the marital act in its unitive and procreative dimension, as wisely regulated by nature itself in its biological rhythms. One can comply with them and use them to advantage, but they cannot be "violated" by artificial interference.[20]

The *Catechism of the Catholic Church* has several paragraphs on this subject. We quote its first paragraph and its quotation from Vatican II.

> A particular aspect of this responsibility concerns the *regulation of births*. For just reasons, spouses may wish to space the births of their children. It is their duty to make certain that their desire is not motivated by selfishness but is in accord with the generosity appropriate to responsible parenthood. Moreover, they should conform their behavior to the objective criteria of morality:
>
> When it is a question of harmonizing married love with the responsible transmission of life, the morality of the behavior does not depend on sincere intention and evaluation of motives alone; but it must be determined by objective criteria, criteria drawn from the nature of the person and his acts, criteria that

respect the total meaning of mutual self-giving and human procreation in the context of true love; this is possible only if the virtue of married chastity is practiced with sincerity of heart.[a21]

Perhaps this whole chapter can be summed up using the above words of the Pope: neither "selfishness" nor "carelessness" but a "prudent, conscious generosity. . ."

In the Couple to Couple League we encourage you to make a periodic review of your own situation. Right now you may feel called to have a baby. One year from now when that baby is only a few months old, you may want more spacing. When that baby is 14-15 months old, you may sense God's call to share life and faith with another child. One last thought as you reflect upon *Gaudium et Spes*, section 50.2: no Western country except Ireland is reproducing itself. Raising a large family in an atmosphere of Christian discipleship can be a real service to your country as well as to God and your other children.

Why not?

We've reviewed the basic principles, but you may very well have good questions about your own situation. We suggest that you can sometimes clarify your questions by asking this basic question: Why not? Why not seek pregnancy at the present time?

At some times in your life you may be almost overwhelmed with reasons not to seek pregnancy right then. It is tremendously clear to you that your reasons have no tinge of selfishness. You know that you have sufficiently serious reasons as indicated above. You are convinced that the Lord is not calling you to conceive at this time.

At other times you may find that when you ask that question, "Why not?" you'll find no good reason to think that the Lord is not calling you to procreate another child. Perhaps the only thing holding you back is some peer pressure from some friends or relatives who can't understand why you would want to raise another child. Say a prayer for them. Ask the Lord for another healthy pregnancy, delivery and baby, and keep praying for all the graces necessary to be good parents.

A warning

"My sister conceived on her honeymoon and had a beautiful baby girl nine months later ... She has never been able to conceive since, and it has been 10 years."

— I.C., IN

Please take this seriously. For some couples, their honeymoon and their first 12 months of married life have been the only times they could conceive. Some couples have expressed extreme disappointment that their NFP teachers and materials did not emphasize this more. The reality is that with each passing year, a certain percentage of couples become infertile. Consider yourselves warned in advance. Don't postpone pregnancy unless you really have a sufficiently serious reason to do so.

Additional reading

"Another Child?"

Chapter 16: Self-Test Questions

The following questions refer to the teaching of the Catholic Church.

1. True____   False____   A couple must have as many children as physically possible.

2. True____   False____   A married couple may postpone pregnancy or limit their family size if there is a sufficiently serious reason to do so.

3. True____   False____   The Catholic Church reaffirms the Christian Tradition calling married couples to be generous in the service of life.

4. True____   False____   The Catholic Church reaffirms the Christian Tradition that it is seriously immoral to use unnatural methods of birth control.

5. True____   False____   The Catholic Church allows the use of natural family planning for sufficiently serious reasons.

6. The Church encourages all couples to _____ natural family planning but not to use it for _____ reasons.

Answers to self-test
1. False 2. True 3. True 4. True 5. True 6. use. . . selfish or trivial

References
(1) Janet E. Smith, "The moral use of natural family planning,"*Why Humanae Vitae Was Right: A Reader*, ed. Janet E. Smith, (San Francisco: Ignatius Press, 1993) 447-471.

(2) The world population was estimated at 5,465,000,000 in 1992. The area of Texas is given as 266,807 square miles. If the world population was all in Texas, there would be 20,483 persons per square mile, or 1,361 square feet per person. It's an unrealistic statistic, but it's an answer about the even more unrealistic fearmongering of "standing room only" from the anti-populationists.

(3) Pius XI, *Casti Connubii*, 31 December 1930, para. 12 in St. Paul Books & Media edition (Boston: Daughters of St. Paul, undated printing).

(4) Pius XII, "Address to the Italian Catholic Union of Midwives" (29 October 1951), in AAS XLIII (1951) 835-854. Ed. and trans. by Vincent A. Yzermans, *The Major Addresses of Pope Pius XII*, Vol I (St. Paul, MN: North Central Publishing, 1961) 168-169. Quoted in Janet E. Smith, *A Reader*, 453-455.

(5) *Gaudium et Spes* or *Pastoral Constitution on the Church in the Modern World*, (7 December 1965) *Vatican Council II*, *The Conciliar and Post-Conciliar Documents*, General Editor, Austin Flannery, O.P. (Boston: St. Paul Editions, 1975) n. 50.

(6) John Paul II, "Homily at Capitol Mall," 7 October 1979. Available in U.S.A.: *The Message of Justice, Peace and Love* (Boston: St. Paul Editions, 1979) 281-282.

(7) *Catechism of the Catholic Church*, English trans. (U.S. Catholic Conference, Inc., 1994) based on Latin text copyright 1994 Libreria Editrice Vaticana, Citta del Vaticano. a: *Familiaris Consortio*, 30; b: *Humanae Vitae*, 12, with further unnumbered reference to Pius XI, *Casti Connubii*.

(8) Pius XI, *Casti Connubii*, para. 59.

(9) Pius XII, "Address to the Italian Catholic Union of Midwives," 29 October 1951.

(10) *Gaudium et Spes*, n. 50.

(11) Paul VI, *Humanae Vitae*, n. 16, trans. by Janet E. Smith (New Hope, Ky: New Hope Publications, ca. 1992).

(12) John Paul II, talk to participants in a course on NFP, 14 December 1990, "Pope calls spouses to a sense of responsibility for love and for life," n. 4, *L'Osservatore Romano* (English ed.) 17 December 1990, 1, 3.

(13) John Paul II, n. 5.

(14) John Paul II, n. 5.

(15) Karol Wojtyla, *Love and Responsibility* (San Francisco: Ignatius Press, 1993) 243; quoted in J.E. Smith, *A Reader*, 463-464. This was first published in Polish in 1960.

(16) Janet E. Smith, *A Reader,* 461.

(17) Ibid, 462.

(18) John F. Kippley, *Marriage Is for Keeps,* wedding edition (Cincinnati: Foundation for the Family, 1994).

(19) *Gaudium et Spes,* n. 48.

(20) John Paul II, "Parents are God's co-workers," Sunday Angelus meditation, 17 July 1994, *L'Osservatore Romano,* 20 July 1994, weekly English edition, 1.

(21) *Catechism,* n. 2368; a = *Gaudium et Spes,* n. 51.3.

17

Your Marriage and NFP

I urge the advocates of artificial methods to consider the consequences. Any large use of the methods is likely to result in the dissolution of the marriage bond and in free love.

—Mahatma Gandhi, 1925[1]

Carried to its logical conclusion, the committee's report [to allow marital contraception] if carried into effect would sound the death-knell of marriage as a holy institution, by establishing degrading practices which would encourage indiscriminate immorality. The suggestion that the use of legalized contraceptives would be "careful and restrained" is preposterous.

—Editorial in the Washington Post, *22 March 1931[2]*

Indeed, it is to be feared that husbands who become accustomed to contraceptive practices will lose respect for their wives. They may come to disregard their wife's psychological and physical equilibrium and use their wives as instruments for serving their own desires. Consequently, they will no longer view their wives as companions who should be treated with attentiveness and love.

—Pope Paul VI, 1968[3]

Building healthy marriages through Natural Family Planning.

—Motto of the Couple to Couple League

In this chapter, you will review some of the elements that can make the practice of natural family planning a very positive factor in your marriage. We make no claims that there's anything automatic about NFP building healthy marriages. Far from it; the whole gist of this chapter is that the periodic abstinence of NFP must be supplemented by courtship and that it needs to be spiritualized. Then, if you have sufficiently serious reasons for avoiding pregnancy, the periodic abstinence of systematic NFP, far from being just a burden, can be a real marriage builder.

Prophets, but why?

Please note: We are not saying contraception is the **only** cause of the terrible increase in the American divorce rate. However, we are convinced that it is either **the** major cause or at least one of the most important causes.

In 1975, we wrote for a previous edition of this book: "Was Mahatma Gandhi, the great Indian leader, a prophet when he spoke the above words in 1925?" With 20 more years of experience, we can say confidently that Mahatma Gandhi, the editorial writer for the *Washington Post*, and Pope Paul VI were all prophetic.

Consider what has happened in the United States. In 1910, there was one divorce for every 11 new marriages;[4] that was the year of the last American census before Margaret Sanger organized the contraception movement in the United States. By 1925 the philosophy of contraception and "companionate marriage" was well circulated, and the divorce rate jumped sharply: there was now one divorce for every seven marriages. In 1965, a few years after the Pill helped to foster the "New Morality," the ratio was about one divorce for every four marriages. As the practice of contraception grew, more and more people began experimenting with all sorts of new sexual "freedoms," and by 1970 there was one divorce for every three marriages. By 1977 the happiness promised by unlimited sex through the Pill and sterilization still had not materialized, and the divorce rate reached the tragic ratio of one divorce for every two new marriages.

Remember that propagandists for contraception have traditionally promised that freedom to have sex at any time without fear of pregnancy will make people happy and build better marriages. The history of the American family since contraception began to be increasingly practiced shows just the opposite. It has made prophets of Gandhi and the others. The question is, why? What is there about using unnatural forms of birth control that contributes to the breakdown of marriages?

We think there are at least four reasons why using unnatural forms of birth control harms marriages.

1. **Overemphasis on sex.** The philosophy behind contraception preaches an unreal, overly erotic idea of marriage and sex. The erotic element of marriage is good, but overemphasis on it leads many people to enter marriage with the utterly unrealistic notion that enough sex will solve all their problems. Current divorce rates prove the size of that error.

2. **Underdevelopment of love.** The unreality of the overly orgiastic concept of marriage leads couples to ignore the proper development of married love. Happily married couples recognize that the words of St. Paul about love apply so well to marital love that they are almost a recipe for marriage: "Love is patient . . . kind . . . ready to endure whatever comes" (1 Cor 13:4-7).

3. **False principle of separation.** Ask yourself who put together in one act what we call "making love" and "making babies." Unless you're an atheist, you answer, "God." Then ask yourself: what is contraception except taking apart what God Himself has put together? That helps to explain why contraception is wrong. It also helps to explain the connection between contraception and marital breakup. Why do a couple resort to contraception? Isn't it because they fear either a pregnancy or abstinence? So they try to "solve" that problem by taking apart what God has put together in the marital embrace.

Why do a couple divorce? They have a problem of some sort. If they have conditioned themselves to "solve" the birth control problem by taking apart what God has put together, they may be all the more inclined to "solve" their marital problem by trying to take apart what God has put together in their marriage.

4. **Non-cooperation with grace.** Couples who practice unnatural forms of birth control are not cooperating with the graces God wants to give

to married couples. They are going against God's will for them every time they have marital relations.

We can't read the state of their consciences; many may be acting out of ignorance and may be in good faith. (If they really are in good faith, then they will want to accept the teaching of *Humanae Vitae* when they learn that it simply reaffirms the teaching of Christ.) But the fact remains that engaging in unnatural, immoral practices, even in ignorance and good faith, doesn't help to build a good marriage. Marriage is both a natural and a supernatural institution. To use unnatural forms of birth control is to engage in unnatural forms of sex. It is, therefore, to act against human nature and the nature of marriage.

This is confirmed by what has happened to the divorce rate among Catholics since *Humanae Vitae*. While the overall American divorce rate began to escalate during the 1920s, the Catholic divorce rate remained generally low. However, after 1968, the Catholic divorce rate skyrocketed as millions of Catholic couples rebelled and joined the search for personal fulfillment and unlimited sex through unnatural forms of birth control.

Priests dealing with broken marriages say that at least 95% of such couples used unnatural forms of birth control and/or started to have sex before they were married. Preaching and really teaching the Christian Tradition against unnatural forms of birth control is one of the best things that priests and ministers can do to reduce the scandalous divorce rate among Christians today. It is an act of true compassion.

Marriage Building

In contrast to the high divorce rate among contracepting couples, the divorce rate among couples practicing NFP is extremely low. One informal survey showed a divorce rate of less than 1% among couples practicing NFP.[5] CCL Central has tracked one small group and found a divorce rate of 1.3%. Since this was a special, dedicated group, we estimate that the rate for the general population of NFP users might be higher, perhaps even two or three times that rate. If so, the rate would still be under 4%. On the basis of the information we have, we think a 5% divorce rate among couples practicing NFP is really the outside maximum limit. More work needs to be done on this, and we have encouraged social scientists to study this in depth.

Apart from statistics, we know from the experience of many couples that NFP has a good effect on marriages. In the very first course we taught in the Fall of 1971, couples who were switching from unnatural methods to NFP asked us: "Why didn't you tell us this was going to improve our marriage?"

Quite frankly, at that point we didn't know. We had only our own experience; we had never used any form of contraception; we had never given any thought to what effect NFP was having on our good marriage. We had just taken it for granted.

Three things happen right away when couples practice natural family planning for the right reasons. First, they discard the old idea that the wife is the immediate relief valve for any and all sexual urges of her husband, but they do not deny that relief of sexual tension can be a valid reason for marital relations.

Second, they start to communicate better. They get involved in mutual decision making. Marital courtship is renewed. They see new meaning to the act of marital relations.

Consider that children are also great marriage-builders when they are properly valued. They help parents to become less self-centered and more other-centered— to become more lovable persons!

Third, when they experience difficulties in abstinence, and most of us have that experience, they are more prepared to accept these difficulties as athletes do theirs—"No pain, no gain." Or, to put it in Christian terms, as the price of discipleship.

Mutual decision making

Natural family planning is built upon mutual fertility awareness and mutual decision making. During each menstrual cycle, both spouses should become aware of changes in the fertility pattern of the wife. We can't lay down fixed rules for every couple, but what follows works well.

1. To the wife: You are responsible for mucus and cervix observations; be sure to make your observations and recordings every day. It's part of your wifely communication.

2. To the husband: You should normally be involved with the temperature taking. Give the thermometer to your wife in the morning; take it back from her a few minutes later; record the reading on the chart when you get up. It's no big deal, but if you refuse to do that little bit, you could be sending a negative message to your wife. Obviously, if you are traveling or get up hours before your wife does, you'll modify this, and your wife will understand.

3. To both: Do your chart interpretation and decision making *together*. The marital embrace is something you do together, and making the decision about *when* to make love is something you should also do together.

Most of the time, interpreting your signs is fairly self-evident, but even a very easy decision is still a decision. If you are inexperienced and need help, get in touch with your teachers. They volunteered to provide such service; they want to help you in every way they can.

Courtship and honeymoon

For most couples, the practice of natural family planning is a period of courtship followed by a period of honeymoon. However, we know that's not a universal experience; so let's take a look at what you can learn from those couples who have a positive outlook on marriage and NFP.

● You need a good reason to be avoiding pregnancy. You both need to agree that you have sufficiently serious reasons—before the Lord—to avoid pregnancy. How can a couple who are attracted to each other not engage in marital relations when the mood hits unless they both agree they have a very good reason not to? How can a man not be hurt if his advances during the fertile time are refused by his wife for reasons that he sincerely believes are unimportant? How can a wife not be hurt if her desires for a baby are thwarted by financial or other concerns of her husband that she sincerely considers to be minor or even trivial? Assuming that you agree that you have sound, just reasons for avoiding pregnancy at this time, you agree to abstain during the fertile times—but you are still married.

● You do not ignore each other during times of abstinence. You are husband and wife. You married for lifelong companionship, not just for sex or for children. You may not think that a group of Irish bishops would have much to say about this, but we submit that the following quotation is the result of some careful listening to married couples as well as reflection on the Gospel:

> Married people's sexual happiness will be the result of their loving care and concern for one another's general happiness. Sexual intercourse will express love only if one's whole way of life expresses love. If couples cease to talk to one another, to listen to one another, to go out together, to share the same interests together, they will become strangers sharing the same house; and sexual intercourse will actually deepen rather than remove the hurt of their estranged silence.[6]

● You renew the pleasantries of courtship. Gentlemen: if you don't know it already, wives just love to talk—and especially with their husbands. Even if you cannot match your wife's conversational abilities, be a good listener and share with her whatever is on your mind.

Her making him a special dinner or his taking her out to dinner provide traditional ways of courtship for the married as well as the unmarried. His performance of some of the household jobs that she wants done or his taking out the garbage without complaint can be most helpful in the art of marital courtship. Also helpful are her verbal thanks for such little things and her compliments for his help with the children.

While you do not need to live as brother and sister during times of abstinence, the point we want to make is this: you need to develop non-genital ways of expressing marital love. Non-married couples with a commitment to purity look for and find non-genital and non-passionate ways to express their love and affection as they look forward to marriage. The fact that they do not have intercourse does not weaken their love for each other; on the contrary, the pleasantries of courtship help to develop their relationship. Tenderness and gentleness instead of passion, and conversation rather than coitus help to broaden and deepen their friendship.

● You will mutually agree upon the degree of romantic activity during your fertile times. Many couples find that a bit of cuddling is very helpful. The wife may feel very much loved for her own sake when her husband puts his arm around her and sprinkles their conversation with a few kisses without coitus— perhaps even more than when they know that all such activity is simply a preliminary to coital gratification.

There is a big difference between a chaste premarital courtship and the regular "courtship" phase of natural family planning. You do not need to live together as brother and sister during times of abstinence, but there are moral and personal limits.

You want to avoid two extremes. In one, spouses treat each other as brother and sister. He says he can't kiss his wife without becoming excessively aroused, etc. So she feels ignored and hurt. A possible solution for this couple may be for him to give her a non-passionate hug and a kiss in the kitchen every day, maybe just before supper. Just a touch of physical affection may go a long way to communicate honest marital love.

The other extreme is where the couple engage in immoral activities during the fertile time or where the husband keeps pestering his wife for a level of activity that she wants only as part of foreplay to complete marital relations. Some couples may be tempted to try to beat the system by using condoms or other barrier methods of contraception during the fertile time. As you will discover more fully in Chapters 18 and 19, such activities are immoral. Other couples may be tempted to engage in masturbation, whether mutual or solitary, or in marital sodomy. (Anatomically, marital sodomy is the same form of anal and oral activity engaged in by those who do homosexual sodomy.) Such activities are really forms of contraceptive behavior and are likewise condemned by the Christian Tradition as seriously immoral. When you are using NFP to avoid pregnancy, you are called to chaste abstinence during the fertile time. A combination of fertility awareness and sexual immorality during the fertile time is *not* natural family planning.

● Permissible behaviors

Among Catholic theologians who accept and teach the Catholic Church's moral teachings about love, sex, and marriage, there is universal agreement that contraceptive behaviors are seriously immoral. You will note that the behaviors listed in the preceding paragraph are clear cut: either a couple use a contraceptive behavior or they don't.

However, there are certain behaviors that are in degrees instead of being "either . . . or." Over the years, we have had many questions about these from married couples of good faith. They want to be chaste; and during times of not having relations, they would prefer to have amorous activity beyond a hug and a kiss in the kitchen. Their questions boil down to this: what is the moral permissibility of kissing and touching not intended as immediate foreplay to completed genital-genital relations? The Magisterium of the Catholic Church has not spoken officially about these matters and the literature is limited,[7] but we have consulted with Catholic moral theologians.

As a result of the need to answer these questions, the Couple to Couple League publishes a leaflet titled *Marital Sexuality: Moral Considerations* which we believe is consistent with Catholic teaching. The leaflet is available at CCL classes and is part of the *CCL Home Study Course*. For a free copy, send CCL headquarters your request and a stamped, self-addressed business-size envelope. Please also state your age and how or where you obtained this book. A few points are as follows:

1. Marital chastity during the fertile time is not the same as pre-marital chastity. A married couple can engage in a degree of kissing and touching that would be objectively sinful for the unmarried. For the married couple, such behavior looks forward to the full sexual union they may morally have now or are postponing until later. If passion should take over, rather obviously they may engage in full marital relations.

2. Activities that are sexually arousing are permissible provided that they do not become excessively arousing. That is, they should be expressions of marital love and affection, but they should not lead to orgasm by either spouse or provide excessive temptation for either spouse to seek relief of sexual tension through masturbation.

3. Spouses should have good reason for engaging in any such activity because it may carry the remote possibility of involuntary orgasm. Such reasons would include a felt need to be held, to be appreciated, and even to take the edge off sexual tension. In every case, the primary intention of the spouses ought to be the promotion of their marriage bond, not just the pleasure to be experienced.

4. Each spouse must remember that marital chastity is a virtue that each must cultivate as a good habit to guide their behavior. You will get no encouragement from Western culture to be chaste. That's why it's important to pray, to frequent the sacraments, and to do regular good spiritual reading.

Keeping in touch with the Word of God in the Bible and as lived out in the lives of saints and their writings is truly important for keeping up your motivation to be pure—as the Lord certainly wants all of us to be. The *CCL Catalog* lists a small number of excellent books that can help you in this regard.

5. In saying these things, we are not trying to encourage you to see how far you can go. There can be dangers in seeking to maximize pleasure, especially on an habitual basis. You can gain spiritual benefits from a certain degree of self-denial in the marital relationship. Furthermore, if you put a heavy emphasis on the erotic during the fertile time, you may be distracting yourselves from the development of the non-erotic marital courtship that is so necessary for building and enriching a good marital relationship. Many find that working on a practical project together is better for them in every way than activities which are sexually arousing.

On the other hand, some couples need to learn that it is not necessary and could be even harmful for them to live strictly as brother and sister during the fertile time. Each spouse needs to be responsive to the other's need to be held, and the responding spouse needs to realize that wanting to be held is not an invitation to intercourse.

Some couples have told us that they've done it both ways—pushing their limits on the one hand and having no more than a hug and a kiss in the kitchen on the other, and they found that the latter was better for their overall marital relationship. Others may find that they can handle some holding and kissing on the couch but not in their bed.

There is no universal recipe for the periodic courtship-without-coitus phase of marriage. For starters, discuss with your spouse what each of you might do for the other in such periods. The important thing is that you show each other that you are friends and truly care about each other. In this way, you can actively work against one of the worst enemies of your marriage— taking each other for granted.

Increased respect

If the feeling of being taken for granted is a prime cause of marital discontent, the feeling of being used must run a close second. For reasons that are probably obvious to most readers, this is particularly true of women. When the frequency and the conditions of intercourse lead a woman to feel that she is being used pretty much just as a means of sexual relief for her husband, her respect for him and her own self-image are hardly increased, no matter how sympathetic she is to his sexual urges. On the other hand when couples give up their practice of contraception and turn to natural family planning, it is a fairly common experience for the wife to develop greater respect for her husband and frequently for herself as well.

A remedy for satiety

In the early Seventies, a popular television show dealt with the subject of spouse-swapping,[8] and this indirectly portrayed the problem of sexual satiation. The spouse-swapping couple explained that they had taken up this way of life because the zip had gone out of their own married life. That was about as close as anyone could get on television (then) to saying, "We became tired of each other as sex partners: we've had so much of each other that we're bored."

Periodic abstinence is good for your marriage because it helps you to avoid the feeling of sexual satiation, the feeling of having too much quantity, and a corresponding lack of joy and meaning. Such voluntary and mutual refraining from intercourse is part of the normal pattern of natural family planning and can help you improve your marriage. For that reason, some couples impose periods of abstinence upon themselves during extended breastfeeding and when they are in the years of menopause. Once a couple resume intercourse after a period of chaste abstinence, it is common for them to enjoy the honeymoon effect.

Spiritual abstinence

Nearly universal contraception, unlimited abortion in much of the West and the Orient, and the growing practice of killing the helpless sick and aged constitute the contemporary culture of death. Thousands of drug-related murders, random shootings, and numerous assaults against both children and the aged fill out the picture.

This is spiritual warfare, and those who believe in God need to use their spiritual weapons to fight for the restoration of a culture of life. Jesus himself has shown us by his own example that prayer and fasting are the first and most effective weapons against the forces of evil (cf. Mt 4:1-11). As he taught his disciples, some demons cannot be driven out except in this way (cf. Mk 9:29).[9]

Voluntary periodic abstinence from marital relations can be a powerful form of prayer and fasting when done for the right spiritual reasons. Therefore, in addition to the Phase II abstinence required by NFP to avoid pregnancy, please consider some additional abstinence—at least occasionally—during other times for purely spiritual reasons: for a stop to abortion; for a rebirth of chastity; in reparation for sins of impurity; for a healing of the divisions within Christianity, at least those dealing with marriage and sexuality.

Also, when you are pregnant or experiencing extended breastfeeding infertility, consider some periodic abstinence for purely spiritual reasons. And, of course, this applies also to those couples who are letting the Lord "plan" their families with ecological breastfeeding but without any systematic Phase II abstinence. Consider some sort of systematic periodic abstinence, and join your prayer and fasting with that of others in the spiritual battle for life and chastity.

Within Christianity, several times have been traditionally associated with prayer and fasting—Advent, Lent, and Fridays throughout the year. Lent starts with a reading from the prophet Joel (2:15-16) which clearly calls for fasting from marital relations:

> Blow the trumpet in Zion;
> sanctify a fast;
> call a solemn assembly;
> gather the people.
> Sanctify the congregation;
> assemble the elders;
> gather the children,
> even the nursing infants.
> Let the bridegroom leave his room,
> and the bride her chamber.

Fasting from marital relations during Lent raises the question of Sundays. They are definitely part of the Lenten season, but in the years of the daily fast under obligation of obedience, Sundays were never obligatory fast days. Couples who fast from marital relations during Lent have to make their own rules about Sundays.

The Catholic Church calls all Christians to practice some form of sacrifice on Fridays in honor of the sacrifice of Jesus. Catholics are urged to abstain from meat but are no longer bound to such abstinence under pain of the sin of disobedience. Friday "marital abstinence" is another form of prayer, fasting and sacrifice to assist the fight for chastity and life. Of course, the practice of abstinence for spiritual reasons must be voluntary on the part of both spouses, never imposed.

Mutual prayer is important for your growth as a married couple. With discussion and proper motivation, some abstinence for purely spiritual reasons can be a real marriage builder as well as helping the cause of chastity and life.

Medical-moral abstinence

Sometimes a woman has a condition that requires medical intervention, and sometimes a physician will prescribe a drug or treatment that can cause abortions or severe birth defects. The morally correct response in these cases is to abstain from relations until the danger is past.

The abstinence will help you to make sure the drug or treatment is truly necessary. Accepted in the right spirit, abstinence for medical-moral reasons can help your marriage and can be offered as a prayer for quick and complete recovery.

Encountering Difficulties

Even with the firmest convictions that natural family planning is the only moral form of spacing babies, you will most likely experience some difficulties, at least occasionally. We have, and we take it for granted that almost everybody does.

Natural family planning involves voluntary sexual self-control, and that can be difficult. Some experienced couples may refrain from relations for only a week; for many it's eight to ten days; for others two weeks, and for some even longer in certain situations. How you approach any difficulty has much to do with your happiness; if you feel sorry for yourself, you're in for a tough time no matter what the difficulty may be. When you accept difficulties in the right spirit, well, that's a different matter. Some of the highest praises of NFP have come from couples who experienced an extended period of abstinence while switching from unnatural methods to NFP. They used the time to grow in marital communication as they had not done since they married, and they grew in love.

Natural family planning demands a certain amount of maturity to begin with, and it helps you develop an even more mature, stable and happy marital relationship. Couples have told us repeatedly that their efforts to make NFP a working part of their marriage have been repaid tenfold in marriage enrichment.

Let's take a look at some ways of using difficulties as stepping stones to growth and greater maturity.

Accept difficulties as an enriching part of life

The famous Jewish psychiatrist, Victor Frankl, reflected deeply upon his experiences as a prisoner in the Nazi concentration camps during World War II. His book, *Man's Search for Meaning,* is the type you can hardly put down, and many read it in one sitting. Frankl writes:

> Suffering is an ineradicable part of life, even as fate and death. Without suffering and death human life cannot be complete. The way in which a man accepts his fate and all the suffering it entails, the way in which he takes up his cross, gives him ample opportunity—even under the most difficult circumstances—to add a deeper meaning to his life. . . Everywhere man is confronted with fate, with the chance of achieving something through his own suffering.[10]

Of course, whatever difficulties you might experience with NFP are far different from the sufferings of Frankl and his associates in the concentration camps. First of all, NFP difficulties are so much less severe that they can hardly be compared with such sufferings. Second, difficulties with abstinence are freely accepted as part of the price of Christian discipleship and/or the pursuit of other values.

Spiritualize your difficulties

Frankl referred to taking up your cross, and that harmonizes well with the teaching of Jesus who said:

> If any man would come after me, let him deny himself and take up his cross daily and follow me. For whoever would save his life will lose it; and whoever loses his life for my sake, he will save it. For what does it profit a man if he gains the whole world and loses or forfeits himself (Luke 9:23-25).

Losing your life for his sake doesn't refer only to ultimate martyrdom. It also applies to those little martyrdoms of everyday life in which you "die" to some expression of self-will and find yourself correspondingly enriched, especially if you have done it for the sake of Christ. And of what value are all the sexual pleasures anyone can imagine if a person loses eternal life in the pursuit of such pleasures?

There's a second way in which you can spiritualize any difficulties you experience with periodic abstinence. You are undoubtedly concerned about the decline of morality in the West. Religious morality has been banned from the United States public school system since the 1950s, and the results are easy to see. William Bennet writes:

> America has lost its sense of civic and moral outrage. Last March [1993], I released through the auspices of the Heritage Foundation the *Index of Leading Cultural Indicators,* the most thorough statistical portrait available of America's cultural health. It showed that since 1960, violent crime has shot up 560%. This is coupled with a 400% increase in illegitimate births, a quadrupling of divorces, a tripling of the percentage of young people in single-parent homes, a more than 200% increase in the teen-age suicide rate, and a drop of 75 points in the average Scholastic Aptitude Test (SAT) score.[11]

To the sexual components of this social decline, the only "answer" a neo-pagan government has is to urge more and more contraception, first the Pill and then the condom. Evidence that this "answer" is a big part of the problem is consistently ignored.

The Christian doctrine of "the communion of saints" means that the prayers, good deeds and sufferings of one person can help someone else through the universal mediation of Jesus Christ. That means that you in your own private life can do something positive to fight against the massive evil of personal immorality that afflicts the world today.

Are you experiencing some difficulty with chaste abstinence? Don't feel sorry for yourself. Instead, give meaning to your sufferings. Join your difficulties with the suffering of the Lord Jesus. Offer them as a special prayer for a stop to abortion and for a rebirth of chastity throughout the Christian churches and throughout the world. Offer those difficulties as a living prayer for the divine guidance and the graces to be good parents. Offer them as a prayer for your children. Do this together as husband and wife, and you have a true marriage builder, a powerful means of growing closer together at the spiritual level.

Count your blessings

One of the worst things you can do to yourself is to feel sorry for yourself, no matter what your situation. Feeling sorry for yourself doesn't make things any better, but it can cripple your abilities to grow as a person, to profit from suffering. When you're tempted to feel sorry for yourself, re-read that brief quotation from Victor Frankl a couple of pages back.

When single persons who want to marry start to feel sorry for themselves, they make it more difficult for themselves to remain chaste, to avoid fornication. When married persons feel sorry for themselves, they weaken their defenses against temptations to adultery. When persons with a homosexual orientation feel sorry for themselves, they weaken their defenses against the temptation to sodomy. And when married couples using NFP start to feel sorry for themselves, they weaken their defenses against the temptation to engage in contraceptive behavior.

> When I was a young boy, my mother took us kids every Christmas holiday to give some cookies to a couple who had been married at least 35 years. The wife was always in a wheelchair. Very early in their marriage, an automobile accident had left her paralyzed from the waist down. They were always happy to see us, and even aside from the initial smiles and greetings, they both looked happy all the time we were there. Mom explained to us that he had to bathe her and take care of all her needs. As an adult it occurred to me that they probably had a sexless marriage after that accident. He remained with her, and he looked happy. What a witness of fidelity to God and to each other! — J.F.K.

In every case, one part of the answer is to count your blessings. If you don't like *periodic* abstinence, thank the Lord you do not have *permanent* abstinence. Either you or your spouse could have a disease or an accident that would make it impossible for you to have marital relations for a very long time—months or even for life.

More positively, in your practice of NFP, you can be glad you are not needlessly endangering each other's health or taking the life of a newly conceived child through various unnatural forms of birth control. You can be proud that you have learned to understand your mutual fertility and infertility. Millions and millions of people don't know where to start; they don't even know it's *possible* to learn their mutual fertility. It's a fundamental rule of life: Count your blessings.

Take one day at a time

It's an important part of Alcoholics Anonymous and of every other 12-step recovery program: take one day at a time. It also applies to married life as a whole and to any difficulties you experience with chaste abstinence. You are married for life, but you have to live your marriage one day at a time. In his famous prayer, Jesus teaches us to pray: "Give us this day our daily bread." God gives you the graces today that are sufficient for any temptations you may experience—today.

Communicate— and have a sense of humor

Open communication is a necessity in every aspect of marriage. You can solve or greatly reduce many problems simply by talking about them, sometimes just by admitting there's a problem. For example, if a husband is feeling a few sexual urges, knows he must exercise self-restraint, but is having a bit of difficulty, he can probably greatly relieve the situation simply by sharing his feelings with his wife. It will probably be more helpful if they are both willing to joke about it: "Honey, I'm feeling oversexed. . ." When you can laugh together about any difficulties of sexual restraint, you are on the road to sexual maturity and miles ahead of the couple who begin to feel sorry for themselves.

Use common sense

Wives, you need to realize how easily men are "turned on" or tempted by appearances. Dress accordingly. Your husband doesn't need to tell you, "When you wear that shorty nightgown, all I can think of is making love with you all the way." It's just a matter of common sense that most husbands will so react, so it's also a matter of common sense not to tease your husband's imagination at times when you have mutually agreed to refrain from marital relations. And husbands should dress modestly, too.

Common sense dictates that you should both avoid TV shows, movies, magazines, and books that have an erotic effect. Most of us, especially husbands, have a sexual drive that receives ample stimulation just from being alive and in the presence of one's spouse. Why complicate life by watching or reading material designed to arouse you? Sometimes the TV ads are the worst part of the whole show!

Eat right

Women, your eating and exercise habits can definitely affect your fertility cycle. Let's put it this way: if you don't eat right or if you exercise too much, you can delay ovulation and frequently give yourself a long mucus patch. That means a much longer Phase II and much more abstinence than might be necessary if you were eating and exercising properly. For example, here's a quotation from a chart that we looked at just the day before writing this paragraph.

> Jogging every day 20-50 minutes per day. Just started jogging again this month. Period has stopped when jogging in the past. —M.P., MA (Nov. '93).

Good cycle patterns not only provide an easier use of NFP but they also promote bone health and other health benefits.

— M. Shannon

Women, you need a minimum of 20% to 22% body fat to maintain normal fertility. M.P. from Massachusetts was 5'3" in height and weighed 115 pounds. That's her "ideal" weight according to this general rule for women of average bone structure: 100 pounds for the first five feet and 5 pounds for every additional inch. Her jogging may not have reduced her weight by much, but she had a record of seriously affecting her fertility cycle with such exercise.

She was most likely converting essential body fat to muscle. Nutrition author Marilyn Shannon writes:

> Note well that women who exercise vigorously (runners, gymnasts, swimmers, ballet dancers, body builders) are converting body mass from fat to muscle, and they may also experience delayed ovulation or complete infertility and amenorrhea when their total body fat drops below the critical level of around twenty percent. I have seen this occur even when body weight has been completely normal. What this means is that a woman needs sufficient weight for her height and a sufficient ratio of fat to muscle in order to have normal fertility-menstrual cycles.[12]

Some weight conscious women eliminate salt from their diets to reduce water retention. However, if your salt is *iodized*, it contains iodine, an essential nutrient. Its absence can affect your fertility cycle. So if you don't use iodized salt, you have to get your iodine from some other source. Seafood is a great source, but for many people, a daily kelp pill provides a cheap and easy way to obtain this important nutrient. (More on this in Chapter 31.)

An iodine deficiency can extend abstinence by delaying ovulation.

The Couple to Couple League wants to help you have the most regular cycles you can have. Therefore we looked for someone to write a book that would relate nutrition to your cycle patterns and problems. We are pleased to publish the book from which the above quotation was taken—*Fertility, Cycles and Nutrition* by Marilyn M. Shannon. The subtitle is "Can what you eat affect your menstrual cycles and your fertility?" and the answer to that question is a resounding YES! You can get it at some bookstores, or you can order it direct from CCL Central (see "Resources"). It may be one of the best investments you will ever make for your own health and that of your family.

Men, the need for good nutrition applies to you as well as to women. Improper diet results in poor body balance and may provide increased difficulties with your nervous system and self-control. In addition, some nutritional supplements can apparently alleviate some sources of infertility.

It is much easier for a wife to practice good nutrition if she is encouraged by the example of her husband.
—M. Shannon

Don't blame NFP for basic marital problems

We address this warning primarily to those who feel that the decision not to practice contraception was more or less imposed on them (or him or her) from the outside or by a spouse. Thus, NFP becomes a convenient scapegoat for all sorts of problems, especially by those who think that more frequent marital relations would solve their problems.

Dr. Max Levin, a Jewish neurologist and clinical professor at the New York Medical College, some time ago addressed an audience that was acquainted with the outlook of some Catholics on this matter.

> In cases where rhythm [periodic abstinence] is a problem, the husband regards sex not as something he can give his wife but as something to give *himself* as a compensation for his various grievances. In cases I have seen where periodic continence was presented as an intolerable burden, there has not been a single case where I didn't find something seriously wrong with the marriage. There was no love, no spirit of devotion. One or both partners were immature, egocentric, selfish. They were wrapped up in themselves, not each other. It was not the frustration of the rhythm method that was disturbing them. Even if the Church were to change the rules and raise all bars, they would still be

miserable living together. What they need is not permission to use other contraceptive methods. They need therapy.[13]

Make the decision your own

If your primary reason for choosing NFP is religious, it's possible that either you or your spouse may see it just as a "rule" you grudgingly accept as part of your faith. There is certainly merit in accepting NFP as part of the daily cross you have to carry. However, we can assure you that sound religious leaders would prefer you to internalize the NFP decision, to make it your own. They would like you to become convinced in your own heart that it is radically dishonest to use unnatural methods of birth control, that contraceptive behaviors fail to uphold the sacredness of human sexuality and the divine order of creation. We hope that Chapters 18 and 19 will help you to understand and internalize the NFP decision.

Remember also that other couples are making the same decision for reasons that have nothing to do with religious faith.

Expand your ideas about making love

9. Where's the best place in your house or apartment to make love?
A. In the kitchen with the children watching.

Obviously, by the term "making love" we don't mean "having sexual relations." We mean doing those things that help to build feelings of being loved and appreciated and respected and wanted. Letting your children see that you like each other and help each other. Talking at meals. Helping each other clean up the kitchen and taking out the garbage. Giving each other a hug and a kiss.

Consider how often the phrase "making love" is misused. Outside marriage the proper terms for heterosexual copulation are adultery, fornication, and prostitution.

Even within marriage, many honest couples will admit that there is no direct and necessary relationship between sexual relations and the "making" or "expression" of love. Sometimes their sexual intercourse is very expressive of love and is truly constructive, a real "making" of marital love. At other times, their marital coitus may be hardly more than a sexual relief mechanism. We are certainly not condemning the idea of marital coitus for relief of concupiscence, as it is called in moral theology, but honesty requires that we admit that "making love" is sometimes just a euphemism to describe what the marital embrace ought to be instead of what it actually is.

Our talk about sex will be more realistic if we eliminate any sort of identity between sexual intercourse and "making love." In this book we have generally avoided the term "making love." Instead we use terms such as marital relations, sexual intercourse, the marital embrace, and the technical "coitus."

On the other hand, we need to see "making love" in a much broader context. There are all sorts of marital "love making" or love building activities that have nothing to with coitus. The following anonymous quotation was given by friends for this manual.

> Each couple will need to find or rediscover for themselves the ways to say, "I love you and I want you to be happy." It is an art that is not acquired without effort. It may include:
> HIS remembering the goodbye kiss or the hello kiss.
> HIS bringing her something occasionally (even a bag of peanuts) to let her know that he thought of her during the day.

HIS sharing the goals and problems of his work with her.

HIS doing at least the masculine jobs around the house.

HIS helping in the physical care and particularly the discipline of the children.

HER preparing his favorite meal even though it is by no means her favorite.

HER sprucing up before he is due home at night.

HER overcoming shyness to give a spontaneous and unexpected physical show of affection.

HER learning enough about it to appreciate his sports or political interests.

HIS asking her how her day has been.

The project may be as subtle and as long-range as HER sensitizing him to the emotional element of love and HIS educating her in sensuality and the physical response.

Cultivating a sense of proportion and sense of humor . . . in all areas including their sexual life. Laughter can relieve tensions. *Love is not necessarily increased by solemnity.*

Expand the meaning of the marital embrace

When you made the commitment of marriage, you and your spouse promised to give of yourselves in a caring love for each other for better and for worse, for the rest of your lives. That's a marriage covenant, a promise of love without reservation. In the perspective of your marriage covenant, what is the meaning of sexual relations?

In God's plan for sex, sexual intercourse is exclusively a marriage act. It is also *the* marriage act, the unique way to reaffirm your original commitment of caring love, for better and for worse.

Look at it this way. Sexual intercourse is intended by God to be at least implicitly a renewal of your marriage covenant. The marital embrace is a *unique* expression of married love. It is a symbolic way to reaffirm or renew your covenant of marriage, your original commitment of giving yourselves totally to each other. In this way, the meaning of the sexual intercourse takes on the meaning of marriage itself.

This understanding of sexual intercourse doesn't rule out the idea of marital relations for the relief of sexual tension, but it certainly goes beyond it. Don't get locked in to the idea that coitus is primarily for the expression of biological urges. Internalize the idea that sexual intercourse is meant to be a marriage act.

This biblical view of sex has no room for contraception. After all, when you married, you pledged your love without reservation. The body language of normal marital relations says, "We take each other again for better and for worse, without reservation." However, the body language of contraception says, "We take each other for better but NOT for the imagined worse of possible pregnancy." This is sex with very serious reservation, covenant contradiction, not at all a renewal of the original marriage covenant.

Then go beyond birth control. Think a little more about the fact that God intends sexual relations to be at least implicitly a renewal of your marriage covenant. That conviction can really be a source of personal examination of conscience and growth. For example, ask yourself: "If I am anticipating marital relations this week or this night, what has there been in my behavior towards my spouse to reflect the caring love I promised when we married?" If you have to answer, "Not much," you are challenging yourself to be more of a lover in the real sense of the word. That sort of personal examination and challenge is lifelong, and it can contribute to a lifetime of marital growth and happiness.

WARNING. Examine only your own conscience, not that of your spouse. Check out Matthew 7:1-5 about seeing the speck in your brother's (or spouse's) eye but not noticing the log in your own.

Be positive about the difference

When you tell contracepting friends or relatives you have decided to use only natural methods of family planning, someone will ask you, "Why? What's the difference? After all, we all have the same purpose."

In Chapter 1, you learned a number of very practical reasons for the NFP choice, and in Chapters 18 and 19 you will review moral and religious reasons for using only natural methods for family planning. Chapter 18 contains a long quotation from Pope John Paul II about the difference between contraception and natural family planning.

There's no need to be bashful about the differences. First, you can challenge such friends. "Do you really think that simply having a common purpose makes all the various means morally equal? Do you really think that wanting to live in a nice house makes selling illicit drugs and selling groceries morally the same?"

Second, you can use this comparison from marriage itself. Imagine two couples who both want to avoid an unhappy marriage. One couple decides that the way to avoid unhappiness is to agree ahead of time to break up if they get unhappy with each other. So they contract with each other for a five year "marriage" with an option to renew; or they make a contract that lists the various conditions under which they will live together or will call it quits.

The other couple do a lot of talking about the important things in life and marriage during their courtship. They are both open to the possibility of discontinuing their relationship before marriage if they find they are really incompatible. They try to have some financial basis for living; perhaps they will postpone the wedding until they reach some milestone such as graduation, military discharge, or employment. In other words, they do their best to reduce the obvious risks of marriage. When they finally marry, they make an unconditional gift of each to the other, for better and for worse, until death parts them. They understand that before God they are married for life even if the sky falls in on their plans a week after they marry.

Does the desire to avoid an unhappy marriage make both of the above scenarios morally equal? Of course not. The first couple are not even married. They never make a marital commitment; they are truly living in sin. The second couple may well have some struggles as they go through life together, but they are married. They have entered into a state in which they can grow in holiness by carrying out their mutual commitments.

Contraception is like the "five year option." It so absolutizes the elimination of risk that it contradicts the meaning of the sexual act as a renewal of the marriage covenant for better and for worse.

On the other hand, the couple who practice NFP to avoid pregnancy do no such absolutizing. When they engage in the marital embrace, they—like our second couple—accept it for all that it is. They keep it as a symbol of that unconditional gift of each to the other, that gift which made them married on their wedding day.

There is a huge difference between using contraception and using NFP. Because sexuality is so important for authentic development as a person, the difference is much greater and more important than the difference between selling cocaine and selling groceries. Be positive about the difference.

False ideas about freedom can bring chaos to marriages and to entire societies. Some people don't want to marry because they feel it will restrict their "sexual freedom," and others pursue freedom and happiness—or just pleasure—in extramarital affairs. Such unfortunate people are more slave then free.

Most of us have found that freedom isn't free. To be free to run a mile or two or five without stopping requires a great deal of training effort. The same is true of sexual freedom. To be sexually free means to have enough sexual self-possession so that we are masters over our urges and can place sex at the service of authentic love. To attain that degree of freedom requires the help of God, and you should not feel ashamed to admit your need for divine help in this area of life.

Recall the frequently quoted words of Jesus, "And the truth will make you free." Then think about the sentence that precedes that one: "If you continue in my word, you are truly my disciples, and you will know the truth" (John 8:31-32). So Jesus teaches that authentic freedom comes from discipleship. That involves learning from the Lord, but it's more than merely intellectual. Discipleship also means walking the narrow road with the Lord and carrying your cross every day.

Do you find it a bit difficult at times to practice chaste abstinence during the fertile time? Maybe sometimes really difficult? If so, you are like most of the rest of us. In one way, that's one of the best things about NFP. If you know you can't do what's right without God's help and you turn to Him regularly in prayer, you are developing the virtue of religion. You are doing something beautiful for God.

Now the great thing about this is that you are developing the habit of turning to God for the grace to be faithful to Him and to each other. That's really important.

You are also developing the very important habit of letting the Lord have dominion over you and your sexual behavior and your marriage. At some time in your marriage—whether you've been married five months or 25 years, you may encounter **marital disillusionment**. That's when you tell yourself: "If I felt this way about my spouse three weeks before we married, there wouldn't have been any marriage." If this happens, you need God's help. If you are in the habit of recognizing the dominion of the Lord over your marriage, then you will also recognize that you don't have the alternative, morally speaking, of divorce and remarriage. (We assume a valid marriage.) Recognizing you are stuck with each other is half the battle in making your marriage work better. Make use of that habit of turning to God for help in your marriage. And don't be afraid to turn to a good priest or minister who truly believes in the permanence of marriage and the evil of marital contraception.

Lastly remember another statement of Jesus: "Apart from Me you can do nothing" (Jn 15:5). That means that if you want to be a disciple of Jesus, you have to admit your need for his help to do anything spiritually worthwhile; and that certainly applies to sex. How can anyone in our fallen condition expect to be sexually pure—and stay married for life—without the help of God?

Additional reading

"Creative Abstinence," CCL brochure.
"Marital Sexuality: Moral Considerations," CCL brochure.
"The Legacy of Contraception," CCL brochure.
"Until death do us part," Foundation for the Family brochure.

***

Whether you are engaged or married for five or ten years, you can benefit from good reading. We recommend *Marriage Is for Keeps*. It's short, easy to read, and addresses the basic questions in Christian marriage. For further information, see page 506.

Chapter 17: Self-test Questions

1. True____   False____   Mahatma Gandhi was a conservative Roman Catholic in the 1920s when he fought the use of unnatural methods of birth control.

2. True____   False____   Having your husband involved in the day to day practice of mutual fertility awareness can help build communication and support.

3. The decision to use only natural methods of conception regulation is
   a) a decision you make only once
   b) a decision you keep on making or reaffirming.

4. True____   False____   Every act of sexual intercourse between husband and wife should reflect the self-giving love they pledged at marriage.

5. True____   False____   Every act of sexual intercourse between husband and wife actually is an act of mutual, self-giving love.

6. True____   False____   The practice of natural family planning excludes barrier methods, masturbation, sodomistic practices, and withdrawal.

7. True____   False____   Couples who practice NFP for the right reasons will never have any difficulties with periodic abstinence.

8. True____   False____   The idea that God intends sex to be a renewal of the marriage covenant provides a challenge to every married couple.

Answers to self-test
1. False 2. True 3. b) a decision you keep on making or reaffirming. 4. True 5. False. 6. True 7. False 8. True

References

(1) Mahatma Gandhi, 1925, quoted in J.F.N. (probably J.F. Noll) *A Catechism on Birth Control,* sixth ed. (Huntington: OSV Press, about 1939) 57-58.

(2) Editorial, *Washington Post,* 22 March 1931. This was a commentary on the action of a committee of the Federal Council of Churches on the previous day. The committee had recommended that its member churches allow marital contraception as morally permissible, thus contradicting 1,900 years of Christian teaching that it is seriously immoral for married couples to use contraception.

(3) Pope Paul VI, *Humanae Vitae,* n. 17, 25 July 1968. Translation by Janet E. Smith, *Humanae Vitae: A Generation Later* (Washington, D.C.: Catholic University of America Press, 1991) 286.

(4) The marriage and divorce statistics from 1910 to 1977 are from the *Statistical Abstract of the United States,* 1978, 59.

(5) Nona Aguilar, *The New No-Pill, No-Risk Birth Control* (New York: Rawson Associates, 1986) 186-190.

(6) Catholic Bishops of Ireland, Pastoral letter titled *Human Life is Sacred,* (Dublin: Cahill Printers, Ltd., 1975) n. 97, p. 49.

(7) The primary treatment of these issues is contained in John Ford, S.J. and Gerald Kelly, S.J., *Contemporary Moral Theology, Volume II, Marriage Questions* (Westminster, MD: Newman Press, 1964). Chapter 10, "Hedonism versus Holiness in Conjugal Intimacy," and Chapter 11, "Special Problems of Conjugal Intimacy," address these and related issues. The issue of moral limits is specifically addressed in John F. Harvey, O.S.F.S., "Expressing marital love during the fertile phase," *International Review of Natural Family Planning* IV:4 (Winter 1980) 279-296. Fr. Harvey was one of the reviewers of the CCL brochure *Marital Sexuality: Moral Considerations* which takes his more extensive article as its starting point. Unfortunately, the Ford and Kelly book is available only in some theological libraries, and the Harvey article is even more difficult to find.

(8) "All in the Family," 28 October 1972.

(9) John Paul II, *Evangelium Vitae* (St. Peter's in Rome; 25 March 1995) n. 100.

(10) Victor Frankl, *Man's Search for Meaning* (New York: Washington Square Press, 1963) 106-107.

(11) William J. Bennett, "Violence a result of social decay," *Cincinnati Enquirer,* (4 January 1994) A-6.

(12) Marilyn M. Shannon, *Fertility, Cycles and Nutrition: Can what you eat affect your menstrual cycles and your fertility?* second ed. (Cincinnati: Couple to Couple League, 1992) 65. Marilyn M. Shannon holds a master's degree in human physiology with a minor in biochemistry from Indiana University's Medical Sciences Program. Her master's thesis involved the effects of the hormone prolactin on kidney function, a topic related to premenstrual syndrome. Since 1984 she has taught an undergraduate course in human anatomy and physiology at Indiana University-Purdue University at Fort Wayne, Indiana. She and her husband, Ronald, have been an NFP teaching couple with the Couple to Couple League since 1982. Her interests in nutrition and reproductive health are an outgrowth of her educational background and experiences as an NFP teacher. She has counseled extensively and lectured widely on nutrition and the fertility cycle.

(13) Max Levin, "Sexual fulfillment with rhythm," *Marriage* (June 1966) 32.

18

Bible and Tradition

The reasons for faith found in Scripture and Tradition constitute the core of this chapter. However, before we can get into the heart of the matter, we need to review a few other issues first.

In the pagan nations surrounding Israel before the time of Christ, religion was not concerned with personal morality. Morality had to do with the practical matters of keeping a society going, keeping people from robbing and killing each other. Religion was strictly concerned with ceremony. It did not entail moral obligations as we understand them, especially regarding chastity. A young woman in a society that worshiped Baal might have felt total revulsion at being a temple prostitute for an appointed time, but that was "religion." One might say that the devil who cooked up such religions knew how to keep some men "interested in religion." The Canaanite religions also included the sacrifice of young children, perhaps a convenient "religious" way to dispose of babies with birth defects. The Prophets of Yahweh, however, condemned all of this as an abomination to the Lord. God is holy, they preached; you are made in the image and likeness of God; you have a covenant with God; you are called to be holy. Because of your relationship with God you have moral obligations to your neighbor. In short, the heritage of the West is religious morality, the notion that true religion makes moral demands upon every believer. It is that heritage which is reflected in this book.

Is there a difference between morality and religion? Strictly speaking, yes. Morality is concerned with this question: Is this action right or wrong? That is, is it in accord with the order of creation? Is it in accord with the very nature of what it means to be a human being? Is it in accord with right reason?

Religion goes beyond reason alone. Religion is concerned with God, his revelation, our relationship with God, and our relationships with other people considering what God has told us. Religion ultimately phrases the morality question a little differently: Is this action in accord with what it means to be a human person *made in the image and likeness of God?* Concerning sexuality, religion asks: Is this action in accord with God's plan for sex?

Religious morality asks the "right or wrong" questions this way: Is there a religious reason to believe that this action is right or wrong? For example, if you say, "It is wrong to commit adultery," that's a statement about morality. If we ask, "**Why** do you believe it is wrong to commit adultery?" you might answer, "My church teaches that way," or "That's in

Morality and religion

the Ten Commandments." Those would be religious reasons for believing that adultery is morally wrong.

Moral *theology* goes a step farther. It asks, "**Why** is adultery wrong? What is there about the nature of man and woman, the nature of marriage, the nature of sexual intercourse that makes it morally wrong for a married person to have relations with someone who is not his or her spouse?" You will notice, if you think about it for a moment, that God did not give us arguments why adultery is wrong. God simply asks for our response in faith. However, the human mind seeks to know why. In short, it seeks to understand the fundamental reasons behind the Commandments, and that's the effort of good moral theology.

The success of moral theology is "more or less." Sometimes it succeeds very well in giving us good reasons; at other times a challenge may arise that forces theologians to dig deeper, to come up with more fundamental reasons. One thing must always be kept in mind. The reasoning of the theologians does not constitute the teaching. For the believer, the force of the Commandment, "Thou shalt not commit adultery" is neither strengthened nor weakened by the arguments put forth by theologians to increase our understanding of it. For the believer, the force of the Commandment rests upon the authority of God. If God has spoken it, we must obey it.

Moral relativism

Let's stick with the subject of adultery for a moment. If someone tells you, "It's wrong for you but not for me," that person is deceived by one of the most prevalent errors of the present age—moral relativism. In moral relativism, there are no absolutes. Whether you are talking about abortion, or fornication, or adultery, or contraception, or incest with one's children, or stealing, or lying, no matter how closely you specify the act, the moral relativist replies, "It all depends." We can understand how an atheist who believes we are nothing more than matter that has evolved strictly by chance might hold such an opinion, but it is incompatible with Christian belief.

We believe that there is a Creator God, that He created the world and all that is in it. We believe that He has a plan for sex as well as for the other relationships between men and women and children. We believe that the Ten Commandments are as good and true and binding on us today as when revealed through Moses.

Many people who are infected with moral relativism really haven't thought it through. For many, it is more or less of a knee-jerk reflex. They hear something which, if it is true, demands that they change the way they are living if they are going to be true to themselves and to God. However, they have no intention of making any changes. So without further thought, they slip into knee-jerk moral relativism—"true for you but not for me." We say that such people haven't thought through the idea of moral relativism because if everyone believed there were no moral absolutes and acted accordingly, our lives, our welfare, and everything we owned would be in constant danger. We would need a police state where there were not only laws against murder, robbery, etc., but also a cop on every block and a huge jail system. When you read about the senseless and multiple killings in the drug infested ghettos of the United States, you are reading about a culture in which moral relativism is being put into practice—with a vengeance.

Someone else might say, "That would be sinful for me to do but I can't say it's wrong for someone else." Well, yes you can. Take the case of murder. Now, not all killing is murder. Murder is the deliberate killing of an innocent person.

What we mean by objective morality is this: it's wrong for me to murder someone, it's wrong for you to murder someone, and it's wrong for Joe Drugfiend and Doctor Bigbucks to murder someone. In God's order of creation, it is morally evil for one human person to murder another human person.

What we mean by subjective guilt is this: We cannot determine the degree of guilt that some other person incurs before God when he or she does something that is morally evil such as deliberately killing an innocent person as is done in abortion. We can rightly say that if **we** did that and then were immediately killed by a bolt of lightning before we had time to repent, we could expect to spend eternity in hell. However, we do not know whether someone else doing exactly the same thing fulfilled the conditions for incurring the guilt of mortal sin. For example, we do not know whether someone else has the advantage of knowing the grave evil of the action. We have to leave to God the judgment of the subjective guilt of every person, no matter how obvious is the evil of the external action.

● **"Judge not lest you be judged"** (Mt 7:1). This teaching of Jesus means what we have explained above: don't try to judge the subjective guilt of anyone. However, it most certainly does not mean that we are not to judge the moral worth of human actions. The Ten Commandments and all the moral teachings of the Bible are judgments of behavior, and it is the responsibility of believers to make these divine judgments known to themselves and to the world at large. The last words of Jesus on earth to his apostles were about going to all nations and teaching them "to observe all that I have commanded you" (Mt 28:20).

A common question is this: "If unnatural methods and natural methods of birth control both have the purpose of avoiding pregnancy, what's the moral difference?"

Let's restate the question: "Does a common purpose make all the means of achieving that purpose morally the same?" If you think about it for a minute, you will quickly conclude that it doesn't. Imagine that two different couples both would like to live in a very nice house. Neither can afford it right now. One couple decides to save every dollar they can; he works hard and goes to night school to improve his earning ability. The other couple decide to sell illicit drugs for a few years. They both have the same purpose—buying that nice house. Does that make hard honest work and the illicit drug trade morally equal? Of course not.

The huge difference between using NFP and using unnatural methods of birth control is the difference between respecting God's order of creation and not respecting it, between honoring the divinely built-in meaning of the marriage act and contradicting that built-in meaning.

● **More on the difference.** Both Paul VI and John Paul II have commented on the difference between using natural and unnatural methods of conception regulation.

To make use of the gift of conjugal love while respecting the laws of the generative process means to acknowledge oneself not to be the arbiter of the sources of human life, but rather the minister of the design established by the Creator (Pope Paul VI, *Humanae Vitae*, n. 13).

In 1981, Pope John Paul II explained this further in *Familiaris Con-sortio*, a teaching on the Christian family.

When couples, by means of recourse to contraception, separate these two meanings that God the creator has inscribed in the being of man and woman and in the dynamism of their sexual communion, they act as "arbiters" of the divine plan and they "manipulate" and degrade human sexuality and with it themselves and their married partner by altering its value of "total" self-giving (n. 32.4).

On the contrary, when couples use chaste NFP,

they are acting as "ministers" of God's plan (n. 32.5).

The Pope went on to note that the difference between contraception and natural family planning

. . . is a difference which is much wider and deeper than is usually thought, one which involves in the final analysis two irreconcilable concepts of the human person and of human sexuality (n. 32.6).

With NFP, the Pope noted, there is "shared responsibility and self control" and sexuality is respected, not used as an object.

Is it NATURAL?

This question asks, "Is it natural for a married couple to abstain if they feel inclined to have marital relations?" Yes. By NATURAL we mean acting in accord with the created human nature God has given us. No one is saying that's easy. The trouble is, we have inherited a fallen human nature, so we experience conflict between what we should do—or should not do—and what we sometimes feel inclined to do. All the Ten Commandments are about acting in accord with our created human nature; many daily newspaper stories are about how people are not doing so. However, with the grace of God—and only with his special help—we can live in accord with what it means to be created in the image and likeness of God.

The Biblical Basis

There are a number of different reasons for believing that God cares about what you do about birth control. We will start with the Bible.

The Onan account

Chapter 38 in Genesis tells the story of Onan. His older brother had died, and he was bound by an ancient Near Eastern custom called the Law of the Levirate to marry his brother's widow, Tamar, and to try to have a son by her. That first son would be considered to be the son of the deceased brother in order to keep alive his name and family line. Onan would go through the motions of intercourse with Tamar but would withdraw and spill his seed on the ground. That's called "withdrawal;" the technical term is "coitus interruptus." God's judgment on this was strong: "And what he did was displeasing in the sight of the Lord, and He slew him also" (Gen 38-10). The death penalty.

Christian commentary has traditionally seen this as God's judgment against all unnatural forms of birth control. St. Augustine wrote: "Intercourse even with one's legitimate wife is unlawful and wicked where the conception of the offspring is prevented. Onan, the son of Judah, did this and the Lord killed him for it."[1]

Many Protestant theologians wrote Bible commentaries, and in commenting on this passage, Martin Luther wrote: "This is a most disgraceful sin. It is far more atrocious than incest and adultery. We call it unchastity, yes, a Sodomitic sin."[2] John Calvin, one of the most dominant figures in early Protestantism, described the sin of Onan as a form of homicide.[3] John Wesley, the father of the Methodist churches, taught that such sins are very displeasing to God and that those who commit them will destroy their souls.[4] An Evangelical Protestant, Charles Provan, did extensive research on this subject and reached this conclusion:

> We have found not one orthodox theologian to defend Birth Control before the 1900s. NOT ONE! On the other hand, we have found that many highly regarded Protestant theologians were enthusiastically opposed to it, all the way back to the very beginning of the Reformation.[5]

As you can well imagine, contracepting Christians have tried to destroy the force of this Biblical teaching. Some say the sin of Onan was *only* the sin of selfishness against his brother, but Biblical scholarship and common sense show the error of this interpretation.

1. Biblical scholarship has pointed out that "in a strict interpretation the text says that what was evil in the sight of the Lord was what Onan actually did; the emphasis . . . of verse 10 does not fall on what he intended to achieve, but on what he **did**."[6] For more on this, see *Birth Control and Christian Discipleship.*[7]

2. The punishment for violating the Law of the Levirate is clearly spelled out in Deuteronomy 25:5-10. An aggrieved widow could bring her offending brother-in-law before the elders. If he still refused to do his duty, she could take a sandal off his foot and spit in his face. Then the offender would be called House of the Unshod. Humiliating, but hardly the death penalty meted out to Onan.

3. In the Onan account, three people are guilty of violating the Law of the Levirate: Onan, his father Judah, and his younger brother Shelah. Judah openly admits his guilt in verse 26. The widow Tamar had tricked Judah into

having intercourse with her and getting her pregnant, and that got Tamar accused of harlotry. Then Judah acknowledged he was the father and further admitted: "She is in the right rather than I. This comes of my not giving her to my son Shelah to be his wife."

When three people are guilty of the same crime but only one of them receives the death penalty from God, common sense requires that we ask if that person did something the others did not do. The answer is obvious: only Onan went through the motions of the covenant act of intercourse but defrauded its purpose and meaning; only Onan engaged in the contraceptive behavior of withdrawal.

4. Onan's sin was a violation of a covenant act. The only place we see God delivering the death penalty in the New Testament is also for a violation of a covenant. In the Acts of the Apostles 5:1-11, Ananias and Sapphira went through the motions of a covenant act but defrauded it, and each was stricken dead for this deception. Marital intercourse is a covenant act. Onan defrauded it and was killed for his dishonest sexual behavior. The Onan account directly supports the Christian Tradition that we are obliged not to defraud the covenantal marriage act by contraception, and the account of Ananias and Sapphira shows how seriously God takes the defrauding of covenant acts.

Chemical birth control

One form of birth control practiced by the pagans in the first century of the Christian era was the mixing of potions—chemical birth control. At that point in history, no one could tell if these potions prevented ovulation or killed the sperm or killed a newly conceived baby or did some combination of all three. In other words, these potions were very much like the modern birth control Pill and raised the same questions: contraceptive or early abortion agent?

The Greek word for such mixing of potions for birth control and other secret purposes was *pharmakeia* (farm-ah-kay-ah), from which we have the modern word "pharmacy." The mixing of medicines for healing purposes would not have been condemned, but that's not what ancient *pharmakeia* was about. *Pharmakeia* is condemned three times in the New Testament (Galatians 5:19-26; Revelations 9:21; 21:8). The context of all three passages is concerned with sexual immorality, and two of the passages also condemn murder. If you check this out in your Bible, you will probably see *pharmakeia* translated as "sorcery," but that word doesn't tell us much. It just raises questions about what the potion mixers were doing.

Therefore, although it is not absolutely certain, it is probable that we have three New Testament passages that condemn unnatural forms of birth control. These would apply first of all to chemical birth control such as the Pill, implants, injections, and some forms of the IUD; then by extension to all other unnatural forms.

The first century Christian teaching document called the *Didache (The Teaching of the Apostles)* also condemns the use of chemical and other forms of birth control, using the words for magic and drugs. "You shall not use magic (*mageia*). You shall not use drugs (*pharmakeia*). You shall not procure abortion. You shall not destroy a newborn child." Father John Hardon, S.J., explains this text:

> Records from the practices of these times tell us that the people would first try some magical rites or resort to sorcery to avoid conception. If this failed, they would use one or another of the medical contraceptives . . . If notwithstanding a woman became pregnant, she would try to abort. And if even this failed, there was always the Roman law that permitted infanticide.[8]

Two things are evident. 1) Chemical birth control was practiced in the pagan world. 2) Early Christian teaching thoroughly condemned chemical and all unnatural forms of birth control.

How does the practice of Natural Family Planning fit in with a life of Christian discipleship? Because periodic abstinence is sometimes difficult, some people have questioned whether it can be required as part of Christian discipleship. The Couple to Couple League publishes a 45 page booklet that examines this question more in depth—*Birth Control and Christian Discipleship*.[9] Here we can be brief.

Christian Discipleship

● **Love.** Is there any place in the Bible where God tells us that love is easy? Of course not. Christians should know that Jesus taught us to love even our enemies (Mt 5:44), and everyone recognizes that as a difficult commandment. However, Jesus carries it further. He commands us to love each other as He has loved us (Jn 15:12). Now, if love was easy, would Jesus have to command us to love each other?

● **The narrow way.** There is much in the Sermon on the Mount that sets the tone for Christian discipleship, and one of those teachings is this: "Enter by the narrow gate, for the gate is wide and the way is easy that leads to destruction, and those who enter by it are many. For the gate is narrow and the way is hard that leads to life, and those who find it are few" ((Mt 7:13-14). Now, even when we understand that "few" is a way of saying "not everyone," that teaching is still a real wake-up call.

● **The daily cross.** The universal symbol of Christianity today is the cross. Is it only a reminder of something that happened on Calvary nearly 2000 years ago or is it something more? Jesus answers that question:

> If anyone would come after me, let him deny himself, and take up his cross daily, and follow me. For whoever would save his life will lose it, and whoever loses his life for my sake, he will save it. For what does it profit a man if he gains the whole world and loses or forfeits himself? (Lk 9:23-25).

There is no question that periodic abstinence is a daily cross for some couples—for about one week each cycle. After all, in a typical cycle, couples who want to avoid pregnancy have to abstain for about 9 to 12 consecutive days. Almost any married person can abstain for two or three days without difficulty unless he or she is really in the chains of sexual addiction. Abstinence doesn't normally become difficult until about the third or fourth day. That's why we can say that the time of difficulty is generally about a week.

Thus the whole question about using NFP or unnatural forms of birth control really gets down to this: can married couples who call themselves Christian be expected to carry the cross of periodic abstinence for a week or so each cycle? Yes, we know there are cases of more extended abstinence, but right now we're talking about the vast majority of cases.

● **The light burden.** What Jesus also teaches is that carrying the cross of discipleship is not impossible or intolerable but is the way to refreshment and happiness even in this life.

> Come to Me, all you who labor and are heavy laden, and I will give you rest. Take my yoke upon you, and learn from Me, for I am gentle and lowly of heart, and you will find rest for your souls. For my yoke is easy and my burden is light" (Mt 11:28-30).

The truth is this: for the Christian, whatever difficulties we might experience in the practice of natural family planning are simply the price of discipleship. Furthermore, the couple who practice NFP for the right reasons and in the right spirit will normally experience a good marriage relationship and an elevation of their spiritual union. They, like millions of Christians over the centuries, will experience that God is not to be outdone in generosity and that the words of Jesus still ring true—His yoke is easy and His burden is light; He gives rest to your soul.

Wouldn't it be helpful if. . .?

Wouldn't it really be helpful if the Bible contained more texts explicitly condemning each and every method of contraception? Not really. Look at the anti-sodomy texts of Genesis 19 (Sodom and Gomorrah), Leviticus 18:22, and Romans 1:24-32. How could Scripture be more explicit in condemning sodomy? Yet those who want to accept sodomy simply shrug off this teaching by saying, for example, that St. Paul was only condemning "promiscuous" sodomy (he made no such distinction). Using another tactic, they dismiss all the texts as simply not relevant to the 20th century.

The point is this: even if the Bible were filled with explicit condemnations of abortion, sterilization and contraception, dissenters would use the same techniques on those texts they have used on the anti-sodomy texts. That's one reason why the Catholic Church teaches that Jesus did not leave us only a book subject to everyone's personal and sometimes contradictory interpretations. Instead, He established his Church as the authoritative teacher guided by the Holy Spirit. The constant teaching of the Church on matters of faith and morals is called Tradition.

The tone of discipleship

Many passages in Sacred Scripture set the tone for discipleship, for walking the narrow way with Jesus (Mt. 7:13). Much is to be found in the Sermon on the Mount (Mt 5-7). When you focus on love and sexuality, you find that the Bible calls us to subordinate romantic or erotic love (eros in Greek) to self-giving love (agape in Greek, pronounced ah-gah-pay).

Look at St. Paul's famous writing on love in 1 Corinthians 13: 4-7. True, he is not writing specifically about birth control, but the morality of birth control has to be evaluated in the light of authentic Christian teaching about love. Note how St. Paul begins and ends this famous passage with two aspects of love that are needed for the happy practice of natural family planning: "Love is always patient and kind. . . It is always ready. . . to endure whatever comes."

On the night before He died, Jesus gave us the New Commandment to love one another as He has loved us (John 15:12). St. Paul picked up on this and told husbands to love their wives as Christ loved the Church and sacrificed Himself for her (Eph. 5:25).

In another tone-setting passage, St. Paul tells Christians that

> the fruit of the Spirit is love, joy, peace, patience, kindness, goodness, faith, modesty and self-control. Against such things there is no law. Those who belong to Christ have crucified their flesh with its passions and desires. If we live by the Spirit, let us also walk by the Spirit (Gal 5:22-26).

The Bible has much more to say about love, but this much shows two things: 1) the religious doctrine of marital non-contraception has a basis in Scripture and 2) the practice of natural family planning with its necessity of a certain amount of sexual self-control fits well within the Christian biblical tradition.

The Christian Tradition

The constant teaching of the same doctrine of faith or morality over the centuries constitutes Tradition. It is Sacred Tradition that enables us to distinguish between Old Testament affirmations of the natural moral law ("Thou shalt not commit adultery") and mere uncleanness rules, between unchangeable truths about human nature and discipline that is open to change. For example, St. Paul spends more words on women's veils in church (1 Cor 11) than he does on sodomy (Romans 1), but the Church has always held that sodomy is a very serious offense against the natural moral law while the wearing of veils is only a matter of changeable discipline.

Sacred Tradition rests primarily upon the word of Christ, but it is also supported by common sense. At the Last Supper, Jesus promised repeatedly that He would send the Holy Spirit to guide the Apostles and their successors into the fullness of the truth (John 14:16-17, 25-26; 15:26-27; 16:12-13). Common sense says that God would not go to such bother and pain to reveal the truth about Himself and Man and then leave it up for grabs and completely contradictory interpretations. Almost all Christians say they believe the Bible is the inspired word of God, but how do they know what belongs in it? All those who say they believe the 27 books of the New Testament are the inspired word of God are making an implicit act of faith that Christ was being faithful to his promises and that the Holy Spirit guided the Catholic Church to accept these writings and reject others in the first three centuries. (See *Where We Got the Bible* by Henry R. Graham.[10])

The early centuries

We have already seen the *biblical* basis for Christian teaching that it is immoral to use unnatural methods of birth control. Non-biblical teaching can be traced back to the *Didache*, "The Teaching of the Twelve Apostles," composed before 80 A.D.[11] Condemnations of oral copulation, which is certainly a contraceptive behavior, are found in a second century work,[12] and that history continues right up to modern times. The Protestant Reformation provided no break in the constant teaching. As mentioned earlier in this chapter, Martin Luther, John Calvin, John Wesley and many other Protestant theologians thoroughly condemned the use of unnatural forms of birth control.

Response to new challenges

In 1798 an English economist named Thomas Malthus wrote a gloomy treatise, *An Essay on the Principle of Population.* This was the first population scare. Malthus thought that population would increase faster than the food supplies and this would cause mass starvation. Malthus was also an Anglican clergyman, and for "population control" he recommended late marriage and total abstinence once a family reached the parents' desired size. In 1823, the neo-Malthusians dropped the morality of Malthus and began to promote contraception. **This was truly revolutionary.** *For the first time in Christian history,* "respectable" persons were openly promoting unnatural forms of birth control in the face of the universal teaching of the churches against such behavior. In 1839 Charles Goodyear accidentally discovered how to vulcanize rubber, and this new technology was soon applied to the making of condoms that had previously been made from animal skins or intestines.

In the 1870s, an American Protestant reformer named Anthony Comstock persuaded the U. S. Congress and many states to pass laws against the sale and distribution of contraceptives. This body of legislation became known as

There is no question: the American anti-contraceptive laws were passed by essentially Protestant legislatures for a basically Protestant America.

the Comstock laws, and it was clearly in response to the neo-Malthusian propaganda for contraception. It is important for the student of religious Tradition to realize that such legislation reflected common Christian belief. There is no question: the American anti-contraceptive laws were passed by essentially Protestant legislatures for a basically Protestant America.

The bishops of the Church of England responded to the neo-Malthusian propaganda. In 1908 and again in 1920 they strongly reaffirmed the traditional teaching against contraception. For example, in 1920 they stated: "We utter an emphatic warning against the use of unnatural means for the avoidance of conception."[13]

The break

Just before World War I, Margaret Sanger began the American organized effort to promote unnatural forms of birth control. She joined forces with like-minded revolutionaries in England, and the continued pressure proved to be too much for the bishops of the Church of England. Although they recognized that they had clearly reaffirmed the Tradition in 1908 and 1920, they capitulated at their Lambeth Conference of 1930. Their statement on August 14, 1930, marked *the first time in Christian history that an organized church body formally permitted the use of unnatural methods of birth control.* In the United States a committee of the Federal Council of Churches made a similar statement on March 21, 1931. Both groups were clearly warned by their own members that accepting contraception would have far ranging disastrous consequences. One of the Anglican bishops said that if they allowed contraception they were opening a Pandora's box.[14] Despite these warnings, they still voted to depart from what had been the universal teaching of Christian churches.

The reaction

Pope Pius XI led the Catholic reaction with an encyclical (teaching letter) titled *Casti Connubii — Concerning Chaste Marriage,* dated December 31, 1930. In very strong and clear language he reaffirmed the Tradition.

> Since, therefore, openly departing from the uninterrupted Christian tradition some recently have judged it possible solemnly to declare another doctrine regarding this question, the Catholic Church, to whom God has entrusted the defense of the integrity and purity of morals, standing erect in the midst of the moral ruin which surrounds her, in order that she may preserve the chastity of the nuptial union from being defiled by this foul stain, raises her voice in token of her divine ambassadorship and through Our mouth proclaims anew: any use whatsoever of matrimony exercised in such a way that the act is deliberately frustrated in its natural power to generate life is an offense against the law of God and of nature, and those who indulge in such are branded with the guilt of a grave sin (para. 56).

To put that in standard Catholic terminology, the Pope was saying that it is the grave matter of mortal sin for a married couple to use unnatural methods of birth control. Those who do so with sufficient reflection and full consent of their wills incur the guilt of mortal sin.

In the very next paragraph he reminded Catholic priests of their obligation to teach the truth:

If any confessor or pastor of souls, which may God forbid, lead the faithful entrusted to him into these errors or should at least confirm them by approval or by guilty silence, let him be mindful of the fact that he must render a strict account to God, the Supreme Judge, for the betrayal of his sacred trust, and let him take to himself the words of Christ: "They are blind and leaders of the blind; and if the blind lead the blind, both fall into the pit" (para. 57).

The language of the Pope was almost mild by comparison with that of others. The day after the Federal Council of Churches' March 21 statement permitting the use of unnatural methods of birth control, a *Washington Post* editorial said this:

Carried to its logical conclusion, the committee's report, if carried into effect, would sound the deathknell of marriage as a holy institution by establishing degrading practices which would encourage indiscriminate immorality. The suggestion that the use of legalized contraceptives would be "careful and restrained" is preposterous.[15]

Lutheran seminary theologian Dr. Walter A. Maier was equally strong: "Birth Control, as popularly understood today and involving the use of contraceptives, is one of the most repugnant of modern aberrations, representing a 20th century renewal of pagan bankruptcy."[16]

Methodist Bishop Warren Chandler was emphatic: "The whole disgusting movement rests on the assumption of man's sameness with the brutes. . ."[17]

The Presbyterian attacked the Federal Council of Churches for allowing such a committee endorsement of contraception: "Its recent pronouncement of birth control should be enough reason, if there were no other, to withdraw support from that body, which declares that it speaks for the Presbyterian and other Protestant churches in ex cathedra statements."[18]

The Sixties to the present

By the Fifties and Sixties, few people remembered that Protestant churches once adamantly opposed the use of unnatural forms of birth control. More and more people thought that birth control was just one of those Catholic *versus* Protestant issues that had been around for 450 years and would stay that way, something no one had to think about.

Catholic teaching on birth control remained firm even at the parish level through the Fifties. Things changed in the Sixties. The Pill came on the market in 1960, and birth control was front page news. The Pope set up a commission to advise him about the Pill because it acted differently from the traditional barrier-type contraceptives. Was it just another unnatural form of birth control? Or did the Pill regulate the time at which a woman ovulated so that it would be easier to practice the calendar rhythm form of natural family planning? (It didn't regulate ovulation then, and it still doesn't.)

The mere fact that the Pope had set up a commission to advise him about the Pill led to all sorts of speculation that he was looking for a way to change Catholic teaching on birth control. Whole books have been written about this, and another CCL book, *Sex and the Marriage Covenant*, goes into this history in some detail.[19]

On 25 July 1968 Pope Paul VI ended such speculation and reaffirmed the Christian Tradition against the use of unnatural forms of birth control. His teaching document was an encyclical titled *Humanae Vitae* (*Concerning*

273

Human Life. Papal documents are named by the first few words of the official Latin text.) In a beautiful but largely unread document, this is the sentence that has received the most attention:

> Nonetheless, the Church, calling men back to the observance of the norms of the natural law, as interpreted by its constant doctrine, teaches that each and every marriage act must remain open to the transmission of life (n. 11).

The Pope made it very clear that this did not exclude recourse to natural family planning when a couple had sufficiently serious reasons to postpone or avoid pregnancy. However, the liberal propaganda machine had led people to believe that the Pope would certainly change the teaching of the Church, and that same propaganda machine now turned directly against the Pope and the Tradition in a verbally violent reaction of dissent that may be without equal in the history of the Church.

When Pope Paul VI died in 1978, his successor, Pope John Paul I, lived only a month. When Pope John Paul II took office on 22 October 1978, there was widespread speculation. Would the new Pope, the first Polish Pope in history, change the teaching?

Pope John Paul II answered the speculation in 1979 by reaffirming the teaching of *Humanae Vitae*. In fact, he reaffirmed this teaching so often and in so many different ways over the next ten years that it became his main teaching effort. He has continued to reaffirm the teaching against marital contraception at least once a year every year since 1988.[20] In 1981 he published *Familiaris Consortio*, an extensive teaching on the family, and in 1993 he published an extensive teaching on moral theology, *Veritatis Splendor*, "The Splendor of the Truth."

The real issue

The real issue at stake in the birth control controversy is **truth.** Are you called to live according to the truth? How can you come to know the truth about love? Is there a divinely built-in meaning to sex? One section of one chapter is hardly the place to give an extensive answer to these questions, but we can make some obvious statements. For more extensive answers, study *Veritatis Splendor*.

1. Are you called to live according to the truth? When you stop to think about it, that's the most basic thing you have in common with every other human person on this earth. What's one of the most damning things you can say about someone else? Isn't it that he or she is dishonest, a fake, a sham, a hypocrite?

2. How can you know the truth about love? The Catholic Church teaches that it is possible to reason to the basic truths about love; however, almost all of us learn from Special Revelation. The Ten Commandments say so much about the truth about love, about what it means to be a human being, that some skeptics have said that they weren't revealed but are just the accumulated wisdom of the Jews. Not so; not at all. Read the Old Testament and see how much they liked those Commandments.

Jesus came to teach us the full truth about love. "For this I was born and for this I have come into the world, to bear witness to the truth. Every one who is of the truth hears my voice" (Jn 18:37).

How could He keep the truth alive? He very deliberately did not leave us anything in writing. He knew that anything He might leave us in print would be interpreted away to nothingness or confusion. Instead, He founded his Church to transmit the truth He had revealed. He promised that the Holy

Spirit would continue to guide it until He returned. In brief, we come to know the truth about love through the vehicle Christ gave us, "the Church of the living God, the pillar and the bulwark of the truth" (1 Tim 3:15).

3. Is there a divinely built-in meaning to sex? The whole of Sacred Scripture from Genesis through the Book of Revelation bears witness that God has a plan for sex. In Exodus, two of the seven Commandments dealing with our neighbor are about sex, both external behavior and lustful desires. Furthermore, Sacred Scripture condemns every form of deliberate genital sexual act except non-contraceptive marital relations.[21] That's certainly good proof that God has a plan for sex.

Pope John Paul II has taught repeatedly that there is a built-in meaning to sex, a nuptial or marital meaning of sexual relations. It is *the* marriage act; it must express the total gift man and wife make to each other when they marry. He has taught repeatedly that when a couple use unnatural forms of birth control, they refuse that total gift of self to the other and they contradict the truth of the marriage act.

Summary

The Christian Tradition against unnatural forms of birth control dates back to the first century, continues to the present, and will continue till the end of time. It is based on the very nature of what it means to be a human person and the meaning of sexual relations, and human nature does not change.

The Tradition was kept alive by all the Christian churches until 1930. Since the break in 1930, every Pope has reaffirmed the Tradition in one way or another, except for the short-lived Pope John Paul I. Pope John Paul II has done more to **explain** the Tradition than any other pope in history.

Additional reading

Birth Control and Christian Discipleship, chapters 1, 2, 4, and 5.

"What Does the Catholic Church Really Teach about Birth Control?" a CCL brochure.

Chapter 18: Self-Test Questions

1. True____ False____ It's "just human nature" to lie, steal, commit adultery, fornicate, etc.

2. True____ False____ Parents who refuse sexual self-control for themselves may have a psychological difficulty in teaching self-control to their children.

3. True____ False____ The American anti-contraception laws of the 1870s were passed by Catholics for a mostly Catholic country.

4. Who made the following statement in 1920?

> *"We utter an emphatic warning against the use of unnatural means for the avoidance of conception, together with the grave dangers—physical, moral and religious—thereby incurred, and against the evils with which the extension of such use threatens the race."*

   a) Bishops of the Church of England b) Roman Catholic bishops

5. The first organized Church approval of unnatural methods of birth control was by the _____ in the year _____.

6. The response by Pope Pius XI was to
   a) accept unnatural methods of birth control
   b) reaffirm the Christian Tradition
   c) call marital contraception "an offense against the law of God and of nature. . ."
   (More than one of the above may be correct.)

7. True____ False____ For 19 centuries unnatural forms of birth control were described by Christians as "Onanism."

8. The whole Biblical teaching on sex supports the idea that God intends that marital relations should be a _____ of your _____.

Answers to self-test
1. False 2. True 3. False 4. a) Bishops of the Church of England 5. Church of England. . . 1930 6. b) reaffirm the Christian Tradition. . . c) call marital contraception "an offense against the law of God and of nature" 7. True 8. renewal. . . marriage covenant.

References

(1) St. Augustine, *De conjug. adult.*, lib II, n. 12. Quoted by Pope Pius XI in *Casti Connubii*, para. 55, 31 December 1931.
(2) Charles D. Provan, *The Bible and Birth Control*, (Monongahela, PA: Zimmer Printing, 1989) 81.
(3) Provan, 68.
(4) Provan, 91.
(5) Provan, 63.
(6) Manuel Miguens, "Biblical thoughts on 'Human Sexuality,' " *Human Sexuality in Our Time*, ed. George A. Kelly (Boston: St. Paul Editions, 1979) 112-115.
(7) John F. Kippley, *Birth Control and Christian Discipleship*, (Cincinnati: Couple to Couple League, 1994) 23-26.
(8) John A. Hardon, S.J., *The Catholic Catechism* (Garden City: Doubleday, 1975) 367-368.
(9) Kippley, *Birth Control and Christian Discipleship*, 31-39.
(10) Henry F. Graham, *Where We Got the Bible* (San Diego: Catholic Answers, 1997; original by Herder, 1911).
(11) Hardon, 334, 367.
(12) John T. Noonan, Jr., *Contraception: A History of Its Treatment by the Catholic Theologians and Canonists*,

enlarged edition (Cambridge: Harvard University Press, 1986) 92. This is the classical work on the historical aspects of this subject.

(13) The Lambeth Conference of 1920, Resolution 68. Quoted in John C. Ford, S.J. and Gerald Kelly, S.J., *Contemporary Moral Theology: Vol. II: Marriage Questions* (Westminster: Newman, 1964) 247.

(14) In Greek mythology, Zeus gave Pandora a box which she was not to open. Curiosity got the better of her; she opened it and all the troubles of the world poured out.

(15) Editorial, *Washington Post*, 22 March 1931.

(16) Walter A. Maier, cited in J.F.N. (probably J.F. Noll) *A Catechism of Birth Control*, Sixth edition, (Huntington: OSV Press, ca. 1939) 31.

(17) Warren Chandler, cited in Noll, 31.

(18) *The Presbyterian*, 2 April 1931, cited in Noll, 30.

(19) John F. Kippley, *Sex and the Marriage Covenant: A Basis for Morality* (Cincinnati: Couple to Couple League, 1991) Chapter 11, "The Historical Context." See also Janet Smith, *Humanae Vitae: A Generation Later*, Chapters One and Two.

(20) *Sex and the Marriage Covenant* assembles much of this teaching.

(21) Kippley, *Sex and the Marriage Covenant*, Chapters 2 and 3.

19

Theology and Ecology

This chapter is about thinking. When it comes to sex and birth control, many people put their thinking abilities into neutral. We have heard otherwise intelligent people argue that if man can invent the Pill with his God-given brains, that makes it morally okay to use it for birth control. As we saw in the last chapter, others ask, "What's the difference between two actions if they both have the same objective?"—as if nothing but the overall purpose really counted.

This chapter contains two major sections. The first section looks at theology; the second reviews the Sexual Revolution.

Theology and Birth Control

Please don't let the word "theology" scare you. Good theology is still what St. Anselm said it was: faith seeking understanding. Theology starts with faith and then seeks to achieve understanding through the use of reason.

Catholic theology makes it clear that the teaching against contraception is based on human nature and on the nature of marriage. Since those don't change, the teaching can't change. If it were a rule made up by the Church such as the discipline of not eating meat on Friday, the Church could change it. But it's not. (By the way, when the Friday abstinence discipline was in effect, the sin of eating meat on Friday was a sin of disobedience. No one ever taught that there was something intrinsically wrong with eating meat on Friday.)

Theologians have developed a number of different ways to show how the teaching of marital non-contraception reflects the demands of human nature. Some explanations are more helpful than others; some may really hit home with one person and leave another cold, and vice versa. What follows is a very limited personal selection. For a much more complete review of the arguments, see Dr. Janet Smith's two books: *Humanae Vitae: A Generation Later* and *Why Humanae Vitae Was Right: A Reader.*[1]

Please note: the moral force of the teaching does not depend on the arguments developed to explain it. The moral force stems from the fact that the teaching is taught with the utmost authority by the Church which we believe is guided by the Holy Spirit to teach the divine truth about human love. However, some explanations can help us to understand better the truth about ourselves and the demands of love, at least if we look at them with an open heart and mind. So let us take a look.

What God has joined together . . .

Christian theology speaks about marital relations as "the marriage act." Both the Bible and Tradition make it very clear that sexual intercourse is intended by God to be a marriage act. Sacred Scripture condemns as immoral every other form of sexual copulation from adultery to sodomy.[2] This has been so much a part of Christian morality that sometimes moral theologians will use the term "marriage act" even when it isn't really a marriage act. For example, "It is the sin of adultery for a married person to engage in the marriage act with someone who is not his or her spouse." It's a way of saying that every act of sexual intercourse is **supposed** to be an act of marital relations.

Jesus taught very clearly about the unbreakable character of true marriage: "What therefore God has joined together, let no man put asunder" (Mt 19:6). The same teaching applies to the marriage act, so we can apply it to birth control.

Pope Paul VI said as much but in different words. First he reaffirmed the Christian Tradition in Section 11 of *Humanae Vitae*: "Each and every marriage act must remain open to the transmission of life." Then he went on to explain why in Section 12:

> That teaching, often set forth by the magisterium, is founded upon the inseparable connection, willed by God and unable to be broken by man on his own initiative, between the two meanings of the conjugal act: the unitive meaning and the procreative meaning.

If you have difficulty absorbing that passage, you are not alone. It has 43 words, and seven key words stem from the Latin language. Let's paraphrase it.

Just ask yourself: Who joined together in the marriage act what we call "making love" and "making babies"? Who else but God? Next question: What is contraception except the effort to take apart what God Himself has joined together? Finally, apply the words of Jesus about marriage to the marriage act: "What God has joined together, let no one take apart."

Let's carry this a step farther. Who made woman in such a way that she is fertile only about one week out of every fertility cycle? Who made woman in such a way that her body signals when she is fertile and when she is infertile? Who has joined together and also provided a natural separation of "making love" and "making babies" at different times in a woman's fertility cycle? Who else but God?

What is natural family planning except the effort to respect what God Himself has joined together and also has taken apart? In other words, what is natural family planning except simple fertility awareness and good stewardship of God's creation? What is NFP except respecting and caring for the gifts He has given us?

In the light of these questions, you might find it easier to read again the quotations from *Humanae Vitae* and *Familiaris Consortio* back in Chapter 18 dealing with the differences between NFP and unnatural forms of birth control.

Sexual intercourse is intended by God to be at least implicitly a renewal of the marriage covenant.

This helps to explain two moral evils—sex outside marriage and marital contraception.

● Sex outside marriage

Both the Bible and Tradition are clear in teaching that it is seriously immoral to have sexual relations outside marriage. The *Catechism of the Catholic Church* puts it succinctly: "Among the sins gravely contrary to chastity are masturbation, fornication, pornography, and homosexual practices" (n.2396). (See *Sex and the Marriage Covenant*[3] for fuller information.) Our explanation is simple. In God's plan, sexual intercourse is exclusively a marriage act. Sexual intercourse ought to be a renewal of the faith and love of the marriage covenant. However, outside marriage, there is no covenant of marriage. A couple absolutely cannot renew a non-existent marriage covenant. Therefore, sex outside marriage is essentially dishonest; it pretends to be what it cannot be. This applies to engaged couples as well as to teenage weekend fornicators.

● Contraception within marriage

Think about it. What makes you married in the first place? Isn't it the public commitment of yourself and your spouse to give yourselves totally and for life to each other—"for better and for worse"? Of course. However, what if a couple stated that they were "marrying" only for better but *not* for worse? Or for five years with a mutually renewable option for another five years? What would you call such an arrangement? You might call it legalized mistressing or prostitution; technically it would be an "invalid marriage"; it is certainly not a true marriage. To live knowingly and willingly in such an arrangement would be living in sin.

The marriage act with your spouse should reflect at least in a minimal way the gift of self you made at marriage. That means that "making love" should be an act of love, an act that you do for the good of the other, not just for self-gratification. Marriage is about love for your spouse and your children, and that combination provides almost endless opportunities for self-giving.

Even if you know in your heart that the primary reason why at least one of you wants to have marital relations is for the relief of concupiscence (sexual desire or tension), you both should have a general intention that this act will be helpful to your marriage, perhaps by increasing your bonding. Sometimes a short prayer might be helpful. "Lord, we thank You for each other; please help us to keep alive the love we pledged at marriage. May our actions now help us to grow in love."

At the very least your acts of "making love" must not contradict the meaning of sex as a marriage act. However, what is the essence of using unnatural methods of birth control? Doesn't the body language of contraceptive birth control make it clear? The body language of contraception says very clearly, "We take each other for better but definitely *not for the imagined worse* of possible pregnancy. We are placing or have placed a positive obstacle (or block or impediment) to the natural consequences of the marriage act."

Contraception makes the marriage act invalid as a renewal or affirmation of the marriage covenant.It is no longer an act that reaffirms "for better and for worse." It is no longer a symbol of the total gift of marriage. It contradicts the meaning and the truth of marriage and of the marriage act.

Humanae Vitae calls the contraceptive marriage act "intrinsically dishonest" (n. 14).

Just as sex outside marriage is essentially dishonest and immoral, so is marital contraception. Contraception contradicts the meaning of the marriage covenant—the gift of self "for better and for worse." It is essentially dishonest, and it is therefore immoral.

The concept that sexual intercourse is intended by God to be at least implicitly a renewal of the marriage covenant is called the covenant theology of sex. It forms the basic thesis of *Sex and the Marriage Covenant* that applies it both to marriage and to sex outside marriage. Many are finding this book helpful for an easy to read yet in-depth treatment of the birth control issue.[4]

Consequences

Pope Paul VI did not base his teaching on the foreseeable consequences of marital contraception. Rather, he based his teaching on the Tradition and on "the inseparable connection. . . between. . . the unitive . . . and the procreative meaning" of the marriage act.

Still, in section 17 of *Humanae Vitae*, the Pope predicted some of the unhappy consequences of using unnatural methods of birth control: Conjugal infidelity. . . the general lowering of morality including that of young people, loss of respect for wives by their husbands. He also predicted that it would be a dangerous weapon in the hands of the State that might even impose unnatural methods of birth control on its citizens.

The Pope was ridiculed at the time. Twenty-five years later he was recognized as a prophet even by those who continued to oppose the teaching. Every dire prediction has been fulfilled—and worse. China has imposed on its citizens not only sterilization and IUDs but also surgical and chemical abortion.

In this chapter's final section, "A Moral Ecology," we review other consequences of the widespread acceptance of unnatural birth control.

The Pro-contraception Arguments

In the American legal system, a person is presumed to be innocent until proven guilty. An accused person does not have to prove he is innocent; the State has to prove he is guilty. That means that the "burden of proof" is on the State. If the State's arguments are full of holes and unconvincing, the accused person cannot be convicted.

A similar thing occurs in the arguments about birth control. The presumption of truth is with the traditional teaching; the burden of proof is upon those who accuse the teaching of being false. In the Christian perspective, when a teaching has been reaffirmed in so many ways over the centuries, the presumption is that the teaching is truly the work of the Holy Spirit and therefore true. If someone wants to challenge it, he has to show that the teaching is false; he also has to show that what he has to offer is better. In that perspective, the arguments *for* contraception actually strengthen the case for the teaching *against* it.

The "can-do" argument

This argument says that since man's mind has figured out *how* to practice unnatural methods of birth control, therefore he can morally do it. Some bring God into the picture by saying that God gave us brains and expects us to use the products of our brain power. People who use this argument seem to be fascinated by the research that went into the Pill.

This argument is truly amazing and shows how sexual desires can cloud the mind. How can the ability to figure out how to do something say anything about the morality of doing it? The mind of man is able to figure out how to make instruments of torture, hydrogen bombs, heroin and cocaine, equipment to dismember and kill babies in the womb, chemicals to cause abortions, and the list could go on indefinitely. "White collar crime" is always the result of someone using his God-given brains to do evil. The ability to do something, no matter how clever, is simply no argument that it is morally right to do it.

The "can't do" argument

This argument says that man and woman are so weak and the sexual urge so strong that it is impossible for them to refrain from sex in the face of desire. This argument looks only at human weakness and ignores the grace of God, and it also argues for the acceptance of every other immoral sexual behavior to which we are inclined.

The Bible has a more optimistic view of man and woman. The Old Law called for 12 to 14 days of abstinence every cycle beginning with menstruation. In the New Testament, St. Paul tells us he was struggling with some temptation and asked God to take the temptation completely away. But the Lord told him: "My grace is sufficient for you, for my power is made perfect in weakness" (2 Cor 12:9). Perhaps the Lord is telling us that we have to recognize our weakness and then to pray, really pray, for his help, and He will give it. Note that He did not tell Paul that he would not have to keep working and struggling, and the same is true for us.

This argument also ignores the fact that countless couples are, with the grace of God, winning the struggle. They *are* practicing chaste NFP. These people are not a sexless elite. They are ordinary married men and women who are "different" in only one respect: they recognize their need for God's help in placing their sex drives at the service of authentic love and in living a good marriage.

"The end justifies the means"

This argument admits that using unnatural methods of birth control is contrary to God's order of creation, but it tries to justify contraception as a means for seeking marital happiness and solving population problems.

Think about it for a moment. If the end or purpose someone has in mind justifies whatever means he uses, what can be wrong? Would building an orphanage justify robbing a bank and killing the guards? Of course not. Almost every thinking person recognizes the truth of the maxim: "The end does *not* justify the means."

Applying this to the birth control issue, Pope Paul VI refers to Romans 3:8 and states: "It is not licit, even for the gravest reasons, to do evil so that good may follow" (*H.V.*, n. 14).

The argument from proportionalism

This argument is simply a more sophisticated version of the previous one. The proponents of proportionalism admit that contraception is a "physical evil" because it takes apart what God has joined together in the marriage act. However, they say, when there is a conflict of values, a physical evil is not a moral evil if there is a proportionate reason for doing it. They say it is permissible to use unnatural forms of birth control if in the long run it fosters the values of marital fidelity, human sexuality, and the permanence of marriage itself.

The whole argument was developed to try to justify marital contraception, but it certainly cannot be restrained to contraception or even to sexuality. It completely undermines universal objective morality, and that's why it was condemned as erroneous by Pope John Paul II in *Veritatis Splendor* (nn. 79 - 83). It can't ever say "absolutely never." For example, we are certain that those who developed this argument would never say that building an orphanage was a proportionate reason for robbing banks and killing some bank guards, but that would be just *their* opinion. Since proportionalism rejects universal objective morality, someone else might decide that helping the poor orphans *would* be a proportionate reason for robbing banks and killing innocent bank guards.

Furthermore, the history of the contraceptive sexual revolution defeats this argument. While an individual couple may say that the practice of contraception has made things easier between them—at least for a while, the wider evidence is against it. Increased non-marital sex, increased divorce, and a general debasing of sexuality are the dominant sexual characteristics of an age marked by an almost universal use of contraception. Proportionalism provides a way to rationalize anything you can imagine—abortion, adultery, contraception, incest, masturbation, sodomy—to limit our list strictly to sex-related behaviors. No wonder the Pope condemned it.

The "lesser of two evils" argument

This argument also admits that contraception is an evil because it directly opposes the order of creation. However, the argument claims it is a greater evil for the couple not to have relations whenever they please if they think they need such frequency for their marital happiness.

Dissident theologians developed this argument specifically to "justify" marital contraception, but it is made to order for anyone who wants to try to "justify" almost any imaginable sexual sin. It is simply a variation of "the end justifies the means" argument and is correspondingly erroneous.

At the practical level it incorporates the damaging view that being able to have sexual relations whenever one or both spouses "feel a need" is necessary for marital happiness. The reality is that this doesn't work. It ends up with many wives feeling used, many husbands developing habits of sexual addiction and insatiable lust, and the 1:2 American divorce:marriage ratio.

Summary

Dissenting theologians developed arguments to try to justify marital contraception, but they have not succeeded. Instead, as you will see in the last major section of this chapter, "A Moral Ecology," those same arguments have been used to "justify" homosexual sodomy and fornication. The general effect of the pro-contraception arguments has been to make a major contribution to the spread of the Sexual Revolution.

Ecumenical Support

The traditional Protestant opposition to marital contraception is still alive and well even if not widespread. The mainline Protestant churches have taken both pro-contraception and pro-abortion stands, but that doesn't mean that all those church members are pro-contraception and pro-abortion. Members of various small Christian churches have written us over the years to say, "Our church teaches against abortion, sterilization and contraception but doesn't provide any practical help. Thanks so much for helping us with NFP."

● German physician and theologian **Dr. Siegfried Ernst** has looked at the birth control issue from a unique perspective. He is a Lutheran in a country that has been the theological hotbed for Catholic dissent from *Humanae Vitae*. He believes in a divinely guided evolution and views the entire sexual revolution as counter-evolutionary, regress instead of progress. According to Ernst, "there is a definite contradiction involved in taking both the 'Pill' and the host" (that is, Holy Communion).[5]

As a Protestant, he had viewed the papacy with suspicion, but *Humanae Vitae* changed his thinking. "Probably no other papal decision in history has helped so much to cancel the old mistrust against the papacy. When Pope Paul remained steadfast against pressure from the entire world, when he chose the cross instead of an easier way, the credibility of the papacy was restored."[6]

● In Australia, **Pastor Daniel Overduin**, a Lutheran theologian, has repeatedly hailed the teaching of *Humanae Vitae* as a vital Christian truth.

● **Ingrid Trobisch** included a chapter on the Sympto-Thermal Method of natural family planning in her book, *The Joy of Being a Woman*.[7] At the time she was the wife and ministerial associate of Austrian Pastor Walter Trobisch, now deceased. The Trobisches were led to look for NFP by the Africans whom they served, people who instinctively knew there was something unnatural and wrong about contraception.

● Another Lutheran couple whose book, *The Christian Family*, entered over a million homes shared their convictions about birth control in another book, *The Christian Couple*. In Chapter Eight, titled "Contraception: Blight or Blessing," **Pastor Larry and Nordis Christenson** explain how they left the practice of contraception and began the practice of natural family planning with the help of Dr. Konald A. Prem. Their extensive work in marriage counseling led them to believe that contraception is definitely a blight upon marriage.

In the Eighties there was a Protestant backlash against birth control.

● **Mary Pride**, in her book, *The Way Home*,[9] was so opposed to any form of family planning for any reason that she condemned NFP right along with the Pill. There was so much other good material in that book that we struck up a dialogue with Mrs. Pride, and she came to agree with the Catholic position that it is permissible to use NFP provided you have a sufficiently serious reason to do so. As a result, in her sequel titled *All the Way Home*,[10] she accepted NFP under such circumstances.

● In *A Full Quiver*, **Rick and Jan Hess** took a very strong position that we call "extreme providentialism." They criticized NFP as "needless tinkering with a system He already controls lock, stock and baby."[11] About the only good thing they had to say about NFP was that Christians who start out using it for

The Seventies

"I would not go back to using a contraceptive device even if the alternative were having twenty-one children."
— *Nordis Christenson*[8]

The Eighties and Nineties

absolute birth control tend to loosen up after a bit and use it for having babies. The position of extreme providentialism is wrong. It seems to deny that there is such a thing as the virtue of Christian prudence when it comes to family planning. We grant that true Christian prudence is difficult; it is hard not to be selfish. However, authentic Christian prudence is possible and is at the heart of Christian acceptance of NFP.

We doubt that the proponents of extreme providentialism reject Christian prudence in any other area of life. We hope they take normal care of their health and that of their children; we trust that they make a reasonable effort to educate their children so they will be employable.

● **Charles D. Provan** also leans to the full quiver approach. The front cover of *The Bible and Birth Control*[12] has a reference to Psalm 127:4 and shows a hand holding nine arrows, and the first two chapters are his biblically based arguments against birth control. However, in personal communication, he appears open to the idea of natural family planning when there are sufficiently serious reasons for avoiding or postponing pregnancy. The third chapter of this book is the resource gem; it contains quotations from 66 Protestant theologians condemning Onanism.

● **Pastor David Prentis** and his wife used contraception when they married in 1973, but his wife became increasingly unhappy with it. In 1978 they stumbled upon *The Joy of Being a Woman* by Ingrid Trobisch and turned to the practice of NFP. In 1988, the 20th anniversary of *Humanae Vitae* brought a new round of criticism of its teaching. In response, Pastor Prentis, while still an ordained minister of the Church of Scotland, wrote to the BBC TV program "Everyman" in London about their experience. In 1989 CCL published his letter as an outreach brochure, "Dear Pastor."[13]

In summary, NFP does not mean "Not For Protestants." In 1995 we learned about a new organization—Protestants Against Birth Control.

A Moral Ecology

Most people are aware of the relationships in nature that we call ecology. Most people are aware that certain pesticides on the fields can run off and cause great and unintended harm to wildlife. In other words, trying to eliminate the problem of bugs can create a huge problem in the environment. Today, American farmers have to use different chemicals for bug control, ones that will not have a disastrous effect on the rest of nature.

The point of this section is that there's a similarity between bug control and birth control.

The idea of a moral ecology is not at all new. **In 1929 Walter Lippmann** reflected on the sexual behaviors of the "roaring twenties," and he blamed the rise of sexual promiscuity squarely upon the availability, acceptance, and use of contraceptives.[14] Lippmann also criticized the idea of "companionate marriage." This was a contraceptive and deliberately childless marriage made to be broken when the spouses no longer felt like close companions. Liberals were promoting this concept in the 1920s as a social advance made possible by efficient contraception. In brief, the advocates of companionate, temporary marriage were saying that contraception enabled them to promote new and radically changed ideas about human sexuality, love, and marriage. Lippmann didn't use the term "moral ecology," but that's what he was writing about.

Shortly after Lippmann's serious book appeared, **Aldous Huxley** published his short novel, *Brave New World*, which is still being reprinted and read today. Readers of that novel soon realize that the whole society of *Brave New World* is built upon the technology of sex. Contraception has almost completely divided coitus from procreation. Any contraceptive "mistakes" are taken care of at the abortion clinic. Just as logically in this novel, procreation (or rather reproduction) of children is done by technology: test tube fertilization and development in bottles (artificial wombs) for nine months.

Huxley carried the idea of companionate, temporary marriages one step farther. Since the reproduction of children was all handled by technology and since the education of these children was in the hands of the State's full-care centers, there was no family and thus no need for parents. Thus, there was no marriage, and everybody was to belong sexually to everyone else.

It's hard to say whether Huxley was serious, at the time he wrote this novel in 1931, or whether he was ridiculing the "new sexuality" that had come out of the 1920s. At any rate, today he looks in many ways, though not completely of course, like a "future-teller."

Ideas have consequences, and the Sexual Revolution is about erroneous ideas and their consequences.

The Sexual Revolution

Every week the American media give us more information about the sad effects of the Sexual Revolution. Maybe it's an article about AIDS; maybe it's about the social problems that stem from the vast increase in single parent families. No one is saying, "This is really great; let's have more of it," as some were saying when "sexual freedom" was such a popular slogan in the Sixties. Ordinary people shake their heads and wonder how we got here and how basic Judeo-Christian morality can be restored.

In our opinion, the Sexual Revolution **started in the 1820s** when the neo-Malthusians began promoting unnatural forms of birth control, implicitly saying it was morally permissible to take apart what God has joined together in the marriage act. This was truly revolutionary at the time. All the Christian churches taught that it was immoral to use withdrawal (Onanism) and other unnatural means of birth control.

The Sexual Revolution was given a tremendous boost in 1930 by the decision of the bishops of the Church of England to permit contraception. It was put into long-standing orbit by the 1931 statement from the Federal Council of Churches. (See Chapter 18 for details.)

In the 1960s the arrival of the Pill put contraception on the front pages of the daily papers and in all the popular magazines. The atmosphere was filled with the idea of men and women being totally in charge of their own sexuality. The idea of an Order of Creation to which we must conform was fading fast. The Sexual Revolution started with married couples, but in the Sixties it spread rapidly to the unmarried. No longer did a boy who wanted sex have to look around for a girl of already damaged reputation; the revolutionaries were telling the "nice girl" next door that she should be his willing partner if she liked him.

The increasing "acting out" of the Sexual Revolution continued throughout the Seventies. In the Eighties it was accompanied by an epidemic of sexually transmitted diseases. Up to this time, "STD" had appeared only after the names of clergy and meant Doctor of Sacred Theology (*Sacrae Theologiae Doctor* in Latin). Now it was all over the newspaper pages and stood for an increasing conglomeration of sexually transmitted diseases that most people had never heard of before. Chlamydia. Herpes II. Genital warts. And AIDS. To say nothing of vastly increased levels of the "traditional" venereal diseases, gonorrhea and syphilis.

During the Eighties and the Nineties, active homosexuals have made increasingly adamant demands that the rest of society should accept sodomy as just another morally legitimate "lifestyle." Some added an extra twist of perversity by advocating that society should lower the legal age of consent or eliminate it altogether. That way, adult homosexuals could legally seek to sodomize young boys, and adult men could legally seduce ever younger girls.

Rising rates of out-of-wedlock births in the United States have led to more sex education in the schools. However, most studies show that such instruction results in increased sexual activity, more contraceptive sex, more contraceptive failures, more pregnancies, more abortions, and generally more births.

In 1930 Anglican Bishop Charles Gore pleaded with his fellow Anglican bishops not to accept contraception. He predicted that the acceptance of unnatural methods of birth control would open a Pandora's box of sexual and social ills. He, too, has been proved right by history.

The divorce rate

The proponents of contraceptive birth control have argued that by using contraception, couples could have unlimited sex and very small families and that they would therefore be happy. The reality is different.

In 1910, the year of the last general census before Margaret Sanger began promoting contraception, the divorce rate was one divorce for every 11.4 marriages. By 1977, there was one divorce for every two marriages. That means that the divorce rate rose by 570% as contraception became more or less universally practiced in the United States. We can't say this *proves* that contraception is bad for marriages, but look at it this way: if contraception were good for marriage, why would the divorce rate go up over five times as more and more couples entered upon the contraceptive way of life?

On the other hand, the divorce rate among couples who practice natural family planning is very low. As mentioned in Chapter 17, we have been able to track one group—CCL Teaching Couples—and have found a divorce rate of 1.3%. This is a special group, so we would guess that the divorce rate among the larger group of couples practicing chaste NFP would be higher. This is an area that needs research; our estimate is that the divorce rate among NFP user-couples is between 2% and 5%, that is, one in 50 marriages to one in 20 marriages. That's between 1/25th and 1/10th of the divorce rate in the United States in the early Nineties; the high end of the estimate is approximately one-half of the American divorce rate in 1910.

These statistics explain why some couples refer to NFP as "marriage insurance."

From contraception to abortion

Every mainline American Protestant church that accepted contraception has also accepted abortion. The process started in 1961. As we have seen, on 21 March 1931 the Federal Council of Churches imitated the Church of England with a grudging acceptance of the "careful and restrained use" of unnatural methods of birth control. Thirty years later on 23 February 1961, the National Council of Churches openly embraced contraception. The statement is worth printing because it has had such widespread effects on unborn babies.

> Most of the Protestant churches hold contraception and periodic abstinence to be morally right when the motives are right. . . The general Protestant conviction is that motives, rather than methods, form the primary moral issue provided the methods are limited to the prevention of conception. Protestant Christians are agreed in condemning abortion or any method which

destroys human life except when the health or life of the mother is at stake.[15]

At first glance, that statement appears to be anti-abortion. However, physical and mental *health* reasons form the primary reasons given for abortion when any reason has to be given. "Health" covers everything from morning sickness to normal pregnancy concerns to schizophrenia. A lawyer once told us that any lawyer who could not get an abortion for a client under "health reason" legislation ought to be disbarred for incompetence.

Note also the emphasis on motives as the primary basis for morality. However, statements about sexual morality are not excused from the normal rules of thought. The deed that you actually do is the first ingredient of morality. Is it imaginable that the National Council of Churches would ever say that "motives rather than methods form the primary moral issue" if the subject was the use of nuclear weapons? Yet more babies are killed through abortion (including abortifacient birth control) *each year* than the total loss of life estimated to occur from a nuclear war between two major world powers.[16]

Very briefly, the acceptance of contraception by the Federal Council of Churches broke the moral authority behind the American anti-contraception laws. The courts sensed this and began finding ways to weaken the laws in the 1930s. For example, in 1936 a federal court allowed doctors to import and distribute contraceptives on the grounds that the law was passed to forbid the "immoral" distribution of contraceptives. However, the judge reasoned, what a doctor did with them was not immoral.[17] In 1965 the U. S. Supreme Court invented a "constitutional right to privacy" and in 1972 it declared all anti-contraception laws to be unconstitutional. Then, on 22 January 1973 the Supreme Court applied this same invention to abortion and declared that all anti-abortion laws were unconstitutional. On 29 June 1992, the Court itself noted the connection between contraception and abortion:

> It should be recognized, moreover, that in some critical respects the abortion decision is of the same character as the decision to use contraception. . .[18]

In *Planned Parenthood versus Casey* quoted above, the Court specifically cited its pro-contraception rulings as laying the precedent for its pro-abortion rulings. There is utterly no question: the social and legal acceptance of contraception led the way to the social and legal acceptance of unrestricted abortion.

Mother Teresa of Calcutta said it well when she addressed the National Prayer Breakfast in Washington, D.C., on February 3, 1994.

> I know that couples have to plan their family and for that there is natural family planning. The way to plan the family is natural family planning, not contraception. In destroying the power of giving life through contraception a husband or wife is doing something to self. This turns the attention to self and so destroys the gift of love in him or her. In loving, the husband and wife must turn the attention to each other, as happens in natural family planning, and not to self, as happens in contraception. Once that living love is destroyed by contraception, abortion follows very easily.
>
> I also know that there are great problems in the world—that many spouses do not love each other enough to practice natural

Statements about sexual morality are not excused from the normal rules of thought. The deed you actually do is the first ingredient of morality.

Theology and Ecology — 19

family planning. We cannot solve all the problems in the world, but let us never bring in the worst problem of all, and that is to destroy love. And this is what happens when we tell people to practice contraception and abortion.[19]

From contraception to sodomy

Thinkers on both sides of the birth control issue have agreed on one point: once a person accepts unnatural birth control as morally permissible, there is no *logical* stopping point. The only norm becomes mutual acceptability among the parties involved.

Among the pro-contraception "logicians," **Michael Valente** stands out for his boldness. First he shows how the logic of marital contraception affects even the idea of sex outside marriage:

> One who permits nonprocreative sexual activity to the married cannot logically forbid it to the unmarried on the traditional grounds that a child might be hurt or that it is always ordered to procreation if, in fact, one can guarantee in advance that a particular act cannot possibly be procreative. Thus, if the use of sexuality outside the married state is to be forbidden, it must be forbidden on grounds apart from the natural law doctrine; for to accept the revisionist position on the liceity [permissibility] of contraceptive use in marriage is not merely to find an exception to the natural law doctrine, but to destroy it.[20]

To understand that, you have to realize that moral theologians have been called to answer the question, "Why is sex wrong outside of marriage?" Traditionally, many have answered, "Because sex is for having babies, and having babies out of wedlock denies a baby its normal right to be raised by two parents." The answer wasn't wrong but it was inadequate. Its emphasis on consequences left it open to attack if the consequences could be avoided. It failed to focus on the inherent dishonesty of having the "marriage act" outside marriage.

What Valente and many other dissenters did is this: they ignored the force of the Scriptural condemnations of sex outside marriage. Instead, they focused on the weakness of certain arguments, saying in effect, "If you can't prove it rationally, then we can ignore the Commandment." We mention this here because you need to know how the Sexual Revolution took hold on allegedly Catholic campuses as well as at big government schools.

Valente also applied his revisionist doctrine to other actions forbidden by the natural moral law. He got very specific and said that to accept contraception *logically* means accepting anal copulation, masturbation, homosexual sodomy, and even bestiality.[21] Why? What all these have in common is that semen is not deposited in the human vagina. Valente is saying that once someone accepts the principle of Onanism—depositing semen someplace other than the natural vagina, the principle applies to all those other acts.

We know of no dissenting theologian who has criticized Valente's logic. He was an embarrassment to them because he spilled the beans and clearly showed the logical consequences of accepting marital contraception, but they couldn't logically disagree.

Seven years after Valente, a group of Catholic dissenting theologians argued that homosexual sodomy was the moral equivalent of marital contraception.[22] In 1989 Father **Charles E. Curran**, the priest who led the dissent against *Humanae Vitae*, carried this one step farther and said that it wasn't just theologians' arguments that were inadequate:

> And while admitting to mistakes in church traditions, the hierarchy should admit that the Bible contains mistakes, too, he said. For example, biblical teachings that sex outside of marriage is sinful must be seen as out of date—evidence of a less sophisticated age, Father Curran said.[23]

In 1991, liberal Presbyterians urged the Presbyterian Church to accept homosexual sodomy as morally good.[24] In 1993, liberal Lutherans urged the Evangelical Lutheran Church in America to accept homosexual sex as simply an extension of the biblical command to "love your neighbor as yourself."[25] Had enough?

We have been trying to show two things that we think are truly obvious once you have the facts. First, historically the Sexual Revolution developed from the promotion and acceptance of marital contraception, and it started in the 1820s. Only after a wide segment of the population accepted contraception was there a major effort to gain social acceptance for fornication, mutually agreed upon adultery, and homosexual sodomy. The contraception battle came first.

Second, there is a built-in logic that most people have never thought about. We think that most people who accepted contraception from the 1930s through the 1980s would have been totally opposed to homosexual sodomy. However, what they didn't know was that after 1968 dissenting Catholic theologians—as well as liberal Protestants—were saying that there is no real moral difference between married couples practicing contraception and homosexuals doing sodomy.

In other words, the acceptance of marital contraception introduces a sexual logic. There is no logical way to say "Yes" to one unnatural form of birth control and "No" to another. Therefore, the logic of contraception cannot say "No" to acts of oral and anal copulation by married couples. Further, such acts make it crystal clear that the whole purpose of all unnatural methods of birth control is to render such acts just as sterile as homosexual copulation. Finally, the logic of marital contraception cannot say a firm and universal "No" to homosexual sodomy or to any imaginable form of sexual activity provided it is mutually acceptable.

In brief, the heart and core of the Sexual Revolution is the acceptance of marital contraception as morally permissible. If you don't like the effects of the Sexual Revolution in today's society, then you will want to do what you can to turn things around.

As a couple, you start with yourselves.

The way home to sexual sanity in society is the narrow way of the Judeo-Christian sexual morality that has been transmitted through the Catholic Church and, to a large degree, by the other Christian churches until 1930. Jesus never promised that it would be an easy road.

The basic principles are simple. Marriage is for keeps.[26] Sexual intercourse is exclusively a marriage act. It is intended by God to be at least implicitly a renewal of the marriage covenant. That is, it is intended by God to affirm your mutual love and affection and to cooperate with Him in bringing babies into existence.

Is there a way home?

The conclusions are clear. No sex outside marriage. Permanent, lifelong marriage, for better and for worse. No contraception. Generosity in the service of life. You and your spouse both working at marital courtship and striving to make marital relations more than just a relief of sexual tensions. When you need to space babies or limit your family size, you practice natural family planning.

The differences today

This has always been true, but today there is a huge difference. There is more practical help available for the practice of natural family planning today than ever before in history. You have unprecedented choices among the various systems of natural family planning. We even know much more about the world's oldest form of baby-spacing, ecological breastfeeding. Today we know we have to point out the big differences between cultural nursing, which has little or no effect upon fertility, and ecological breastfeeding which spaces babies about two years apart, on the average, without any fertility awareness or abstinence.

There's another big difference. In the 1960s some Catholics could rightfully claim they were confused because the sight of theologians questioning the traditional teaching and even teaching dissent was new. However, today's Catholics have unprecedented certainty about the truth and force of Catholic teaching. The arguments of the dissenters have been exposed as simply rationalizations for a cross-less Christianity, and the disastrous consequences of the logic of contraception are there for all to see. More positively, the teaching of *Casti Connubii* (1930) and *Humanae Vitae* (1968) has been reaffirmed by Pope John Paul II many times since 1978. Of special note are *Familiaris Consortio* (1981), *The Universal Catechism of the Catholic Church* (1993), *Veritatis Splendor* (1993), and *Evangelium Vitae* (1995). There is no longer any room or reason for dissent or doubt.

You can be certain that only the natural methods are in accord with God's plan for sex, love and marriage. You can be certain that using unnatural methods of birth control is the grave matter of mortal sin. When you really need some baby spacing or finally need to keep your family at its present size, having that certainty makes the practice of NFP a lot easier.

Additional reading

Birth Control and Christian Discipleship, pp. 8-9, 15-18, 23-26.
"The Legacy of Margaret Sanger"
"Until death do us part"

Chapter 19: Self-Test Questions

1. True____   False____   The fact that you can figure out *how* to do something means that it is morally okay to do it.

2. True____   False____   As the rate of contraceptive usage has risen, the divorce rate in the United States has fallen.

3. True____   False____   "The end justifies the means" is a slogan stating that you can do anything if you have a sufficient or proportionate reason for doing so.

4. True____   False____   "The end justifies the means" argument can be reconciled with Christian morality.

5. True____   False____   There is a logical connection between the acceptance of contraception and the acceptance of homosexual sodomy.

6. True____   False____   Advocates of companionate marriage in the 1920s founded their radical ideas on the practical cornerstone of efficient contraception.

7. One reason why pre-marital _____ is immoral is that God intends that sex should be a _____ act, at least implicitly a _____ of your marriage covenant, and _____ marriage, there is obviously no _____ to renew.

8. A committee of the Federal Council of Churches (USA) accepted marital contraception in the year _____.

9. The National Council of Churches accepted abortion for the health of the mother in the year _____.

The next two questions are based on material in Birth Control and Christian Discipleship.

10. True____   False____   Michael Valente and Raymond Dennehy agree about the morality of contraception.

11. True____   False____   Valente and Dennehy agree that the acceptance of contraception leads *logically* to the acceptance of any imaginable sexual behavior agreeable to both parties.

Answers to self-test
1. False 2. False 3. True 4. False 5. True 6. True 7. intercourse. . . marriage . . . renewal . . . outside . . . covenant
8. 1931 9. 1961 10. False 11. True.

References

(1) Janet E. Smith, *Humanae Vitae: A Generation Later* (Washington: Catholic University of America Press, 1991) especially chapters three and four. *Why Humanae Vitae Was Right: A Reader*, edited by Janet Smith, Foreword by John Cardinal O'Connor (San Francisco: Ignatius Press, 1993).

(2) Kippley, *SMC*, Chapter 2, "Sex outside marriage."

(3) Kippley, *SMC*, 25-49.

(4) Kippley, *SMC*, see "Resources."

(5) Siegfried Ernst, *Man: The Greatest of Miracles* (Collegeville: Liturgical Press, 1976) 143.

(6) Ernst, 132.

(7) Ingrid Trobisch, *The Joy of Being a Woman, and What a Man Can Do* (New York: Harper and Row, 1975).

(8) Larry and Nordis Christenson, *The Christian Couple* (Minneapolis: Bethany Fellowship, 1977) 74.

(9) Mary Pride, *The Way Home* (Westchester, IL: Crossway, 1985).

(10) Mary Pride, *All the Way Home* (Westchester, IL: Crossway, 1989) 35.

(11) Rick and Jan Hess, *A Full Quiver: Family Planning and the Lordship of Christ* (Brentwood, TN: Wolgemuth & Hyatt, 1989) 94.

(12) Charles D. Provan, *The Bible and Birth Control* (Monongahela, PA: Zimmer Printing, 1989).

(13) David Prentis, "Dear Pastor . . .: A message from a minister of the Church of Scotland about Natural Family Planning" (Cincinnati: Couple to Couple League, 1989). David Prentis and his family entered into full communion with the Catholic Church at Easter time, 1995.

(14) Walter Lippman, *A Preface to Morals* New York: Macmillan, 1929).

(15) *New York Times,* 24 February 1961, 16.

(16) John F. Kippley, "Abortifacient birth control," *Birth Control and Christian Discipleship,* second ed., (Cincinnati: Couple to Couple League, 1994) 12-15.

(17) Noonan, 413.

(18) U.S. Supreme Court, *Planned Parenthood of Southeastern Pennsylvania v. Casey,* 29 June 1992.

(19) Mother Teresa of Calcutta, speech to the annual National Prayer Breakfast, Washington, D.C. 3 February 1994. Among some 4,000 people were President and Mrs. Clinton, Vice President and Mrs. Gore, numerous other government officials, and the media. She also said, "Any country that accepts abortion is not teaching its people to love, but to use any violence to get what they want."

In his coverage of the event, columnist Cal Thomas said the following: "At that line, most of those in attendance erupted in a standing ovation, something that rarely occurs at these sedate events. At that moment, President Clinton quickly reached for his water glass, and Mrs. Clinton and Vice President and Mrs. Gore stared without expression at Mother Teresa. They did not applaud. It was clearly an uncomfortable moment on the dias."

(20) Michael F. Valente, *Sex: The Radical View of a Catholic Theologian* (New York: Bruce: 1970) 126. At the time of his writing, Valente was chairman of the theology department at Seton Hall University in New Jersey. Such a prestigious position may help to account for his boldness in openly stating the logical consequences of revisionist thinking.

(21) Valente, 126.

(22) Anthony Kosnik, William Carroll, Agnes Cunningham, Ronald Modras and James Schulte, *Human Sexuality: New Directions in American Catholic Thought* (New York: Paulist Press, 1977) 216.

(23) Terry Mattingly, "Fighting an Uphill Battle," *The Cincinnati Post,* 25 February 1989, 4A. Usually Fr. Curran is more subtle, so when we read this, we immediately phoned the original reporter in Denver. He assured us that he had spoken with Fr. Curran after the lecture to make sure the quotation was correct.

(24) The General Assembly Special Committee on Human Sexuality, *Keeping Body and Soul Together: Sexuality, Spirituality, and Social Justice,* a document prepared for the 203rd general assembly (1991) (Louisville: Presbyterian Church U.S.A., 1991).

(25) *The Church and Human Sexuality: A Lutheran Perspective,* First Draft of a Social Statement (Chicago: Division for Church in Society, Department for Studies of the Evangelical Lutheran Church in America, October 1993) 15. The document represented the thinking of Lutheran liberals but was not accepted by the membership.

(26) John F. Kippley, *Marriage Is for Keeps* (Cincinnati: Couple to Couple League, 1994). This is a small book to help couples prepare for Christian marriage (student edition, 125 pages; wedding edition, 168 pages). See also *Until death do us part,* a CCL brochure.

Part IV: Pregnancy and Postpartum

This part of the book has six chapters—from seeking pregnancy to the return of your fertility after childbirth. Chapter 20 reviews the normal case of seeking pregnancy and setting your due date. Chapter 21 deals with the frustrating situation that every young couple thinks can't happen to them—difficulty in achieving pregnancy. We have a number of practical hints that singly or in combination help some couples to increase their mutual fertility and achieve pregnancy. However, not everything that is physically possible is morally right to do, and that's the subject of Chapter 22. In Chapter 23, you will learn how different forms of baby care affect the return of your fertility. In Chapter 24 you will learn about ecological breastfeeding, the only form of baby care that will space your babies to any extent. Chapter 25 teaches you how to detect the return of fertility after childbirth.

If you turned immediately to this part of the book for help to have a baby, be sure to review the first eight chapters, preferably all of Part I. You need those chapters to understand your fertility signs and our terminology. It's critical to know that your temperatures are lower before ovulation and higher afterwards and that before ovulation you have a mucus discharge which generally disappears after ovulation.

We remind you of the style we have adopted in this manual. Although this book is addressed to both husbands and wives, for the easiest reading we generally address the wife.

20

Achieving Pregnancy

The first thing to be said about pregnancy is that you are a mother as soon as you become pregnant, not just when your baby is born. You will want to give good care to your baby, and the best time to start is before you become pregnant.

If you eat right before and during pregnancy, you have a better chance of a healthy pregnancy and a healthy baby.

If you have been smoking cigarettes, stop.

If you have been using marijuana, cocaine, crack cocaine, heroin or any other mind altering drug, stop. Of course, you will need to get help if you have a real addiction.

If you use alcohol, either stop or reduce your consumption to no more than a small glass of wine at your main meal of the day.

If you are consuming large amounts of caffeine, reduce your daily consumption to no more than one or two cups of coffee or tea.

If you are taking any medications, check with your physician even before you start to seek pregnancy so you can eliminate all but essential medications.

If you are consuming products that contain aspartame (NutraSweet®), stop.

More positively, eat right. For many women in the United States and Europe, eating right may mean consuming some dietary supplements along with eating well-balanced meals because foods lose some—or much—of their nutritional value when they are processed, or stored for long periods, or cooked too long.

We recommend taking 400—800 micrograms (mcg) of **folic acid** daily if you are anticipating pregnancy. Research indicates that folic acid can significantly decrease the rate of spina bifida and other "neural tube defects." It may also help prevent miscarriages.

Folic acid is one of the B vitamins. Researchers compared mothers who supplemented folic acid (100 to 1,000 mcg daily) in the first six weeks after conception with those who didn't. The babies of the supplementers had only one-fourth as many neural tube defects.[2] Granted, those defects are uncommon anyway, but why not reduce the incidence as much as is humanly possible? (Many people, including ourselves, take 400 mcg of folic acid every day as part of their nutritional regimen in hopes of some extra energy.)

Pre-pregnancy nutrition

The case against aspartame is, we think, well made by Dr. H. J. Roberts in Aspartame (NutraSweet®) Is It Safe?[1] We're not going to review his arguments, but we have found them persuasive enough that we do not allow products containing that chemical into our home. NutraSweet® is a registered trademark of the Merisant Corporation which also produces Equal®, another aspartame product.

Vitamin E, other **B vitamins, vitamin C** and other nutrients such as the bioflavinoids, iodine, zinc, and adequate protein may also be related to the prevention of miscarriages.[3]

It's definitely best to start proper supplements at least three months before pregnancy, but even if you wait until you are pregnant, it's not too late.

Become better educated about nutrition. The Couple to Couple League leadership is so convinced that nutrition can have a big influence on the fertility cycle that it publishes a small but highly informative and well-researched book on the subject. *Fertility, Cycles and Nutrition* is a book every woman, homemaker, and mother should have. (See *Resources* at the end of the book.) Author Marilyn Shannon makes specific recommendations about pre-pregnancy and pregnancy dietary supplements.[4]

Immediately reversible

One of the great things about Natural Family Planning is that it is immediately reversible: you simply change the timing of marital relations.

This does not guarantee that you will achieve pregnancy in the very first cycle, as you will see in the next chapter. What we mean by *immediately* reversible is this: you don't have to *wait* to seek pregnancy as women should if they're coming off chemical birth control such as the Pill, Norplant, and some IUDs. You don't have to wonder if an IUD has damaged your uterus or if it gave you pelvic inflammatory disease that frequently causes permanent sterility. With NFP for spacing, you respect your body and therefore increase your chances of achieving your desired pregnancy when you reverse your timing.

● Knowing your maximum fertility

Your overall fertile time starts as soon as your mucus discharge starts, even the less-fertile mucus. The time of your maximum fertility is when you have the more-fertile mucus and frequently includes the first day of drying up. More-fertile mucus shows that you are close to ovulation, and the raw egg white or watery mucus provides the best environment for the sperm. Frequently, your temperature pattern may be a little lower during your most fertile time; the low temperatures reflect high levels of estrogen. In some cycles you may notice a further dip in your waking temperature toward the end of your mucus patch; in some cases that may be an especially fertile day. At your time of maximum fertility, your cervix will generally be as high and open as it gets.

However, you **cannot pinpoint** the exact day of ovulation with your fertility signs. To pinpoint ovulation, you actually have to see it occurring. A physician can do that in two ways: by sonogram and by laparoscopic examination. Both are utterly impractical for ordinary use.

Peak Day does **not** identify the day of ovulation.

Ovulation sometimes occurs as early as three days before Peak Day (P - 3) and sometimes as late as three days after Peak Day (P + 3). Ovulation often occurs on Peak Day, about 37% of the time according to one study.[5] According to the same estimates, ovulation occurs about 38.5% of the time on P - 1 and P - 2 combined, about 20% of the time on P + 1 and P + 2 combined, and about 3% of the time on P - 3 and P + 3 combined. (In this study, no Peak Day was observed in 1.5% of the cycles.) These are estimates based on hormones in blood specimens. What these estimates show is that in normal cycles Peak Day is close to ovulation but certainly cannot be used to pinpoint the day of ovulation. In abnormal cycles, the variation can be even larger.

The start of your thermal shift pattern is also **not** a precise indicator of the exact day of ovulation.

When Peak Day and the start of your thermal shift occur on the same day, or next to each other, or even separated by a day, you can reasonably estimate that ovulation has occurred within a two or three day range, and that's good enough. To repeat, you cannot pinpoint the exact day of ovulation with the signs you can observe and chart.

The proper timing

To maximize the supply of sperm, abstain in Phase I. Begin having marital relations in Phase II when you notice your more-fertile mucus. Abstaining every other day during the more-fertile mucus provides a little more time for the sperm supply to be replenished, but coitus every day during the most-fertile mucus may be best in some cases.

Abstinence during Phase I and early Phase II is generally not necessary for a couple of normal fertility. However, if you do not achieve pregnancy within a few cycles of proper timing, such abstinence is part of the self-help package described in the next chapter.

Knowing you are pregnant

Keep taking your waking temperatures when you are seeking pregnancy. When your temperature pattern stays elevated for 21 days, you have about a 99% certainty that the Lord has blessed you with pregnancy.

That assumes you normally have no more than 16 days of elevated temperatures. If you typically have longer luteal phases, to know you are pregnant, just add 7 days of elevated temperatures to your usual number. Example: if you usually have 17 days of elevated temperatures, add 7, and on the 24th day of elevated temperatures, you would have that 99% probability you are pregnant.

Your temperature record provides you with an excellent confirmation of pregnancy. You would be wasting money to take a pregnancy test, except in a very rare case. A suggestion: donate the money you save to a good pro-life cause.

When you decide to visit your doctor, you can tell him two things: 1) that you are pregnant and 2) your estimated due date. Bring him a copy of your sympto-thermal chart. If he is not well informed about its value, let him read these pages.

Estimating your due date

The temperature pattern in your pregnancy cycle gives you the most accurate way to estimate when your baby's birth is due. Use the rule developed by Dr. Konald A. Prem when he was professor of Obstetrics and Gynecology at the University of Minnesota School of Medicine. Here is his rule for your Estimated Date of Childbirth (EDC):

EDC = First day of overall thermal shift minus 7 days plus 9 months.

The process is simple.
1. Identify the first day of your upward thermal shift pattern.
2. Subtract 7 days.
3. Add 9 months.
The result is your Estimated Date of Childbirth (EDC) by the Prem Rule.

The Prem EDC is calculated in Figure 20.1. The secondary rise in temperature starting on Day 19 is typical for pregnant women. By Cycle Day 33, the couple have a 99% certainty that they have achieved pregnancy.

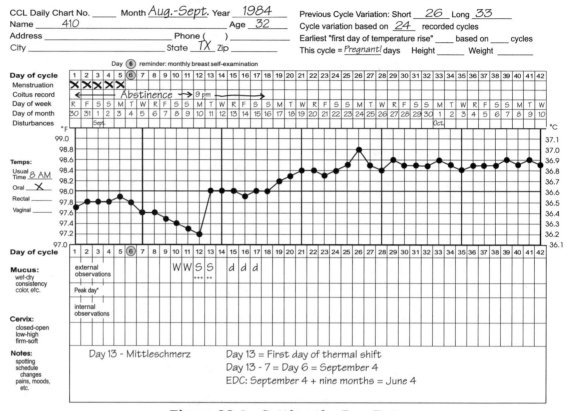

Figure 20.1   Setting the Due Date

● Accuracy of the Prem Rule for the EDC

No formula can be 100% exact; there are normal variations in the time of gestation. We conducted a small study of 26 deliveries and found these results: 69% (18) were within 7 days before or after the Prem EDC; 81% (21) were within 10 days before or after, and 100% were within 12 days before and 9 days after the Prem EDC.[6] A slightly more conservative generalization would be as follows:

Actual Date of Delivery	Probability
Within 7 days before or after EDC	65%
Within 10 days before or after EDC	80%
Within 14 days before or after EDC	99%

Despite these normal variations, your upward thermal shift gives you the **single most accurate way** of dating the time of conception, the age of your pre-born baby, and the estimated date of childbirth. It's even better than ultrasound. As Dr. Prem has written, it is **more accurate** than much more elaborate and expensive procedures such as "estimation of uterine size by palpation or measurement, the dates of quickening and engagement of the fetal head and auscultation of the fetal heart tones with the head stethoscope. . ." or "biochemical and biophysical methods such as estriol, ultrasound, and phospholipids. . ."[7]

We are emphasizing the accuracy of the Prem Rule because your doctor may not know it. He deals mostly with women who do not take their temperatures so he generally uses the Naegele Rule which dates from the 19th century. That rule starts with the first day of the last-menstrual-period (LMP), adds seven days, and then adds nine months to arrive at the EDC. The Naegele Rule works well when ovulation occurs around Day 14. It becomes increasingly inaccurate when ovulation is either very early or is delayed by a week or more.

By comparison, in our study of 26 pregnancies, the deliveries ranged from 9 days before the Naegele EDC to 18 days after it. Physicians rightfully are concerned if you're more than two weeks "overdue"; some get anxious if you're one week beyond the estimated due date. The advantage of the Prem temperature-based EDC is obvious and is illustrated by the following two incidents.

● A Midwest woman using CCL charting took her sympto-thermal pregnancy chart to her physician who was reluctant to give it any credit. Instead, he turned to sonograms at about seven months. These indicated a head size about typical for delivery. He wanted to induce labor immediately. The woman, however, had delivered other babies with head sizes larger than average, and she trusted her temperature graph. We sent the woman a copy of the article by Dr. Prem that we quoted above.[8] Faced with this scientific information from a recognized medical expert and with the definite possibility of inducing labor two months prematurely, the physician decided to wait on a week by week basis. The baby came naturally within three days of the temperature-based EDC with no signs of being post-mature; this was a good six weeks after the time originally planned for induced labor.

● In another case, a woman coming off the Pill had no periods after her initial withdrawal bleeding. She finally achieved a much desired pregnancy around the time her thermal shift started—Cycle Day 115!

In our opinion, **every** woman who is seeking pregnancy should take her waking temperatures and continue to take them for at least three weeks after the upward thermal shift begins. This is particularly true of women who have any health condition that might be affected by pregnancy (for example, diabetes) or who have irregular cycles. The most exact knowledge of the date of conception can be helpful to her physicians. Furthermore, since any woman *could* develop a medical condition during pregnancy, we think it's advisable for every couple to maintain both the mucus and the temperature records while seeking pregnancy.

Sex during pregnancy

If you, the wife, are having a healthy pregnancy, and if your husband has no diseases that can be transmitted sexually, there is no reason for any special abstinence during pregnancy.

That also applies to the final weeks of pregnancy. At one time physicians routinely told couples to refrain from relations from six weeks before the due date and for six weeks after childbirth. Add an extra week for a delayed childbirth and you have a routine "doctor's order" for a quarter of a year of abstinence. Certainly situations may arise in any marriage where the couple may have to refrain from coitus for much longer periods, but in the case of a healthy pregnancy and healthy parents, it is not necessary to refrain from coitus until the beginning of labor. (Postpartum abstinence is discussed in Chapter 23.)

On the other hand, if you have problems with your pregnancy, consult your physician and follow his advice about any abstinence.

While there may be no *medical* reasons to refrain from relations during pregnancy, there may be other reasons—the wife's comfort, personal discipline, and so forth.

Preparation for childbirth

There are customs that appear totally innocent but which can irreversibly destroy the breastfeeding relationship; e.g., artificial nipples are a cultural custom which can cause nipple confusion and eliminate breastfeeding.
—*Joy Kondash, M.D.*

Having your first baby will be one of the biggest moments of your life. Prepare well for it.

Attend prepared childbirth classes and plan to have as non-medicated delivery as you can. As you will learn in childbirth classes, medications go from the mother's blood supply through the placenta into her baby.

Attend the breastfeeding classes of the La Leche League or other qualified nursing mother associations. Yes, there is no doubt that breastfeeding is the natural way to feed your baby, but that doesn't mean that there are never any little problems. Your association with experienced nursing moms helps you to get off to your best possible start and to know where to get help if you need it.

Select a pro-life doctor or midwife who will help you have the type of childbirth experience you want to have. Use what you learn in the childbirth and breastfeeding classes to help you determine what sort of doctor or midwife you want and where you can find him or her.

Speak up if your instructors push contraception, downgrade NFP, or ridicule the idea that breastfeeding can space babies. There's much ignorance, and if you speak up in a convincing way, you can educate everyone in the class.

Sustaining your pregnancy

No one likes to think about miscarriages, but it is commonly estimated that about one in six babies die *in utero*. There is nothing you can do about many of these, but there are some things that are known to increase the chances of birth defects and miscarriages. We have briefly noted a few of these in the previous section on "Preparation for childbirth," but our more extensive treatment of this subject is in Chapter 32 on miscarriages. Please read the sections in that chapter dealing with "Causes in general," "Specific causes," and "Prevention."

Trying to pre-select the sex of your baby

We bring up this subject reluctantly because too much concern about sex selection can detract from the "gift-ness" of each child. The most important aspect of this subject is this: whatever the sex of your new baby, accept her or him as a gift from God.

● One theory

For years, there has been talk how the timing of intercourse can influence the sex of your baby. One popular theory (associated with Dr. Landrum Shettles) has been that the smaller, male-bearing sperm are faster swimmers but live for only a short time, while the larger, female-bearing sperm are slower swimmers but live longer.

On that basis, if you want a girl, you have relations in the early part of Phase II and then abstain until Phase III. If you want a boy, you abstain until you think you are very close to ovulation. As you develop experience with your own cycle pattern, you will be able to estimate when you are close to ovulation.

The longer the theory is around, the more controversial it becomes, and some researchers claim it is totally wrong. For example, "The birth sex ratio favored males when intercourse preceded ovulation/fertilization by two days or longer."[9] The same authors concluded that their results "clearly refute the theory proposed by Shettles."[10]

Current status

In December 1995 a study published in a major American medical journal stated the following: "We found no association between the sex of the baby and the time of intercourse in relation to ovulation. We conclude that the deliberate timing of intercourse around the day of ovulation has no practical value in sex selection."[11]

Selective spermicides

Some have suggested different kinds of douches; one kind supposedly kills the male-bearing sperm, the other kills the female-bearing sperm. We definitely discourage this practice. Our objection is not based on this being a partial contraceptive because plenty of sperm are unaffected. However, first there is the possibility that a douche-damaged sperm could cause fertilization and contribute to birth defects, a problem that has been associated with spermicides in general. Second, the process is morally ambiguous at best because the deliberate destruction of sperm raises questions about the limits of biotechnology and the manipulation of the life processes. For these reasons, we ourselves would never use selective spermicides, and we do not teach how to use them.

Self-Test Questions: Chapter 20

1. True_____   False_____   The most fertile time is about a week that includes several days before ovulation to the day after ovulation.

2. The temperature pattern in the week before ovulation is:
   a) higher b) lower than it is after ovulation.

3. True_____   False_____   For some women, by the time the temperature starts to go up, they may already be in postovulation infertility.

4. True_____   False_____   You can pinpoint the exact day of ovulation with your natural signs of fertility and infertility.

5. True_____   False_____   In some cycles, the first day of drying-up may be the day of ovulation.

Questions 6-10 refer to Example 1.
   Example 1:

	D	D	T	T	S	S	S	S	W	T	T	D	D
Cycle day	6	7	8	9	10	11	12	13	14	15	16	17	18

6. In the above example, which cycle day is the first day of the more-fertile mucus? _____

7. Which day is "Peak + 1"? _____

8. What are the limits of the overall fertile time to be avoided by a couple seeking to avoid pregnancy? Days _____ through _____.

9. What are the days of maximum fertility to be used by a couple seeking pregnancy? Days _____ through _____.

10. With the advantage of hindsight, which consecutive three days do you think were most likely the very best days for seeking pregnancy? Days _____.

11. True____   False____   By Peak Day plus 4, you can be absolutely certain that you have ovulated.

12. True____   False____   The single best indicator of both pregnancy and your due date is the temperature pattern.

13. You can have a _____% certainty that you will deliver within one week before or after the Prem EDC.

14. According to the limited study reported in this text, you can have a _____% certainty that you will deliver within two weeks of your Prem EDC.

15. True____   False____   A physician can calculate the Prem EDC for a woman who has not taken her temperatures during the pregnancy cycle.

Answers to self-test
1. True 2. b) lower 3. True 4. False 5. True 6. Day 10 7. Day 15 8. Days 8 through 17, until evening of Day 18 9. Days 10 through 15 10. Days 12, 13, and 14 11. False 12. True 13. 65% 14. 99% 15. False

References

(1) H.J. Roberts, M.D., *Aspartame (Nutrasweet®) Is It Safe?* (Philadelphia: Charles Press, 1990). See especially ch. 23, "Pregnant women; nursing mothers" 181-183.

(2) Shannon, 102.

(3) Marilyn M. Shannon, *Fertility, Cycles and Nutrition* 2nd Ed. (Cincinnati: Couple to Couple League, 1992) 101-102.

(4) There are many pre-natal formulas. Our nutrition advisor, M. Shannon, recommends Professional Prenatal Formula (Life Time, 1015 East Katella Avenue, Unit D, Anaheim, CA 92805). Says Shannon: "It is ideal for pregnant and breastfeeding women and for women preparing to conceive. Professional Prenatal Formula is far better balanced and far more potent than prescription prenatal vitamins—I suggest you compare labels. Women (or men) who are attempting to overcome anemia or fatigue will also find it ideal." (Shannon, *Fertility, Cycles and nutrition*, 145). If your local health food shop does not stock this product, you can order it through the American Pro-Life Enterprise, P.O. Box 1281, Powell, OH 43065-1281, USA; 800-227-8359; FAX and international phone, (614) 881-5520. Service is quick—same day or next day shipment after receipt of order.

(5) Thomas W. Hilgers, Guy E. Abraham, and Denis Cavanagh, "Natural Family Planning: I. The peak symptom and estimated time of ovulation," *Obstetrics and Gynecology* 52:5 (November 1978) 579.

(6) "Temperatures during pregnancy," *The CCL News*, XII:1 (July-August 1985) 2ff.

(7) Konald A. Prem, "Assessment of Gestational Age," *Minnesota Medicine*, September 1976, 623.

(8) Prem, 623.

(9) John T. France, Frederick M. Graham, Leonie Gosling, Philip Hair and Bruce S. Knox, "Characteristics of natural conceptual cycles occurring in a prospective study of sex preselection: fertility awareness symptoms, hormone levels, sperm survivial, and pregnancy outcome," *International Journal of Fertility* 37:4 (1992) 244.

(10) France, 253.

(11) Allen J. Wilcox, Clarice R. Weinberg and Donna D. Baird, "Timing of sexual intercourse in relation to ovulation," *New England Journal of Medicine* 333:23 (7 December 1995) 1521 plus editorial. For responses, see the series of letters in *NEJM* (9 May 1996) 1266-1268.

21

If You Don't Succeed at First...

If you have personal experience with infertility, you certainly have our sympathies. We regularly get requests for more information, more help on overcoming this problem; we know it can bring both sadness and frustration. In this chapter, we will be discussing ways to reduce or overcome some causes of infertility. Some may apply to you; some may not. At any rate, please do not use this chapter to stir up a batch of "what if" or "if only" memories. Let us look to the present and the future.

On the other hand, if you think that this subject doesn't apply to you because you're not planning to have children for several years, think again. Even if your cycles appear perfectly normal—normal periods, mucus, temperature shifts, and luteal phases—you *still* could have an infertility problem. In addition, none of these things say anything about your husband's fertility and your *mutual* fertility.

Delayed childbearing is definitely a factor in reduced fertility. We urge you: don't postpone pregnancy unless you have a serious reason to do so. Endometriosis can start early, and it gets worse with age. It causes infertility in one-third of the women who develop it.

Fertility: a matter of degrees

If you are a couple with normal high fertility, you are likely to achieve pregnancy within three cycles with the right timing of intercourse. If you are a couple with somewhat lower fertility, you will generally achieve pregnancy within four to six cycles. If you are a couple with low mutual fertility, it may take you up to twelve cycles to achieve pregnancy. If you are not pregnant within a year even with good timing, you would be regarded as having an infertility problem.

In the 1950s, approximately one out of ten couples had some sort of infertility problem. In the 1990s, that rate is nearly double. Reasons include delayed childbearing, poor health habits, and even environmental causes.

Another big reason for this astounding increase in infertility is the Sexual Revolution. Abortion, the IUD, the Pill, sexually transmitted diseases (STDs), and early and promiscuous sexual relations all can reduce fertility and even cause permanent sterility. The IUD can cause sterility through scarring of the uterus and pelvic inflammatory disease; the Pill can cause a woman to be infertile for months after discontinuing it; chlamydia and gonorrhea are among the sexually transmitted diseases that can leave a woman permanently sterile.

Infertility can be due to either or both male or female factors. Male factors would include insufficient numbers of sperm or sperm that do not move fast or with enough vigor. Female factors include failure to ovulate, blocked Fallopian tubes, insufficient cervical mucus, and hormonal imbalances.

Primary infertility refers to couples who have never been able to achieve pregnancy. *Secondary* infertility refers to couples who have had at least one pregnancy but are currently not able to conceive and bear more children.

The good news is that perhaps 80 percent of couples with reduced fertility have no apparent cause that absolutely prevents pregnancy. Many of them can be helped to achieve pregnancy by low-tech, cost-free or very inexpensive natural methods. Therefore, the emphasis in this chapter is going to be on the low-tech natural things you can do to improve your fertility. However, first we need to mention two medical practices dealing with sperm collection.

Medical tests

Many physicians dealing with couples with low fertility routinely tell the husband to masturbate for seminal analysis. The Couple to Couple League accepts and transmits the traditional teaching of the Catholic Church that masturbation for any reason, including seminal analysis, violates the natural moral law and is therefore a serious moral evil.[1]

Traditional Christian teaching against masturbation raises another question. Are there any morally acceptable methods of semen collection that are also medically useful? The answer is "Yes."

The Huhner test

The Huhner test (sometimes called the Sims-Huhner test) is a sperm-gathering process that is morally and medically acceptable because it simply involves gathering a sample of semen from the vagina after normal intercourse. For the Huhner test to be valid, intercourse must take place during the flow of the most-fertile mucus because this is the mucus that is most favorable to sperm life. If the test is performed during the infertile times (when the vaginal environment is hostile to sperm life), a false low count will occur.

The Huhner test has the additional advantage of showing how the sperm and cervical mucus interact. In some cases of infertility, there may be a normal sperm count, but the sperm are immobilized by contact with the cervical mucus.

The perforated condom

If your physician needs a sample of semen that has not been in contact with cervical mucus, you can use a perforated condom during normal intercourse. (A special silicone condom must be used because contraceptive condoms are treated with spermicides. If your physician is unaware where to buy the silicone condom, you or he can contact CCL for a current supplier.) Make two or three pinholes at the end of the condom; some sperm will go through the pinholes and remain in the vagina; most sperm will remain in the condom for analysis.

This process respects the requirements of the natural moral law that deliberate orgasm (as contrasted with nocturnal emission) should occur only with sexual intercourse in which the semen is deposited in the wife's vagina. This may sound like hairsplitting to some, but you can understand it more easily in the context of the birth control controversy.

Back in the early 1960s, some moral theologians began to argue for masturbation for seminal analysis. Then they used *their* acceptance of masturbation to "justify" any voluntary sexual act you can imagine. "For the good purpose of achieving pregnancy, we have 'justified' masturbation which previously had always been condemned. *Therefore* we have justified departing from the natural moral law if we think there is a sufficient reason. *Our* conclusion is that if a couple think they have a sufficient reason to avoid pregnancy, we can accept contraception, oral and anal sodomy, as well as mutual masturbation, all of which also violate the natural moral law." This is a summary, not a direct quotation.

This is not a prediction of a theological domino theory. This is what has already happened, and the first steps were to ridicule the perforated condom and to accept masturbation for seminal analysis.

Practical helps for seeking pregnancy

You may be surprised at how much you can do to improve your fertility.[2] We divide these practices into three sections—for wives, for husbands, and for both of you together.

Wives: have good health habits

Most of the following recommendations will be good for you regardless of your fertility status.

1. Don't smoke

Women who smoke are estimated to have only 72% of the fertility of non-smokers; they are three and one-half times more likely to take a whole year to conceive.[3] Smoking one pack of cigarettes per day is enough to impair fertility; starting to smoke before age 18 also has negative effects on fertility.[4]

2. Don't over-exercise

You need a minimum of 20% of your weight in body fat to maintain normal fertility. Excessive exercise can reduce your body fat below this critical ratio and cause infertile cycles even though you are still having periods. It can also cause "runner's amenorrhea"—the absence of both ovulation and menstrual periods.

3. Don't over-diet—for the same reason

A general rule for a healthy ratio of your weight for your height is this: 100 pounds for the first five feet and 5 pounds for every additional inch. This assumes average bone structure. For example, on that basis, if you are 5 feet 6 inches tall, your "ideal" weight would be 130 pounds. If you restrict your eating so you can weigh less than your "ideal" weight, don't be surprised if your cycles range from long to very long with delayed ovulation and perhaps extended ambiguous mucus patterns. In the extreme eating disorder of anorexia nervosa, a woman stops ovulating and having periods.

4. Don't be excessively overweight

Too much body fat upsets the balance of estrogen and progesterone in some women. Ten to twenty pounds of excess weight does not impair fertility, but if you are obese and are having irregular cycles or difficulty in achieving pregnancy, your excess body fat might be an important factor.

If this applies to you, lose weight *sensibly*. Crash diets can also have adverse effects on your fertility even when your weight is still well above your "ideal" for your height. If you stop having periods after dieting sensibly to your "ideal" weight, try gaining a few pounds again. Your best weight may be a bit higher than the average for your height.

5. Eat properly

Eat nutritionally well balanced meals. Vitamins and minerals affect the synthesis of your reproductive hormones, the functioning of your reproductive organs, and even the cervical mucus. Certain vitamins can normalize the levels of estrogen, progesterone, and prolactin during the luteal phase. Vitamin A is necessary for the proper functioning of mucus membranes throughout your body, and that applies to the membranes that secrete cervical mucus. Green and yellow vegetables are good sources of vitamin A. (One woman reported going from scanty mucus to a five-inch stretch when she began eating raw carrots every day. For most women, one well-chewed carrot per day would be sufficient.) The B vitamins are essential for good nutrition and normal fertility. Vitamin B6 helps some infertile women to conceive; it should be taken in some form of a B-complex supplement. Folic acid, part of the vitamin B family, reduces the incidence of certain birth defects.

Eliminate caffeine consumption or greatly reduce it. "Coffee and other sources of caffeine can cause *cycle irregularity and even infertility in some women.*"[5] Caffeine is also associated with an increased risk of miscarriage.[6] Eliminate food additives as much as possible. Completely eliminate products sweetened with NutraSweet®.[7]

If you don't cook with iodized salt or use it daily to salt your food, make sure you get iodine daily from some other reliable source such as kelp tablets. Iodine is essential for the proper functioning of your thyroid gland, and your thyroid functioning affects your fertility.

6. Educate yourself

Go beyond this brief treatment of nutrition and fertility. Read *Fertility, Cycles and Nutrition* by Marilyn Shannon (see "Resources"). It's the best book we know of for relating nutrition to fertility and infertility. You will find informative chapters on cycle irregularities and female infertility, inadequate luteal phase, repeated miscarriages and birth defects, other problems related to pregnancy, male infertility—and, of course, what you can do to try to alleviate these and other problems.

7. Consider taking dietary supplements

A well-balanced multi-vitamin/mineral supplement not only covers many potential needs, but it also increases the effectiveness of interacting nutrients and reduces the possibility of overdose.

Most American physicians will tell you to supplement folic acid for a few months before and after seeking pregnancy to reduce the incidence of neural tube defects such as spina bifida.

Fertility, Cycles and Nutrition recommends certain dietary supplements which other women have found helpful for various problems. The Couple to Couple League publishes this book as part of CCL's continuing effort to assist the practice of NFP—both for achieving and for postponing pregnancy. If you

In the morbidly obese woman, abnormal menses can occur without ovulation.
— Konald A. Prem, M.D.

A woman experiencing secondary infertility of about 18 months asked me about her problem. I suggested that she cut out sugar and caffeine, improve her nutrition, and try to drop a few pounds, as she was rather overweight. She conceived two months later, and reported that the only change she had made was to reduce her coffee consumption from six or seven mugs per day to one or one and a half cups daily.
— M. Shannon[8]

are having difficulty in achieving pregnancy, or if you are experiencing irregular cycles (and "irregular" covers a wide variety of matters), you will do well to study this book.

8. Consider guaifenesin

During the fertile time, if you have scanty or thick cervical mucus that does not improve with better nutrition, consider taking guaifenesin. Guaifenesin is a pharmaceutical product used in many cough syrups to increase the fluidity of bronchial mucus, and it can have the same effect on cervical mucus. Ask your pharmacist to help you find a product in which guaifenesin is the only active ingredient.

Infertility experts now use guaifenesin. Its value has definitely been established.
—Konald A. Prem, M.D.

Begin taking this product after your period ends or when your mucus discharge begins or at least five days before your usual Peak Day. Stop taking it on the second day after Peak Day. Follow the directions on the container for quantity and frequency.

Personal friends of ours adopted five children during thirteen infertile years. Then they heard about guaifenesin and had two of their own babies while using it. Coincidence or partial causality—who can say? However the bottle of cough syrup was much less expensive than the battery of infertility tests the wife had taken ten years previously.

If you use guaifenesin, try to find a product that is not made by companies which have become notorious for their involvement with abortifacient forms of birth control—the Pill, implants, and the IUD. Such companies include A. H. Robins, G. D. Searle, Johnson and Johnson (which owns Ortho Pharmaceutical), Mead Johnson, Parke-Davis, Syntex, Wyeth-Ayerst, and Pharmacia-Upjohn.

9. If you have short luteal phases. . .

If you are having short luteal phases with less than nine days of elevated temperatures, be aware that such cycles are probably not fertile. *Fertility, Cycles and Nutrition* describes a supplement (Optivite) specifically formulated to balance a woman's hormones and to lengthen the time from ovulation to the start of the next period (the luteal phase). We think it would be sensible to take this supplement according to package directions to try to lengthen your luteal phase to the range of 12 to 14 days.

10. If you are nursing. . .

If you are nursing and can't get pregnant, the situation is not entirely clear.

a. If you are having short luteal phases, the above section applies. Some breastfeeding research by K. K. Singh and associates indicates that the earlier you have your first postpartum period, the more likely it is you will have, at first, luteal phases too short to sustain pregnancy.[9]

b. If you are having normal cycles with good mucus patches and with elevated temperature patterns of 9 to 14 days, and if you're still not getting pregnant, be aware that some nursing mothers simply do not become pregnant until the baby weans completely. (Also be aware that your experience after the next baby may be entirely different.) The above-mentioned research by Singh suggests that, for whatever reasons, breastfeeding after the return of menstruation reduces the rate of conception by 41% compared to women who stop nursing after the first postpartum period.[10] You may want to wait a few months simply to save yourself frustration every time you have a period.

11. Darken your bedroom

Believe it or not, light during sleep affects the balance of hormones in some women. Even the light from a digital clock face can affect some women. The reasons for this are explained in *Fertility, Cycles and Nutrition*. The conclusion is this: eliminate light from your bedroom while you sleep.

12. Slow down

A full-time job outside the home doesn't directly cause infertility, but it can cause you to eat a poor diet due to time pressures, to depend on caffeine, and to get insufficient sleep. On the other hand, part-time work or volunteer activities may help you to keep from dwelling unnecessarily on your desire for a child.

Husbands, take these practical steps

These practices will be good for your health, regardless of your fertility status. We recommend them even if your fertility is normal.

1. Wear boxer shorts

Your testicles are outside your body, so to speak, to maintain a slightly cooler temperature. Close fitting (jockey style) underwear forces the testicles close to your body, making them subject to higher temperatures. So wear boxer shorts instead of close fitting underpants. A number of couples have solved their "infertility" problem by the husband switching from tight to loose fitting underwear.

By the same token, avoid hot tubs and be aware that a very hot working environment can damage your fertility. Note: the process of bringing sperm cells to maturity takes about 70 days. Therefore, if your fertility is damaged by hot tubs, it will take that time for normal fertility to return.

2. Don't smoke; limit alcohol

Nicotine may impair sexual function, and a government report has stated that smokers are 50 percent more likely to suffer from impotence than non-smokers.[11] The long term use of marijuana also can cause impotency. Excess alcohol can cause infertility that may be irreversible.[12]

3. Eat properly

Eat a well-balanced diet, and consider taking a multi-vitamin/mineral supplement. Be sure to read the chapter on "The Male Connection" in *Fertility, Cycles and Nutrition* where you will find out about the need for Vitamin C, zinc, the B vitamins and other nutrients for proper male fertility. Please note: it may take three to six months of changed environment or better nutrition before your fertility improves.

Sometimes the effects of a dietary supplement are simply spectacular. When sperm cells clump together, it is called sperm agglutination. According to Earl B. Dawson, research professor at the University of Texas at Galveston, when more than 25% of a man's sperm clump together, his sperm cannot fertilize the ovum.[13] Dawson tested Vitamin C with a group of such men against a control group receiving placebo pills. Within two months, the wives in the Vitamin C group were all pregnant, but none in the control group had conceived. The men in the study group took one gram of Vitamin C daily.

The Androvite dietary supplement contains the nutrients needed for proper male fertility. The maximum daily dosage includes 1,000 mg of Vitamin C.

These recommendations apply to both of you.

1. Don't try too hard

To build up sperm count, abstain for *at least* five days before having relations in Phase II. Better yet, abstain from the beginning of the cycle until you are into your most fertile, stretchy mucus patch. Then have relations every other day until the start of Phase III. Once in Phase III, continue to have relations every three or four days since this may help to stimulate sperm production.

The normal advice is not to have coitus on consecutive days or more than once a day since the extra times may deplete sperm count. However, some physicians recommend having relations daily during the time of the most fertile mucus. You might want to try the not-on-consecutive-days regimen in one cycle, the daily regimen in the next.

Another exception to the general rule is the advice sometimes given to have a second coitus about 45 minutes after the first. In some men, apparently, the first ejaculation opens up the pathways, so to speak, and the second delivers the sperm with a much higher sperm count than the first. This is the opposite of what happens with men of normal fertility. Or possibly the semen of the first ejaculation has many older or less motile sperm while the second has fresher, more motile sperm.

2. Assist sperm migration

After relations during the fertile time, the wife should be on her back with a pillow under her buttocks for about 30 minutes. This may help sperm to enter the uterus in greater numbers.

3. Use the self-helps simultaneously

Utilize all the self-help means to increase your fertility before you go to an infertility specialist. Use all the self-help aids simultaneously. That confuses things from a research perspective, but you're interested in having a baby, not research.

4. Seek help if you don't achieve pregnancy soon

If you don't achieve pregnancy within three months, contact your local CCL teaching couple; they may refer you to CCL Central. If you are a CCL member, we can send you a Fertility Data Form that can help us to evaluate your situation.

If you're not pregnant within six to twelve months despite good mucus, good timing, good thermal shifts indicating that you have been ovulating, and the self-helps above, it may be time to seek medical help from an infertility specialist. Blocked tubes and other physical obstacles to conception and/or the continuation of pregnancy can be examined.

A competent infertility specialist will be able to evaluate correctly your sympto-thermal charts. If he says you're not ovulating in the face of well-defined thermal shifts of 9 to 15 days in every cycle, you should certainly ask him for the basis of such an evaluation, and you may want to go elsewhere. If you are substantially overweight, or if you're experiencing runner's amenorrhea or anorexia nervosa and obviously not ovulating, and if he doesn't treat your basic health problem but instead wants you to use ovulation stimulating drugs, you should question your own prudence and his too. This is not meant to detract from the fact that a good infertility specialist can sometimes be very helpful.

If a physician cannot interpret a normal thermal shift pattern as indicative of ovulation, go elsewhere. He is not knowledgeable enough to investigate the problem.
—Konald A. Prem, M.D.

As this section was being written, we received a phone call from a young newlywed woman.[14] She was confused by her irregular cycle pattern with delayed ovulation and ambiguous mucus. Very quickly, we determined that she was 15 pounds under the "ideal" weight for her height and that she exercised vigorously. In fact, the same day she called, we read that her favorite winter exercise—cross-country skiing—is the "best" for burning up calories—1,100 per hour! Those two factors were tip-offs that she may not be eating enough of the right foods and/or that she may have worked off so much body fat that she was below the critical level of 20%. Medical tests had shown a low estrogen level, and that's consistent with insufficient body fat because you need body fat to hold estrogen.

Her physician did not recognize the possible connection between her physical condition and her complaints of cycle irregularities. He suggested either doing nothing, or taking an estrogen supplement, or taking the Pill for three months, or using Clomid to stimulate ovulation. We are not criticizing legitimate hormone therapy where it is truly the only remedy, but certainly the low tech, cost free avenues of improved body balance and nutrition need to be explored and used first.

In such a case, estrogen supplements or the Pill might make matters worse. Clomid might work immediately.
—Konald A. Prem, M.D.

5. Do not resort to immoral methods in seeking pregnancy

We are all called to marital chastity whether we are seeking to achieve or avoid pregnancy. That means we are called to cooperate with God in the procreation and education of children whom we hope will give glory to God. That process starts with respect for God's laws in our personal lives.

Therefore, husbands, refuse to masturbate for seminal analysis. Likewise refuse to attempt artificial insemination whether using the husband's sperm or that of another donor, and avoid *in vitro* fertilization ("test tube babies"). It is the teaching of Popes Pius XII and John Paul II and contemporary orthodox theologians that such actions depersonalize the marital act and offend against its true unitive meaning.

In addition, in vitro fertilization involves masturbation and the killing of the newly conceived lives when they are not all implanted. The moral status of such actions is explained more fully in the next chapter.

6. Consider adoption

The combination of increased infertility and the vast increase in the number of babies being killed by abortion has resulted in long waiting periods for adoption in many areas of the country. Offer your best talents to the pro-chastity and pro-life movement. Get involved. Consider joining the ranks of sidewalk counselors or prayerful picketers outside the modern Auschwitzes called abortion clinics. You may not get the baby you save, but maybe somebody else in your situation will be so blessed.

Look into the adoption of foreign or other disadvantaged or orphaned children. Look into the adoption of a special child. Their needs are very real, and they will probably take special care, but maybe you as a childless couple will have that extra time and patience called love to be real parents to such children.

7. First and last, pray

Pray for the gift of your own conceived child. Pray also for the gifts of discernment, prudence and wisdom regarding the various adoption possibilities. Should you spend $3,500—or more—on fertility testing when a similar amount might pay many of the expenses of adoption? That's a question only you as a couple can answer and a subject certainly worthy of prayer.

May God bless all of you who are struggling with this. As we learn more about self-help or medical treatments for infertility, we will pass on the information in the CCL magazine, *CCL Family Foundations*. Marilyn Shannon and CCL are also committed to keeping her book, *Fertility, Cycles and Nutrition*, up to date. It is definitely the place to start.

8. When your baby comes, practice full-time mothering

In some parts of the United States, foster care laws require the foster mother of a child under three to practice full-time mothering. This is based on the very real needs of the child. We suspect there may be another element as well. The agency people may well think, "Why should we screen the couple, get references, check out their home, etc., to try to ensure the welfare of the child, if the parents are going to turn over the care of the child during most of its waking hours to someone else?"

We believe that your baby deserves the full-time mothering that only you can give it. For more information about the reasons for this conviction, read our leaflet, *The First Three Years*,[15] and our booklet, *The Crucial First Three Years*.[16]

Fertility, Cycles and Nutrition, Chapter 6 ("Cycle Irregularities and Female Infertility") and Chapter 12 ("The Male Connection").

Additional reading

Self-Test Questions: Chapter 21

1. True____   False____   For some couples of marginal mutual fertility, too frequent intercourse may hinder their becoming pregnant.

2. For couples of marginal mutual fertility and seeking pregnancy, the purpose of abstinence in Phase I and early Phase II is to _____.

3. Two more general suggestions for not depleting his sperm supply unnecessarily are:
   a) don't have relations on _____ and
   b) don't have relations more than _____ a day.

4. However, in some cases of low sperm count, it may be helpful to have a second intercourse about _____ after the first one.

5. A Texas researcher found that the sperm _____ of some husbands increases when the husband takes one gram of Vitamin ____ each day.

6. Nature intends that a man's testicles should be
   a) the same temperature as
   b) warmer than
   c) cooler than
   the rest of his body.

7. For the Huhner test to be valid, it must be made shortly after intercourse
   a) before the mucus patch starts
   b) when the most fertile mucus is present
   c) during Phase III.

8. True____ False____ Vitamin A is necessary for the proper functioning of mucus membranes throughout your body.

9. True____ False____ Some women find that an adequate intake of vitamin A increases the quantity and stretchiness of their cervical mucus during the fertile time.

10. The drug called _____, when taken during the mucus patch, can make cervical mucus more fluid.

11. For normal fertility, a woman needs a minimum of _____% of her weight in body fat.

12. A handy rule for estimating your "ideal" weight is this: 100 pounds for the first five feet and _____ pounds per additional inch (assuming average bone structure).

13. Nutrition is concerned about _____ you eat and drink just as much as about _____ _____ you eat and drink.

14. True____ False____ Inadequate nutrition can reduce your fertility.

15. True____ False____ Too much exercise can reduce a woman's fertility.

16. True____ False____ Gonorrhea can make a woman sterile.

17. True____ False____ An IUD can make a woman sterile through pelvic inflammatory disease and/or scarring of the uterus.

18. True____ False____ An induced abortion can make a woman sterile.

19. True____ False____ The Pill, implants, and birth control injections can make a woman sterile for months after discontinuing them.

20. True____ False____ Six cycles of well-recorded sympto-thermal daily observations can help a competent infertility specialist with his initial diagnostic review.

Answers to self-test
1. True 2. maximize sperm count 3. consecutive days. . . once 4. 45 minutes 5. motility. . . C 6. c) cooler than 7. b) when the most fertile mucus is present 8. True 9. True 10. guaifenesin 11. 20% - 22% 12. five 13. what. . . how much 14. True 15. True 16. True 17. True 18. True 19. True 20. True

References

(1) Sacred Congregation for the Doctrine of the Faith, *Declaration on Certain Questions concerning Sexual Ethics*, (Rome, 29 December 1975) n. 9. Printed by St. Paul Books & Media, Boston MA 02130.

(2) This section is adapted from a CCL brochure, "Practical Helps for Seeking Pregnancy," (Cincinnati: CCL, 1992).

(3) Associated Press report, "Women smokers at risk," *Cincinnati Enquirer* 24 May 1985, reporting on article in *Journal of the American Medical Association*, same date. The study also reported that "women who smoke 25 cigarettes or more daily and take the pill had 23 times the risk of a heart attack" compared to non-smokers on the pill.

(4) S.L. Laurent et al., "An epidemiologic study of smoking and primary infertility in women," *Fertility and Sterility* 57 (1992) 565-572. Reviewed by Hanna Klaus, M.D. in DDP *Science Notes*, March/April 1992, 6.

(5) Marilyn M. Shannon, *Fertility, Cycles and Nutrition: Can what you eat affect your menstrual cycles and your fertility?* Second ed. (Cincinnati: CCL, 1992) 68.

(6) Claire Infante-Rivard, "Fetal loss associated with caffeine intake before and during pregnancy," *JAMA* 270:24 (22/29 December 1993) 2940. Contradicting an earlier study, this one found that the caffeine in 1.5 to 3 cups of coffee may nearly double the risk of miscarriage. Consumption of 3 or more cups of coffee daily in the month before conception can have a similar effect on pregnancy and miscarriage.

(7) Nutrasweet® is the trademark of the Merisant Corporation for the chemical aspartame. For the health dangers of consuming this chemical, see H.J. Roberts, M.D., *Aspartame (NutraSweet®) Is It Safe?* (Philadelphia: The Charles Press, 1990).

In his practice, Dr. Roberts has found a whole list of ailments associated with the consumption of aspartame. Examples include "unexplained headaches, seizures, learning disabilities, [and] hysterectomy." The table of contents in his book lists chapters dealing with convulsions, headache, confusion and memory loss, eye and ear complaints, excessive weight gain and loss, heart and chest problems, and more. If you read Dr. Roberts' book, it's doubtful you will consume aspartame-containing products.

(8) Shannon, 68.

(9) K.K. Singh et al., "Effects of breastfeeding after resumption of menstruation on waiting time to next conception," *Human Biology* 65 (1993) 71-86. Reported in La Leche League, *Breastfeeding Abstracts* 13:4 (May 1994) 30.

(10) Singh, above.

(11) Associated Press, "Smoker impotence cited," *Cincinnati Enquirer* 02 December 1994, A-11. "Smokers are 50 percent more likely to suffer from impotence than non-smokers, the government said Thursday [01 Dec.]. Researchers at the Centers for Disease Control and Prevention said the rate may be even slightly higher, because their study was based on men willing to acknowledge the sexual disorder. 'It's more bad news for smokers,' said Dr. David Mannino of the CDC's National Center for Environmental Health. Researchers estimate that up to 10 million U.S. men are impotent and that half of the cases are caused by such factors as diet, diabetes, aging, alcohol and medication. Smoking has long been suspected."

(12) P. Weathersbee and J. Lodge, "A review of ethanol's effects on the reproductive process." *J. Reproductive Medicine* 21 (1978) 63. From Shannon, *Fertility, Cycles and Nutrition,* 115. "Alcohol decreases the levels of testosterone, ultimately contributing to lowered sperm production *which may be irreversible*" (emphasis in Shannon text).

(13) Earl B. Dawson, reported at the 1983 annual meeting of the Federation of American Societies of Experimental Biology. "New claim for vitamin C," *The Cincinnati Enquirer,* 17 April 1983, D-2.

(14) Phone call received by John F. Kippley, 5:05 p.m. 2 March 1994.

(15) John and Sheila Kippley, *The First Three Years: the importance of mother/child togetherness* (Cincinnati: Foundation for the Family, 1988) leaflet.

(16) Sheila Matgen Kippley, *The Crucial First Three Years* (Cincinnati: The Couple to Couple League, 1998) booklet. Updates 1988 leaflet with research from the Nineties.

22

Thy Will Be Done

Not everything which is *physically* possible in the pursuit of pregnancy is *morally* permissible. This is simply the application of the basic moral principle that the end or purpose does not justify the means. For example, if a husband is infertile, the couple may not invite another man of known fertility to have sex with the wife to achieve pregnancy. That would be adultery, and most people understand the immorality of such an action.

If you agree that a couple may not commit adultery to have a baby, then you agree in principle that there are moral limits to what you—or anyone else—may do in the pursuit of this human good. That is true about every human good.

Marriage endures

Marriage endures despite infertility. That may seem obvious in the American culture, but in some cultures where children are highly valued, childless husbands have divorced their wives in order to try to have children by another woman. The Fathers of the Second Vatican Council specifically addressed this issue:

> But marriage is not merely for the procreation of children: its nature as an indissoluble compact between two people and the good of the children demand that the mutual love of the partners be properly shown. Even in cases where despite the intense desire of the spouses there are no children, marriage still retains its character of being a whole manner and communion of life and preserves its value and indissolubility.[1]

Donum Vitae

The Catholic Church has addressed also the morality of different methods of seeking to achieve pregnancy in a document titled *Donum Vitae* in Latin.[2] The English title is more informative but very long: *Instruction on*

Respect for Human Life in Its Origin and on the Dignity of Procreation. So we will use the Latin title.

The English document is 40 pages (about 4.5 x 7 inches). If you want to study it, we strongly recommend you also get the 22 page commentary by Father Lorenzo Albacete;[3] this makes it much easier to read and to understand *Donum Vitae*. The encyclical, but not the commentary, is available from the Couple to Couple League.

Five principles

Donum Vitae sets out five principles in its "Introduction."

1. Human life is a gift from God. "Donum Vitae" means "The gift of life," and those are the opening words of this teaching. As Father Albacete summarizes it: "Human persons are not created by humans; they are to be welcomed, recognized, appreciated, accepted and respected as gifts."[4] Parents supply the matter, but only God creates the human person endowed with an immortal, spiritual soul.

2. Science and technology are to serve the human person. God has entrusted to us the task of "having dominion over the earth" (Gen 1:28). There is, however, a world of difference between *dominion* and *domination*. Dominion means respecting God's order of creation. Domination means trying to impose man's will upon creation without regard for the natural moral law and sometimes even without regard for physical nature. Dominion involves good stewardship of both the material world and sexuality. However, almost every environmental disaster is a result of wrongheaded domination instead of stewardship. The moral disasters involved in abortion, freezing embryos, sperm banks, artificial insemination, "test-tube" babies, and surrogate motherhood are all results of ignoring the natural moral law regarding sexuality. "Science without conscience can only lead to man's ruin" (*D. V.* n. 2).

3. Man is more than matter. Any sort of intervention on the human body "affects not only the tissues, the organs and their functions but also involves the person himself on different levels" (*D. V.* n. 3). Interventions dealing with fertility "must be given a moral evaluation in reference to the dignity of the human person, who is called to realize his vocation from God to the gift of love and the gift of life" (*D. V.* n. 3).

4. Technique does not equal morality. "What is technically possible is not for that very reason morally admissible" (*D. V.* n. 4). No one has any problem seeing that truth when it is applied to nuclear bombs. Obviously, several countries have the technical capability of bombing others, but everyone except the proverbial "mad scientist" recognizes that capability does not make such actions morally right. We must apply moral principles to technical capability.

5. "The Magisterium of the Church offers to human reason in this field, too, the light of Revelation" (*D. V.* n. 5.).

Almost nobody will have any trouble with the first four principles; they are more or less self evident. However, the last principle needs further explanation.

Consider what's involved in some high-tech ways of seeking pregnancy. In some, there is masturbation, glass-dish fertilization of several eggs, implantation of one or more embryos, and freezing or destruction of the other embryos. In other procedures, there is masturbation, considerable manipulation of the sperm and the eggs, and then re-insertion into the woman prior to conception.

How can we come to certain knowledge about the morality of such actions? The biblical judgment on the sin of Onan is also a condemnation of masturbation. However, it is obvious that artificial insemination, test-tube conception, and manipulation of the eggs and sperm were not even thought about during biblical times.

That's why, the Catholic Church teaches, Christ Himself did not leave us a book but rather founded a living teaching authority through which God can continue to teach about new questions. It is Catholic teaching that when the Pope speaks authoritatively on matters of faith and morals, he is a real authority about what is right and wrong, and is to be heeded. In biblical terms, he holds a prophetic office through which God can communicate as He did through the biblical prophets (Mt 16: 18-19). A text from the Second Vatican Council sets forth Catholic teaching:

> Bishops who teach in communion with the Roman Pontiff are to be revered by all as witnesses of divine and Catholic truth; the faithful, for their part, are obliged to submit to their bishops' decision, made in the name of Christ, in matters of faith and morals, and to adhere to it with a ready and respectful allegiance of mind.
>
> This loyal submission of the will and intellect must be given, in a special way, to the authentic teaching authority of the Roman Pontiff, even when he does not speak *ex cathedra*, in such wise, indeed, that his supreme teaching authority be acknowledged with respect, and that one sincerely adhere to decisions made by him, conformably with his manifest mind and intention, which is made known principally either by the character of the documents in question, or by the frequency with which a certain doctrine is proposed, or by the manner in which the doctrine is formulated" (*Lumen Gentium* 25.1).[5]

That's the background for understanding *Donum Vitae.* In the face of growing publicity about "test-tube babies" and surrogate motherhood, clear moral teaching was necessary.

Terminology

The text of *Donum Vitae* uses several technical terms.
Heterologous: either the sperm or eggs are *not* from the spouses
Homologous: both the sperm and the eggs are from the spouses
In vitro: in a glass dish
In vivo: in the living body

Respect for human embryos

After the "Introduction," the first major section teaches that "The human being must be respected—as a person—from the very first instant of his existence" (*D. V.* "I. Respect for human embryos" n. 1). The first right of a person is the right to life.

Therefore it is a grave moral evil to destroy or freeze or experiment upon embryonic persons, regardless of the place of their conception, whether in the mother's fallopian tube or in a glass-dish. Directly therapeutic procedures are morally permissible, but "keeping human embryos alive *in vivo* or *in vitro* for experimental or commercial purposes is totally opposed to human dignity" (n. 4).

Artificial interventions

The second and longest part of *Donum Vitae* is titled "II. Interventions upon Human Procreation." It first reminds us that the abortion mentality has made possible the acceptance of *in vitro* (glass dish) fertilization. With the *in vitro* procedure, multiple ova are fertilized with masturbated sperm. Some of the embryos are placed in the woman's reproductive tract. Others, generally called "spare," are destroyed or frozen. "On occasion, some of the implanted embryos are sacrificed for various eugenic, economic or psychological reasons."

There is a tragic irony here: those who are seeking one human life willfully participate in the destruction of other human lives. What is happening is a "dynamic of violence and domination," and this is a grave moral evil.

● Various means of artificial fertilization

At this point, the subject matter becomes highly technical, and we will be relatively brief.

1. Children are to be the fruit *only* of the marriage act of husband and wife. It is wrong to use a third person's eggs or sperm, and it is wrong for a man to provide sperm for such use. (Technically, that's called "heterologous" artificial fertilization.) The document also carefully defines surrogate motherhood and applies the same negative judgment to it.

2. What about *in vitro* fertilization (IVF) and embryo transport (ET) which use only the ovum and sperm of the spouses? (Technically, that's called "homologous" artificial fertilization.) What if this could be done without masturbation and without killing or freezing unwanted embryos? This is one of the two really tough questions which some married couples face.

Catholic teaching insists that procreation must not be separated from the marriage act. To repeat, children are to be the fruit only of the marriage act. However,

> homologous IVF and ET is brought about outside the bodies of the couple through actions of third parties whose competence and technical activity determine the success of the procedure. Such fertilization entrusts the life and the identity of the embryo into the power of doctors and biologists and establishes the domination of technology over the origin and destiny of the human person. . . The generation of the human person is objectively deprived of its proper perfection: namely, that of being the result and fruit of a conjugal act in which the spouses can become "cooperators with God for giving life to a new person" (*D.V.*, II, B, n. 5).

Therefore, *in vitro* fertilization is morally wrong, even if it could be done without masturbation and the killing or freezing of the unwanted embryos.

3. What about procedures in which the egg and/or sperm are manipulated outside the body and then reinserted so that actual fertilization/conception occurs within the body of the wife?

> Homologous artificial insemination within marriage cannot be admitted except for those cases in which the technical means is not a substitute for the conjugal act but serves to facilitate and to help so that the act attains its natural purpose (*D.V.*, II, B, n. 6).

That rules out what is commonly called "artificial insemination." However, it does not rule out the physician trying to assist migration of the sperm after a normal marriage act.

Donum Vitae concludes this section by encouraging scientists to "continue their research with the aim of preventing the causes of sterility and of being able to remedy them so that sterile couples will be able to procreate in full respect for their own personal dignity and that of the child to be born" (*D.V.,* II, B, n. 8).

Different procedures have been suggested that will respect these moral principles, and the situation is too fluid for comment in this manual. Some procedures appear to have such serious technological intervention on sperm and eggs taken out of the body that they seem to substitute for the marriage act. Others may merely serve to facilitate the natural consequences of the marriage act.

The procedure known as GIFT—gamete intra-fallopian transfer—is frequently mentioned. However, as of this writing, it remains highly controversial. Some theologians think it is morally acceptable. Others think it is immoral because it involves excessive technological manipulation including removal of both sperm and ovum from the woman's body. Critics also note that in the GIFT procedure a technician could use an egg or sperm that are not from the spouses. We are persuaded by the arguments of the critics, but in mid-1995 there was no authoritative teaching addressed to this particular procedure.

Theologians are addressing these questions. As more information becomes available about acceptable means of assisting the normal conception process, we will review it in *CCL Family Foundations*, the magazine of the Couple to Couple League.

We trust that it is clear that the Couple to Couple League is opposed to any form of artificial insemination, masturbation for seminal analysis, or attempted "test-tube" conceptions. The basic reason is that every act of sexual intercourse is intended by God to be an act of *personal* love between husband and wife performed in the natural way which carries the possibility of conception according to the state of their natural mutual fertility. Procreation involves husband and wife and God.

When procreation becomes "making babies in glass dishes" or some other highly technical laboratory procedure, it becomes depersonalized. Such actions do not respect the dignity of the baby or of the married couple.

At the same time, we need to recognize that the moral fault is with the people doing such procedures, not with the baby who is conceived. Once a child is conceived, he or she has the dignity of human personhood, and that dignity must be respected.

In brief, God intends that sexual intercourse should be a marriage act. Babies ought to be conceived only through the marriage act. The words of Jesus about marriage and divorce apply both to contraception and to efforts to achieve pregnancy: "What therefore God has joined together, let no man put asunder" (Mt 19:6).

Self-Test Questions: Chapter 22

1. True____   False____   When some Catholic writers accepted masturbation for seminal analysis, it was the beginning of a logical chain of accepting contraception and marital sodomy (completed oral or anal copulation).

2. True____   False____   "The end justifies the means" provides a sound principle for making moral decisions.

3. True____   False____   The Catholic Church teaches that contraception, sterilized intercourse, mutual and/or solitary masturbation, marital sodomy, and "withdrawal" are immoral means of avoiding pregnancy.

4. True____   False____   The Catholic Church teaches that artificial insemination, masturbation for seminal analysis, "test-tube" conception, embryo transplants, and surrogate motherhood are immoral means of seeking pregnancy.

5. The basic reason behind this teaching of the Catholic Church is that God intends that every deliberate sex act should be a _____ act of love between _____ _____ _____, an act which is fertile or infertile according to their state of natural fertility or infertility.

6. True____   False____   The dignity of the human person is present from the first moment of conception and must be respected.

7. True____   False____   Respect for the dignity of the human person demands that even when newly conceived and tiny, such persons should not be frozen, manipulated, experimented with, or otherwise treated as material objects at the disposal of older and larger persons.

8. True____   False____   Respect for the dignity of the human sexual act and the dignity of the human persons involved—husband and wife and the child to be conceived—prohibit the application to human procreation of some procedures that are acceptable in veterinary medicine.

Answers to self-test
1. True 2. False 3. True 4. True 5. personal. . . husband and wife 6. True 7. True 8. True

References

(1) Vatican Council II, *Gaudium et Spes* or *The Church in the Modern World*, 7 December 1965 (Boston: St. Paul Editions, Austin Flannery, O.P. General editor, 1981) n. 50.

(2) Joseph Cardinal Ratzinger, Congregation for the Doctrine of the Faith, *Donum Vitae* or *Instruction on Respect for Human Life in Its Origin and on the Dignity of Procreation: Replies to Certain Questions of the Day*, 22 February 1987 (Boston: St. Paul Books and Media, 1987).

(3) Lorenzo M. Albacete, *Commentary on Instruction on Respect for Human Life in Its Origin and on the Dignity of Procreation* (Boston: St. Paul Editions, 1987).

(4) Albacete, 8-9.

(5) Vatican II, *Lumen Gentium*, n. 25.1. as translated in *Vatican Council II: The Conciliar and Post Conciliar Documents*, Austin Flannery, O.P. general editor (Boston: St. Paul Editions, 1975).

23

The Return of Fertility after Childbirth

When will your fertility return after childbirth? It depends largely on the kind of care you give your baby.

1. If you do ecological breastfeeding (and we'll describe that in just a bit), you can expect an extended delay in the return of your fertility. For a number of reasons, we strongly recommend this form of baby care.

2. If you do cultural breastfeeding (and we'll also describe that), you can expect an early return of fertility.

3. If you bottlefeed your baby, you can expect a very early return of fertility.

As usual, we refer to babies and doctors as male to keep straight the pronouns representing mother and baby.

Postpartum abstinence

In the United States, it was common in the past for doctors to tell new parents to abstain until after the mother comes in for a checkup at six weeks postpartum. This abstinence may be necessary if the woman is having difficulty with the healing of an episiotomy, but it is not a universal necessity. The more appropriate advice to the medically healthy couple would be to refrain from coitus until the wife feels physically comfortable. For many women, that will be about three to four weeks postpartum.

We write on the strength of statements made by Konald A. Prem, M.D., while a professor of obstetrics and gynecology at the University of Minnesota School of Medicine. If your doctor disagrees, politely ask him for the medical evidence that contradicts this. You may also want to read up on childbirth practices because your childbirth process can make a big difference in your postpartum healing.

Terminology

Amenorrhea: the extended absence of menstruation.

Breastfeeding amenorrhea: the extended absence of periods due to breastfeeding.

Baby Care and the Return of Fertility

The biggest factor in the return of fertility after childbirth is the form of baby care. We describe five different situations and their usual effects on the return of fertility.

1. Ecological breastfeeding

When a mother does ecological breastfeeding, her baby gets 100% of his liquids, nourishment, and pacification directly from her breasts for the first six months or so. Her baby nurses frequently during the day and a few times during the night. Once her baby starts solids at six to eight months, she continues to let him nurse as often as he wants. She can continue to let him nurse frequently until he weans himself.

Only ecological breastfeeding brings any significant delay in the return of fertility. It is definitely part of God's plan for spacing babies.

The baby's frequency of suckling is the most important factor in the natural delay of fertility. We have conducted two studies which show that mothers who follow the simple rules of ecological breastfeeding will experience the return of menstruation and presumed fertility around 14.5 months, on the average. There is no question: ecological breastfeeding is the world's oldest form of natural family planning. In areas of the world not yet on the bottlefeeding economy, ecological breastfeeding postpones more births than all the contraceptives and abortifacients shipped into those countries by the so-called developed countries.

● **Practical advice**

Ecological breastfeeding was the form of baby care practiced all throughout history and pre-history. Unfortunately, it has become somewhat counter-cultural in the West. Therefore, we use the entire next chapter to explain both how to do it and its many benefits to mother and baby alike. The Couple to Couple League also publishes *Breastfeeding and Natural Child Spacing: How Ecological Breastfeeding Spaces Babies.*[2] See "Resources."

> "Exclusive breastfeeding is ideal nutrition and sufficient to support optimal growth and development for approximately the first six months after birth ... In the first six months, water, juice, and other foods are generally unnecessary for breastfed infants ... Flouride should not be administered to infants during the first six months after birth, whether they are breast- or formula-fed."
> — *American Academy of Pediatrics*[1]

2. Cultural breastfeeding

Cultural breastfeeding is the form of nursing that is common in Western culture. The breastfeeding mother supplements in the early months with bottles of liquids—including her own milk, and with formulas, baby foods, cereals or other solids. She frequently tries to get her baby to nurse on a schedule similar to that of a bottlefeeding baby. She goes for several hours without nursing. She typically uses pacifiers and babysitters, and she does her best to get her baby to sleep all through the night as soon as possible.

All of these practices limit the frequency and the total amount of the baby's suckling at the breast. Since the frequency of suckling is the biggest factor in postponing the return of fertility, these practices encourage the early return of fertility.

● **Practical advice**

If you do cultural breastfeeding, you can expect your fertility to return quickly, usually just as soon as for the bottlefeeding mother. Therefore, follow the rules below for the bottlefeeding mother.

Do not be surprised if your baby weans quite early. Without frequent nursing, you may lose your milk supply, or your baby may simply lose interest in nursing.

The biggest difference in the return of fertility between bottlefeeding and cultural breastfeeding is this: the latter has a much wider range. With cultural breastfeeding, fertility may return anywhere from four weeks postpartum until after weaning. This variation is due mostly to big differences in the frequency and the amount of nursing among different cultural-nursing mothers. Physical differences among mothers may also influence the return of fertility.

● Advantages of cultural breastfeeding

The many advantages of breastfeeding are described in the next chapter. Cultural nursing will give your baby some important benefits of breastfeeding such as certain immunities and a reduction in allergies. It is much better for your baby than formulas and the early introduction of solid baby foods. However, cultural nursing will not provide the extended infertility of ecological breastfeeding, and it tends to be relatively short-term.

3. Exclusive breastfeeding

Exclusive breastfeeding means that the mother is feeding her baby only her breastmilk: no other liquids or solids. However, exclusive breastfeeding is NOT the same as ecological breastfeeding. With exclusive breastfeeding, the mother might be expressing her milk so the baby takes it in a bottle. She might be using pacifiers, schedules, and having long absences from her baby. All of these factors reduce the frequency of suckling at the breast and therefore encourage the return of fertility. Therefore, "exclusive breastfeeding" is frequently a form of cultural nursing.

Exclusive breastfeeding can take place only for six to eight months. Once the baby starts taking solids or other liquids, breastfeeding is no longer "exclusive."

● Practical advice

Do not expect exclusive breastfeeding by itself to provide the extended breastfeeding infertility that is a natural side effect of ecological breastfeeding, and do not be surprised if your nursing experience is shorter than you wanted.

4. Deliberate weaning

By deliberate weaning we mean that the mother stops her nursing over a very short period of time. The effect on the return of fertility is the same whether she weans her baby in one day or ten days. However, weaning in a one or two day period can be extremely uncomfortable for the mother because she may have an ample milk supply and engorged breasts for several days. Quick weaning is also hard on babies, and parents who wean their baby off the breast should continue to hold and cuddle him often, especially during his feeding times.

● A ten-day weaning program

We do not recommend short-term weaning for optimal baby care. Rather, we offer this to those in difficult situations who think that baby-led weaning is impossible in their case.

As far as the weaning process itself, be prepared. Your baby most likely would prefer to nurse. You might start by eliminating one of the baby's typical nursing times each day. Be sure you give your baby lots of holding and cuddling during this time of transition.

Please note: a quick weaning process such as this does not guarantee a quick return of fertility and regular cycles. We have seen cases of fairly long intervals between the end of a short weaning and the return of fertility.

5. Bottlefeeding

Ovulation has been detected after childbirth as early as 27 days postpartum.[3] Other evidence indicates that when the first menstruation occurs at 42 days, there is only about a five percent chance that it has been preceded by ovulation.[4]

If you bottlefeed your baby, your fertility will return within a few weeks postpartum. The evidence suggests that the first six weeks postpartum are quite infertile; that is, in about 95% of cases when menstruation occurs at or before six weeks, it is not preceded by fertility. After six weeks, ovulation before the first period becomes increasingly common.

● Practical advice

During the first three weeks postpartum, there is almost no possibility of conception. Abstinence and coitus during this time would be dependent upon the wife's health and comfort.

By the fourth week, the bottlefeeding mother enters the range of recorded fertility. Thus the practical advice for avoiding immediate pregnancy in this case is as follows:

1. Do **not** take any pills or shots after childbirth or later to dry up your milk supply. Some may contain hormones that will interfere with your normal signs of fertility and infertility; others may have serious side effects. Hand express to relieve engorgement and discomfort, not to empty your breasts. Without nursing, your milk production will stop in a few days without any medication.

One product to dry up mother's milk, Parlodel (bromocriptine mesylate), has been linked to serious medical effects. "In 1987, seven years after the drug was first marketed as a lactation suppressant, Parlodel's principal manufacturer, Sandoz Pharmaceuticals, placed a warning on its package insert that reported 38 cases of seizures and 15 cases of strokes 'mostly in postpartum patients whose prenatal and obstetric courses had been uncomplicated.' "[5] In 1993 the Public Citizen Health Research Group complained to the FDA that since 1989 there had been over 220 reports of adverse side effects and 13 deaths linked to Parlodel; the FDA promised an investigation.[6]

2. Begin taking your waking temperatures at least by Day 15 after childbirth. Take and record your temperatures even if you want to become pregnant soon. Your temperature record is the single best indicator of when ovulation occurred and pregnancy started.

3. Begin mucus and cervix observations as soon as possible. However,

the after-childbirth bloody discharge called the **lochia** will obscure mucus observations for several weeks. Do not make the cervix examinations until your vaginal tissues are completely healed from childbirth.

4. After the lochia disappears: if you have no mucus or cervix signs of fertility, you are in Phase I infertility. If you choose to have marital relations, be sure to follow the Phase I rules of not-in-the-mornings and not-on-consecutive-days. We continue to recommend the internal exam for mucus at the cervical os once your vaginal tissues are thoroughly healed.

5. If you have no experience with the mucus observations or if you are confused, we recommend that you abstain until you have a sympto-thermal indication you are in Phase III. Normally it will not be a long abstinence.

Probably the majority of bottlefeeding mothers experience six or more weeks of postpartum discharges. Therefore, the most common practice will be to refrain from coitus until after the first menstruation, generally until the first Phase III.

6. If you have relations during your Phase I infertility, be sure to consider yourselves in Phase II as soon as you notice any type of mucus. Then abstain until you have a sympto-thermal certainty of being in Phase III. (Having relations in your Phase I infertility assumes that you have enough experience to know what you are looking for in your mucus observations.)

7. After your first menstruation, consider yourselves back into your normal fertility cycle. Use the regular rules of NFP for fertility awareness. (Sometimes a second menstruation will occur without a preceding ovulation, but this is rare in the bottlefeeding mother.)

The Return of Menstruation

Generally the return of menstruation signals the return of fertility, and the couple must consider themselves back in a cyclic pattern of fertility and infertility. However, this is not always the case.

The early "period"

Within the first eight weeks postpartum, some mothers doing ecological or exclusive nursing have a bleeding episode that has nothing to do with fertility. The cause is still not fully known. However, some call it "hormonal bleeding" because they think it reflects a change from pregnancy and immediate postpartum hormone levels to hormone levels more typical for mothers doing ecological and exclusive breastfeeding.[7]

● **Practical advice**
If you are doing ecological or exclusive breastfeeding, you can treat any bleeding episode that occurs in the first 56 days postpartum as unrelated to fertility, according to a consensus of breastfeeding experts.[8] Consider yourself still in breastfeeding infertility.

If you are doing exclusive breastfeeding that very closely resembles ecological breastfeeding, you can follow the advice for ecological nursing. If you are doing exclusive breastfeeding that is really a form of cultural nursing, follow the advice for bottlefeeding and cultural nursing.

If you are bottlefeeding or doing cultural nursing, consider any bleeding episode as a possible menstruation marking the return of fertility, and consider yourself in Phase I.

The first menstruation

When true menstruation occurs as early as six weeks postpartum, it is rarely preceded by ovulation. However, after six weeks, fertility returns quickly for bottlefeeding and cultural nursing mothers. By ten weeks postpartum, a bottlefeeding mother almost always ovulates before her first period.

● Practical advice

Whether bottlefeeding or breastfeeding, consider the beginning of a true menstruation as the beginning of a fertile cycle. Consider yourselves in Phase I and follow the standard Phase I rules.

If you are experienced in making the mucus observations, you can apply the standard Last Dry Day rules once dryness has been established after the bleeding episode.

If you want to apply the 21-Day Rule, use the shortest cycle among your pre-pregnancy cycles of the past two years.

Whether bottlefeeding or breastfeeding, chart your sympto-thermal observations as soon as you experience a bleeding episode or any other sign of fertility. Even if you generally rely only on the mucus sign, be sure to take and record your waking temperatures until you are well established in your postpartum cycles. Only your upward thermal shift pattern will tell you whether a mucus patch was associated with ovulation and whether a bleeding episode was preceded by ovulation.

Q. What if amenorrhea returns after a first period?
A. This would be very unusual except for a woman doing ecological breastfeeding. See this question in Chapter 25.

Transition cycles

The first few cycles after the first menstruation are frequently irregular because they are part of an overall transition from infertility to regular cycles. No matter what kind of care you give your baby, for a short time you might experience delayed ovulation, longer cycles with an extended Phase II, and/or short luteal phases.

Figure 23.1 (two charts) illustrates a somewhat delayed ovulation for a bottlefeeding mother. Her baby was two weeks old when she began charting on January 19. Her first period started on Day 80 postpartum and was preceded by ovulation and 14 days of obvious thermal shift. (With the LTL at 97.9°, Rule B yields Day 68 postpartum as the start of Phase III.)

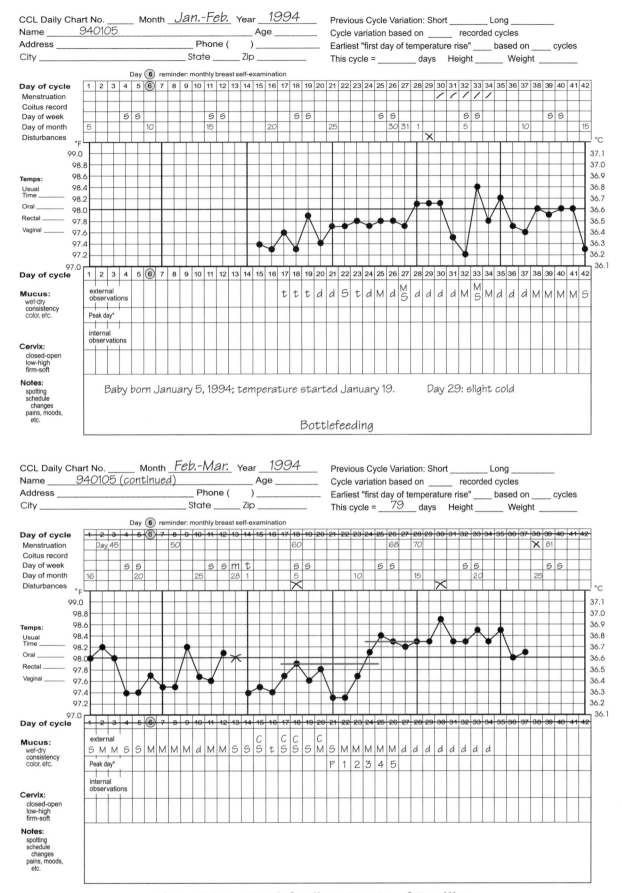

Figure 23.1 Bottlefeeding; Return of Fertility

Figure 23.2 illustrates the same sort of thing for a breastfeeding mother.

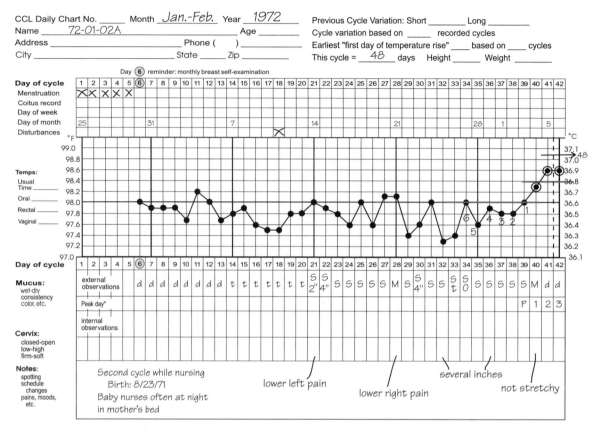

Figure 23.2   Breastfeeding: Return of Fertility

In the case illustrated by Figure 23.2, the breastfeeding mother had an early return of fertility. Roughly two weeks before the menstruation at the beginning of this chart, she had ovulated as indicated by a mucus patch and 12 days of well-elevated temperatures. The baby continued a heavy pattern of ecological breastfeeding. We suspect that the delayed ovulation and extended Phase II (which began on Cycle Day 14) was the result of conflicting signals—"let's have another ovulation" from part of her hormonal system versus "let's suppress ovulation" from the breastfeeding.

Ovulation finally occurred, probably between Days 38 and 40. With an LTL of 98.0°, Rule R indicates the start of Phase III on the evening of Day 42. The nine-day luteal phase (as measured by elevated temperatures on Days 40-48) is a bit on the short side, but many women will experience an even shorter luteal phase during the first one or two postpartum cycles.

● *For how long?* The length of the transition phase will vary. During the transition time, Phase I and Phase II will become shorter and Phase III will become longer as your cycle pattern shortens to its normal range.

● *The 21 Day Rule and the Doering Rule.* Do not use the length of your first half dozen postpartum cycles for applying the 21 Day Rule. Each cycle may be shorter than the previous one. To use the 21 Day Rule, base it on the shortest cycle in the last two years before you conceived your new baby. The same holds true for the Doering Rule. Use your pre-pregnancy cycles as your basis for applying it in the first six cycles postpartum.

Self-Test Questions: Chapter 23

1. The world's oldest form of natural family planning is

   _____.

2. True____   False____   Fertility returns much sooner for the bottlefeeding mother than for the mother who does ecological breastfeeding.

3. True____   False____   If you breastfeed and also give supplements in the first six months, your fertility may return as soon as it does for the bottlefeeding mother.

4. There's a greater range in the return of fertility among mothers who do cultural breast-feeding because of a)_____ and
   b)_____.

5. True____   False____   "Dry-up" pills and shots for bottlefeeding mothers contain hormones that can affect the signs of fertility, and there-fore they should be avoided.

6. Bottlefeeding and cultural nursing mothers should start taking their temperatures at about _____ days postpartum, and they should start making their mucus observations as soon as the _____ no longer obscures such observations.

7. True____   False____   With ecological breastfeeding, your baby receives *all* his liquids, nourishment, and suckling pacification from your breasts for the first six to eight months.

8. Compared to bottlefeeding, breastfeeding offers your baby several health advantages such as fewer _____ and some _____.

9. A bleeding episode at six to eight weeks postpartum may be either the last of the _____, or your _____ _____, or what is called _____
   _____.

10. You can consider yourself in Phase I infertility during your postpartum weeks and months provided two conditions are met:
    a)_____.
    b)_____.

11. If you use the 21 Day Rule during your postpartum cycles, it should be based on:
    a) your postpartum cycles   b) your pre-pregnancy cycles.

12. True____   False____   More than the usual abstinence is sometimes required during your postpartum transition cycles.

Answers to self-test
1. ecological breastfeeding 2. True 3. True 4. differences in the amount and frequency of nursing. . . b) normal bodily differences between mothers 5. True 6. fifteen. . . lochia (postpartum bloody discharge) 7. True 8. allergies. . . immunities 9. lochia. . . first period. . . "hormonal bleeding" 10. a) you know what you are looking for. . . b) you have no signs of fertility, i.e., you haven't had a period yet, you're still dry, and there's been no upward thermal shift 11. b) your pre-pregnancy cycles 12. True

References

(1) American Academy of Pediatrics, Work Group on Breastfeeding, "Breastfeeding and the Use of Human Milk," *Pediatrics* 100:6 (December 1997) 1037.

(2) Sheila Matgen Kippley, *Breastfeeding and Natural Child Spacing: How Ecological Breastfeeding Spaces Babies,* Fourth ed. (Cincinnati: Couple to Couple League, 1999).

(3) T.J. Cronin, "Influence of lactation upon ovulation," *Lancet* (1968) 422.

(4) Konald A. Prem, "Post-partum ovulation," unpublished paper delivered at La Leche League International Convention, Chicago, July 1971.

(5) Pamela Newkirk, "Did their mother die from a 'safe' drug?" *McCalls* (May 1994).

(6) Newkirk.

(7) Kathy I. Kennedy, Roberto Rivera, and Alan S. McNeilly, "Consensus statement on the use of breastfeeding as a family planning method," *Contraception* 39:5 (May 1989) 485. This statement is known as the "Bellagio Consensus" after the conference site, Bellagio, Italy. The authors noted that 56 days postpartum is "a reasonable upper limit at which this normal postpartum bleeding episode would occur." The cause is not known; not everyone experiences it; and it has been recognized for a long time in some societies.

(8) Kennedy et al., Bellagio Consensus, 485.

24

Ecological Breastfeeding

Nothing is simpler or more joyful than ecological breastfeeding. It also spaces babies. Unfortunately, over the years Western culture has gotten away from it, and a number of questions have come up. So this chapter is longer than it would be in a culture where ecological breastfeeding is the norm.

In this chapter we address the woman who wants to do this form of baby care—or is at least considering it. We encourage every husband and wife to read it so they can appreciate better the advantages of breastfeeding in general and of ecological breastfeeding in particular. To repeat, to keep the pronouns straight, we treat babies and physicians as male.

Ecological breastfeeding is the type of nursing that respects and follows the natural order. Your nursing provides all your baby's nourishment, liquids, and pacification for the first six to eight months. You let your baby have some of your soft table foods when he shows a real interest. Once your baby starts solids, you continue to nurse your baby frequently—day and night, and you continue to take him with you wherever you go.

Full ecological breastfeeding excludes bottles, mother substitutes, pacifiers, strict schedules, and abrupt weaning. The keys to ecological breast-feeding are mother-baby togetherness and frequent suckling. A mother can take care of her baby easily when she is with him.

We coined the term "ecological breastfeeding" in 1968. We needed a term to distinguish two forms of nursing that have extremely different effects upon the return of fertility—cultural nursing and ecological breastfeeding. Ecology is concerned with natural interrelationships, so "ecological breast-feeding" is an appropriate name.

In this balance of nature, you give your baby the best nourishment both physically and emotionally, and his frequent suckling normally provides you with more than a year of infertility. Because this pattern of baby care is so much more than just feeding, we also call it **natural mothering**.

● Not just "exclusive breastfeeding"

As we noted in Chapter 23, ecological breastfeeding is different from "exclusive breastfeeding." The latter term means that you are giving your baby nothing but your own milk. However, with "exclusive breastfeeding" you could be expressing your milk on a regular basis so that someone else could

Definition

bottlefeed your baby with your milk. That form of baby care gives a baby *some* important nutritional benefits of breastmilk, but it is **not** ecological breastfeeding. With ecological breastfeeding, your baby stays with you, nurses frequently, and gets his nourishment directly from your breasts.

> When you express your milk for later bottlefeeding, it's not the same as breastfeeding. Proteins, enzymes, hormones, and live cells may be destroyed during handling, freezing or heating. The timing between foremilk and hindmilk is lost. Also lost are the daily changes in composition in response to the baby's changing needs and the external secretions of the areolar Montgomery glands. Therefore, bottlefeeding breastmilk is not the emotional or nutritional equivalent of breastfeeding.
>
> — Joy Kondash, M.D.[1]

Reasons to Breastfeed

You and your baby can gain some of the following advantages with any form of nursing, but both of you will benefit the most from extended, ecological breastfeeding. We want what's best for both you and your baby; that's why we promote ecological breastfeeding.

Bonding

Breastfeeding is a biological device of nature to keep the mother with her baby.
—*Herbert Ratner, M.D.[2]*

God knows that good mothering requires effort. Therefore the Lord gives you prolactin through breastfeeding to make it easier.

It is beyond question that breastfeeding gives the best start for the baby; it is equally true that breastfeeding is the best start for mother. Her joy and happiness in being intimately wrapped up in her baby give her warm feelings of total love and caring.

It's a relationship unlike any other. Her small infant is helpless and completely dependent. The mother alone can best take care of her infant's needs for love and nourishment. Breastfeeding helps a mother to feel very special because she knows she is giving her baby the best there is. In turn, breastfeeding greatly increases prolactin, the "mothering hormone" that helps the mother to bond with her baby. Through breastfeeding, nature provides an easy learning environment for the new mother, and she gradually builds her self-confidence.

Bonding is a mysterious process by which a mother accepts her baby as "my baby" at every level of her being. Bonding is what makes baby care a labor of love and joy, and breastfeeding is God's plan for bonding. This may be hard to comprehend for the person who has never experienced it. One young mother told us that she started breastfeeding only to keep her own mother happy. Once she was into it, she loved it and couldn't figure out why every mother didn't breastfeed.

Expert observers tell us that the best way to start the bonding process is to breastfeed *right after delivery* and to have unrestricted nursing and plenty of skin to skin contact during the first five days.[3]

The baby's nursing releases two maternal hormones—oxytocin and prolactin. Oxytocin is very important right after delivery because it causes the mother's uterus to contract, to expel the placenta, and to reduce blood loss. (If your baby nurses right after delivery, you do NOT need a shot of hormones.) Prolactin is the hormone that helps a mother feel good about mothering, and thus it is a great help for bonding—both short term and long term.

The combination of frequent suckling and mother-baby togetherness yields the blessing of bonding. It's the pattern of baby care instituted by the Author of Nature, and it definitely helps a mother experience real joy with her child.

Breastfed babies normally are healthier than bottlefed babies. They have more built-in immunities and therefore they have fewer allergies, fewer chronic ear infections, fewer intestinal diseases, less obesity, less asthma, less diabetes, less SIDS, and an overall lower infant mortality rate. Dr. David Stewart sums up the importance of breastmilk for the infant in his book, *The Five Standards for Safe Childbearing.*

> Breast milk is the best possible nutrition for all babies—full term, premature, healthy or ill. It is more than just a standard. It is the only truly compatible, truly nutritious food a newborn baby can eat. Adults can quarrel over the pros and cons of breastfeeding and breast milk. For adults, breastfeeding can have both advantages and disadvantages. . . For the baby, breastfeeding has all the advantages.[4]

The medical evidence is overwhelming in favor of breastfeeding, and some of it is summarized in the following list compiled by Barbara Heiser, R.N.[5]

● Breastfed children are half as likely to have any illness during the first year of life.

● Breastfeeding for 4 months reduces the occurrence of *otitis media* [middle ear infection] by 50 percent and of recurrent *otitis media* by 61 percent.

● Children breastfed for one year or longer have half the risk of becoming diabetic.

● Breastfed infants are 10 times less likely to be admitted to the hospital during their first year of life.

● Breastfed children are 4 times less likely to contract the infections which cause meningitis.

● Children who are exclusively breastfed for at least 6 months are half as likely to develop cancer before age 15 than children not breastfed.

● Breastfed infants are 5 times less likely to contract *Giardia* [a gastro-intestinal infection] during the time they are breastfed.

● Breastfed infants are 5 times less likely to be diagnosed with urinary tract infections between 0 and 6 months of age.

● Breastfed babies are one-third less likely to die of SIDS.

That list came from an article about the economics of breastfeeding during a time of increasing concern about the costs of health care. The author concluded that "universal breastfeeding for only three months could decrease hospitalization costs for infants in the U. S. by $2 to $4 billion per year."[6]

In the mid-Nineties, many mothers and their doctors, however, were still acting as if formula feeding was just as good as breastfeeding in developed

Health of your baby

countries with high standards of hygiene. (It's common knowledge that poor hygiene makes bottlefeeding dangerous in many areas of the world.) Thus the American Academy of Pediatrics (AAP) issued a policy statement on breastfeeding to emphasize the benefits of breastfeeding for American babies and their mothers.

The AAP policy statement is not bashful about the benefits of breastfeeding. "Extensive research, especially in recent years, documents diverse and compelling advantages to infants, mothers, families, and society from breastfeeding and the use of human milk for infant feeding . . . Human milk is uniquely superior for infant feeding and is species-specific; all substitute feeding options differ markedly from it."[7]

What are these compelling advantages? "Research in the United States, Canada, Europe, and other **developed** countries, among predominantly middle-class populations provides strong evidence that human milk decreases the incidence and/or severity" of the following disorders (emphasis in original):

Diarrhea	Bacterial meningitis
Lower respiratory infection	Botulism
Otitis media [inner ear infection]	Urinary tract infection
Bacteremia	Necrotizing entercolitis

Those are the *proven* benefits. Next come the *possible* benefits. "There are a number of studies that show a possible protective effect of human milk feeding" against the following disorders:

Suddent infant death syndrome	Lymphoma
Insulin-dependent diabetes mellitus	Crohn's disease
Other chronic digestive diseases	Allergic diseases

"Breastfeeding has also been related to possible enhancement of cognitive development."

Psychological health

In 1971 a landmark symposium on breastfeeding established beyond question the health, economic, emotional, and maternal benefits of breastfeeding. It also succeeded in bringing these facts to the attention of the scientific community.[8]

At this conference the evidence showed that an ecological breastfeeding relationship of over one year may have long term psychosocial benefits for the child in later years.[9]

Brain food

The human brain approximately doubles in size during the first year of postpartum life, and most of that takes place in the first nine months postpartum. Therefore we can say that the human brain takes 21 months to develop—nine months in the womb and twelve months after birth. Brain development is particularly important for the human person because everything we do that is distinctly human—such as writing and reading this book—is dependent upon our brains.

Once you know these things, it is easy to understand the value of optimum nourishment for brain development. The milk of every mammal is designed by the Author of Nature specifically for the needs of that particular species. For example, calves thrive on cow's milk which is rich in the calcium needed for rapid bone growth and strength. The Lord designed only one food specifically for optimum human brain development—human mother's breastmilk. In fact, "the breast itself synthesizes some neural hormones."[10] Therefore, human babies thrive on breastmilk. Father William Virtue has noted in *Mother and Infant*:

> As species-specific, breastmilk provides nutriments and especially neural hormones that are irreplaceable for neonatal development and brain growth that continues at a fetal rate in the first year following birth.[11]

There is no question: breastfeeding for nine months to a year is by far the best thing a mother can do for the optimum brain development of her child. The value of your breastmilk for your baby's optimum development is shown by some evidence that breastfed children are smarter. "Children who were breastfed (for months, not days) are more likely to score higher on IQ tests, read sooner and have fewer learning disabilities than their formula-fed counterparts."[12] Another study concluded that breastfeeding during those early months gives the child an eight point advantage as measured by IQ tests.[13]

An 18-year New Zealand study found a positive relationship between the duration of exclusive breastfeeding and academic success even in high school.[14]

Dental health

Breastfed children have fewer dental problems than bottlefed babies. In areas where prolonged breastfeeding is common, thumbsucking does not seem to be a problem among older children.

Nursing stimulates the growth of the whole facial area. There is less need for orthodontic work in cultures where women nurse for several years than in areas where breastfeeding is limited.[15] Breastfeeding helps prevent tongue-thrusting, incorrect swallowing, and speech problems—all of which are common dental problems associated with bottlefeeding.

Dental decay is less frequent among breastfed children.[16] Many formulas contain sugar which can do serious harm to a baby's teeth. This is particularly the case when parents go against medical advice and put their baby in a crib with a bottle. Breastfeeding has occasionally been blamed incorrectly for dental caries. Parents and dentists must look elsewhere for the cause of dental decay in a breastfed child.

Health of the mother

Breastfeeding that begins right after delivery reduces the amount of postpartum bleeding; breastfeeding immediately after delivery causes uterine contractions that assist the delivery of the placenta. Regular breast-feeding helps your uterus to regain its non-pregnant size more quickly. In brief, breastfeeding helps a mother to recuperate from the demands of pregnancy and childbirth.

The AAP statement also specifies a number of well-researched benefits of breastfeeding for mothers. In addition to the immediate postpartum healing mentioned above, it names two benefits that have to do with natural child spacing: "delayed resumption of ovulation with increased child spacing" and "lactation amenorrhea [that] causes less menstrual blood loss over the months after delivery." It also lists "an earlier return to prepregnant weight, . . . improved bone remineralization postpartum with reduction in hip fractures in the postmenopausal period, and reduced risk of ovarian cancer and premenopausal breast cancer."[17]

"Breast cancer is the most frequent cancer in the Western world. . . The National Cancer Institute in 1993 stated that the incidence has doubled over the last 30 years—now one woman in eight will develop breast cancer during her lifetime."[18]

You may hear that there is nothing you can do to prevent breast cancer; all you can do is try to detect it as early as possible. That's wrong. Having an abortion and using the Pill both raise the risk of breast cancer,[19] so never having an abortion and never using chemical birth control (the Pill, shots, implants) are two ways of not increasing your risk of breast cancer.

Extended breastfeeding can help prevent breast cancer, but short-term breastfeeding has not been associated with anti-cancer protective effects.

More positively, extended breastfeeding is the best thing you can do to reduce significantly your risk of developing breast cancer. This statement is *not* an old wives' tale, nor is it just theory. It is based on the experience of countries where prolonged breastfeeding is common.[20] It has been confirmed by the scientific observations of physicians working among populations where extended breastfeeding is the norm, as well as among American mothers.

Working among the Canadian Eskimos who did extended ecological breastfeeding, Dr. Otto Schaefer found only one case of breast cancer. That woman had one breast on which she could not nurse ("nipple on that side didn't work"), and that was where the cancer developed.[21] Dr. Roy Ing as a medical student in Hong Kong was amazed to see that the Tanka fisherwomen had lopsided breasts: they nursed only on the right breast for convenience because their dresses opened up on the right side. Returning later as a public health physician, Dr. Ing found that among the women over age 55, 79% of the breast cancers were in the left, unused breast.[22]

Other researchers have found a 40% reduction in breast cancer among women who breastfed a total of two years;[23] others found a 66% reduction when mothers breastfeed for a total of six years.[24]

Studies that have found no anti-cancer effects of breastfeeding have confined their research to women who breastfed for only a few weeks, and they are probably correct. We are not aware of any evidence showing that short term nursing has any anti-cancer protective effect.

Such studies show the absolute importance of defining the type (cultural or ecological) and the duration of breastfeeding. Amazingly, cancer researchers have not yet quantified the amount of suckling. The world still awaits a breast cancer study which measures suckling frequency as well as duration of breastfeeding.

Money saved

Add up how much money you will save if you don't buy any bottles, bottle bags, formula, juices, sterilizers, bottle warmers, baby foods, or pacifiers—probably at least $500 in the first six months. By not buying any formula or baby foods in the next six months, you will save a similar amount. So, in terms of mid-1990s dollars, you will save about $1,000 in the first year—just on baby foods while giving your baby the best nourishment at your breast. (And don't forget, those are after-tax dollars. To earn $1,000.00 to *spend* on artificial feeding, the average American with a total tax load of 35% has to *earn* $1,538 before federal, state, and local income taxes, social security, and sales taxes.) Even more significant, you will probably have additional savings by having a healthier baby.

"I debated a long time before deciding to send you this list [of expenses]. I have a six-month old baby with a stomach disorder. He can only drink a meat-based formula and cannot have many solids. I did not fully realize the cost of all this, $1,301.31, until I sat down to add it up for you.

The sad part about this is: if I only would have breastfed him, I could have completely eliminated the hurt and pain he has had, the cost of the meat-base formula, the medicine, the bottle warmers, bottles, extra nipples, and the two hospital visits. . . I have learned a great lesson here. God gave women a cheap and easy way to feed our infants, and the rewards of it I hear are so great." —North Dakota mother.[25]

The natural spacing of babies

Why does the Couple to Couple League promote ecological breast-feeding? The answer is simple. The League exists to promote God's plan for families and to provide the best practical help for living up to that plan. That's why we teach Natural Family Planning. In ecological breastfeeding, the Author of Nature—God Himself—has given Mankind a built-in form of natural family planning. The evidence is overwhelming: ecological breastfeeding spaces babies. It is the world's oldest form of natural family planning. We take the following quotation from a 1989 doctoral thesis:

> A recent survey [not including China] revealed that breast-feeding contributes more to birth regulation worldwide than the sum of all public and private contraceptive programs. The magnitude of the natural effect has been estimated to be at least thirty-six million couple-years of protection against pregnancy, compared with twenty-seven million couple-years afforded by contraception.[26]

In August 1988, a group of scientists with a special interest in breast-feeding and population met in Bellagio, Italy and issued a statement that is now called the "Bellagio Consensus."

> There is abundant evidence to show that a birth interval of two or more years significantly enhances infant survival and re-duces maternal morbidity, particularly in less developed coun-tries. Demographic data indicate that in many developing countries, the protection from pregnancy provided by breastfeed-ing alone is greater than that given by all other reversible means of family planning combined, and that breastfeeding makes a considerable contribution to securing a two-year birth inter-val.[27]

We don't like the "protection from pregnancy" terminology, but it's common in scientific literature.

● Striking contrasts

The contrast in the return of fertility between ecological breastfeeding and other forms of baby care is sometimes striking. Doctors Otto Schaefer and J.A. Hildes found that the Igloolik Eskimo mothers who did traditional, ecological breastfeeding conceived 20 to 30 months postpartum. However, when the trading post brought in practices of bottlefeeding and Western cultural nursing, the mothers who adopted these practices were conceiving two to four months postpartum![28]

A Boston study of approximately 450 nursing mothers illustrates a classic example of cultural nursing.[29] Only one-fifth of the mothers were still nursing at six months, and 60% of those mothers had already had a return of menstruation. That means that only 8% were still having breastfeeding amenorrhea at six months postpartum. In striking contrast, in our study of 98 mothers doing ecological breastfeeding, 93% were having breastfeeding amen-orrhea at six months postpartum! In addition, 56% were still having breastfeeding amenorrhea at 12 months, and one-third had 18 months or more of amenorrhea.[30]

Mother-baby togetherness

Here is where the ecology comes in. Babies have a real built-in psychological need to be with their mothers. With ecological breastfeeding, you satisfy this need. Your baby is always near you at home, and you take your baby with you wherever you go. In turn, your baby will nurse frequently, and that's the key factor in the baby-spacing effect of breastfeeding. Frequently this close mother-baby relationship will extend beyond the breast-feeding relationship.

We have been criticized for advocating both ecological breastfeeding and mother-baby togetherness. Critics say we are trying to make mothers feel guilty, but that is certainly not the case. No one ever feels guilty about doing what he or she truly believes to be right. Nor will anyone feel guilty about mother-child separation if it is absolutely needed for family survival. However, if we did not share what we have learned over the last 30 years on these subjects, we would certainly be guilty of withholding precious information.

The Foundation for the Family, a sister organization of the Couple to Couple League, publishes a leaflet titled *The First Three Years: They're Important.*[31] It is simply a collection of 21 powerful quotations from experts in child development. We quote just two of them.

● **Maria Montessori, M. D.,** author and educator:
> For it is not at all paradoxical to say that, while adults suffer among the poor, children suffer among the rich. . .Let us think, for a moment, of the many peoples of the world who live at different cultural levels from our own. In the matter of child rearing, almost all of these seem to be more enlightened than ourselves—with all our Western ultramodern ideals. Nowhere else, in fact, do we find children treated in a fashion so opposed to their natural needs. In almost all countries, the baby accompanies his mother wherever she goes. Mother and child are inseparable. . . Mother and child are one. Except where civilization has broken down this custom, no mother ever entrusts her child to someone else.[32]

● **Theodore Hellbrügge,** Director of The Children's Center, Munich.
> The child's social development is always retarded if the child does not have a single main mother figure constantly about him, i.e., a person who has enough time and motherly love for the child. In this sentence, every word is equally important. *Single* does not mean two, three or four persons. *Constant* means always the same person. *Motherly* means a person who shows all of the behavior toward the child which we designate as "motherly." *Main mother figure* means that secondary mother figures (father, brothers, sisters, grandparents) may support the main mother figure but may not substitute for her. *Person* means that the respective adult has to support the child with her whole being and has to have time for the child.[33]

Religion and morality

Consider all the blessings to both baby and mother that flow from breastfeeding. Then consider all the social pressures that work against breastfeeding. With those two considerations, it will be less of a surprise to learn that breastfeeding has been a matter of religious and moral concern—for centuries.

Recent papal statements

● Pope Pius XII

In 1941, Pope Pius XII urged all mothers to breastfeed their babies. He was addressing Women of Italian Catholic Action about doing their best to develop the character of their children. It is clear from the context that he thought that character formation could start right at the breast.

> This is the reason why, except where it is quite impossible, it is more desirable that the mother should feed her child at her own breast. Who shall say what mysterious influences are exerted upon the growth of that little creature by the mother upon whom it depends entirely for its development.[34]

Today, however, many of these influences, both physical and psychological, are no longer mysteries; many of the benefits are scientifically validated.

● Pope John Paul II

In May 1995, Pope John Paul II encouraged breastfeeding in comments to the Pontifical Academy of Sciences. He noted "two major benefits to the child: protection against disease and proper nourishment." Then he added: "In addition to these immunological and nutritional effects, this natural way of feeding can create a bond of love and security between mother and child, and enable the child to assert its *presence as a person* through interaction with the mother." The Pope continued:

> All of this is obviously a matter of immediate concern to countless women and children, and something which clearly has general importance for every society, rich or poor. One hopes that your studies will serve to *heighten public awareness of how much this natural activity benefits the child and helps to create the closeness and maternal bonding* so necessary for healthy child development. So human and natural is this bond that the Psalms use the image of the infant at its mother's breast as a picture of God's care for man (cf. Ps. 22.9). So vital is this interaction between mother and child that my predecessor Pope Pius XII urged Catholic mothers, if at all possible, to nourish their children themselves (cf. *Allocution to Mothers,* 26 October 1941). From various perspectives therefore the theme is of interest to the Church, called as she is to concern herself with sanctity of life and of the family.[35]

The Holy Father also commented favorably upon efforts to encourage extended breastfeeding:

> . . . The overwhelming body of research is in favor of natural feeding rather than its substitutes. Responsible international agencies are calling on governments to ensure that women are

enabled to breastfeed their children for four to six months from birth and to continue this practice, supplemented by other foods, up to the second year of life or beyond.*

The Pope also noted the social pressures against breastfeeding:

> *Mothers need time, information, and support.* So much is expected of women in many societies that time to devote to breastfeeding and early care is not always available.

He therefore called for a critical review of contemporary social policies which drive women from their homes and children. He quoted from his encyclical, *Evangelium Vitae*:

> *A family policy must be the basis and driving force of all social policies. . .* It is also necessary to rethink labor, urban, residential and social service policies so as to harmonize working schedules with time available for the family, so that it becomes effectively possible to take care of children and the elderly.[38]

An obligation?

Is there a moral obligation to breastfeed your baby? That question has been raised in recent years from two sources at opposite ends of the moral spectrum—one a pro-abortion doctor and the other a faithful Catholic priest-theologian.

● The Potts-Harvey exchange

In 1984 a rather amazing exchange between a pro-abortion doctor and an orthodox Catholic theologian took place in the *International Review of Natural Family Planning*.[39] Malcolm Potts at the time was the head of Family Health International in North Carolina, an organization known for its promotion of contraception and abortion. However, he had become well acquainted with the benefits of breastfeeding and the hazards of bottlefeeding in developing countries. What was amazing was not his praise of breastfeeding but that he indirectly asserted a moral obligation to breastfeed:

> Should the moralist conclude that since breastfeeding is obviously part of the natural process of begetting and nurturing offspring, not to employ this method is wrong and therefore sinful, unless it proves gravely inconvenient or is physically impossible?[40]

In the same issue of that journal, Father John F. Harvey, OSFS, refuted the argument of Potts that refusal to breastfeed was like the sin of contraception. He also wrote two things of special interest to people who want to do what God wants them to do. First:

> If these benefits of breastfeeding [listed by Potts] can be further substantiated, then it would seem that it is time to formulate a strong moral argument in favor of breastfeeding.

---

* The Pope here referred to a 1990 UNICEF document which urged "all women exclusively to breastfeed their children for four to six months and to continue breastfeeding, with complementary food, well into the second year.[36] By 1994 the World Health Organization (WHO) and UNICEF were saying this: "About six months of exclusive breastfeeding is encouraged, not four-to-six as previously recommended. Breastfeeding from complementary foods continues from six months to two years."[37]

We responded in the next issue that "further research, while perhaps helpful for additional confirmation, is really not needed."[41] In short, Potts was on well-proven ground concerning the benefits of breastfeeding.

Second, Father Harvey noted that the moral argument in favor of breastfeeding should not be in terms of a moral absolute like that against contraception.

> In no way is it [bottlefeeding] comparable to contraception, a proven [moral] evil. At the same time, however, parents, teachers, doctors, nurses, and priests should make known to young women the tremendous advantages which breastfeeding can have for the child, the mother, and the father. The young will respond to this approach much more willingly than they would to an imposition of a moral obligation not really demonstrated. Meanwhile, thanks to Dr. Potts, and many others, moralists will study the question of breastfeeding.[42]

● A dissertation thesis

A Catholic priest did such a study. In 1995 Father William D. Virtue published a doctoral dissertation book, *Mother and Infant*, in which he closely examined the mother-infant relationship. His study of the health benefits led him to this conclusion:

> In sum, breastfeeding is best because breastmilk is fresh and available, convenient at night, digests easily and gives soft stool; it is biochemically the perfect food for the body and brain of the infant; it is a source of immunity, of respiratory and skin health, and of facial and dental arch development. In light of these facts, *breastfeeding is the normal and perfect food for the first nine months.* Conversely, the lack of breastfeeding in modern society means lost physical benefits and unrealized intellectual potential.[43]

Then Fr. Virtue explored the psychological aspects of the mother-infant relationship—the needs of the baby for the physical presence and contact with his mother and the need of the mother for the bonding hormones that come only from breastfeeding. Here he quotes from Dr. Herbert Ratner: "Ratner wisely says it is not the breasts or the bottle but the woman behind them that matters most."[44]

In his fourth chapter, "Breastfeeding and Bonding," he shows well that breastfeeding is the natural and best way to meet the baby's very real needs for love—for affection and for being held.

Finally, Fr. Virtue addresses the question of moral duty. Reading this was a real eye-opener for us. Previously we had no idea that moral theologians over the centuries taught that mothers had a moral duty to breastfeed their own babies. Nor would we have guessed in a thousand years that some late-20th-century feminists have criticized the Catholic Church for not having done more to curb the practice of wetnursing 100 to 1000 years ago.

Such criticism raises an interesting question. How will the Church today be judged 100 and 200 years from now? Today we know more about the nutritional and emotional needs of the baby than ever before. We know more about the unique advantages of human breastmilk and the mother-infant bonding that is hormonally facilitated only by breastfeeding. We also know that some people are "turned off" by any talk about moral obligation. Should we therefore just stress the positive benefits of breastfeeding and be silent about any obligation of mothers to breastfeed their babies?

Quite frankly, that was our approach for 25 years—from 1971 to the publication of this edition in 1996. However, that was before we knew there was a long history of teaching a maternal obligation to breastfeed. That was before we knew that Pope Pius XII had urged mothers to breastfeed. Then within a two week period in May 1995 we read the statement of Pope John Paul II and received the book by Fr. William D. Virtue, S.T.D., from which we have been quoting. We no longer feel free to avoid the issue of a moral obligation for a mother to breastfeed her babies.

● A positive obligation

Any duty to breastfeed your own baby would be a *positive* obligation as contrasted with a universal *negative* obligation such as "Thou shalt not commit adultery." Universal negative laws have no exceptions. Positive obligations can and do have exceptions. Moral theologians have always recognized exceptions regarding breastfeeding. The principal ones are the inability to nurse or the true need of the mother to work outside the home to support the family.

● Two bases

The traditional theological teaching, as explained early in the 20th century, is that the duty of maternal nursing stems from both the natural law and the Fourth Commandment dealing with parental duties.[45]

● Degree

Is there a serious obligation to breastfeed or is the obligation only a small one? Fr. Virtue notes that the seriousness of the obligation rests upon "the material benefits of human milk and the moral value of maternal nursing as forming the infant in love."[46] Before the day of modern formulas and good hygiene, the refusal to breastfeed subjected the baby to a high risk of dying, and that made the duty very serious indeed. This is undoubtedly still the case in many less-developed parts of the world. In much of the developed world today, however, the risk of infant mortality is greatly reduced. Nevertheless, the nutritional benefits of breastmilk remain so superior to artificial foods that Fr. Virtue thinks the "physiological value of human milk remains a basis of obligation."[47]

Just as we know much more today about the superiority of breastmilk to any substitute, so we also know much more about the psychological needs of the baby. We have not done even partial justice to Fr. Virtue's arguments for breastfeeding "as the optimum presence whereby mother becomes the infant's private tutor of love."[48] However, much of his argument is common knowledge in the field of good child care.

A baby's psychological needs to be held, cuddled, and loved are just as real as his nutritional needs. Modern baby slings, front carriers, and back carriers are not just trendy. They respect the baby's need for physical contact and the baby's desire to be upright and close to his mother when he's awake. They can and ought to be used by breastfeeding and bottlefeeding mothers alike.

Fr. Virtue concludes:

> In my judgment, the testimony of the Magisterium and moral experts confirms that *it has been the constant teaching of the Church that there is a serious obligation of maternal nursing.*[50]

Because it imposes continuous contact, breastfeeding fosters good mothering by leading her to give herself completely to the needs of her infant.
—Herbert Ratner, M.D.[49]

In personal communication, Fr. Virtue has clarified this terminology.[51] By "serious obligation" he does not mean the matter of serious or mortal sin. To repeat, he does not mean that the knowledgeable and able woman who chooses not to nurse thereby falls from the life of grace.

● An opposing opinion

In true scholarly fashion, Fr. Virtue quotes a contrary opinion from Fr. Thomas O'Donnell:

> While the nutritional, psychological, and humanistic advantages which are claimed for breastfeeding may well make it a preferable method in most cases, I do not believe they can support a maternal obligation to choose breastfeeding in preference to bottlefeeding under medically approved conditions, with proper hygienic precautions, and in a manner manifesting a loving intimacy between mother and child.[52]

● Our opinion

We think that Fr. Virtue is on rock solid ground when he teaches the rights of the baby to proper nutrition and maternal love. We agree with him that those rights of the baby translate into duties of the mother whom God has endowed with the natural abilities to provide the best food and loving care. We further agree that there is no question that in ordinary circumstances a mother can best fulfill these duties through breastfeeding.

We can agree with Father O'Donnell (about the lack of obligation) if he is thinking in terms of obligation under pain of mortal sin. You will note that he carefully describes conditions which are conducive to the physical and emotional health of the baby. No moral theologian would assert a "mortal sin" obligation under those circumstances.

We've been asked, "Is there an obligation to breastfeed under pain of *venial* sin?" We don't know. We are not aware of any specific teaching on this point. We conclude that it is best to talk about any obligation to breastfeed in more general terms.

However, the fact that an obligation doesn't register at the mortal sin level on the moral scale, or even as a venial sin, doesn't mean that it is a trifle. We think most parents recognize this. We think most parents recognize that parenthood brings them real obligations to their children. Our children have basic rights to the best care we can reasonably provide, and we have the corresponding duty to provide it.

We know that many people shrink from hearing about moral obligation today, but in a time of social decline, maybe it's time to recognize that any reform of society must include the fulfillment of family obligations. After all, the family is the basic unit of society.

We have met couples who have chosen to bottlefeed as if the choice were no different than deciding to dress the baby in green or red. Knowing what we know, we have been literally shocked by such decisions. We have been unable to understand the completely casual acceptance of decreased health benefits for baby and mother alike along with increased costs. Therefore, we have tried to provide a more thorough explanation of the many benefits of breastfeeding.

Whether it's because you want your baby to have the optimum brain food or because you want to greatly reduce the risks of infant diarrhea and juvenile diabetes, you have good reasons to breastfeed.[53]

We conclude that the obligation to breastfeed our children is real and not trivial. We think it is an important part of the general obligations that all of us recognize: to do what is best for our children within the constraints of our abilities, to make sacrifices for our children, and to love our neighbor as ourselves—and who are closer neighbors than a mother and her baby?

Most parents want to go beyond just the bare minimum of legal and "sin" obligations to their children. Most parents want to do what is really best for them. However, so often what people think is "best" is too expensive or otherwise out of reach for ordinary people. So they have to settle for second-best.

However, that's not true when it comes to rearing children. Under ordinary circumstances, ordinary people can do what's best for their young children simply by breastfeeding and being with them. Anything else is second best, no matter how much more it costs.

Breastfeeding failures

Some mothers try to breastfeed but it doesn't work. In fact, some mothers try amazingly hard to breastfeed their babies before they finally give up. They know well the benefits of breastfeeding, and they really make a tremendous effort to give them to their babies. Sometimes the problem is more with the mother's breasts or milk supply; at other times the problem is more with the baby.

The number of women who experience a breastfeeding failure is small, but such mothers are not to be ignored. We have nothing but the greatest sympathy for them, and we want to make three comments.

1. If you made every reasonable effort to breastfeed your baby but suffered a breastfeeding failure, *you* are not a failure. You gave it your best shot, and no one expects you to do any more. We commend you for your efforts. So don't be down on yourself.

Look at it this way. If your husband fails at some particular job, *he* is not a personal failure, but he will need your support. If you experience a breastfeeding failure, *you* are not a personal failure, and you definitely deserve your husband's support in coping with your disappointment.

2. Continue to be the best mother you can be. As we mention elsewhere, one of the good things about ecological breastfeeding is that it requires mother-baby attachment. You can give your baby that same togetherness. So enjoy your baby. Hold him when you feed him. Carry him. Bring him with you wherever you go.

3. Some breastfeeding failures are related to practice. People who should know better—such as nurses and others in hospital maternity wards—sometimes give bad advice. A friend who gave birth in May 1995 told us that the advice she received in the hospital was not helpful and would have led a first-time mother to a nursing failure. Therefore we include the following section on how to do ecological breastfeeding. We hope you find it helpful.

How to Do Ecological Breastfeeding

We continue to emphasize "ecological" breastfeeding for three reasons. 1) It's the only form of breastfeeding about which we can be precise. 2) It offers you the best chance of having an extended nursing relationship. 3) It is the only form associated with extended breastfeeding infertility.

The basic principles of ecological breastfeeding are mother-baby togetherness and frequent suckling. Imagine that you, your husband, and your baby are on a deserted island with plenty of fresh water and food just waiting to be plucked from bushes and trees. Now: how are you going to take care of your baby? You will take your baby with you when you gather your food. When he gets restless, you'll let him nurse. When you're tired, your baby will be lying at your side.

With that sort of living and baby care, when will your next baby arrive? There are still people living like that, and researchers have found that among the **!Kung* tribe** of hunter-gatherers, the nursing is frequent and the babies are spaced about 44 months apart.[54] Their average family size is 4.4 children. According to a Dr. Peter Howie, a professor of obstetrics and gynecology at the University of Dundee in Scotland, "With loss through infant mortality, that produces an exact replacement level for the population, and that is certainly how the human species reproduced itself over the greatest part of human history."[55]

You might say: "I'm not a hunter-gatherer. I gather my food at the local market." The principle still holds. Ecological breastfeeding is still the best care for baby in the most modern technological society.

The Seven Standards of ecological breastfeeding

To find out if the extended infertility found in less developed cultures was also part of ecological breastfeeding in modern America, we have conducted two studies. In this research, we had to be specific about the form of baby care. Therefore we used what we now call the Seven Standards of ecological breastfeeding:

1. Do exclusive breastfeeding for the first six months of life; don't use other liquids and solids.

2. Pacify your baby at your breasts.

3. Don't use bottles and pacifiers.

4. Sleep with your baby for night feedings.

5. Sleep with your baby for a daily-nap feeding.

6. Nurse frequently day and night, and avoid schedules.

7. Avoid any practice that restricts nursing or separates you from your baby.

In both of our studies, the American mothers who did this form of ecological breastfeeding averaged 14.5 months of amenorrhea (that is, 14.5 months between childbirth and the first postpartum period).[56] For further information, see Chapter 21 of *Breastfeeding and Natural Child Spacing*.[57] These Standards can be better understood with a list of do's and don'ts.

The do's and don'ts of ecological breastfeeding

Frequency of suckling is the key factor in breastfeeding's spacing of babies. You can readily see how each of the following mothering practices affects the frequency of suckling. These practices all ensure that the mother will have an adequate milk supply because milk production depends upon the frequency of suckling.

---

* The ! before the Kung indicates a clucking sound.

Research in Central Africa shows how cultural practices can affect the duration of breastfeeding infertility. The researchers looked at two groups—rural and urban. Among bottlefeeding mothers they found no differences in the return of fertility in the two groups. However, they found big differences among the breastfeeding mothers. Why? The rural mothers kept their babies with them all the time and nursed at any time; the urban mothers used baby-sitters and schedules. In the rural group, 75% of conceptions occurred between 24 and 29 months postpartum; in the urban group, 75% of conceptions occurred between 6 and 15 months postpartum.[58] Nursing patterns make a difference.

1. **Do** let your baby nurse as often as he wants. Since human milk is much easier for baby to digest than anything else, and since your baby will enjoy pacification at the breast, it is quite natural for your breastfed baby to nurse often.

2. **Don't** allow any artificial nipples in your baby's mouth. Sucking on artifacts subtracts from the suckling at the breast. In addition, it frequently results in nipple confusion, a common cause of breastfeeding failure. See more on this subject in the next list, "The do's and don'ts of getting started well."

3. **Don't** set a time limit for nursing at each breast. **Don't** time the feedings. The best environment for delaying ovulation is the combination of short feedings and short intervals between feeds, as contrasted with long feedings and long intervals. Unrestricted nursing at the breast for naps and during the night also contributes to longer amenorrhea.

4. **Don't** set up a nursing schedule of so many feedings per day. Schedules are strictly for bottlefeeders—to avoid either stuffing or starving. Adults often eat when they feel like it. Human milk is digested in two hours. Why expect babies who are growing rapidly to wait three or four hours?

Realize that it is perfectly natural and normal for your baby to nurse frequently—sometimes every hour, sometimes more and sometimes less. That knowledge frees you from the highly erroneous old wives' tale that frequent nursing means you don't have enough milk. We can't emphasize this enough: four-hour schedules were invented by doctors for bottlefeeding mothers—to keep them from overfeeding or starving their babies. Babies can't read schedules or clocks, and frequent nursing is the norm. It's nature's way of keeping mother and baby together and spacing babies.

5. **Do** be one with your baby. Avoid situations that separate the two of you. Take your baby with you, and **don't** leave him with baby-sitters. If you absolutely cannot avoid a separation, don't let it be for more than one or two hours.

If you understand the importance of mother-baby togetherness, you will not have a goal of getting away from your baby once a week or taking a vacation apart from your baby. We can assure you: if you do these things, your baby will sadden and really miss you, and you will miss your baby. With ecological breastfeeding, the goal is togetherness, not separateness.

6. **Don't** try to get your baby to sleep all through the night without nursing. Remember: it is frequent, unrestricted suckling that is so important for providing normal postpartum infertility. You can easily provide such nursing during the night when you lie near your baby. Going eight to twelve hours between nursings is too long and can reduce your milk supply.

7. **Do** let your baby nurse while you are sleeping. At the least, put your baby to breast before you go to sleep. When he wakes up during the night, bring him to bed with you and let him nurse while you and he sleep. It's the one thing you can do well while you're sleeping!

Better yet, bring your baby to bed when you are ready to go to sleep. When your baby is sleeping with you and your husband, one of you is likely to hear your baby start making suckling noises before he wakes up and starts to cry. In that way, you can put him to breast without having to get out of bed, and no one gets fully aroused from sleep. When a baby learns that his needs are met without crying, he cries far less, day or night.

Two cautions:

1) Do not sleep next to your baby if you are intoxicated, on drugs, or taking sleeping pills. However, if you are sober, you do not need to worry about rolling over on your baby any more than you worry about rolling out of bed. If you don't believe us, place a life-size doll in bed to prove to yourself that you do not roll over on it.

2) Do not lay an infant face-down on a waterbed or on soft, deep bedding. There have been reports of face-down babies smothering on adult beds, and in most cases the infants became trapped face-down between the mattress and the headboard, footboard, or wall. With waterbeds there is the additional hazard of being trapped between the mattress and the bed frame. Fortunately, the breastfeeding baby who falls asleep at the breast usually sleeps on his back or side.

If your bed is too small for the three of you, have the baby's crib right next to your bed. Or put your mattresses side by side on the floor.

Better yet, use a king-size bed with a firm mattress. Get it with the money you will save by not buying formula and baby foods with your first baby, and you'll reap the benefits all during your child-rearing years. To save money, don't buy a headboard or a footboard.

If your husband is a light sleeper and cannot tolerate the baby next to him, place a barrier next to your side of the bed and let your baby sleep between you and the barrier.

Note well: Sleeping with your baby, besides its good emotional effects for both baby and mother, is an extremely important factor in the natural spacing of babies with ecological breastfeeding. It is at these times—during naps and during the night—that your baby will suckle often and contentedly to satisfy both his appetite and his suckling needs.

If this sounds different or strange, read *Nighttime Parenting*[59] by Doctor William Sears, a California pediatrician, and *The Family Bed*[60] by Tine Thevenin. Sleeping with your baby is also the single most important thing you can do to prevent infant death through SIDS (Sudden Infant Death Syndrome). The theory is that your baby unconsciously patterns his breathing after yours.

According to mother-baby sleep researcher Dr. James McKenna, "When sleeping alone, babies sleep too long, and in much too deep of a sleep." In a continuing study, he and Dr. Sarah Mosko have found that "the heart rates, breathing patterns, and sleep stages of the babies and their mothers largely coincide when they sleep side by side. Mothers and babies tend to wake each other up during the night." McKenna suggests that this prevents the babies from having long breathing pauses that in some cases may result in sudden infant death syndrome.[61]

8. **Do** take a daily nap with your baby. Fatigue can reduce your milk supply and hasten the return of menstruation and fertility. In addition, your napping baby usually will nurse to his heart's content. Such unrestricted nursing is important to maintain the natural spacing mechanism. Sleep times may be the only times you experience unrestricted nursing. (Have your older small children lie down with you at the same time for their naps.)

9. **Don't** use a pacifier. Your breasts are wonderful for mothering and are the best pacifiers for your baby. Suckling at the breast has a calming effect upon babies—and moms too—and a tired baby falls asleep easily at his mother's breast. Suckling for pacification is important for the emotional well-being of your baby; it also plays a significant part in the natural spacing effect of ecological breastfeeding.

Another "Do" —

*If you would like to find support and experience the extended infertility side effect of ecological breastfeeding, read the only book on the subject — **Breastfeeding and Natural Child Spacing.** Subtitled, "How Ecological Breastfeeding Spaces Babies," it is much more complete than our discussion here. Its 4th edition has more on night feedings and naptime nursings, and whole chapters are devoted to some of the Seven Standards. See "Resources."*

10. **Don't** give your baby any solids, juices, cereals, or water during his early months. His only source of nourishment should be your milk until he's big enough to take food off the table and feed himself. With ecological breastfeeding, there is no reason to have baby bottles in the house. Some babies want solids at six months; others are not ready until a few months later.

11. **Do** drink plenty of liquids yourself and eat a balanced diet. You may also want to take some extra vitamin supplements.

12. **Do** keep nursing after your baby starts solids. His table foods should be simply a supplement to your milk for some months; you can start other liquids some months after he starts solids. This means that once your baby starts solids, the amount and frequency of nursing are not decreased at all at first; later he will gradually decrease both the amount and the frequency.

Remember: ecological breastfeeding after six to eight months no longer refers to "exclusive breastfeeding" in which the only food or drink is mother's milk. Rather, it refers to the continuing practice of complete mother-baby togetherness with the baby nursing whenever he desires but also taking gradually increasing amounts of food from the table. This type of breastfeeding generally provides another six months—or more—of natural infertility *after* the baby starts solids.

13. **Don't** force weaning. Natural weaning occurs gradually and usually over a period of many months or a few years at baby's pace—not society's. The appearance of baby teeth in no way signals weaning.

The do's and don'ts of getting started well

To do extended ecological breastfeeding, you first have to get off to a good start with your nursing experience. Here's a short list that applies to every form of nursing experience, short-term or long-term.

1. **Do** attend meetings of La Leche League or other nursing mother associations if available where you live, or write the nearest La Leche League representative for information or to have your questions answered. Read the excellent LLL manual, *The Womanly Art of Breastfeeding.*[62] If at all possible, attend the meetings during pregnancy, even if you have had successful nursing experiences in the past.

2. **Do** attend prepared childbirth classes and have your childbirth experience as unmedicated as possible. Problems with breastfeeding can sometimes be traced to the type of childbirth. For example, a medicated delivery can leave a baby drugged and unable to get off to a good nursing start, and a good start can make a big difference in some cases. At the same time, do not be surprised if your childbirth educator pushes contraception and discounts the spacing effects of ecological breastfeeding. Be prepared to educate them in a light-handed and winsome way.

3. **Do** keep your baby with you after childbirth. If you have a hospital birth, have your physician or midwife give strict orders that your baby is not to have any bottles, pacifiers, or nipple shields. You need your baby's nursings. Even more important, if your baby gets exposed to the artificial sucking pattern of a bottle-nipple or pacifier, he may suffer "nipple confusion" and not put forth the entirely different effort required at your breast. (And it's that greater effort that develops his facial muscles and helps prevent some dental problems.)

Nipple confusion is a big cause of breastfeeding failure. Sometimes even a single exposure to a bottle nipple, a pacifier, or a nipple shield can seriously impair or permanently destroy your breastfeeding relationship.[63] More commonly, nipple confusion leads to a gradual erosion of breastfeeding and causes an insufficient milk supply.

4. **Do** be prepared to inform your doctor and some well meaning but misinformed friends and relatives. Let your doctor check your baby's blood if he questions your baby's iron supply. Anemia in the exclusively breastfed baby up to six months is extremely rare.[64]

Doctors are better informed about the health benefits of breastfeeding than they were in the Seventies, but frequently they are not helpful when it comes to common "how to do it right" questions. A mid-1995 article noted that among doctors surveyed, "Many doctors gave incorrect answers to common questions, answers that could lead a mother to needlessly stop nursing."[65] Remember that the average doctor learned very little about breastfeeding in medical school and even less about the child-spacing effects of ecological breastfeeding. His own wife probably used bottles or did cultural breastfeeding.

5. **Don't** be discouraged if some of your friends and relatives think you're strange for doing ecological breastfeeding. (Many of them will secretly admire you for it.) Instead, reach for the support that you can find in La Leche League, the Couple to Couple League, and in *Breastfeeding and Natural Child Spacing*. Review all the advantages of breastfeeding and be comforted in the knowledge that nature's food is best. Be proud that in the early months you alone can provide your baby with the best.

"Play it by ear"

To some prospective mothers, this may sound demanding, so we say, "Play it by ear." You don't have to make any prior commitment to your baby or to yourself to continue with ecological breastfeeding for any set number of months. Keep in mind, however, that many mothers are exquisitely happy with this type of mothering and only regret not caring for previous babies this way.

Remember also that the benefits to your baby are both emotional and nutritional. After six months, the emotional benefits play a much greater role, and the nutritional benefits still remain and are supplemented by the normal expansion of baby's diet at this time.

You can always change from ecological breastfeeding to the patterns of baby care more common in Western culture, but once you have lost your milk supply through bottlefeeding or cultural nursing, it will be quite difficult, though not impossible, to establish a pattern of ecological breastfeeding.

The Return of Fertility

No matter how frequently and for how many months you nurse, your fertility will eventually return even with continued breastfeeding. Detecting the return of your fertility while doing ecological breastfeeding is the subject of the next chapter.

Self-Test Questions: Chapter 24

1. True____   False____   If your baby wants to nurse every hour, it's a sign that you don't have enough milk.

2. True____   False____   One of the most important elements in postpartum infertility is how often your baby nurses.

3. True____   False____   Exclusive breastfeeding is the same as ecological breastfeeding.

4. True____   False____   There is good evidence that extended breastfeeding helps to prevent breast cancer.

5. True____   False____   There is general agreement among pediatricians that breastfeeding provides the best nutrition for a baby.

6. True____   False____   In 1941 Pope Pius XII urged mothers to breastfeed except when it is quite impossible.

7. The world's oldest form of natural family planning is _____ _____.

8. Not letting your baby nurse during the _____ is one of the most frequent departures from the rules of ecological breastfeeding.

9. A _____ _____ can make sleeping with your baby much easier.

10. Sleeping next to your baby seems to assist your baby's _____ _____ and therefore may be the best thing you can do to prevent _____.

11. True____   False____   Nursing for pacification plays an important part in the suckling pattern of ecological breastfeeding.

12. In their two studies, the Kippleys found that American mothers who did ecological breastfeeding averaged _____ months of postpartum amenorrhea.

13. The most important factor in providing the natural spacing of ecological breastfeeding is _____ _____.

14. The use of pacifiers and bottles can cause _____ _____.

15. Ecological breastfeeding for the first year can save you approximately $_____ (in mid-Nineties dollars).

Answers to self-test
1. False   2. True   3. False   4. True   5. True   6. True   7. ecological breastfeeding   8. night   9. king-sized bed
10. breathing pattern. . . Sudden Infant Death Syndrome   11. True   12. 14.5   13. frequent suckling   14. nipple confusion   15. $1000, and these are after-tax dollars

References

(1) Joy Kondash, M.D., review comments on this chapter, February 1995.

(2) Herbert Ratner, M.D., personal communication by phone, 14 June 1995.

(3) William D. Virtue, *The Moral Theology of Embodied Self-Giving in Motherhood in Light of the Exemplar Couplet Mary and Jesus Christ*, (Peoria: William D. Virtue, 1995) 231. Fr. Virtue refers to the work of Marshal Klaus and John Kennel, *Maternal-Infant Bonding: The Impact of Early Separation or Loss on Family Development* (St. Louis: Mosby, 1976) and their revision, *Parent-Infant Bonding* (St. Louis: Mosby, 1982).

(4) David Stewart, Ph.D., *The Five Standards for Safe Childbearing* (P.O. Box 267, Marble Hill, MO: Napsac Reproductions, 1981) 281.

(5) Barbara Heiser, R.N., "Affordable health care begins with breastfeeding," *Breastfeeding Abstracts* 14:2 (November 1994) 11-12.

(6) Heiser, referencing M.H. Labbock press conference, Georgetown University, 05 August 1994.

(7) AAP statement, p. 1035. For complete reference, see Chapter 23.

(8) Derrick B. Jelliffe and E.F. Patrice Jelliffe, symposium guest editors, "The Uniqueness of Human Milk," *The American Journal of Clinical Nutrition* 24 (August 1971) 968-1024. Six scientific papers plus an introduction and concluding overview constitute the symposium papers.

(9) Niles Newton, "Psychologic differences between breast and bottle feeding," *The American Journal of Clinical Nutrition* 24 (August 1971) 993-1004.

(10) Virtue, *Mother and Infant*, 240, referencing Natalie Angier, "Mother's milk found to be potent cocktail of hormones," *New York Times*, 24 May 1994.

(11) Virtue, 244.

(12) Rita Laws, "The real brain food: breastfeeding and IQ," *Mensa Bulletin*, May, 1987.

(13) A. Lucas, R. Morley, T.J. Cole, G. Lister, C. Lesson-Payne, "Breast milk and subsequent intelligence quotient in children born preterm," *The Lancet* 339 (01 Feb 1992) 261-264.

(14) L. John Horwood and David M. Ferguson, "Breastfeeding and later cognitive and academic outcomes," *Pediatrics*, 101:1 (January 1998).

(15) Mary White, "Breastfeeding: first step toward preventive dentistry," *La Leche League News* (July-August 1972) 57.

(16) White, above.

(17) AAP, 1035.

(18) Joy Kondash, M.D., "NFP, breastfeeding, and breast cancer," paper delivered at the bi-annual convention of The Couple to Couple League, Omaha NE, 25 June 1994.

(19) Chris Kahlenborn, M.D., *Breast Cancer: Its Link with Abortion and the Birth Control Pill* (Dayton, OH: One More Soul, 2000). See also J.C. Willke, M.D., *The deadly after effect of abortion: Breast Cancer* (Cincinnati: Hayes, 1993) brochure; Paul Weckenbrock, R.Ph., The Pill: how does it work? Is it safe? (Cincinnati: Couple to Couple League, 1993) leaflet.

(20) Newton, "Mammary effects," *Am J Cl Nu*, 989.

(21) Otto Schaeffer, "Cancer of the breast and lactation," *Canadian Medical Association Journal*, 100 (05 April 1969) 625-626.

(22) "Hong Kong's Medical Mystery," *The Washington Post*, 26 July 1977.

(23) D.M. Layde, et al., "The independent association of parity, age at first full-term pregnancy, and duration of breastfeeding with the risk of breast cancer," *Journal of Clinical Epidemiology* 42 (1989) 763-773.

(24) J.M. Yuan, et al., "Risk factors for breast cancer in Chinese women in Shanghai," *Cancer Research* 48 (1988) 1949-1953.

(25) North Dakota mother, *The CCL News*, 6:4 (Jan-Feb 1979).

(26) Harry William Taylor, Jr., *Effect of nursing pattern on postpartum anovulatory interval*, Doctoral dissertation (Davis: Univ. of California, 1989) 4. The survey Taylor quotes: Franz W. Rosa, "Breast feeding: a motive for family planning," *People*, vol. 3 (1976) 10-13.

(27) Kathy I. Kennedy, Roberto Rivera, and Alan S. McNeilly, "Consensus statement on the use of breastfeeding as a family planning method," *Contraception* 39:5 (May 1989) 477-496. From the Bellagio Consensus Conference on Lactational Infertility, Bellagio, Italy, August 1988.

(28) J.A. Hildes and Otto Schaefer, "Health of Igloolik Eskimos and changes with urbanization," paper presented at the Circumpolar Health Symposium, Oulu, Finland (June 1971).

(29) E. Salber, M. Feinleib, and B. Macmahon, "The duration of postpartum amenorrhea," *American Journal of Epidemiology* 82 (1966) 347.

(30) Sheila K. and John F. Kippley, "The spacing of babies with ecological breastfeeding," *International Review* XIII: 1&2 (Spring-Summer 1989) 112.

(31) *The First Three Years: They're Important* (Cincinnati: Foundation for the Family, 1988).

(32) Maria Montessori, *The Absorbent Mind* (New York: Dell, 1967) 99, 104-105.

(33) Theodore Hellbrügge, "Early social development and proficiency in later life," *Child and Family* 18:2 (1979) 122.

(34) Pope Pius XII, "Guiding Christ's little ones," address to the Women of Italian Catholic Action, Feast of Christ the King, 26 October 1941. In *The Major Addresses of Pope Pius XII: Vol I Selected Addresses*, edited by Vincent A. Yzermans, (St. Paul: North Central Publishing, 1961) 44.

(35) John Paul II, Address to the Pontifical Academy of Sciences, 12 May 1995. The Academy was concluding a conference on breastfeeding sponsored by the Royal Academy and the Pontifical Academy of Sciences.

(36) UNICEF, *Children and Development in the 1990s*, on the occasion of the World Summit for Children, New York, 29-30 September 1990.

(37) Forty-seventh World Health Assembly, "Infant and young child nutrition," Agenda item 19, 9 May 1994, p. 2.

(38) John Paul II, *Evangelium Vitae* (25 March 1995) n. 90.

(39) Malcolm Potts and John F. Harvey, OSFS, "Letters," *International Review of Natural Family Planning* VIII:2 (Summer 1984) 174-180.

(40) Potts, 177-178.

(41) John F. Kippley, "Letters," *International Review of Natural Family Planning* VIII:3 (Fall 1984) 277.

(42) Harvey, 180.

(43) Rev. William D. Virtue, *Mother and Infant: The Moral Theology of Embodied Self-Giving in Motherhood in Light of the Exemplar Couplet Mary and Jesus Christ* (Rome: Pontifical University of Saint Thomas, 1995) 244.

(44) Virtue, 251.

(45) Virtue, 270.

(46) Virtue, 270.

(47) Virtue, 277.

(48) Virtue, 245.

(49) Virtue, 276.

(50) Virtue, 278.

(51) Fr. William Virtue, phone conversation, 08 June 1995.

(52) Thomas O'Donnell, S.J., "Breast-feeding and bottle feeding: Business ethics and medical ethics," *The Medical-Moral Newsletter* 29:5 (1992) Ayd Medical Communications.

(53) C.F. Verge and others, "Environmental factors in childhood IDDM [insulin dependent diabetes mellitus]: A population-based, case-control study," *Diabetes Care* 17:12 (Deember 1994) 1381-9. Study reported a 52% increase in IDDM related to introduction of formula based on cow's milk before three months.

(54) Melvin Konner and Carol Worthman, "Nursing frequency, gonadal function, and birth spacing among !Kung hunter-gatherers," *Science* 207 (15 February 1980) 788-791.

(55) Peter W. Howie, "Synopsis of research on breastfeeding and infertility," in *Breastfeeding and Natural Family Planning*, selected papers from the fourth national and international symposium on natural family planning, Chevy Chase, MD, November 1985, ed. Mary Shivanandan (Bethesda, MD: KM Associates, 1986) 17.

(56) Sheila K. Kippley and John F. Kippley, "The relation between breastfeeding and amenorrhea: report of a survey," *JOGN Nursing* 1:4 (Nov-Dec 1972) 15-21; "The spacing of babies with ecological breastfeeding," *International Review* XIII: 1 and 2 (Spring-Summer, 1989) 107-116.

(57) Sheila K. Kippley, *Breastfeeding and Natural Child Spacing*, Fourth ed., 191.

(58) Monique Bonte, Emmanuel Akingeneye, Mathias Gashakamba, Etienne Mbarutso and Marc Nolens, "Influence of the socio-economic level on the conception rate during lactation," *International Journal of Fertility* (1974) 15-21. The research was done in Rwanda.

(59) William Sears, M.D., *Nighttime Parenting* (New York: Plume, 1985). Available from CCL.

(60) Tine Thevenin, *The Family Bed* (Wayne, NJ: Avery, 1987).

(61) "Bring baby in bed, new study suggests," *New York Times,* reported in *Cincinnati Enquirer,* 31 March 1994, A9.

(62) *The Womanly Art of Breastfeeding* 5th edition, revised and edited by Judy Torgus (New York: Plume, 1991). Available from CCL and LLLI.

(63) Mary Jozwiak, "Nipple confusion: a common problem," *Leaven* (Nov.-Dec. 1993) 85-86.

(64) *Anemia: rare in breastfed babies* (Franklin Park, IL: La Leche League) pamphlet.

(65) Elizabeth Neus, "Doctors' knowledge of breast-feeding found lacking," New Jersey *Courier-Post* (14 May 1995) 2C. Neus referred to a study in *JAMA* which showed that doctors "don't know much about the mechanics of breast-feeding."

25

Ecological Breastfeeding: Return of Fertility

Duration of natural infertility

In the previous chapter we mentioned several reports and studies of extended breastfeeding infertility—the !Kung tribe, the Canadian Eskimos, the Rwanda mothers, and some American women. Here we focus on the findings of the two studies we conducted among American mothers living ordinary lives.[1,2]

The marker of fertility we used was the first postpartum bleeding of any kind. In both of our studies, the average duration of breastfeeding amenorrhea (no periods) was 14.5 months. In other words, on the average, the women had 14.5 months between childbirth and their first period.

This was a very solid average figure. However, there was a range from 2 to 30 months. (Three women reported "periods" in the first two months, but we now think those were most likely "hormonal bleeding" as indicated in Chapter 23.) As you can see from Table 1, 33% of the first periods were between 13 and 18 months postpartum, and 85% were between 7 and 24 months.

Table 1
Return of Menstruation with Ecological Breastfeeding

Months of Amenorrhea	Number	Percent of experiences
1-6	7	7%
7-12	36	37%
13-18	32	33%
19-24	15	15%
25-30	8	8%
	Total = 98	

Data: 1989 report[3]

Table 1 makes it obvious that 44 percent of the nursing experiences had 12 months or less of amenorrhea. On the other hand, the remaining 56% had more than a year of breastfeeding amenorrhea.

There are a couple things of interest which are not evident in Table 1. Only 16% of these 98 cases had less than nine months of amenorrhea. Second, among the mothers who continued with extended ecological breast-feeding, 34% had 18 months or more of amenorrhea. (That includes 10 experiences of 18 months plus 23 experiences of 19 to 30 months amenorrhea.)

Assuming that our sample was representative of American women, what these numbers mean is this: without any fertility awareness or planned abstinence, ecological breastfeeding spaces babies about 24 months apart, on the average. About 77% of babies will be spaced between 18 and 33 months apart, and a few more will be spaced between 34 and 39 months apart. A few mothers will have an earlier return of fertility, and for them it may be more important to detect the return of their fertility whether it occurs before or after the return of menstruation.

● No periods: is it natural?

Yes, it is perfectly natural for the mother who is doing ecological breast-feeding to go months and months without having a period. The absence of periods helps you to regain your strength after pregnancy and childbirth. You lose a small amount of iron through breastfeeding, but amenorrhea saves the iron you would otherwise lose through menstruations.

Do not take any medication to "bring on your period." Some physicians do not understand that breastfeeding amenorrhea is normal and healthy. If you appear worried about the absence of periods while breastfeeding, your physician might suggest taking some hormone pills for a few days to cause a bleeding. For years the U.S. Food and Drug Administration has had a rule against giving progestin pills to women who might be pregnant because they might harm the baby.

● Temperatures: any value?

If you start to wonder if you might be pregnant, take your waking temperatures. Continued low temperatures in your typical pre-shift range are a positive sign you are not pregnant. On the other hand, three weeks of temperatures in your typical thermal shift range are a good sign you might be pregnant.

Chances of pregnancy with ecological breastfeeding

The chances of becoming pregnant **before** your first period while doing ecological breastfeeding vary according to two main factors: 1) age of your baby and 2) your fertility awareness.

● During your first three months postpartum, the chances of pregnancy are **practically nil** (even if you have mucus signs of fertility) if you do ecological breastfeeding and remain in amenorrhea.

● During the next three months, there is only **about a 1% chance** of becoming pregnant before your first period if you are following the Seven Standards of ecological breastfeeding listed in Chapter 24. However, if you have mucus and cervix signs of being fertile, you should consider yourself to be in Phase II.

Note that the requirements of "fully or nearly fully breastfeeding" in the Bellagio consensus do **not** meet the *frequency* or the *exclusive breastfeeding* standards of ecological breastfeeding. Women who follow the Bellagio "fully or nearly fully" rule should not be surprised to have their periods return prior to six months postpartum. The scientists at the Bellagio conference also agreed that when a mother was fully or nearly fully breastfeeding, any bleeding in the first 56 days could be ignored, i. e., that she should not consider it to be her first postpartum period.

> ### The Bellagio Consensus:
>
> *Fully or nearly fully breastfeeding women who are not menstruating have less than a two percent chance of becoming pregnant in the first six months postpartum.*[4]
>
> "Fully or nearly fully" allows slight supplementation—from a few swallows up to less than one feeding per day. This consensus applies only to the first six months postpartum.

● After six months, there's **about a six percent chance** of becoming pregnant before your first period, and that assumes no systematic abstinence.[5,6,7] Babies generally start taking solids in a small way around six months, and fertility starts to return as indicated in Table 1 above.

● After 12 months, the possibility increases that you will ovulate before your first period.

Lastly, some women will not be able to become pregnant until after weaning. This may not repeat itself with subsequent babies.

Detecting fertility before your first period

We repeat: the above chances of conception before your first period assume that the couples are not practicing systematic abstinence before the first postpartum menstruation or using any form of contraception.

If you want to **detect** the possible return of your fertility before your first period, then you need to make your standard sympto-thermal observations and recordings.

Most women get ample return-of-fertility signs from their cervical mucus. The first postpartum ovulation is almost always preceded by a mucus discharge, and the mucus flow is typically—but not always—longer and more abundant than it is in regular cycles.

If you want to **postpone** pregnancy, use the standard Phase I rules: dry days only, not on consecutive days, and not in the morning. Ordinarily you do not need to apply these rules in the first six months postpartum of ecological breastfeeding because there is such a small possibility of achieving pregnancy in this time. After six months postpartum, it's a good idea to use the Phase I rules.

● When to start your mucus and cervix charting

Start to make your external mucus observations after your postpartum discharge (the lochia) has stopped. However, don't bother to start actual charting until you notice mucus. No need to fill up pages with "dry" notations.

After three months, if you have a very serious reason to avoid pregnancy, you might want to start the internal observation once a day in the evening. However, most women get plenty of advance warning of fertility from their external mucus.

After six months, you enter a time when fertility starts to return more frequently with each passing month even though it remains very low until after the first menstruation. Keep up your daily observations and start charting when you notice mucus or when you have any of the events listed in the following section on waking temperatures.

Start your cervix charting when you start your internal mucus observations.

Q. If I detect the mucus sign and then have a period some days later, does that mean I ovulated?

A. Not necessarily. Most women do *not* ovulate before their first period. After your first period, you might have another one or two periods which are not preceded by ovulation. Here's where your daily waking temperature pattern helps. If it stays low, you haven't ovulated. If it rises, then you know you have ovulated and can apply a Phase III rule.

In addition, you may notice mucus for one or two days before your period starts, even if these periods are not preceded by ovulation.

● When to start recording your temperature

Start taking and recording your waking temperatures when you have any of the following events:

1. The appearance of cervical mucus and/or changes in the cervix.

2. Menstruation or spotting, even if light.

3. Any sudden decrease in suckling (perhaps due to illness of your baby or yourself). This is very important.

4. The start of bottle-liquids or solid foods if this has been followed by an early return of periods with previous nursing babies.

5. The start of the ninth month postpartum. This is optional and is based only on the fact that fertility starts to return more frequently starting in the ninth month postpartum.

If you take your waking temperatures by these rules, you will have a good base for your first Low Temperature Level. In the event of pregnancy, your temperature pattern will determine the baby's age.

Don't be concerned if your waking temperatures while nursing tend to be somewhat up-and-down more than usual and for no apparent reason. That's typical. Since it can be confusing, we do not strongly urge you to take temperatures until you experience one of the events listed above. However, we've done it, and the temperature variations were no problem.

● Secondary signs

Some mothers have reported sore nipples before their first postpartum ovulation. Some report feeling several weeks of uterine "bloating" or slight "crampiness" before the first postpartum ovulation. These signs are not universal, but some mothers may find them helpful for fertility awareness.

● Early fertility detection: two examples

1. The cycle history in Figure 25.1 came from a *well experienced* woman; it shows her detection of fertility with ovulation occurring approximately 15 months postpartum and *before* her first period. (We're using a chart from 1970 to show you that this information has been around awhile.)

Figure 25.1
***Experienced
Nursing Mother:
Detection of Fertility
Before First Postpartum
Menstruation***

October-November 1970
Chart 70-10-1

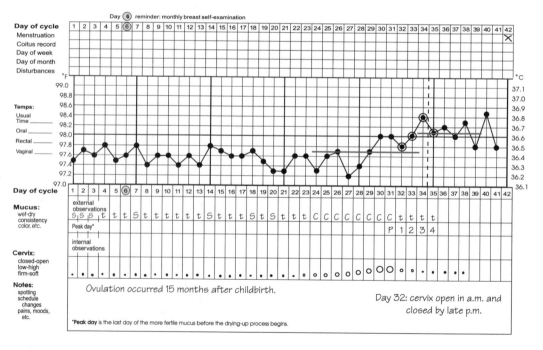

There was a long period of mucus that was tacky and small in quantity, and it was not accompanied by any significant opening of the cervix. The onset of more-fertile clear mucus ("C") was accompanied by the opening of the cervix. The eight day patch of the more-fertile mucus was followed by ovulation as indicated by the thermal shift.

Interpretation: Set the Low Temperature Level (LTL) at 97.7° and the High Temperature Level at 98.1°. An overall shift pattern begins on Day 30. Peak Day is Day 31. Count only the post-peak temperatures as part of an overall thermal shift. On Day 35, the four day overall thermal shift cross-checks the four day drying-up pattern. Rule B indicates the evening of Day 35 as the start of Phase III.

2. The cycle history in Figure 25.2 came from a *very inexperienced* woman who had learned about NFP and CCL just a few weeks before the first temperature recorded here. She had no previous experience in observing mucus.

When her baby was four months old (day 13 on the chart), she observed a mucus-like discharge; she wondered if it was the cervical mucus, and she had a knowledgeable physician examine her. He helped her to identify the thick and sticky mucus then present and advised her to refrain from marital relations. Five days later the mucus was clear and would stretch six inches. The next day her temperature rose, and two days later (Day 21) the mucus began to disappear. Eleven days after the Peak Day (20), her first postpartum men-struation occurred.

Interpretation: Pre-shift six: 13-18. Low Temperature Level: 97.9°. High Temperature Level: 98.3°. Peak Day: 20. Three consecutive days of full thermal shift: 21-23. Three days of drying-up after Peak Day: 21 - 23. Rule K yields the evening of Day 23 as the start of Phase III.

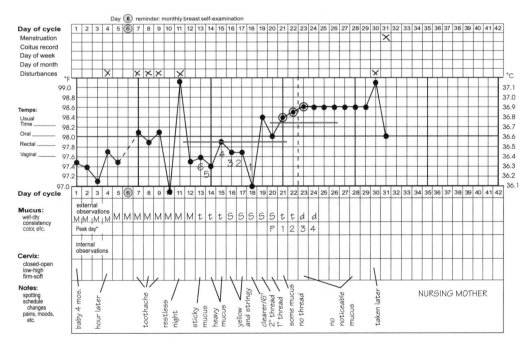

Figure 25.2
Inexperienced
Nursing Mother:
Detection of Fertility
Before First Postpartum
Menstruation

November-December 1971
Chart 71-12-01A

This chart (Figure 25.2) shows the importance of recording mucus and temperature observations as soon as the mucus begins to appear even while doing full ecological breastfeeding day and night. This was definitely an early return of fertility for ecological breastfeeding, but it was typical for this particular woman. However, by observing her mucus, this woman became aware that her fertility might be returning, and by taking her waking temperatures she knew that ovulation had definitely occurred.

We stress the importance of temperature recording because a breastfeeding mother may experience a long period of mucus of various qualities before her first menstruation.

We cannot guarantee that *every* inexperienced woman will observe the signs of fertility if they occur before her first postpartum menstruation, but the evidence certainly shows that inexperienced women *can* detect them. We mention again that most women have a longer and more abundant mucus patch before their first postpartum ovulation than they do during regular cycles.

Ambiguous signs: the transition phase

We repeat: both bottlefeeding and breastfeeding mothers typically experience a period of transition from postpartum infertility to regular cycles, and ambiguous signs of fertility are common in this transition phase. The bottle-feeding mother will experience the transition soon after childbirth; the mother doing ecological breastfeeding will have her transition later, and it may last longer.

Ambiguity can entail abstinence for couples who have a serious need to avoid pregnancy. For those who have a "life or death" reason to avoid pregnancy, we have to counsel to abstain during ambiguous times until you have a definite sign of being infertile, preferably a full sympto-thermal sign you are in Phase III.

Whenever transition ambiguity calls for abstinence, you need to remember that the transition phase is only temporary and that normal fertility patterns will soon return.

Where there is less than a "life or death" reason to postpone pregnancy, sometimes abstinence can be significantly reduced. The following comments are addressed primarily to the couple doing ecological breastfeeding and experiencing an extended transition phase, but anyone can apply what fits.

1. Time of first appearance of mucus before your first period

1. First 12 weeks of postpartum amenorrhea. For all practical purposes, if you are doing ecological breastfeeding, you can ignore mucus of any kind that appears in the first 12 weeks postpartum. See "Chances of pregnancy with ecological breastfeeding" above.

2. Second 12 weeks of postpartum amenorrhea. Any less-fertile mucus in this time is probably "false alarm" mucus. It most likely has nothing to do with the return of your fertility. (See "Chances of pregnancy with ecological breastfeeding" above.) However, if you are quite concerned about postponing pregnancy, then consider the first appearance of less-fertile mucus as the start of Phase II—at least for a while.

If you have the more-fertile mucus, there's a higher chance you might be the exception such as the mother who gave us the chart in Figure 25.2. Consider yourselves to be in Phase II.

3. After six months, consider any mucus, even the less-fertile type, as the start of Phase II when if first appears. However, if it continues for some time, see the next section on continuous, less-fertile mucus.

2. Continuous less-fertile mucus before your first period

Some women have less-fertile mucus all the time while they are still in breastfeeding amenorrhea. Doctors John and Lyn Billings have called this the Basic Infertile Pattern (BIP); another term is "background mucus." It can start very early in your breastfeeding experience; it can also start after months of no mucus whatsoever.

If you experience this change from no mucus to a less-fertile mucus, at first treat it as a sign of possible fertility. However, after you experience less-fertile mucus for three weeks, you might want to do what many others have done: treat all-the-time less-fertile mucus as a Basic Infertile Pattern or "background mucus." Then consider yourselves in Phase II when you notice a *change* to the more-fertile mucus.

In other words, treat a background mucus pattern during breastfeeding as an extended Phase I. Follow the standard rules for Phase I: not in the morning, not on consecutive days, internal observation if possible. Abstain as soon as the mucus changes toward a more-fertile type.

● What are your chances of a surprise pregnancy with the practice of treating background mucus as Phase I and abstaining when you notice the more-fertile mucus? We aren't aware of any studies specifically on this point, but we estimate that such a practice would have an effectiveness between 95% and 97% in postponing pregnancy. Keep in mind that without *any* fertility awareness or *any* systematic abstinence, you have only about a slight chance of becoming pregnant before your first period while you are doing ecological breastfeeding—1% prior to six months and 6% after six months.

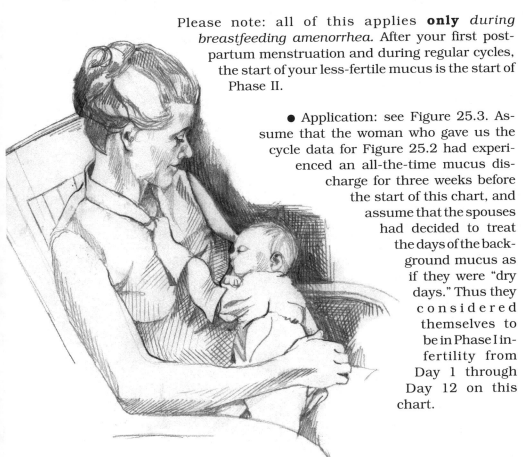

Please note: all of this applies **only** *during breastfeeding amenorrhea.* After your first postpartum menstruation and during regular cycles, the start of your less-fertile mucus is the start of Phase II.

● Application: see Figure 25.3. Assume that the woman who gave us the cycle data for Figure 25.2 had experienced an all-the-time mucus discharge for three weeks before the start of this chart, and assume that the spouses had decided to treat the days of the background mucus as if they were "dry days." Thus they considered themselves to be in Phase I infertility from Day 1 through Day 12 on this chart.

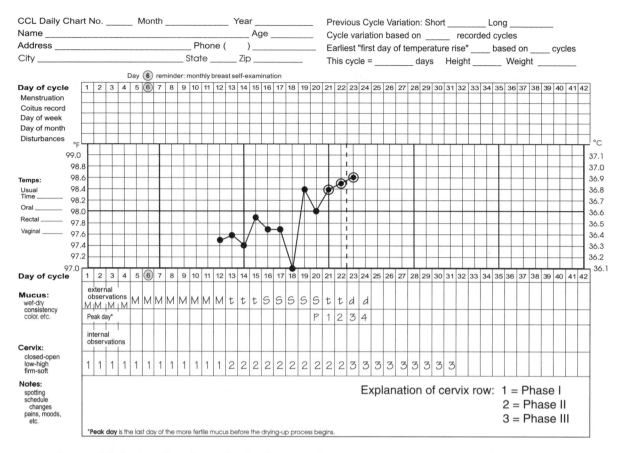

CCL Daily Chart No. _____ Month _____ Year _____   Previous Cycle Variation: Short _____ Long _____
Name _____ Age _____   Cycle variation based on _____ recorded cycles
Address _____ Phone (   ) _____   Earliest "first day of temperature rise" ____ based on ____ cycles
City _____ State _____ Zip _____   This cycle = _____ days   Height _____   Weight _____

Figure 25.3 Application of "Background Mucus" Rules to Data of Figure 25.2

Beginning on Day 13, *the mucus changed* and they considered themselves to be in Phase II. This is very important. Even though the mucus on Day 13 was not yet the more-fertile type, it was a definite and noticeable *change* from the all-the-time mucus discharge she had experienced for weeks. That change signaled a possible change in estrogen activity, and thus the spouses had to interpret the change as the start of Phase II.

The mucus soon changed again to the more-fertile type. After a few more days, it dried up, the temperature rose, and there was a sympto-thermal start of Phase III by Day 23.

3. Patches of mucus

During breastfeeding amenorrhea, you might also experience patches of mucus that come and go. The patches can be two types: 1) patches of less-fertile or more-fertile mucus against a background of dryness; 2) patches of the more-fertile mucus against a background of continuous less-fertile mucus. The following rules or guidelines refer to both kinds of mucus patches.

● **Patches of three days or more.** Begin abstinence on the first day of the mucus patch. If your waking temperature starts to rise during the drying-up process, wait for a full sympto-thermal start of Phase III.

If your temperature pattern remains low, wait for four days of drying-up past Peak Day (the last day of the mucus patch). Consider yourselves in Phase I infertility on the evening of Peak Day plus 4. Continue to apply the standard Phase I rules (not in the morning, not on consecutive days, internal observations if possible) until your first postpartum period or until another mucus patch begins.

● **Patches of one or two days.** The more conservative course: treat these as above.

However, if you know from you own experience that you always experience at least three or four days of continuous mucus discharge when you ovulate during normal cycles, then you can presume that a mucus patch of only one or two days during ecological breastfeeding is not associated with ovulation.

The real presumption is this: there must be several days of higher estrogen activity to make ovulation occur. Normally this is reflected by more than two days of the more-fertile mucus, especially among breastfeeding mothers.

Begin abstinence when the mucus patch starts because you cannot know at the start how long it will be. When the drying-up starts, cross-check it with your temperature pattern.

If your temperature rises (very unlikely after a patch of only one or two days), wait for a sympto-thermal start of Phase III.

If your temperature stays low, consider yourselves back into Phase I on the night of the second day of drying-up (Peak Day + 2).

Use these "patch rules" **only** during breastfeeding amenorrhea. After your first period and during regular cycles, treat the beginning of any sort of mucus discharge as the start of Phase II. (During regular cycles, a second patch might be too short to give sufficient notice.)

● Application. In Figure 25.4 we have applied the patch rules to the mucus pattern in Figure 25.1.

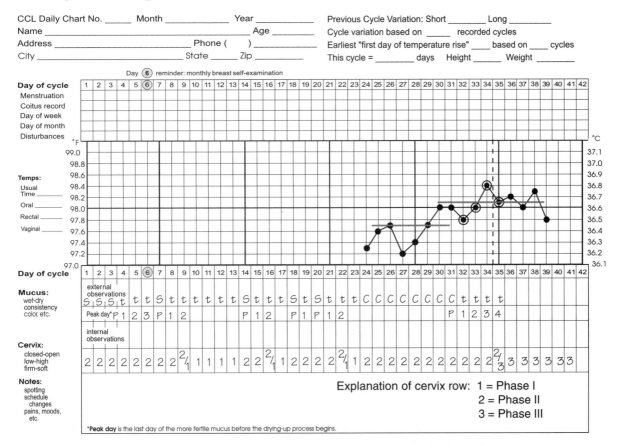

Figure 25.4 Application of Patch Rules to Figure 25.1

The three-day more-fertile mucus patch on Days 1, 2 and 3 is followed by three days of "drying-up." However, on what *might* have been Peak Day + 4 (Day 7) the more-fertile mucus returns for a one day patch. We restarted the dry-up count. Phase I infertility restarts on the evening of Day 9 indicated by 2/1 in the cervix row. Day 14 is a one day patch; Phase I resumes on Day 16. Day 18 is a one day patch but is not followed by two days of drying up. After a one day patch on Day 20, Phase I resumes on Day 22. More-fertile mucus reappears on Day 24 and remains for eight days. Peak Day + 4 is cross-checked by four days of overall thermal shift, and the start of Phase III is established on Day 35.

● What are your chances of a surprise pregnancy while using the patch rules? We have no definite proof derived from careful studies. However, what we wrote above in the section on "Continuous less-fertile mucus" would apply here. Wide experience indicates that most nursing mothers have a fairly long more-fertile mucus patch before their first postpartum ovulation. Therefore, if they abstain according to the patch rules, there should be very few surprise pregnancies.

Apply these rules to the cases in Figures 25.3 and 25.4, and assume that ovulation might occur as early as Peak Day-2. Even with that assumption, there would have to be a sperm life of more than five days for conception to occur. Not impossible but very rare.

4. Help from the cervix

Experience with your cervix signs of fertility and infertility can be a big help if you have ambiguous or on-and-off mucus. If your cervix remains low, firm and closed during such times, you will have much more confidence in recognizing the infertility of a continuing less-fertile mucus discharge and in applying the patch rules. If you apply this to Figure 25.1, with hindsight you can see that the cervix provided a better indicator of infertility than the mucus; however, you could not ignore the patches of the more-fertile mucus.

Fertility after your first period

If you have an *early* return of menstruation—say 6 to 10 months, you might have one or two more periods before you ovulate. If your first period is *more* than a year postpartum, there is a higher chance that you will ovulate before the period. There's also a higher probability that you will have normal, fertile cycles after that first period. Furthermore, some breastfeeding mothers have difficulty achieving pregnancy while still doing frequent nursing after their periods have returned. Despite these differences, for couples seeking to avoid pregnancy, the general rule has to be this:

Consider yourself to have normal fertility as soon as you have your first period. Count the first day of your first period to be Day 1 of a regular cycle. Apply the standard Phase I rules if you intend to postpone your next pregnancy.

Q. What if I have a period and return to amenorrhea?
A. Chart for six weeks after the first bleeding episode, even if it occurs during the first 56 days postpartum. Consider yourselves in Phase I during those six weeks.

If you have no more signs of fertility during those six weeks of observing and charting, you can discontinue your charting. Consider yourselves back into normal breastfeeding infertility; keep up your observations even if you don't record them.

When you get your first mucus, consider yourselves in Phase II. Make and record your full sympto-thermal observations.

● Short luteal phase

It is common for the early postpartum cycles to have short luteal phases. Occasionally the luteal phase is so short that menses starts on the first day of Phase III. In such a case, it may be helpful to remember that the first six days of the new cycle are highly infertile. (See Chapter 11.)

An unusual return of fertility

Over the years, we have encountered some couples for whom the return of fertility was marked by a number of ambiguities and occasions for abstinence. Sometimes they would complain that their charts looked something like the following series of charts which appeared anonymously in the previous editions of *The Art of Natural Family Planning*. They seemed to be relieved when they learned that these charts are ours.

You might ask, what went wrong? Sheila was certainly doing ecological breastfeeding, but the problem was this: the week the baby was born (14 September 1972) she signed a contract with Harper and Row for the publication of *Breastfeeding and Natural Child Spacing*. That put her under deadlines. She spent every spare moment working on the book, she stayed up later than usual, and fatigue took its toll. We can't prove it, but we think it was the fatigue and the stress of the deadlines that brought back her periods so early.

How's that for irony? While Sheila was working on the book that would free thousands of women to relax and enjoy natural mothering, the stress of writing it gave us a year of off-and-on ambiguity instead of a year of clear infertility. Would we do it over again? Certainly.

With other experiences of ecological breastfeeding, her periods returned when the babies were a year old. At least one thing should be obvious: we write from the generalized experience of our studies, not just our own personal experience.

● Evaluation of charts

The absence of any thermal shift in the first two cycles (January-March and March-April) shows that they were definitely anovulatory (without ovulation).

In the third cycle (April-May), ovulation may have occurred, followed by a very short luteal phase and thermal shift pattern. Cycles with luteal phases of less than nine days are sometimes called "infertile" because it is possible that the lining of the uterus might not be maintained long enough for implantation to take place. However, if conception should take place, it is also possible that the HCG from the newly conceived life can maintain the corpus luteum and thus the endometrium. We evaluate cycle 3 as possibly fertile.

Cycle 4 postpartum was anovulatory.

Cycle 5 was probably anovulatory.

Cycles 6 and 7 seem to indicate infertile ovulations.

Cycle 8 was a fertile ovulatory cycle.

Cycle 9 was an ovulatory cycle; the length of the luteal phase is unclear.

Cycles 10, 11, and 12 were fertile ovulatory cycles.

Throughout the year covered by this sequence of charts, the baby continued to nurse regularly day and night. In this sequence, the cycles beginning with cycle 4 were of typical length with a relatively short luteal phase when ovulation occurred. In the ensuing months, Phase II shortened and the luteal phase gradually lengthened while the overall cycle length remained about the same.

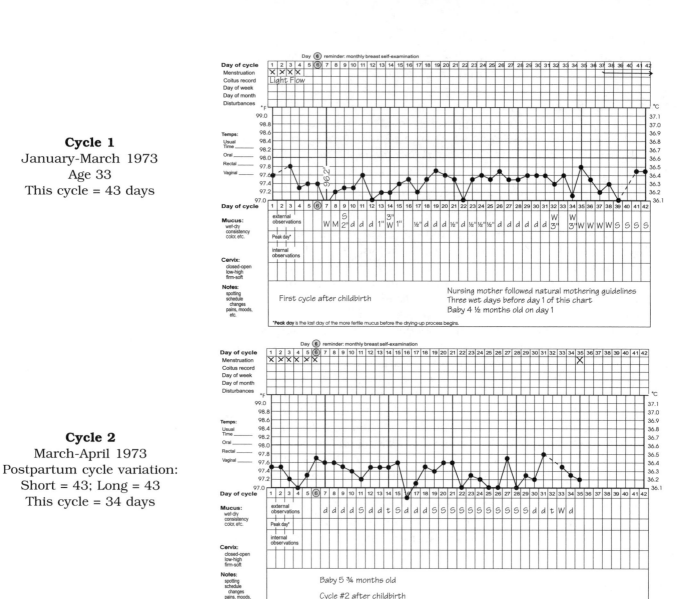

Cycle 1
January-March 1973
Age 33
This cycle = 43 days

Cycle 2
March-April 1973
Postpartum cycle variation:
Short = 43; Long = 43
This cycle = 34 days

Cycle 3
April-May 1973
Postpartum cycle variation:
Short = 34; Long = 43
This cycle = 40 days

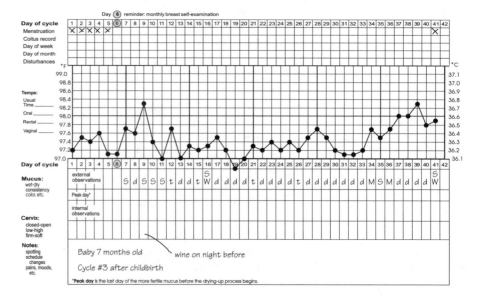

Figure 25.5 Nursing Mother: First 12 Cycles After Return of Menstruation (page 1 of 4)

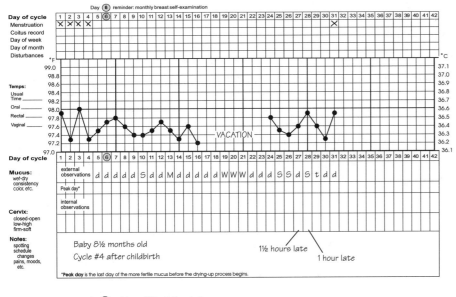

Cycle 4
May-June 1973
Postpartum cycle variation:
Short = 34; Long = 43
This cycle = 30 days

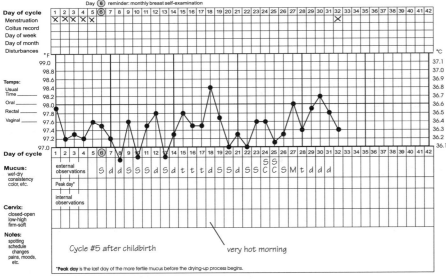

Cycle 5
June-July 1973
Postpartum cycle variation:
Short = 30; Long = 43
This cycle = 31 days

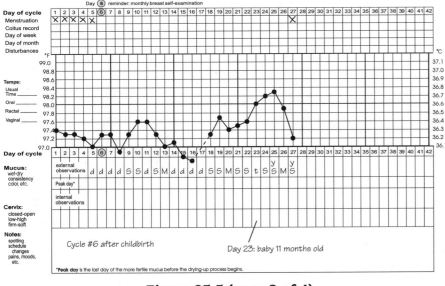

Cycle 6
July-August 1973
Postpartum cycle variation:
Short = 30; Long = 43
This cycle = 26 days

Figure 25.5 (page 2 of 4)

Cycle 7
August-September 1973
Postpartum cycle variation:
Short = 26; Long = 43
This cycle = 30 days

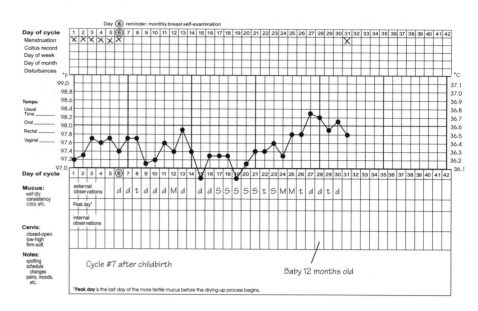

Cycle 8
September-October 1973
Postpartum cycle variation:
Short = 26; Long = 43
This cycle = 28 days

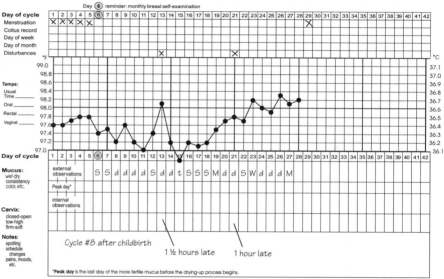

Cycle 9
October-November 1973
Postpartum cycle variation:
Short = 26; Long = 43
This cycle = 25 days

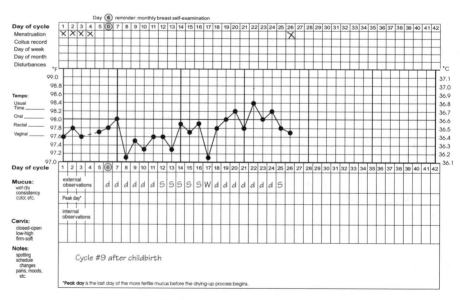

Figure 25.5 (page 3 of 4)

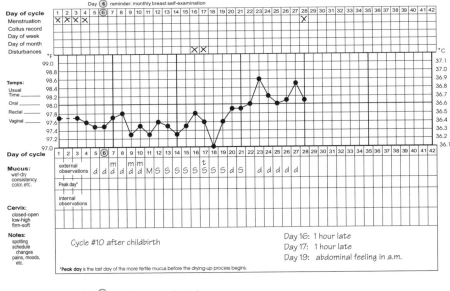

Cycle 10

November-December 1973
Postpartum cycle variation:
Short = 25; Long = 43
This cycle = 27 days

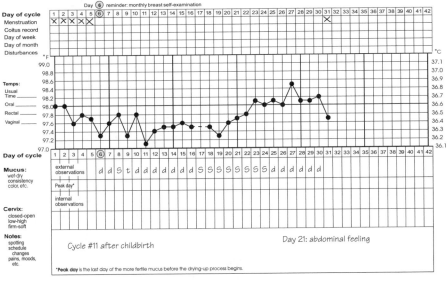

Cycle 11

December-January 1974
Postpartum cycle variation:
Short = 25; Long = 43
This cycle = 30 days

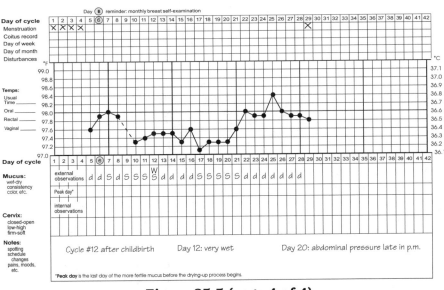

Cycle 12

January-February 1974
Postpartum cycle variation:
Short = 25; Long = 43
This cycle = 28 days

Figure 25.5 (page 4 of 4)

Temperature-only interpretations

Sometimes while breastfeeding and having ovulatory cycles, the temperature goes up but the mucus doesn't go away. For example, look at the "Cycle 6" chart in Figure 25.5, page 367. Here we would set the LTL at 97.3° based on the pre-shift six temperatures on Days 12-18. After some middle range temperatures, there were three days well above the HTL of 97.7°. The Temperature-only Rule would yield Day 25 as the start of Phase III. With such a strong temperature pattern, we would ignore the mucus sign and use the Temperature-only interpretation. Please note: This applies only to frequently nursing mothers.

Abstinence with breastfeeding

Breastfeeding has given rise to several questions. The first two reflect entirely different experiences.

1. In the typical case, ecological breastfeeding continues the deep infertility of pregnancy so the total infertile time may be around two years. The combination has raised this question: Can sexual satiation be a problem during pregnancy and extended breastfeeding infertility?

Sometimes yes. The periodic abstinence in normal cycles for couples postponing pregnancy is psychologically healthy but is lost as a "necessity" during pregnancy and postpartum infertility. Some couples mutually agree upon periods of abstinence during these times in order to avoid sexual satiation.

2. The opposite question arises from ambiguities. Are there periods of extended abstinence with breastfeeding and baby-led weaning?

Sometimes yes. If a couple are very serious about postponing pregnancy, if they experience ambiguous signs of fertility, and if they follow the most conservative practice, they will sometimes experience extended abstinence. We certainly had that experience in the series of 12 cycles illustrated in Figure 25.5. Unfortunately for sharing our experience, we did not record coitus, but we recall that in those cycles there was considerable abstinence.

3. What effect will occasional extended abstinence have on our marriage?

We think the most accurate answer is this: it all depends on you and your spouse. If one spouse is totally convinced that a little more than usual sexual self-control is going to have a bad effect, it probably will.

On the other hand, we know from experience that many relationships improve during times of extended abstinence. The following quotation is not at all unusual.

> The baby had pneumonia in early December. She had to be put in the hospital for a time. My good doctor got us a private room so I could stay with her. Molly, however, went on a nursing strike, and after we got home things began to happen. We noticed all sorts of signs pointing to menstruation, and although Molly started breastfeeding when we got home, I got my period about six weeks later. We did pretty well though—Molly was then 11¾ months old. We are following the manual like a bible. We are now in a cycle and no signs of anything! Temps show nothing and there has been very little mucus. Thus far we have abstained for ten weeks—I do hope I get that second period! Actually, all is going very well and I am wondering if we are abnormal; it isn't bothering us. In fact, we are closer than ever before.

No, they weren't abnormal, but they may have been following a course more conservative than that described in the previous sections on ambiguous mucus and mucus patches.

Many difficulties with sexual abstinence are mostly psychological. If you spend time thinking about the next time you plan to enjoy marital relations, you are going to have a rough time with any abstinence, brief or extended. On the other hand, if you mentally and spiritually accept a period of abstinence ahead of time—whether it be ten days or a month—you will have a much easier time.

Early in the year of cycles illustrated by the charts in Figure 25.5, we realized that we might be in for some extended abstinence. We found that once we accepted the *idea* of three to four weeks of abstinence ahead of time, the *reality* was relatively easy to handle.

4. Can our practice of chaste abstinence help our baby?

Yes. You can rest assured that about 15 years from now, your baby is going to be having temptations of a sexual nature. You can begin your prayers for his or her teenage chastity right now by offering any difficulties you experience with marital chastity as a living sacrifice and prayer for your children.

"Breastfeeding: Does It Really Space Babies?"

Additional reading

Workbook chart 21

Workbook exercise

Self-Test Questions: Chapter 25

1. In the two Kippley studies, American mothers who did ecological breastfeeding averaged _____ months of amenorrhea before their periods returned.

2. Several studies have shown that with ecological breastfeeding there is only about a _____% chance of becoming pregnant before your first period in the first six months postpartum and a _____% chance before your first period after six months postpartum.

3. With true ecological breastfeeding, the chances of becoming pregnant in the first 12 weeks postpartum are _____.

4. True____ False____ Both bottlefeeding and breastfeeding mothers typically experience a transition phase from postpartum infertility to more or less regular cycles.

5. True____ False____ The transition phase is frequently characterized by an irregular mucus pattern.

6. Imagine that you start to experience an all-the-time, less-fertile mucus while nursing and before your periods have returned. After _____ weeks of this, you can regard it as having no immediate connection with fertility, i.e., as sort of a breastfeeding "background mucus," and you can treat it as "dry days."

7. If you treat the time of "background mucus" as Phase I, which two standard Phase I rules should you be sure to follow?
   a. _____
   b. _____

8. True____ False____ During extended breastfeeding amenorrhea, you should consider any change from dry days to mucus days as a potential start of Phase II, even if only temporary.

9. True____ False____ Any change in a nursing "background mucus" pattern to a different, more-fertile type of mucus must be regarded as a potential start of Phase II, even if only temporary.

The following questions assume you are doing ecological breastfeeding and that you need to postpone your next pregnancy.

10. If you have a mucus patch of three days or more, you should begin abstinence on the _____ day of the patch and continue until the evening of the _____ day after its disappearance, assuming your waking temperatures remain low.

11. If you have a mucus patch of only one or two days, you should begin abstinence on the _____ of the patch and continue until the evening of the _____ day after it has disappeared, again assuming your waking temperatures remain low.

12. If your waking temperatures go up and stay up during the mucus patch or during its drying-up, you should wait for a full _____ sign of being in Phase III, i.e., that you are in Phase III according to one of the standard Phase III _____.

Answers to self-test
1. 14.5 2. one . . . six 3. practically nil 4. True 5. True 6. three 7. a) not in the morning. . . b) not on consecutive days 8. True 9. True 10. first. . . fourth 11. first. . . second 12. sympto-thermal. . . rules.

References

(1) Sheila K. Kippley and John F. Kippley, "The relation between breastfeeding and amenorrhea: report of a survey," *JOGN Nursing* 1:4 (November-December 1972) 15-21.

(2) Sheila K. and John F. Kippley, "The spacing of babies with ecological breastfeeding," *International Review* XIII: 1 & 2 (Spring-Summer 1989) 107-116.

(3) Kippley and Kippley, *International Review*, 1989.

(4) Kennedy, *Contraception*, 479.

(5) Leonard Remfry, "The effects of lactation on menstruation and pregnation," *Transactions of the Obstetrical Society of London* 38 (1897) 22-27. Found a pregnancy rate of 5% prior to the first period among breastfeeding mothers.

(6) Prem, op cit. Found a pregnancy rate of 6% prior to the first period among fully breastfeeding mothers.

(7) Monique Bonte and H. van Balem, "Prolonged lactation and family spacing in Rwanda," *Journal of Biosocial Science* 1:2 (April 1969) 97-100. Conceptions during breastfeeding prior to the first period were on the order of 5.4%.

Part V: Beyond the Basics

The chapters in Part I took you through the basics of the Sympto-Thermal Method, and many thousands of couples have successfully practiced NFP with less instruction and knowledge than you have already. However, there are several variations that can be confusing if you are not prepared for them.

The first variation, which we call "Shaving irregular temperatures," is more common, so we have already described it in Chapter 6.

Although we do not highly recommend the single-sign systems of NFP, we explain the mucus-only and temperature-only approaches in Chapter 26, and in Chapter 14 you learned about calendar rhythm.

Irregular mucus patterns and irregular temperature patterns are not very common. What follows in Chapters 27 and 28 are truly some fine points. You are not expected to remember the details, but if you experience these patterns, you will know where to find help in your manual.

By knowing about the various options within the overall field of Natural Family Planning, you are all the more free to choose which system you want to use. *Learning* the full Sympto-Thermal Method and ecological breastfeeding gives you the maximum freedom of choice among morally acceptable choices.

26

Mucus-only; Temperature-only

The Mucus-only System

Our experience is that it is easier to start NFP by using the combination of the mucus and temperature together than by using the mucus sign alone. However, once you have learned the different options, you may want to use a single sign system.

An Australian husband-wife team, Dr. John J. Billings and Dr. Lyn Billings, have popularized a system of NFP that uses only the mucus sign. Not surprisingly, their system is known as "the Billings method." The Billings themselves call it "The Ovulation Method" although it does not give the positive assurance of ovulation that you get from an elevated temperature pattern.

The Mucus-only System

Start of Phase I: The first dry day after menstruation.

End of Phase I: The last dry day before the mucus starts.

Start of Phase III: The evening of the fourth day of drying-up past Peak Day.

● Explanation

If you want to follow a mucus-only system, it is important to follow the rules. Most of these are the standard Phase I rules. The ones that are different are numbered with bold-face italic type.

1. Abstain during menstruation and any other bleeding episode.

2. Make your external observations after each urination and bowel movement. Begin your observations as soon as your period has ended.

3. Last Dry Day Rule: Consider the dry days after menstruation to be infertile up to the beginning of the mucus discharge. Any mucus—less-fertile or more-fertile—counts for the start of the mucus discharge.

The mucus-only rules

4. Not-on-consecutive-days: Do not have relations on consecutive days in Phase I unless you are perfectly dry the day after relations; that is, you notice no mucus and no seminal residue.

5. Not in the mornings: Do not have relations in the morning during Phase I. A dry day is dry all day long, and you need to make your observations all day.

6. Phase II begins when the mucus begins.

7. Phase III begins on the evening of the fourth day of drying-up past Peak Day (Peak Day + 4).

8. If any mucus reappears after Peak Day, begin to abstain again through that mucus patch until the evening of the new Peak Day + 4.

9. In our opinion, to rely upon the Last Dry Day Rule, you ought to be having mucus patches that are at least five days long from the first day of mucus up through and including Peak Day.

Mucus-only or Sympto-Thermal?

Ever since the Doctors Billings began to say in 1970 that their mucus-only system was both simpler and just as effective as the cross-checking sympto-thermal system, there has been debate about the Billings' claims. In the United States, the "Los Angeles study" was undertaken in 1976 to answer the questions about simplicity and effectiveness.[1]

● Effectiveness
Very briefly, the Los Angeles study found a 100% "perfect-use" effectiveness rate among those couples following the rules for a conservative version of the Sympto-Thermal Method (the 21 Day Rule for Phase I and essentially Rule C for Phase III). It found a 94% "perfect-use" effectiveness rate among those following the rules for the mucus-only Ovulation Method. The claim to equal effectiveness was not sustained in this study, the only comparative test that has been conducted in the United States.

A greater disparity was found in the *user*-effectiveness rates—13.7 per 100 woman-years in the STM group and 39.7 in the OM group. There are several reasons for "user-surprise pregnancies"—misunderstanding, poor teaching, wrong interpretations, and "taking chances." For whatever reasons, the couples in the OM group had a user-effectiveness unplanned pregnancy rate 2.9 times higher than the couples in the STM group.

● Simplicity
The simplicity claim was rebuffed by the fact that the teachers found that it took 50% more time to teach the mucus-only learners than those learning the cross-checking mucus-and-temperature system. Learning only one sign *sounds* more simple than learning two or three signs, but consider this comparison: a tricycle is easier to learn to ride than a bicycle, and a bicycle is much easier to learn to ride than a unicycle.

1. The mucus-only system works well for many couples. Method effectiveness rates as high as 97.8% have been reported for couples with regular cycles.[2] User-effectiveness rates are somewhat lower in some studies (see previous page).

2. It is not clear to us whether couples who use the Phase I rules in the high effectiveness studies of the mucus-only method have regularly pushed the rules to the limit or whether they have set for themselves a more conservative practice such as this: "The mucus almost always starts by Day 9; let's never go beyond the night of Day 7." The Last Dry Day Rule needs more research.

3. With the Sympto-Thermal Method, it is usually not necessary to abstain during the days of menstruation. A primary reason for abstinence during menstruation is a cycle irregularity called "breakthrough bleeding" which is described in Chapter 30 of this book. In brief, when a bloody discharge has been preceded by a thermal shift, you know the bleeding is the beginning of menstruation. Without that preceding elevated temperature pattern, you cannot be sure; it might be breakthrough bleeding, a very fertile time.

4. The drying-up of the mucus after Peak Day is only a *negative* sign that you are past the fertile time. By "negative" we mean that it is a going-away, a disappearance. Such a disappearance can happen even when ovulation has not occurred. By contrast, the presence of mucus is a positive sign of fertility, and the elevated temperature pattern is a positive sign of infertility.

Usually the disappearance of mucus is sufficient. However, stress— both physical (e.g., sickness) and psychological—can interrupt the process of ovulation. When this happens, the mucus starts, then goes away, and then returns for just a few days before ovulation. This is described more fully as "the double mucus patch" in Chapter 27, "Irregular mucus patterns." In such cases, the temperature pattern remains low during the mucus dryup, and you are alerted that you do not yet have the positive sign of being past ovulation.

5. With a mucus-only system, you must continue to make your mucus observations with just as much diligence after you think you are in Phase III as you do in the early part of the cycle. The reason: without the elevated temperature pattern, you do not have the positive sign of being past ovulation; you could experience the "double mucus patch" described in the next chapter.

● It's your choice

After you have learned how each fertility sign works in your cycle pattern, you are in a good position to judge whether you want to continue to use the full STM or whether you want to use a mucus-only or temperature-only approach.

In general:

If your shortest mucus patch in the last 6-24 cycles has been 5 to 8 days long, you are a good candidate for the Last Dry Day Rule (5 days is minimum).

If your drying-up coincides very closely with your thermal shift, you are a fairly good candidate for the mucus-only Phase III rule.

If you have any significant stress during Phase I or Phase II, you should start taking your temperature immediately and insist on a full STM start for Phase III. Otherwise, in stress cycles, continue to abstain after Peak Day + 4 and expect a second mucus patch.

See page 107 for more data on cycle experience.

The Doering system

The only temperature-only system that covers both ends of the cycle was developed by a German physician, G. K. Doering. The rules are simple once you understand the terminology.

> **The Doering System**
>
> **End of Phase I:** Earliest first day of thermal shift (in previous cycles) minus 7 yields the last day of Phase I.
>
> **Start of Phase III:** The evening of the third day of full thermal shift is the start of Phase III.

Two cautions:

1. Do not shave pre-shift temperatures when you use the 3-day Doering Rule. If you need to shave, use the CCL Four-Day Temperature-Only Rule.

2. If you have usable mucus patterns, use the cross-checking Sympto-Thermal rules. The Temperature-Only rules are for women who do not have an identifiable Peak Day and dry-up pattern.

● Explanation

End of Phase I. You determine your "earliest first day of thermal shift" by reviewing your last six charts. (Twelve is better, but do not go back more than two years.) In these cycles, mark or note the *first day of sustained thermal shift.* That's the first day that your temperature pattern started to go up and stayed up. Then select the earliest "first day of sustained thermal shift." If you should experience an earlier first day of sustained thermal shift in a new cycle, then *that* day becomes your "earliest first day" for subsequent calculations.

Subtract 7 days from your earliest "first day of thermal shift." The result is the "last day of Phase I" according to the Doering system. So, if your earliest "first day of thermal shift" was Day 15, subtract 7, and your last day of Phase I would be Day 8.

Start of Phase III. Use the standard CCL system for determining the pre-shift six, the Low Temperature Level, and the High Temperature Level. Phase III starts on the evening of the third consecutive day of full thermal shift according to the Doering system.

● Effectiveness

The very high effectiveness reported by Dr. Doering is described in Chapter 13.

● Comment

We do not recommend routinely ignoring the mucus if it should start before the day indicated by the Doering Phase I rule.

We see the chief value of the Doering Phase I rule for two cases:

1) as a substitute for the 21 Day Rule in cases where a history of short luteal phases—the postovulation time of the cycle—makes the 21 Day Rule excessively conservative;

2) with delayed-ovulation patterns and extended days of less-fertile mucus.

With our preference for cross-checking, we normally modify the Doering Phase I rule as indicated on the next page.

● Modifications

The high effectiveness rates reported by Doering were achieved without giving any attention to the mucus sign. Yet, they can probably be improved if you pay some attention to the mucus or add an extra day to help make up for the lack of a mucus cross-check.

1. First modification:

> **End of Phase I:** Earliest first day of sustained thermal shift (in previous cycles) minus 7 yields the last day of Phase I *provided that day is still a dry day.*

2. Second modification: If you have all-the-time mucus during Phase I, you can possibly use the Doering rule during the distinctly less-fertile mucus, but we would *never* suggest ignoring the more-fertile mucus. Also, since "less-fertile" mucus is more conducive to sperm life than "no mucus," the number to subtract is **8**. In other words, you would modify the rule as follows:

> **End of Phase I:** Earliest first day of sustained thermal shift (in previous cycles) **minus 8** yields the last day of Phase I *provided* that day has no *more-fertile* mucus.

Limitations. We stress that this application of the Doering rule is only for the experienced woman (at least 6 cycles of charted experience) who consistently has all-the-time less-fertile mucus *and* who consistently has mucus patches of at least five days of the more-fertile mucus. This is a rule for couples who have a good reason for spacing; it is not for couples who have a most serious reason to avoid pregnancy.

- To determine your "earliest first day of thermal shift" —
  Do not count your first 6 postpartum cycles.
  Do not count your first 6 cycles of coming off hormonal birth control (HBC).
- Do not *apply* this modification in your first 12 postpartum cycles.
- Do not *apply* this modification in your first 12 post-HBC cycles.

3. The third modification would be to use the standard CCL four-day temperature-only rule described below.

The CCL four-day temperature-only rule

We prefer having the signs cross-check each other. When there is no cross-check, we greatly prefer adding one day to help make up for the lack of the cross-check. Thus CCL has taught this standard 4-day temperature-only rule for many years.

> **Four-Day Temperature-Only Rule**
>
> **Phase III starts** on the evening of the *fourth* day of thermal shift in which the last three days are consecutively at the full thermal shift level. The first day can be a day of partial elevation.

The temperature-shaving principle in Chapter 6 can be used with the Four-Day and Five-Day Temperature-Only Rules.

A slight modification can be made in some cases where all four temperatures are well elevated even if the last three are not all at the full thermal shift level. We have in mind a pattern such as Example 1 (on next page):

Mucus-only; Temperature-only — 26

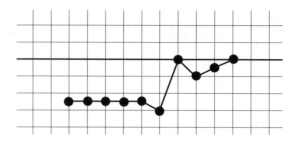

Example 1   Modified Four-day Temperature-only Pattern

This would be a judgment call you could make in the light of the Doering experience and your own previous cycle patterns.

The Marshall five day temperature-only rule

The two previous temperature-only rules called for three days of *full* thermal shift or at least four days of *very strong* thermal shift as indicated in the modification of the standard four-day rule just above.

The rule developed by England's Dr. John Marshall makes use of the weaker "overall thermal shift" pattern and calls for five days of such a pattern.[3] In CCL terminology:

> ### The Marshall Five-Day Temperature-Only Rule
>
> **Phase III starts** on the evening of the fifth day of an overall thermal shift in which at least one temperature has reached the High Temperature Level.

Note: Dr. Marshall cautions that when a couple have the most serious reasons to avoid pregnancy, they should wait for three temperatures at the full thermal shift level.

An application of this rule is made in Chapter 28.

Commentary

There is no question: some mucus-only and temperature-only studies have shown excellent effectiveness results. However, our experience leads us to think that most couples will find it easiest and most effective to use a cross-checking system.

● *Easiest.* You can have an occasional confusing mucus pattern or a confusing temperature pattern. Frequently the cross-checking sign makes the situation clear.

If you do not want to take your temperature every day, you will still get valuable help if you start taking it by Day 6 or at least when you first notice mucus and continuing it through a standard STM Phase III interpretation. We have even seen charts in which the temperature charting didn't start until the more-fertile mucus started. We don't recommend such a practice because usually you would not get six pre-shift temperatures, but it's generally better than nothing.

If you do not want to make the internal observation for cervix and mucus, at least make and record your external observations. It doesn't require any extra effort or time, merely an awareness each time you use the bathroom.

● *Most effective.* Our preference for a cross-checking system was confirmed by an Italian study reported in 1988.[4] In this study, 460 couples contributed 8140 cycles in which they charted mucus, temperature and intercourse. The couples were relatively experienced; they had completed at least six cycles before entering the study. The 25 unplanned pregnancies yielded an effectiveness rate of 96.4% using the Pearl Index (P.I.). The pregnancies were analyzed according to the part of the cycle in which they occurred. NOTE: The reported analysis does not conform to the highest statistical standards explained in Chapter 13, but they still illustrate our preference for a cross-checking system.

● None occurred from Phase I intercourse using a 20-Day Rule to determine the end of Phase I.

● Ten occurred from Phase I intercourse using the Last Dry Day Rule (Pearl Index = 1.47 = 98.53% effectiveness).

● Two pregnancies occurred from relations on Peak Day + 4 or later but before the third day of thermal shift (Pearl Index = 0.29 = 99.71% effectiveness).

● None occurred when the couples waited for three days of sustained thermal shift. It is not clear whether all three days had to be at the High Temperature Level and if all three had to be beyond Peak Day.

The 10 pregnancies while using the Last Dry Day Rule confirm what we have long thought about this rule. It is very effective, but it is less effective than the more conservative end-of-Phase-I rules. You *may* make it more effective if you make the internal observation.

Recommendations

By way of cross-reference, check also "The Most Conservative Approach" on page 134.

1. We encourage you to be generous in the service of life. We caution you against using NFP for selfish and/or materialistic reasons. But when you do have sufficiently serious reasons to postpone pregnancy or to keep your family at its present size, we recommend using the system that provides the most confidence and the highest effectiveness, the cross-checking full Sympto-Thermal Method. Make sure that your mucus drying-up pattern is cross-checked by at least three days of thermal shift. Make sure your thermal shift is cross-checked by the required number of dry days.

2. If you choose to use a mucus-only approach, we recommend:

● Do the internal mucus examination in Phase I to detect mucus as early as possible.

● Add one day to the mucus-only Phase III rule. That is, Phase III would start on the night of P + 5 (the *fifth* day after Peak Day).

3. If you choose to use a Doering temperature-only approach, we recommend that you add a day at each end.

That is, the end of Phase I would be this: earliest first day of thermal shift minus **8** yields the last day of Phase I.

The Phase III rule would be this: Phase III starts on the fourth day of thermal shift in which the last three temperatures are at the High Temperature Level. That's the standard CCL Temperature-only Rule which already includes the extra day to help make up for the lack of a cross-check.

4. Do **not** use a mucus-only or temperature-only rule to advance the start of Phase III just because your obvious mucus and temperature signs are not coinciding very well. (Review Workbook charts 6 and 7 again.) It is precisely in such cases of non-coinciding that you need the benefit of the STM cross-checking system.

5. We encourage you to share the knowledge of the full Sympto-Thermal Method with others. We encourage you not to limit the freedom of others by sharing with them the knowledge of just a single sign. Let them have the same freedom of choice that you have.

6. This manual has not prepared you to teach NFP to others. If you would like to volunteer to teach natural family planning, please get in touch with your local CCL chapter or with the CCL international headquarters. It is one thing to know and practice NFP; it is something else to teach and counsel others in unusual or difficult situations. The League has developed a separate program for training teachers, and then it provides an organized teaching program for all certified teachers. This program includes backup for teachers and various levels of support for client couples.

Self-Test Questions: Chapter 26

1. True_____   False_____   In learning the full Sympto-Thermal Method, you can learn each sign well enough to use it by itself if necessary.

2. The leadership of the League is convinced the full Sympto-Thermal Method gives you
   a) a higher _____ according to comparative statistics
   b) greater _____ with its cross-checking indicators
   c) greater _____ of choice.

3. Dr. G. K. Doering used the temperature pattern to establish both the end of Phase I and the start of Phase III; therefore his system can be called a true _____ _____ system.

4. The Billings Ovulation Method is an example of a _____ _____ system.

5. True_____   False_____   You get the same positive assurance of postovulation infertility from a mucus-only system as when you have a mucus-temperature cross-check.

6. True_____   False_____   Any single sign system works well for some women.

7. Proponents of mucus-only systems generally say that Phase III starts on the evening of Peak Day plus _____.

8. If you use a mucus-only system, CCL recommends adding _____ day (or days) to the above mucus-only rules; thus, the start of Phase III would be on the evening of Peak Day plus _____.

9. For determining the start of Phase III, the CCL temperature-only rule calls for _____ days of thermal shift in which the last _____ days are consecutively at the full thermal shift level.

10. According to CCL, you need a mucus patch history of at least _____ cycles before you can reliably use the Last Dry Day Rule.

11. Also, your shortest mucus patch in those previous cycles should be at least _____ days long from the start of the _____ fertile mucus through _____ Day.

12. True_____   False_____   If you always have a mucus patch of at least 7 days from start through Peak Day, you can use the Last Dry Day Rule with a greater confidence than if you have five day mucus patches.

13. The Doering temperature-based rule (not modified) for the end of Phase I is this: "Earliest first day of thermal shift minus _____ yields the last day of Phase I.

14. Imagine that your shortest cycle has been 22 days long and that in your short cycles you have been having only nine days of elevated temperatures. The earliest your temperature pattern has started its thermal shift is Day 14. In such a situation, the 21 Day Rule would yield Day _____ as the end of Phase I. The Doering Rule (not modified) would yield Day _____ as the last day of Phase I.

15. Continue with the above situation. Imagine that you have a four day menstrual flow. Days 5 and 6 are dry days. You notice a less-fertile mucus on Day 7. According to the most conservative modification of the Doering rule, you should consider Day 7 as
    a) the last day of Phase I   b) already in Phase II.

Answers to self-test
1. True 2. a) effectiveness. . . b) confidence. . . c) freedom 3. temperature-only 4. mucus-only 5. False 6. True 7. four—and without any cross-check from the temperature sign. 8. one. . . five 9. four. . . three 10. six 11. five. . . less. . . Peak 12. True 13. seven 14. one. . . seven 15. b) already in Phase II.

References

(1) Maclyn E. Wade, Phyllis McCarthy, et al., "A randomized prospective study of the use-effectiveness of two methods of natural family planning," *American Journal of Obstetrics and Gynecology* 141:4 (15 October 1981) 368-376.

(2) World Health Organization Task Force on Methods for the Determination of the Fertile Period, November 1981, "A prospective multicentre trial of the ovulation method of natural family planning. II. The effectiveness phase," *Fertility and Sterility* 36:5, 591-598.

(3) John Marshall, M.D., *The Infertile Period: Principles and Practice,* revised edition (Baltimore: Helicon, 1969) 34-36.

(4) Michele Barbato, M.D., and Giancarlo Bertolotti, M.D., "Natural methods for fertility control: a prospective study—first part," *International Journal of Fertility,* Supplement (1988) 48-51.

27

Irregular Mucus Patterns

Some women experience a continuous mucus discharge during the entire cycle, and others experience this all-the-time mucus only during the pre-ovulatory part of the cycle.

Continuous mucus

● **Causes**

The causes vary from poor nutrition and yeast infections to night lighting and causes that are still unknown.

● **What to do**

To try to eliminate or reduce a continuous mucus discharge, we currently have only two recommendations.

1. Improve your nutrition as needed to bring it up to an optimum level. Give yourself a thorough nutritional check. Follow the recommendations in *Fertility, Cycles and Nutrition*. Perhaps take dietary supplements as recommended in that book. See also Chapter 31, "Cycle Irregularities."

2. Darken your bedroom. Keep even the light from a digital clock away from your face. See more on this in Chapter 31 and *Fertility, Cycles and Nutrition* (see "Resources").

Those two procedures work for some women, but we cannot guarantee they will work for you. Nevertheless, they are easy steps to follow, so they are certainly worth trying.

● **How to cope**

Phase III. All-the-time mucus does not cause a big problem for the determination of the start of Phase III. Even if you have a mucus discharge the entire cycle, you will most likely be able to notice the presence and the disappearance of the more-fertile mucus.

If you notice a distinct change from the more-fertile to the less-fertile mucus, establish your Peak Day, and use a standard sympto-thermal rule to determine the start of Phase III.

If you cannot determine any change in the mucus pattern but you are experiencing a thermal shift pattern, use one of the standard temperature-only rules. Use either the CCL four-day temperature-only rule or the Marshall five-day temperature-only rule. Both of these are in the preceding chapter.

Phase I. Rather obviously, the most conservative practice would be to abstain from relations during Phase I if you are having all-the-time mucus. That program, however, is made more difficult by the fact that in some cases of all-the-time mucus, ovulation is delayed and the mucus discharge is quite long. If that is your situation, we urge you even more emphatically to review your nutrition, your weight-to-height ratio, and your exercise program. Better yet, study Chapter 31 in this book and *Fertility, Cycles and Nutrition.*

There are two other alternatives for having relations during Phase I.

1. Modify the Doering Rule as described in the previous chapter: "Earliest first day of sustained thermal shift minus 8 yields the last day of Phase I, provided that day has no *more-fertile* mucus." Be **sure** to check the limitations stated on page 379.

2. Make the internal observations — both mucus and cervix — and modify the Last Dry Day Rule as follows: "If you consistently have SIX or more days of the more-fertile mucus from its start through Peak Day, then you can treat the earlier days of the less-fertile mucus as 'dry days.' Consider yourselves in Phase II as soon as the cervix starts to open or rise or the more-fertile mucus starts, even if it should disappear for a day or so."

We cannot quote any effectiveness figures for this more liberal practice. The Last Dry Day Rule normally requires that you consistently have a mucus patch of at least *five* days from start through Peak Day. We have added an extra day since we assume that the less-fertile mucus is more conducive to sperm life than a mucus-dry vagina. We would **not** recommend this plan for a couple with a life or death reason to avoid pregnancy, but it is what we would probably use during our spacing years if we were in this situation.

We would also be doing everything we could to remedy the overall cycle problem. Something might well be improved when the mucus discharge consistently drags out beyond ten days.

The double peak pattern

When a Peak Day is followed by four or more days of drying-up and then the more-fertile mucus reappears, we call it the "double peak" or "double patch" pattern. In the true double peak situation, your waking temperatures remain low after the first Peak Day, and that warns you that ovulation has **not yet** occurred. Remember: after ovulation, progesterone causes your temperature to rise.

Q. Does this mean that I can have a mucus patch without ovulating?

A. Yes. You can have one mucus patch in which you do **not** ovulate, followed by some drying-up days, and then followed by another mucus patch in which you **do** ovulate. Generally the second mucus patch is very short.

● **Key elements in a double peak pattern**
1. You have a mucus patch and a Peak Day.
2. You have four or more days of drying-up.
3. Your temperature pattern stays low.
4. More-fertile mucus returns, usually just for a few days.
5. You have a second Peak Day.
6. Your temperature pattern rises near the second Peak Day.
7. You enter Phase III only when you have at least three days of elevated temperatures to cross-check the drying-up after the second Peak Day.

Analysis
● Why does this happen? **Stress** can delay ovulation. You can have the

mucus and cervix signs of fertility, but considerable stress can postpone ovulation. There are two kinds of stress that can delay ovulation: 1) bodily stress such as sickness and 2) psychological stress such as people experience from the death of a parent, a child or a close friend. Sometimes the stress of college examinations and/or wedding preparations can delay ovulation. Even a big change in life such as entering college away from home can affect a woman's fertility-menstrual cycle.

Take a look at the mucus pattern in Figure 27.1.

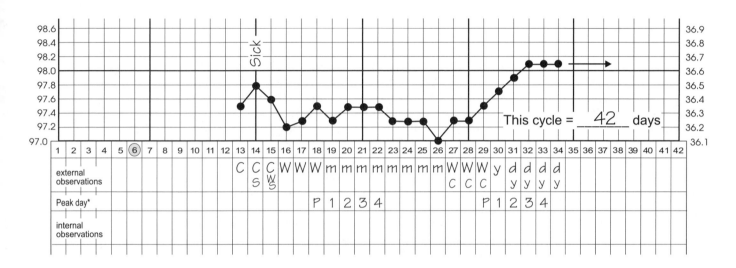

Figure 27.1   Double Peak Mucus Pattern

● What happened here? The woman was sick on Day 14, and we think that is what delayed her ovulation. First there was a normal six-day mucus patch ending with a true Peak Day on Day 18. It was followed by this woman's typical drying-up pattern—never all the way dry, as you can see by the drying-up pattern after her second Peak Day on Day 29. However, her temperature pattern after the first Peak Day stayed low instead of rising as it does after ovulation. Then the more-fertile mucus reappeared for three days (27 - 29) with another true Peak Day on Day 29. This time, her temperature rose and stayed up for 14 days. There is no question here: she ovulated in connection with the second mucus patch, not the first.

Note well: this is **not** a case of double ovulation because she did **not** ovulate in connection with the first mucus patch. Ovulation most likely occurred between Days 28 and 30 inclusive.

● How often does this happen? The frequency has not been scientifically documented, but our experience suggests it is neither quite common nor extremely rare. It's a "sometimes" type of thing.

As you can well imagine, the Calendar Rhythm method has great difficulty with delayed ovulation. When doctors were teaching Calendar Rhythm in the 1930s, the better instructors told their patients that if they experienced real stress in the cycle, they should abstain until the start of their next menstruation. How do we know what the better rhythm teachers were saying in the 1930s? Around 1978 the mother of a CCL teacher sent her a doctor-authored article which made that point. The mother had saved it from a 1938 issue of Ladies Home Journal!

● What to do:

1. The double peak or double mucus patch offers no problem of interpretation if you are practicing the cross-checking Sympto-Thermal Method. When your temperature fails to rise after the first mucus patch, you know that something is out of order. You know that you have not yet ovulated. Your conclusion is that you are **not** into Phase III on Peak Day + 4 or Peak Day + 5. Therefore, wait until your temperature rises for three days to have a positive assurance that you are into postovulation infertility.

2. Mucus-only systems have a problem with the double mucus patch. First, if you use only the mucus sign, you must keep making your mucus observations in every cycle just as diligently after the first mucus patch (even though you presume that ovulation had occurred). If you find any of the more-fertile mucus, you must abstain again. The problem is that *the second mucus patch tends to be very short*. In almost every case of this we have seen, the second mucus patch was only three days long. If you have coitus on the day before the start of a three-day mucus patch, the sperm would require only a very ordinary lifespan to be present at the time of ovulation.

Second, if you experience unusual stress during your mucus patch, you may not want to trust the first dry-up pattern just by itself. Start to take your temperatures immediately.

● **The delayed ovulation associated with the double mucus patch provides a very sound reason for using the cross-checking Sympto-Thermal Method.** The mucus patch (or the cervix changes) provides you with a *positive* sign you are *fertile*, but only the elevated temperature pattern provides you with a *positive* sign you have ovulated and are into postovulation *infertility*.

The split peak

The "split peak" pattern is the same as the "double peak pattern" with one exception: after the first Peak Day, there are only one, two or three days of drying-up (instead of four or more) before the more-fertile mucus returns. See Figure 27.2.

We make a distinction for two reasons: First, we want you to be able to distinguish this from the "split dry-up" pattern that we explain next. Second, we need to emphasize that even if you have only one, two or three days of drying-up after a Peak Day, or a second mucus patch that's only a day or two long, you have to treat a second patch as a "double peak" situation and restart the drying-up count after the last Peak Day. The bold-faced items 2 and 4 on the next page highlight the distinctions between the double peak and the split peak patterns.

We do not expect you to remember these distinctions. They are too complicated. But if you experience this sort of irregular mucus pattern, you know where to look. The important thing to remember is that you need at least three days of thermal shift to cross-check your drying-up pattern.

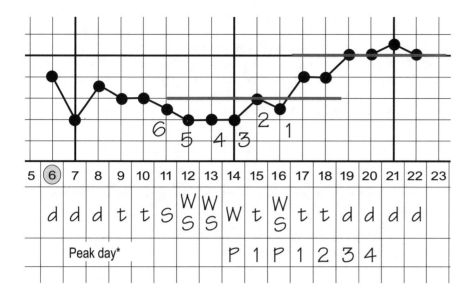

Figure 27.2 A Split Peak Pattern

● **Key elements in a split peak pattern**
1. You have a mucus patch and a Peak Day.
2. You have **one, two** or **three** days of drying-up.
3. Your temperature pattern stays low.
4. Mucus returns, sometimes just for one or two days.
5. You have a second Peak Day and a normal drying-up pattern.
6. Your temperature pattern rises near the second Peak Day.

● What to do: Consider yourselves into Phase III only when you have at least three days of elevated temperatures to cross-check the drying-up after the second Peak Day. In Figure 27.2, Rule R yields Day 19 as the start of Phase III.

The split dry-up

However, what if the temperature pattern starts to rise before or during the second mucus patch? If the second mucus patch is only one day long and if it occurs while the temperature pattern is rising, then you can apply the next rule: the split dry-up rule. You need all the key elements as follows.

● **Key elements in a split dry-up pattern**

1. The Peak Day is followed by **two or three days** of drying-up.

2. Your more-fertile mucus reappears **only for one day** and then is followed by dry days.

3. An **obvious thermal shift pattern** has been established after Peak Day.

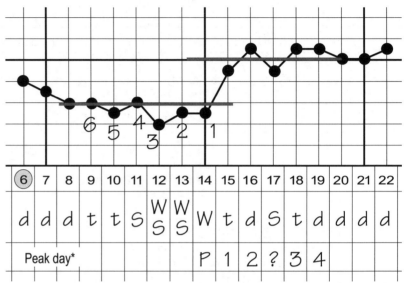

Figure 27.3 The Split Dry-up Pattern

● What to do:

When those three conditions are met, label the single day of more-fertile mucus with a question mark and continue the drying-up count on the next day, as in Figure 27.3. Then use a standard interpretation for the start of Phase III.

● Why does this happen? We don't know for sure. We *think* it may be due to the slight post-ovulation increase in estrogen that is illustrated in Figure 9.5 in Chapter 9.

Workbook exercises

Workbook charts 9, 17, 18, 19, and 23.

Self-Test Questions: Chapter 27

1. True____ False____   The double mucus patch indicates that ovulation occurred twice in that cycle.

2. In the double mucus patch pattern, the second mucus patch is typically
   a) longer than usual
   b) quite short
   c) about the same as the first patch.

3. If you arrive at "Peak Day + 4" without any sign of an upward thermal shift, you should
   a) assume that something is wrong with your thermometer
   b) consider yourselves still in Phase II
   c) consider yourselves back into Phase I and use the Phase I rules, hoping to catch the start of the second mucus patch in time.

4. When a first Peak Day is followed by four or more days of drying-up and then there's a second mucus patch, it is called
   a) the split dry-up
   b) the split peak
   c) the double mucus patch

5. In the double mucus patch pattern, the temperature pattern on the days between the patches
   a) remains low
   b) becomes elevated.

6. If you have a pattern like this—P d P d d—it is always called
   a) the split peak
   b) the split dry-up.

7. True____ False____   In the split dry-up situation, the second "patch" is always only one day long.

8. Consider this pattern: P d d P d d d d. If the temperature pattern remains low, it's a _____ _____. If the temperatures establish a good upward thermal shift pattern right after the first Peak Day, this pattern would be called a _____ _____.

9. If the second patch of more-fertile mucus after two or three days of drying-up is two or more days long, it is always called a _____ _____ pattern.

10. In the split dry-up pattern, how many days of drying-up can there be between the first Peak Day and the return of the more-fertile mucus?
    a) one
    b) two or three
    c) four or more.

As we said earlier, you aren't expected to remember these fine points, but now you know where to find them.

Answers to self-test
1. False   2. b) quite short   3. b) consider yourselves still in Phase II.   4. c) the double mucus patch   5. a) remains low   6. a) the split peak, because there is only one dry day between the two Peak Days   7. True   8. split peak. . . split dry-up   9. split peak   10. b) two or three

28

Irregular Temperature Patterns

In Chapter 5 you learned about *disturbed* temperatures. They were generally one or two distinctly out-of-line temperatures. Most of them were from easily explained false rises; some were unexplained rises. The focus was on their effect on the Low Temperature Level. In this chapter we focus first on some unusual thermal shift *patterns*; then we look at a variety of unusual *temperatures*.

Unusual Thermal Shift Patterns

In general, when you have a very difficult temperature pattern but also have a usable mucus pattern, you turn to Rule B. When you reach "Peak Day + 4," you ask, "Does the temperature pattern now offer a valid cross-check?" Usually it does, sometimes with shaving, but occasionally you have to wait as in *Workbook* Chart 6.

We offer the temperature-only interpretations because they may be helpful for those few women who find very little mucus or have continuous mucus and are unable to establish a Peak Day. The Marshall Five-day Temperature-only Rule is sufficiently conservative for most cases.

In the first three cases, we have used real-life charts. First we interpret them according to the standard sympto-thermal rules. Then we pretend there are no usable mucus or cervix signs, and we provide two temperature-only interpretations. One is the standard CCL Temperature-only Rule you learned in Chapter 26. The other is the five-day Marshall rule that is also described in Chapter 26. We remind you that Dr. Marshall cautions that when you have a most serious reason to avoid pregnancy, you should have at least three days of temperatures at the High Temperature Level as in the standard CCL Temperature-only Rule.

For your convenience we repeat those rules here.

> **Four-day Temperature-only Rule:** Phase III begins on the evening of the fourth day of thermal shift in which the last three days are consecutively at or above the High Temperature Level. (To repeat, the High Temperature Level is 4/10 of 1° F. above the Low Temperature Level, the LTL.)

Marshall Five-day Temperature-only Rule: Phase III begins on the evening of the fifth day of **overall** thermal shift. Use the standard requirements of an overall thermal shift. (All the temperatures are at least 1/10 of 1° F. above the LTL; they are all in a general rising pattern; at least one of them reaches the normal High Temperature Level of 4/10 of 1° F. above the LTL.)

The slow rise

In some cycles (14% according to Marshall[1]) a slow temperature rise takes several days to reach the normal High Temperature Level of 4/10 of 1° F. above the Low Temperature Level (LTL).

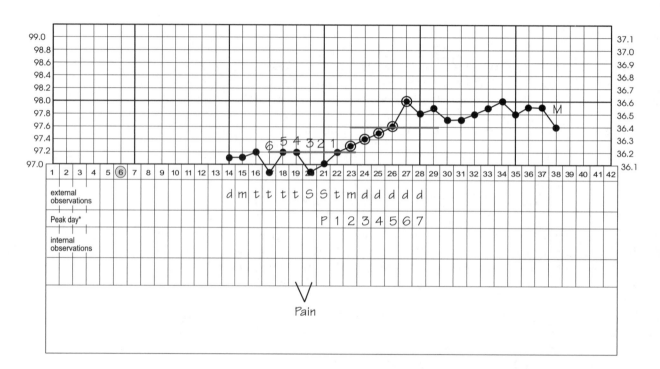

Figure 28.1 The Slow Rise Pattern

In Figure 28.1, the LTL is easily set at 97.2°, and sympto-thermal Rule B yields Day 26 as the start of Phase III.

Now pretend there are no mucus signs.

1. The standard Four-day Temperature-only Rule yields Day 28 as the start of Phase III.

2. The Marshall Five-day Temperature-only Rule yields Day 27 as the start of Phase III.

A small percentage of charts (3% according to Marshall[2]) show a step-like upward progression. See Figure 28.2.

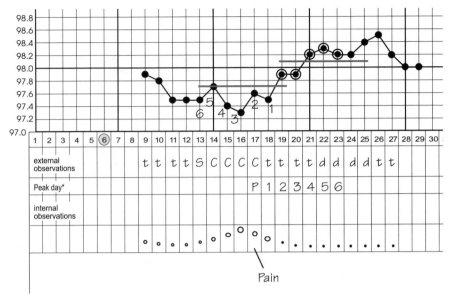

Figure 28.2 The Step Rise Pattern

Set the LTL at 97.7° and the High Temperature Level at 98.1°. Sympto-thermal Rule B yields Day 21 as the start of Phase III.

Now pretend there are no mucus signs.
1. The Five-day Temperature-only Rule yields Day 23 as the start of Phase III. If the temperatures on days 21 and 22 had been at 97.9°, 98.0° or 98.1°, the five-day rule would still have been fulfilled on Day 23.
2. The standard Four-day Temperature-only Rule yields the same result because the last three temperatures are at the High Temperature Level.

The zigzag rise is similar to the step rise except that the temperatures rise in a zigzag pattern. See Figure 28.3.

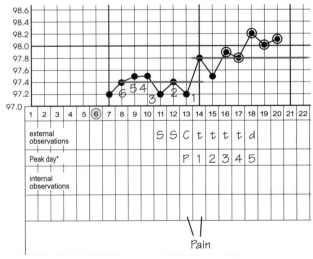

Figure 28.3 The Zigzag Rise

The mucus pattern helps us to see that the rising temperature pattern starts on Day 14. Therefore the pre-shift six temperatures are Days 8 - 13. Shave Days 9 and 10; set the LTL at 97.4° and the HTL at 97.8°. Sympto-thermal Rule B yields Day 17 as the start of Phase III.

Again, imagine no help from the mucus signs.
The Five-day Temperature-only Rule would yield Day 18 as the start of Phase III.
The standard Four-day Temperature-only Rule yields the same day because the last three days are all at the High Temperature Level.

Premature temperature rise

The essence of the Sympto-Thermal Method is the cross-check. In the double peak situation, you have to wait for the temperature cross-check (see previous chapter). It also works the other way around.

In the cycle illustrated in Figure 28.4, the temperature pattern starts to rise on the same day the most-fertile mucus *starts*. You know something isn't quite right. The couple sought and achieved pregnancy during those days of most-fertile mucus and rising temperatures. Then after Peak Day, the temperatures became further elevated.

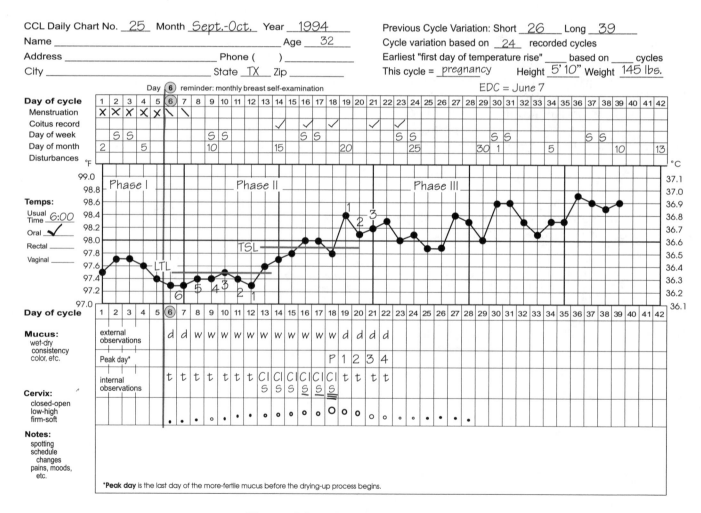

Figure 28.4 Premature Temperature Rise

Q. Why does this happen?

A. Sometimes the ovaries produce small amounts of progesterone before ovulation. However, even with that knowledge, the case in Figure 28.4 is highly unusual. We don't know *how* the ovaries produce progesterone before ovulation, but in most cases where we suspect that might be the case, the pre-peak temperature rise is very slight and only for one or two days. The case illustrated is exceptional. (Variations in bedroom temperatures can also cause very slight temperature rises, but generally you will be aware of such changes.)

● What to do. You can interpret this chart in several ways. Using Days 6-12 as the pre-shift six, you can set the LTL at 97.5°, the HTL at 97.9°, and have a Rule K interpretation on Day 21. Or you could shave the LTL to 97.4° and find another Rule K interpretation on Day 20 with the minimum two days of drying-up. Alternatively, you could consider this an "ambiguous temperature rise" and use Peak Day to help set the last day of the pre-shift six (see Example 1 later in this chapter). In that case, the pre-shift six would be Days 13-18. With an unshaved LTL of 98.0°, Rule B yields Day 22 as the start of Phase III. With an *averaged* LTL of 97.8°, Rule K yields Day 21 as the start of Phase III.

In general, you may find that the mucus pattern and the requirement of the sympto-thermal cross-check are very helpful for interpreting difficult temperature patterns.

Unusual Temperatures

The pre-shift spike

Some women experience a high, unexplained temperature rise for one or two days, usually right before or including Peak Day. Then the temperature pattern drops back to the previous level for one or two days before starting a normal thermal shift pattern. We call this a "pre-shift spike." **Note:** It is the drop back to the previous level that makes the spike temperatures stand out.

● **When to treat temperatures as spikes**

The general rule is this: when you get to Peak Day + 4 and a sympto-thermal interpretation cannot be made because of one or two spiked temperatures, treat those temperatures as a pre-shift spike.

● **What to do**

1. Remember that the pre-shift six are your six temperatures immediately before the start of your *sustained* thermal shift; and "sustained" means that the thermal shift pattern isn't broken by any dips down to or below the Low Temperature Level before the start of Phase III.

For shaving and averaging, see page 64.

2. Include the spiked temperatures among the pre-shift six.

3. If you have only one spiked temperature, you can shave it, or you can average it as with two spikes.

4. With two spiked temperatures, calculate the arithmetic average including the spikes.

5. Select as your Low Temperature Level whichever is higher—the arithmetic average or the highest of the pre-shift six apart from the spiked temperatures.

Look at the charts in Figures 28.5a and 28.5b. They are consecutive charts from the same woman.

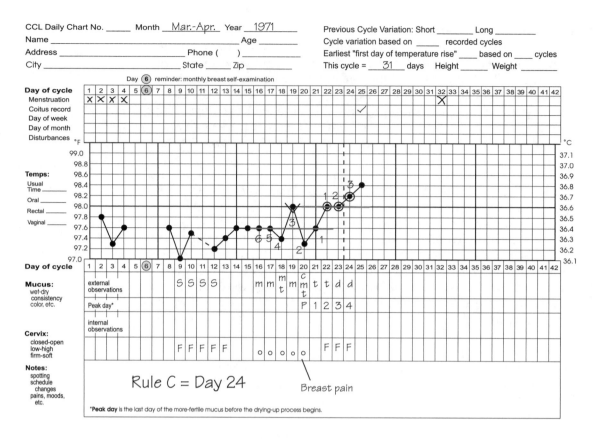

Figure 28.5a Pre-shift Spike of One Day

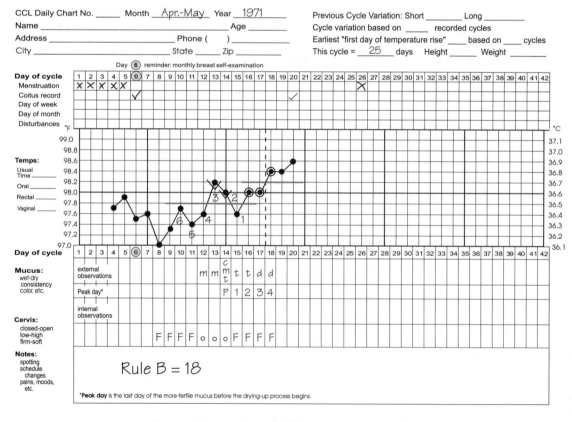

Figure 28.5b Pre-shift Spike of Two Days

In Figure 28.5a, the arithmetic average of the pre-shift six is 97.58° (which rounds up to 97.6°, the same as the next highest level apart from the spike temperature). With a Low Temperature Level of 97.6° and a Peak Day on Day 20, Rule C yields Day 24 as the start of Phase III.

The chart in Figure 28.5b looks a little more difficult to interpret at first glance, but just apply the above principles and everything works out. A two-day spike on Days 13 and 14 is followed by a drop to the previous level on Day 15. By Day 18, there are three temperatures above the previous six if you shave the two spike temperatures. The arithmetic average of the pre-shift six (10-15) is 97.75° which rounds up to 97.8°. The temperatures on 16, 17 and 18 constitute an overall thermal shift to cross-check the drying-up pattern. Rule B yields Day 18 as the start of Phase III.

The post-shift dip

Sometimes the temperature pattern will dip back to or below the Low Temperature Level soon **after** a Phase III interpretation has been established. This happens very rarely, and we have no scientific explanation for it. We can only speculate that this might be caused by an unusually large postovulation surge in estrogen, especially if mucus reappears that day or the next. (The normal surge is illustrated in Chapter 9, Figure 9.5.) The true post-shift dip lasts only for one or two days.

● **What to do**

If your waking temperature drops to or below your Low Temperature Level *after* the start of Phase III (as indicated by the mucus and temperature signs), the situation is unclear. Therefore, abstain until the temperature rises again.

If the dip is a true post-shift dip, the temperature will return the next day to the level of the previous thermal shift temperatures. It does not necessarily have to be at the High Temperature Level. Once the temperature has risen again from a one-day dip, you are immediately back into Phase III. No further abstinence is required. The same thing holds for a two-day dip.

The mid-shift dip

Sometimes your upward temperature shift may be very uneven, and sometimes it may be broken by a dip to or below the pre-shift Low Temperature Level.

● **What to do**

1. If your temperature dips during the thermal shift process, but it does not return to (or below) your pre-shift Low Temperature Level, there is no problem. Just treat it as part of the thermal shift pattern. See Day 15 in Figure 28.3, "The zigzag rise pattern."

2. If your temperature starts to rise and then dips down to or below the pre-shift Low Temperature Level, the *normal* rule is this: restart your thermal shift count. Wait for three elevated temperatures beyond the dip for the temperature indication of the start of Phase III. If you have a most serious reason to avoid pregnancy, you would want to follow this rule.

On the other hand, if your reason for postponing pregnancy is good but not crucial, you might be able to follow a more relaxed interpretation. If you are well experienced in your mucus and cervix signs, and if these indicate P + 5 or more, you might not need to wait for a full three days past the dip. This would be a judgment call, and in a manual such as this we cannot describe every possible situation. At the least you would need enough temperature cross-check to show that you were not experiencing a relative dryness before a second mucus patch as described in the last chapter. In brief, you would be treating such a mid-shift dip more like the post-shift dip described above.

Post-shift return to low temperatures

There is an extremely rare possibility that temperatures may drop back to pre-shift levels soon after a thermal shift has already been established. We have seen less than a handful of these situations since 1971.

We don't know why this happens—even very rarely. We can only speculate. It might be caused by a defective corpus luteum with poor production of progesterone. Or the *first* thermal shift might have been caused by a slight infection or other unnoticed sickness, or perhaps by unrecorded environmental changes.

The situation is this: your temperatures and your mucus have already indicated you are in Phase III. Then the temperatures drop to or below your Low Temperature Level. If it is simply a post-shift dip, the temperatures will rise immediately, but in this case the temperatures stay low for **three or more days.**

● What to do

1. Consider yourselves back into Phase II on the first day of temperatures at or below the LTL, and abstain accordingly.

2. Check your mucus and/or cervix signs very carefully.

3. If you have any mucus or cervix signs of fertility, treat this as a double mucus patch, and wait for a full sympto-thermal indication of being in Phase III.

4. Even if you find no mucus or cervix signs of fertility, wait for three days of thermal shift before considering yourselves back into Phase III.

As indicated above, this is such a rare situation that we have almost no experience with it. Therefore we have to offer conservative counsel.

● Declining temperature pattern

The normal thermal shift pattern is elevated or rising. If your temperature goes up sharply and then clearly declines almost to the LTL when you reach a Phase III interpretation, consider waiting one more day unless this is your regular pattern. If the temperature rises slightly, you are in Phase III. If it becomes a post-shift dip or a post-shift return to low temperatures, follow the advice given in those sections above.

Sometimes a temperature rise is so ambiguous that it is difficult to decide which temperatures to count as your pre-shift six. If that happens the general rule is this: the last day of the pre-shift six should be on Peak Day or as close to it as the situation permits.

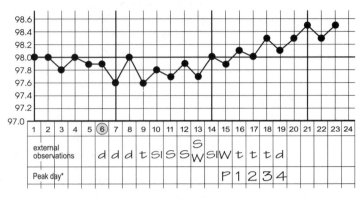

Example 1

In Example 1 above, the zigzag pattern makes it obvious you will have to shave a temperature—but which one? Go to Peak Day and use it as the last day of the pre-shift six temperatures. With a shaved LTL of 97.9°, it is easy to see an overall thermal shift; Rule B yields Day 19 as the start of Phase III.

We deliberately made the temperature pattern in Example 1 difficult to interpret in order to make the point. For a real life situation, see Workbook Chart 20. See also Figure 28.4.

You have seen irregular patterns of mucus and temperature in these last three chapters (26, 27 and 28). And we're not done yet: Chapter 30 contains some more irregular cycle patterns.

What's the point of all these examples? You will probably never see most of them in your own charting history, but if you do experience any one of them, you will be able to know what's happening.

When confronting an unusual situation, you take these factors into account:
1. Your previous cycle patterns, especially the last two or three cycles
2. The overall temperature pattern, sometimes excluding any questionable temperatures
3. The mucus pattern
4. The cervix pattern.

In most cases of unusual cycle patterns, you will be able to use the principles in these and other chapters to determine where you are in your cycle. If it is not clear to you, contact your local NFP teachers. If you are learning through the *CCL Home Study Course*, contact your local CCL teachers. If they are not available, contact CCL Headquarters for help.

Workbook charts 6, 7, 13, and 20.

Self-Test Questions: Chapter 28

These questions also contain some review.

1. The normal amount of upward thermal shift from the Low Temperature Level is _____ of 1° Fahrenheit.

2. A person, female or male, normally experiences a rise and a fall in her/his temperature during each 24 hour period. This periodic rising and falling is called a _____ rhythm.

3. In this daily rhythm, your body temperature reaches its lowest point in the wee hours of the morning, and it begins to rise during your normal waking hours at the rate of approximately _____ of 1° F. every *half* hour.

4. Therefore, if you took your temperature *two* hours later than your usual time, your later temperature might be _____ of 1° F. higher than it was at your normal waking time.

5. True____   False____   The circadian rhythm is so rigid and precise that you can reliably "discount" up and down if you take your temperature an hour or two late or early.

6. True____   False____   Taking your temperature within a half-hour of your normal waking time shouldn't affect your temperature by more than 1/10 of 1° F.

7. Disturbed temperatures among the pre-shift six are:
   a) shaved and used in the pre-shift six
   b) ignored, and you go backwards for additional valid temps for your pre-shift six.

8. True____   False____   Assume undisturbed temperatures. If you experience a pre-shift spike of one or two days, you can shave those temperatures to the next highest level or to the arithmetic average, whichever is higher.

9. True____   False____   If you shave one or two pre-shift temperatures, you include them among the pre-shift six temperatures.

10. True____   False____   A *sustained* thermal shift consists of the temperature readings that start upward and stay above the LTL level.

11. The pre-shift six temperatures are the six temperatures—
   a) just after menstruation
   b) which form a visual grouping someplace early in the cycle
   c) immediately before the start of the sustained thermal shift.

12. Consider this situation. You have one or two days of rising temperatures; then a valid temperature dips *to or below* your LTL level. What do you do?
   a) Skip the low temp and continue your thermal shift count with the next elevated temperature.
   b) Include the one or two rising temperatures and the low temperature among the pre-shift six and restart your thermal shift count with the next three elevated temperatures.
   c) Count the low temp among your thermal shift temperatures.

13. If you experience a difficult temperature pattern but have an easily interpreted mucus pattern, you will most likely use Rule _____.

14. If you have three days of *strong* thermal shift simultaneously cross-checked by three days of drying-up past your Peak Day, the rule to use is Rule _____.

If you are having any problems with charting, please review Chapter 4. When you draw your phase division lines, start at the very top of the graph, right between the boxes for the Cycle Day numbers. For example, if the last possible day of Phase I is Day 7, draw your Phase I/II line between the boxes for Days 7 and 8; then draw the line downward *between* the temperature lines, ending up between the bottom boxes for Days 7 and 8. If the first day of Phase III is Cycle Day 17, then the last day of Phase II was Day 16. Draw your Phase II/III division line between the top boxes for Days 16 and 17 and continue downward.

Answers to self-test
1. 4/10 2. circadian 3. 1/10 4. 4/10 5. False 6. True 7. b) ignored, and you go backwards for additional valid temps for your pre-shift six. 8. True 9. True 10. True 11. c) immediately before the start of the sustained thermal shift. 12. b) include the one or two rising temperatures and the low temperature among the pre-shift six, and restart your thermal shift count with the next three elevated temperatures. 13. B 14. R

(1) John Marshall, M.D., *The Infertile Period* (Baltimore: Helicon Press, 1969) 30.
(2) Marshall, 30.

Part VI

Special Situations

29

Coming Off the Pill

If you have been using the Pill for birth control and have now made the decision to abandon that form of birth control and to use only the natural methods of conception regulation, we congratulate you. If you have never used the Pill, even for a therapeutic reason, we rejoice with you. Chapter 1 lists some of the effects of the Pill, and those effects hold true regardless of the reason for which it was taken.

If you are currently taking the Pill (or any other estrogen or progesterone medication),you have to stop taking it to obtain true sympto-thermal observations. If you are on the Pill, your mucus, cervix, and temperature signs will reflect the artificial hormones, not your naturally produced fertility and infertility hormones. That is, you can expect the synthetic estrogen in the combination Pill to produce a mucus discharge, and you can expect the synthetic progesterone to produce a relatively high and flat temperature pattern.

The artificial hormones from the Pill may remain in your system for several months, and this hormonal residue may affect your mucus signs for the first one to three cycles. Therefore, we recommend using a special temperature-only rule to determine the start of postovulation infertility.

In mid-1999 we learned about a group of young teenage girls who completed a medical history form required for attending summer camp. Reviewing the forms, a counselor was shocked. Every girl was taking the Pill, supposedly for the control of acne. According to reliable research, that means that every one of those girls is at increased risk of breast cancer later in life.

— John & Sheila K.

Standard Post-Pill Rules

1. Abstain during Phase I and Phase II for the first three cycles.

2. **Phase III starts** on the evening of the fifth day of upward thermal shift in which the last three temperatures are on consecutive days and are at or above the High Temperature Level, with at least the last day of temperature rise also dry or drying-up.

The standard post-pill rules

● Explanations

1. The Pill manufacturers recommend that you do not become pregnant for three cycles after discontinuing the Pill; they fear lawsuits alleging birth defects due to the hormonal residues of the Pill. The evidence on that point is apparently vague, but we report their recommendations. Therefore we strongly advise that you abstain during Phases I and II for the first three cycles off-the-Pill even if you want to become pregnant.

This recommendation is just slightly more conservative than our standard recommendation for all beginners, that is, to abstain in Phases I and II for the first one to three cycles.

2. The Post-Pill Rule assumes that the more-fertile mucus does not extend into Phase III as determined by the five-day thermal shift. The more-fertile mucus may extend into the first three or four days on which the temperature is rising, but it has to disappear for you to be in Phase III. You can, however, apply the Post-Pill Rule even though you notice the distinctly less-fertile tacky or sticky mucus. Such less-fertile mucus may last for the entire Phase III of the first one or two cycles.

The Post-Pill Rule takes the standard CCL four-day temperature-only rule and adds one extra day for beginners. See examples in Figure 29.1.

Common questions

Question: What if I should have a good Peak Day and drying-up in those first three cycles? Should we apply the regular STM rules if they will give us an earlier start of Phase III?

Answer: If you think you can determine a definite Peak Day, chart it. However, we still recommend using the five-day temperature-only rule for the first three cycles off-the-Pill. We are unsure of the value of the mucus sign when the Pill residues may still be having some effect on your cycle.

Q: Should I finish taking my current Pill regimen?
A: There *might* be a bit more initial cycle regularity if you complete the 21 or 28 day regimen.

Q: When should we begin abstinence?
A: Immediately. Every form of the Pill has abortifacient powers. So, whether you finish the Pill regimen or never take another Pill, you should begin immediately to abstain from sexual relations so that you do not cause an early abortion with the chemicals of the Pill. Most likely, the sooner you stop the Pill, the sooner you will be in Phase III by the CCL Post-Pill Rule.

Q: Once I have a normal cycle, will I go on to have consistently normal cycles?
A: Generally yes, but not necessarily. We have seen a few instances in which a woman had one to three normal cycles and then had a highly unusual cycle with extended mucus and delayed ovulation. Such a cycle provides a test of conviction, but it soon passes into history.

If your cycles before taking the Pill were irregular, it's likely they will be irregular again after you discontinue the Pill, in some cases even more irregular. If that's your situation, you may find help in Chapter 31.

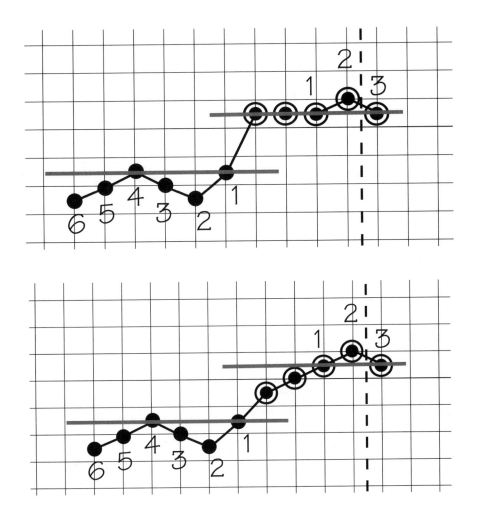

Figure 29.1   Just-off-the-pill Five-day Temperature-only Patterns

In Figure 29.1, the circled temperatures make up the post-pill thermal shift pattern. In the upper graph, all five elevated temperatures are at the High Temperature Level. In the lower graph, the first two days of elevated temperatures are not yet at the HTL, but they can still be counted as the first part of the five-day off-the-pill temperature-only rule since they are followed immediately by three more temperatures at the High Temperature Level. The last three temperatures consecutively at the High Temperature Level are numbered in each example.

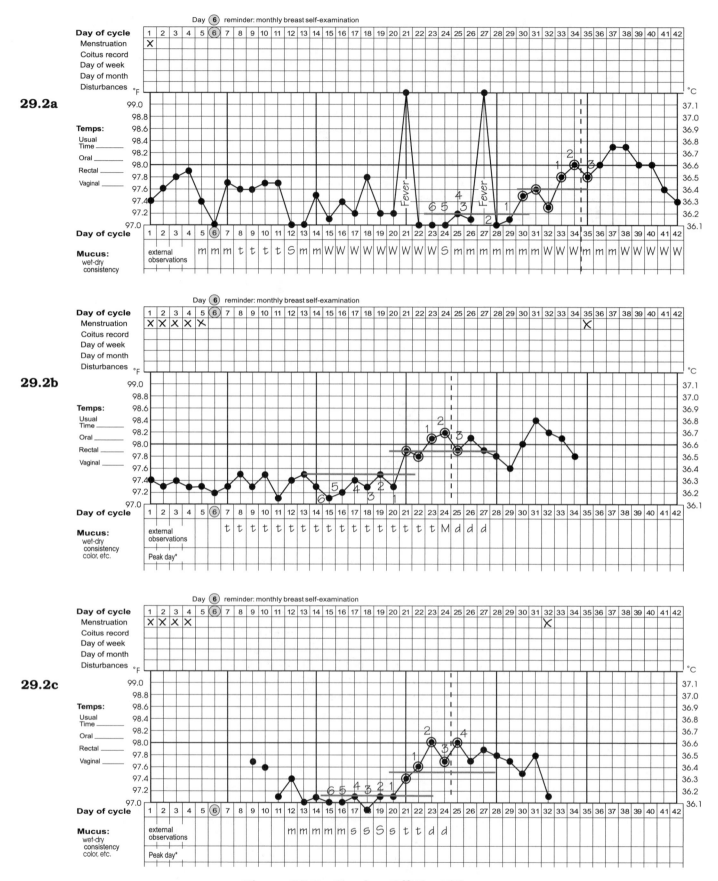

Figure 29.2   Coming Off the Pill

Q: What will happen in my first cycles off-the-pill?

A: Experience with the lower dosage Pills indicates that you may well have a cycle similar to that which is illustrated in Figure 29.2c. However, you might also have one more like those illustrated in Figures 29.2a, 29.2b, and Chart 5 in the Workbook section. The cycles in 29.2a and 29.2b are consecutive from the same woman; the cycle in 29.2c is from her sister who came off the Pill at the same time.

Sometimes temperatures may be erratic for one or more cycles before they settle down. Look at the differences between 29.2a and 29.2b. Sometimes the mucus flow will be heavy and/or continuous before it becomes normal. Again check those same two charts.

Most of the time fertility returns quickly, but sometimes fertility is permanently damaged by the Pill, and at other times the return of fertility is greatly delayed. We recall one woman who wanted to achieve pregnancy shortly after stopping the Pill. Month after month, she never experienced a period but did take daily temperatures. Finally, at about six months a thermal shift confirmed ovulation. She became pregnant at that time and, fortunately for her, the thermal shift enabled her to inform her physician when she conceived.

Because of the variety of the drugs used and because of the variety of effects they have on different women, it is difficult to make any certain generalizations about cycles coming-off-the-Pill. Nevertheless, we provide three examples in Figure 29.2.

Compare Figures 29.2a and 29.2b, one woman's first two cycles off-the-Pill. In the first cycle, the mucus pattern is confusing, to say the least. Perhaps it reflects the hormonal residues. In the second cycle, it is less confusing and dries up after ovulation.

The temperature pattern in the first cycle is erratic in the early part of the cycle. However, apply the standard rule of "looking for three above the previous six" and you will see a thermal shift starting on Day 30. Since the last three temperatures have to be *consecutively* at the High Temperature Level, the Post-Pill Rule yields Day 35 as the start of Phase III.

The temperature pattern in the second cycle is stable. Set the Low Temperature Level at 97.5° and the High Temperature Level at 97.9°, and the Post-Pill Rule yields Day 25 as the start of Phase III.

The cycle in Figure 29.2c is also a first cycle off-the-Pill; it shows that some women have clearly defined patterns right away. The Low Temperature Level is set at 97.1°, and Peak Day occurs on Day 20. If this were a normal cycle, the CCL Rule R would yield Day 23 as the start of Phase III. However, we strongly recommend using the Post-Pill Rule for the first three cycles off the Pill, and that rule yields Day 25 as the start of Phase III.

Psycho-sexual adjustments

Couples just coming off the Pill sometimes experience difficulties in the adjustment of their sexual activity, and this should be no surprise. They sometimes have come from a pattern of unlimited sex and are now committed to respecting the natural patterns of fertility and infertility. For some, this is no problem, and they may soon be having sexual relations more frequently than when using the Pill because then the wife had been feeling used and had been using every excuse to avoid marital relations. But for others, the change is a challenge. Because sex is so greatly psychological (your brain is your primary sex organ) and because your sexual attitudes are so important in the regulation of your sexual activity, perhaps it might be helpful to reflect on some ideas that can influence attitudes.

Those who think in terms of nature and ecology might reflect on the fact that contraceptive drugs and devices do a certain violence to nature. They know that any violence against nature calls for some sort of restoration and that this always comes at a price, usually at the price of some form of self-control.

Those who think in psychological terms of maturity certainly know that maturity does not come automatically with age but only at the price of growing pains. This is also true of sexual maturity and the growth in self-control that is needed for mature sexuality.

Those who think in moral terms and have come to regard the practice of contraception as immoral know that their past mistakes or sins call for some sort of penance or work of reconciliation with God and nature.

Those who think in Christian religious terms can see in the suffering of Christ something that gives meaning to their own difficulties or sufferings in the effort to be faithful to Him.

In the last analysis, almost any difficulties can be borne if they can be seen as meaningful, and the above meanings can enrich the process and pain of human growth.

Workbook exercise

Workbook chart 5.

Self-Test Questions: Chapter 29

1. True____ False____ Couples coming off the Pill should abstain in Phase I as well as in Phase II for the first three cycles.

2. In the CCL Temperature-only Rule for coming off the Pill, _____ days of thermal shift are required.

3. In the Post-Pill Rule, the _____ _____ of those temperatures must be consecutively at the High Temperature Level.

4. Residues from the synthetic hormone _____ may cause a confusing mucus pattern for two or three cycles.

5. True____ False____ In the Christian perspective, difficulties with abstinence can be offered in union with the sufferings of Christ as reparation for one's own sins and those of others.

Answers
1. True   2. five   3. last three   4. estrogen   5. True

30

Breakthrough Bleeding

In long cycles, bleeding may occur which begins like menstruation but really isn't. This "breakthrough bleeding" is a fertile time because it generally occurs just before ovulation.

What happens is this. The endometrium builds up so much that the top layer cannot be sustained just by estrogen, so it breaks down. It may be only spotting, or it may be like a normal menstrual flow. Generally, a mucus discharge occurs at the same time.

Breakthrough bleeding occurs infrequently during the most fertile years. It is less rare during the premenopausal years. However, the chart in Figure 30.1 shows breakthrough bleeding in a 22 year-old woman. Charts from a 40 year-old woman are used in the "Workbook" section, Chart 10.

● **What to do**

How can you distinguish breakthrough bleeding from a true menstruation?

1. Record waking temperatures at least until a thermal shift is established for Phase III. (Breakthrough bleeding is an excellent reason to record your waking temperatures.)

2. Regard a bloody discharge as a true menstruation **only** when it has been preceded by a thermal shift.

3. Interpret a bloody discharge **not** preceded by a thermal shift as possible breakthrough bleeding and therefore a fertile time.

4. Apply the standard Phase I rules to a true menstruation. The first day of bleeding is Day 1 of the new cycle.

5. Do not extend Phase I beyond Day 6 during a long menstruation: an extended bloody discharge may obscure the beginning of your mucus discharge.

6. If you experience a bloody discharge that has *not* been preceded by a thermal shift, keep charting on the same chart during the bleeding episode and for a week afterwards. If it's breakthrough bleeding, you will most likely experience something close to what's illustrated in Figure 30.1—mucus during and after the bloody discharge, followed shortly by a thermal shift. If that's what you experience, keep on charting for the rest of the cycle on the same chart.

7. On the other hand, a bloody discharge *not* preceded by a thermal shift could be a menstruation at the end of an *anovulatory cycle*—a cycle in which no ovulation occurred (see Chapter 31). If that's the case, you may or may not have any noticeable mucus during the discharge and will have your usual post-menstruation dry days. In such a case, start a new chart by copying the data beginning with the first day of menstruation and regard it as Day 1 of your new cycle.

Remember: when you have a bloody discharge that's *not preceded by a thermal shift*, you can't tell at first whether it's breakthrough bleeding or menstruation at the end of an anovulatory cycle. You don't know at first if it's a very fertile time or the start of Phase I in your next cycle. The only way you can tell the difference for sure is by hindsight. So the rule is this: *Assume* that it might be breakthrough bleeding and a fertile time and abstain if you are seeking to avoid pregnancy. If it turns out to be a normal menstrual flow without mucus and is followed by dry days and continuing low temperatures, then you have the hindsight to call it an anovulatory menstruation, and you copy those days onto your new cycle-chart.

We repeat: both breakthrough bleeding and anovulatory cycles are relatively rare events.

We are not aware of anything you can do to prevent breakthrough bleeding. It's just something to be aware of during long cycles. Keep in mind the usual things that can delay ovulation—stress, inadequate nutrition, excessive exercise, and both obesity and too little fat. However, sometimes this infrequent condition happens without any obvious causes.

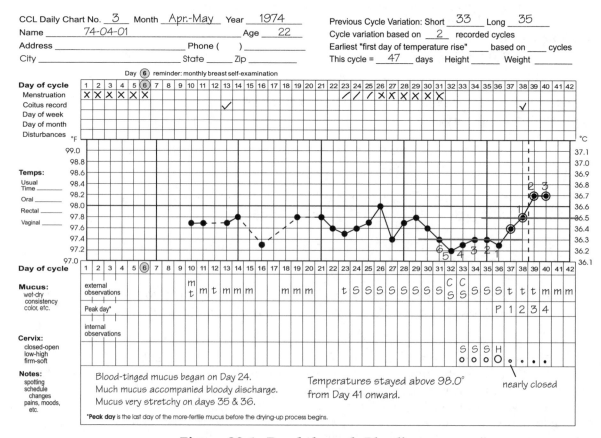

Figure 30.1 Breakthrough Bleeding

The chart in Figure 30.1 is a classic example of breakthrough bleeding occurring near ovulation. The young couple were only in their third cycle of sympto-thermal observations. When they reached the time they had previously been in Phase III (around Day 19), they saw no signs of being in Phase III yet in this cycle. On Day 23 she noticed a slight blood-tinged mucus, and this quickly developed into more than a week of mucus and bloody discharge. Then the bleeding stopped while the more-fertile mucus continued, and the temperature began to rise right after Peak Day.

Set the LTL at 97.4° based on the pre-shift six temperatures on Days 31 - 36. Rule R yields Day 39 as the start of Phase III. The cycle continued through Day 47. Coitus on Day 38 was too soon by any of the rules, but the couple was planning a pregnancy in a few months and decided to cut down gradually the days of abstinence.

You can see that in this cycle, the couple had two indications that the bleeding was not menstruation. First there was no thermal shift preceding it. Second, the presence of mucus indicated possible fertility.

Continuous bleeding

In contrast to breakthrough bleeding, there's another type of bleeding that requires medical attention according to Dr. Konald A. Prem. He writes:

> In some forms of anovulatory bleeding episodes, especially in premenopausal years when endometrial hyperplasia is more common, mucus may be present all through the bleeding because the cause of the hyperplasia is continuous estrogen production. In these cases, bleeding is also prolonged and may be continuous. In such cases, an endometrial biopsy or a D & C is recommended.[1]

For your own practical use, the medical terms are not necessary. Just remember that if you have very long or continuous bleeding episodes, you should get a checkup.

Workbook exercise

Workbook chart 10.

When you do Chart 10 in the Workbook, note that the X on Day 27 in the top graph marks the start of a bloody discharge and is the same day as Cycle Day 1 of the middle graph. The X on Day 30 of the middle graph marks the start of a bloody discharge and is the same day as Day 1 of the bottom graph. Note also the circle around the temperature dot for "Day 4" in the bottom graph: it indicates intercourse. The couple didn't know about breakthrough bleeding and had assumed that the bloody discharge on Day 30 of the middle graph was the start of a new cycle. As you can see, the "Day 4" was really Cycle Day 33, the fourth day of breakthrough bleeding; it was a fertile time. Why didn't she become pregnant? Not every act of intercourse during the fertile time results in pregnancy.

Self-Test Questions: Chapter 30

1. The days of breakthrough bleeding are
   a) highly fertile
   b) very infertile

2. A bloody discharge that is preceded by a thermal shift is properly interpreted as

   _____.

3. A bloody discharge that is not preceded by a thermal shift must be regarded at the time as possible _____ _____.

4. A cycle in which ovulation does not occur is called an _____ cycle.

5. Breakthrough bleeding is typically followed by some days of _____ _____ and by a thermal shift.

6. True____   False____   It is impossible to become pregnant from relations during a true menstruation.

7. True____   False____   If you experience a bloody discharge not preceded by a thermal shift, you should assume that it might be break-through bleeding and you should keep on using the same chart.

Answers
1. a) highly fertile 2. menstruation 3. breakthrough bleeding 4. anovulatory   5. cervical mucus 6. False 7. True

References
(1) Konald A. Prem, M.D., personal correspondence, December 1986.

31

Cycle Irregularities

"Cycle irregularity" means different things, so we start with a list:
- cycles that swing from short to long without apparent reason
- cycles that are consistently very long and which have extended discharges of mucus
- cycles with all-the-time mucus that provides no clear Peak Day
- cycles with short luteal phases
- cycles in which there is no evidence of ovulation between one period and the next (anovulatory cycles)
- cycles with unusual bleeding episodes.

Causes of Cycle Irregularities

Things don't "just happen." Regular cycles are caused by the normal pattern of fertility hormones acting in a normal body. Cycle irregularities are caused by something that's not 100% normal. That doesn't mean that a cycle irregularity is abnormal in the sense of being caused by a disease. A pathological cause is possible but it's also extremely rare. Most of the time cycle irregularities reflect something that is out of adjustment but is not a threat to your overall health. At other times, cycle irregularity may simply reflect an already existing condition that may be more obvious to someone besides the woman herself. We're thinking here of eating disorders (anorexia nervosa and bulimia) and excessive exercise.

Stress can also cause ovulation to be delayed, and stress comes in two kinds: bodily stress such as sickness, and psychological stress such as is caused by the death of a loved one, earthquakes, job losses, etc.

Our experience suggests that the causes of cycle irregularity are as follows:
- improper nutrition
- improper body balance
- stress
- environment
- something pathological

"Body balance" refers to the ratio of weight to height and to the ratio of body fat to total weight.

417

● Normal cycle irregularity

Few women have 28 day cycles, one after another. The woman who has a 28 day cycle every cycle is a statistical rarity. Cycle variation is the range between your shortest cycle and your longest cycle, and almost every woman has a certain amount of cycle variation. Even if you have very regular cycles, you can expect an occasional shorter or longer cycle.

Our primary concern is with cycle variations of more than two weeks, especially when this sort of variation happens frequently, but the suggestions in this chapter may also help women with lesser cycle variations.

Help for Irregular Cycles

The practical question is this: what can you do to make your cycle more normal? Our answer is fourfold. Eat right. Exercise right. Consider night light. Have a medical checkup.

In what follows, we offer suggestions that can help you in three ways: to stay healthy; to keep your cycles more or less regular; and to improve them if you're experiencing cycle irregularities.

Eat right

Poor nutrition can cause all six examples of irregular cycles listed at the beginning of the chapter. It may also cause breakthrough bleeding which was discussed in the last chapter.

It is definitely established that very poor nutrition affects fertility. Women imprisoned and starved in concentration camps stop menstruating and ovulating. The same is true of young women afflicted with anorexia nervosa and/or bulimia, the semi-starvation experiences in which girls, fearing to add an ounce of weight, stop eating or deliberately vomit up their meals and stay very skinny, occasionally dying of malnutrition or its long-term effects as did the famous singer Karen Carpenter.

Please note that if your system doesn't do a good job of absorbing some nutrient, you can have a nutritional deficiency even if you are eating well-balanced meals.

● Overall diet

We have long suspected that even moderate defects in nutrition can influence a woman's fertility and cycle pattern. In 1976 we ran an article in *the CCL News* (November-December) by Pierre Slightam, M.D., and our experience suggests that his advice is still valid.

> People who are insulting themselves nutritionally . . . with a diet high in empty refined calories (nutritionless — without vitamins and minerals) will find it is impossible for their bodies to function in a healthy manner . . . [and] to have good balance and control of their nervous systems. . .Many women would have more regularly spaced natural periods and menstrual cycles if they would eat better.

Dr. Slightam went on to note that the woman who consumes too much caffeine, sugar, white flour and refined or "factory foods" is more likely to develop B-complex deficiencies that cause a chronic vaginal discharge which in turn complicates the mucus observation.

● Some basic nutrition suggestions

Most of the following ideas are adapted from the article of Dr. Slightam, and variations of these can be found in almost any health book or magazine.

1. Eat "natural" foods. Fresh is better than frozen, and frozen is better than canned or otherwise processed. Fresh fruit is better than processed juices.

2. Adopt a generally high fiber and low fat diet.

3. Eat plenty of fruits and vegetables, and eat them raw or cooked as lightly as possible; use the vegetable cooking juices.

4. Drink pure water (if you can get it), milk, and unsweetened fruit juices.

5. Avoid refined (white) flour and sugar and factory foods containing these because most of the nutrition has been refined away.

6. Avoid artificial preservatives and dyes.

7. Avoid or sharply limit caffeine. This comes in coffee, tea, chocolate and cocoa, and cola drinks.

8. Avoid the empty calories of soft drinks and alcohol.

9. Avoid products containing the chemical aspartame (NutraSweet®).

Once you read that list, you may think it's impossible to live that way in middle-class America. Our suggestion: follow the recommendations in *Fertility, Cycles and Nutrition* including the realistic 80/20 rule (eat right at least 80% of the time). CCL publishes this book so that you can have much more complete answers to a number of questions, much more complete than is possible in this manual. See "Resources" near the end of this manual.

Here's an anecdote that illustrates the benefits of improved nutrition.

I personally have seen improvements in my own cycles after making some suggested dietary changes that Mrs. Shannon outlines in the first section of her book. I have a history of painful periods (requiring extra-strength Tylenol every three to four hours the first day in order to get around), and I decided to avoid caffeine and sugar while emphasizing more fresh fruits and vegetables. I also made sure I drank six to eight glasses of water a day.

I've had two periods since making these simple changes, and each month I needed to take Tylenol only once. I've also noticed a secondary benefit: a marked improvement in the quality of my mucus pattern. I've gained three to four more dry days at the end of Phase I, and it is much easier to detect the changes in the quality of mucus. I now experience the wet, raw-egg white type of mucus; previously my more-fertile type mucus stretched only about an inch.

Fertility, Cycles and Nutrition is not just for women with obvious fertility problems; it can ease the practice of NFP for the more "typical" NFP user as well. My cycles were improved with very little effort. — A. G.[1]

● Dietary supplements

The use of dietary supplements—vitamins, minerals and foods—to alleviate various forms of cycle irregularities is admittedly controversial. However, the accumulation of experience and research leaves no doubt in our minds that some supplements help some women with some sorts of irregularities.

You may think that's a rather general and weak statement, and you're right. We don't know of any panacea—something that works equally well for everybody. However, that doesn't negate the value of dietary supplements. Even if there were some powerful drug that could be used to treat some of these irregularities, it is doubtful that it would be effective for all women and for all irregularities. On the other hand, something very simple can sometimes make a big difference. Consider the anecdote at the right.

"Low fat" does not mean "no fat." The essential fatty acids found in fresh, "expeller-pressed" salad oils and flax oil are just that—essential to life and health. Be sure to get a tablespoon or two of good quality salad oil daily. Consider a capsule of flax oil daily.
—Marilyn Shannon

*A woman went on a self-directed diet that included the total exclusion of salt. Soon she was having a cycle like she had never had before with a very much delayed ovulation. In eliminating the salt, she had likewise eliminated her only source of **iodine** that is needed for proper functioning of the thyroid gland. We suggested that she might get help by taking a kelp tablet each day; she did so and promptly got back into clockwork cycles. Her case is by no means unique.*

Dr. Guy Abraham, among others, has done considerable research on nutrition to try to alleviate the symptoms of pre-menstrual syndrome. He's convinced that nutrition—whether good or bad—affects the female cycle, and he has developed a dietary supplement aimed at normalizing the cycle by enabling the hormones to function properly. *Fertility, Cycles and Nutrition* puts the results of this research into readable form. For sound ideas about dietary supplements and well balanced eating, we again recommend this book.

If you decide to use dietary supplements, please buy from companies whose primary business is dietary supplements rather than the products of companies involved in the manufacture of abortifacient and contraceptive devices and drugs. For example, the Pharmacia-Upjohn Company manufactures a prostaglandin product whose only government-approved use is for abortions. Why use their vitamins (Unicaps) and other products?

● **Weight to height balance**

Most women experience their best cycle regularity if their weight is approximately right for their height and if they have sufficient but not too much body fat. Women who are significantly underweight or who have too little fat may experience very long cycles, perhaps only three to six per year. Furthermore, you could be at your "ideal weight," but if you were all muscle and bone, you would most likely have cycle problems because you need a certain amount of your weight in fat to have normal fertility. That's the way the Lord made women.

At the other end of the scale, truly obese women have more cycle irregularity and generally more menstrual problems than women with normal ratios of weight to height.

Why? The ovarian hormones are fat soluble. On the one hand, they need a certain amount of body fat—**20% to 22%** of your weight is the minimum—to accomplish their functions. On the other hand, an excess of fat may absorb the ovulation-inducing hormones sufficiently to delay ovulation.

So be sensible about your weight. If you are overweight, eat right and exercise sensibly. Eliminate desserts and between-meal snacks except for raw vegetables such as carrots and celery. Eat 100% whole wheat bread and toast—without any butter or jelly. Follow the general nutritional guidance in *Fertility, Cycles and Nutrition* including suggestions about dietary supplements.

If you decide to go on a weight-loss program that will cost you a fair amount of money, we suggest doing so only after working with the above common sense means of safely reducing your intake of fat and unnecessary calories. Join a support group. Certainly, avoid "wonder diets" that would have you losing large amounts of weight in a short time. There are programs that promote gradual weight loss through proper eating at three meals a day. Be aware that any sudden loss of weight may affect your signs of fertility.

Exercise right

For proper body balance, exercise right. It is common knowledge today that **excessive exercise** can reduce a woman's body fat below the critical point needed for normal fertility resulting in "runner's amenorrhea" — the complete or partial absence of periods due to such exercise.

Exercise moderately. Everyone should try to get some exercise every day, even if it's only walking briskly for 20 minutes. On the other hand, if you are really "working out" and/or doing aerobic exercise for more than two hours a week, don't be surprised if it affects your fertility. Being trim is nice, but if you exercise to the point where your body fat drops below 20%-22% of your weight, your Phase II may be very extended—a long mucus patch with greatly delayed ovulation. Or ambiguous, off-and-on mucus. To repeat, this is true even if your weight stays the same and is correct for your height.

At the second NFP class, "Shirley" showed us a chart that indicated delayed ovulation. We talked about eating and exercise. She was not underweight, but she had been a competitive swimmer and still swam every day for exercise. She reduced her swimming to three times a week and achieved a much desired pregnancy.

Consider night light

Some women are affected by the light in their sleeping environment. Therefore, if you should ever experience an all-the-time mucus discharge, consider making your bedroom darker at night.

We know this sounds weird, but for some women, sleep-time light is the apparent cause of some forms of cycle irregularity. A Spokane nurse, Joy De Felice, has researched this, and in her experience, total darkness during sleep-time is the key to eliminating problems of chronic mucus discharge.[2] She has also seen night darkness improve short luteal phases, infertility, the ambiguous mucus of the breastfeeding or bottlefeeding mother, heavy bleeding, prolonged bleeding, and constant spotting. Some women are affected even by the light from a digital clock-face or the control device of an electric blanket!

There's more on this in *Fertility, Cycles and Nutrition* which raises an interesting question: could sensitivity to sleep-time light reflect a nutritional deficiency?[3]

At the other extreme are women who can induce a more regular cycle pattern by keeping a bedroom light on all night for several nights each cycle.

Scientists have long known that in some lower forms of life there is a definite connection between light and fertility. Furthermore, in some primitive tribes, there was some evidence that all the women (or nearly all) were ovulating at about the same time—during the full moon. On the other hand, some CCL members from Tanzania report that their expression for menstruation is to be "in the moon."

Operating on the theory that ovulation occurs at the time of light, E. M. Dewan had some women use a 100 watt bulb at the end of the bed and reported on his experiment in 1967.[4] A few years later a woman built this theory into a book in which she claimed that a small amount of light in the bedroom on nights 14-17 of the cycle produces very regular cycles.[5] However, she did not start with women who had already recorded irregular cycles. De Felice found that a combination of total darkness for most of the cycle plus light on a few days provided the best cycle regularity results.[6] It is not clear *why* different degrees of sleep-time light and darkness can affect a woman's fertility, but speculation focuses on the pineal gland which in turn influences the hypothalamus, etc.

We repeated some of this research and found that 22 out of 24 women (92%) experienced some reduction in cycle irregularity by using the "silvery moon" rules listed below.[7] This is no panacea, but it may be helpful for some.

Did you know melatonin is marketed as a "natural" sleep inducer? The pineal gland produces it—in the dark!
— Marilyn Shannon

Silvery moon rules.

1. Beginning with menstruation, keep your bedroom very dark. Use heavy curtains or opaque shades to block out street light.

2. Turn on a light all night long on Cycle Days 14 through 17. Dewan used a 100 watt light bulb placed on the floor at the base of the bed, but we think that's excessive brightness. After all, the idea is to duplicate the light of the full moon. All you need is enough light so you can notice it with your eyelids closed. A light in the closet meets that requirement.

3. Then go back to darkness for the rest of the cycle.

4. Expect any change to be gradual, taking several cycles.

● Other environmental factors

It is entirely possible that other environmental factors may influence the fertility cycles of some women. We have heard a few anecdotes in which air-borne smoke and other fumes apparently affected a sensitive woman, but we are not aware of any research that has been done. We think the scientific community has to be open to this possibility.

Medical checkup

We mention a medical checkup last because for the most part cycle irregularity is not caused by anything pathological.

● Possible diseases and disorders

Cycle irregularity can be caused by malfunctioning of the glands and organs associated with the whole process of fertility—in alphabetical sequence: adrenal glands, hypothalamus, the liver, the pineal gland, the pituitary gland, the ovaries, and the thyroid gland.

The **adrenal glands** secrete male hormones in both men and women. Excess secretion of male hormones in women can disrupt the menstrual cycle.

The **hypothalamus** is the part of your brain that controls your fertility cycle. In our ordinary discussion of the fertility cycle, we describe the pituitary gland as the master controller of the cycle, but that's a simplified version of reality. The hypothalamus secretes hormones called "releasing factors" that allow the pituitary to release the FSH and LH at the appropriate times. Some think that an underweight condition affects fertility through decreased hypothalamic releasing factors.

The **liver** breaks down the hormones of the fertility cycle. Adequate vitamins are necessary for the liver to process the sex hormones. Excessive alcohol has bad effects on your liver, and some medications also affect liver function.

The **ovaries** have to secrete estrogen and progesterone for the proper functioning of the fertility cycle. Rather obviously, if something interferes with either of these functions, cycle regularity will be affected.

The **pineal gland** is located in the brain and is usually not mentioned in standard texts dealing with the fertility cycle. However, the pineal gland is at the heart of a theory that light while you are sleeping can affect your cycle. (See the preceding section, "Consider night light.")

The **pituitary gland** regulates the ovulation process since it secretes both FSH which starts the process and LH which triggers ovulation. If you've forgotten the terms, review them in Chapter 9, "Basic Fertility Data."

Your **thyroid gland** is located in your neck and is one of the master controlling glands of your body. Slight decreases or slight increases in thyroid secretions can affect your fertility. We've seen repeated evidence that minor malfunctioning of the thyroid can have major effects on your fertility cycle.

If something is wrong with any one of those glands or organs, it may seriously affect your cycles. In our experience, this is quite rare. We have seen one case in which a cancer was detected because of cycle irregularity, but *only* one such case has come to our attention.

The couple were young and newly married. She felt fine, but her charted cycle went on and on and on. They knew that something was wrong. A medical examination revealed cancer of the thyroid gland. After surgery, she took thyroid replacement medication and returned to a classic cycle pattern.

A minor disorder known as *hypothyroidism* (too little thyroid or thyroid stimulating hormone) can cause major cycle problems. If you have a pre-shift temperature pattern around 97.2° F. or below, delayed ovulation, and are feeling tired much of the time, you might benefit from a checkup. Note: it appears that levels of thyroid that are within the "medically normal" range may sometimes be too low for normal fertility functioning. Keep in mind that the "medically normal" range of thyroid is concerned with levels known to be sufficient to avoid goiter. If you have tried the nutritional strategies described earlier in this chapter and in *Fertility, Cycles and Nutrition* and still have the above symptoms, you might discuss this with your doctor. Perhaps he might prescribe a weak thyroid supplement as an experiment.

Remember that you can have low thyroid levels simply because you aren't eating right. Reread the sidebar in the previous section titled "Dietary supplements."

Cycle Irregularities

In this section, we are providing some examples of cycle irregularities. Where there is anything you can do about reducing these irregularities, we offer suggestions.

An anovulatory cycle is one in which you go from one menstruation to the next without ovulating. You may have a mucus discharge, but you will not have an elevated temperature pattern.

For women of normal fertility, anovulatory cycles are extremely rare during the normal years of fertility. They are common only when a young girl first starts to menstruate and when a woman is approaching menopause. They may occur occasionally in the first few postpartum cycles and among women with certain hormonal disorders. They may also occur with overdieting, with overexercise, with being underweight, and with excess secretion of prolactin.

Anovulatory cycles

The chart in Figure 31.1 shows the pattern. This particular chart came from a breastfeeding mother and shows that the return of fertility after childbirth is probably near, but the temperature pattern would be similar in any anovulatory cycle. Most anovulatory cycles would contain many more dry days.

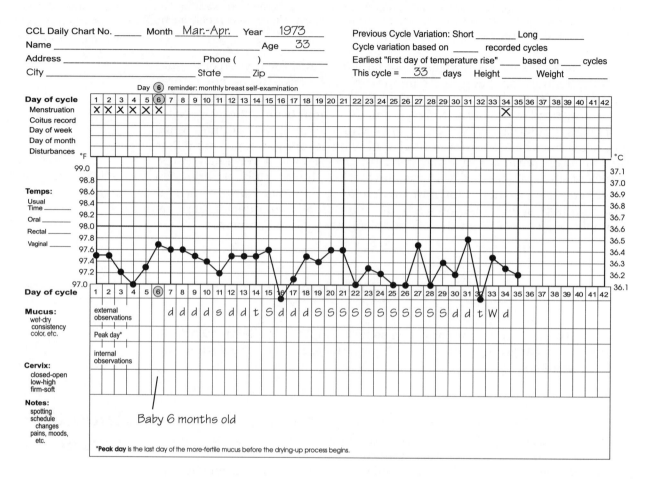

Figure 31.1   An Anovulatory Cycle

Since there was no ovulation, there was no thermal shift. However, there was the appearance of mucus, and this sometimes happens in anovulatory cycles. The absence of a temperature rise after a mucus patch indicates that ovulation did not occur.

What about coitus during an anovulatory cycle? With the advantage of hindsight, you can see that marital relations on any day would have been infertile, but you would know that only after the next menstruation. Couples who have decided to have relations only in Phase III as indicated by cross-checking signs would abstain throughout such a cycle. Couples who rely upon the Last Dry Day Rule would typically find a Phase I. If there are patches of mucus, much would depend upon the woman's cycle history and her experience. See questions at the end of Chapter 11 dealing with Phase I.

If you are postponing pregnancy, do not have relations during any "menstruation" that has not been preceded by a thermal shift. Without that preceding elevated temperature pattern, you cannot determine whether the bleeding is a true menstruation or "breakthrough bleeding" discussed in the previous chapter.

Usually anovulatory cycles occur as a continuum beginning with delayed ovulation and ending with amenorrhea when a woman 1) loses weight, 2) loses fat, 3) diets excessively, or 4) has elevated prolactin.

— Marilyn Shannon

● What to do

About the only time a married woman will normally experience anovulatory cycles is when fertility is returning after childbirth, during premenopause, and if her body fat approaches the minimum 20% required for fertility. The first two are normal happenings; there is nothing special to do. For the third, the women should reduce her exercise to allow a normal accumulation of body fat.

If you should experience anovulatory cycles somewhat frequently during normal cycling, give your health care a good check—nutrition, exercise, ratios of weight-to-height and fat-to-weight, and stress. If those are normal, have a medical checkup to find out if your hormone system is working properly. If no disorders are found, you might try the dietary supplement (Optivite) which Dr. Guy Abraham formulated to help a woman's fertility hormone system function at its best. See "Resources."

Sometimes a woman will have spotting or start her menstrual flow while the temperature is still elevated. The temperature pattern remains elevated for several days after menstruation begins and drops to pre-shift levels only toward the end of the menstrual flow. This is called "irregular shedding." It always develops into a menstrual period; it does not leave, only to have a menstrual flow appear sometime later.

Irregular shedding is infrequent during the most fertile years; you have an increased possibility of this during your premenopausal years. In women in their fertile years, it is a sign of luteal phase inadequacy. Vitamin supplements designed to improve luteal phase hormones (e.g., Optivite) can be effective in eliminating this premenstrual spotting.

Premenstrual spotting

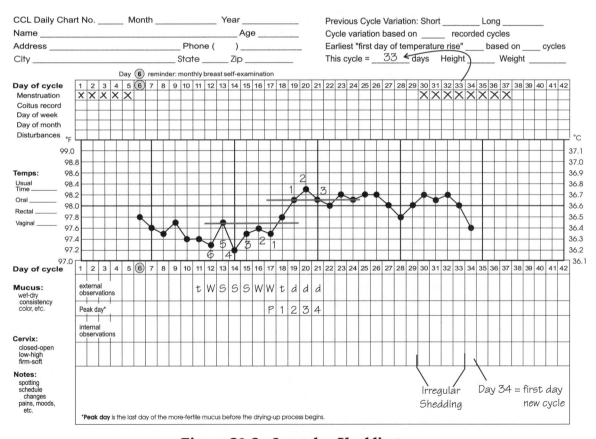

Figure 31.2 Irregular Shedding

● What to do

If you experience irregular shedding, count the first day of temperature drop to the LTL as the first day of Phase I. In Figure 31.2, some bleeding started on Day 30 and the temperature stayed elevated. The temperature dropped on Day 34, so Day 34 is the first day of the new cycle.

Continuous mucus

Another form of cycle irregularity is a more or less continuous mucus discharge—no dry days after menstruation and generally continuing into the next menstruation. Two questions arise: 1) What should you do about NFP signs and interpretation? and 2) Is there anything you can do to cause a more normal mucus pattern?

● Signs and interpretation

1. Without any postmenstrual dry days, you cannot use the Last Dry Day rules for the end of Phase I.

2. For the application of other Phase I rules, check the specific rule in Chapter 11.

3. Record your waking temperatures. You may be able to notice a change between your more-fertile and less-fertile mucus even when you have a continuous mucus discharge, but you will really need your temperature pattern to determine the start of Phase III.

4. In some cases, your cervix signs might still be very clear and can be used as a substitute for the mucus in applying the STM rules.

5. Use either true STM cross-checking rules or a temperature-only rule for the start of Phase III.

Other suggestions:
—More water
—More milk, though milk has been associated with infertility in some cases
—Optivite
—Capsules of flax oil.
*   —Marilyn Shannon*

● A more normal mucus pattern?

Is there anything you can do to stop an all-the-time mucus discharge? Perhaps. It all depends upon the cause.

1. In the "Eat right" section early in this chapter, Dr. Slightam suggests that a deficiency of the vitamin B complex can cause a chronic vaginal discharge. Eating 100% whole wheat bread (watch the labels to make sure it's 100%) is a healthy way to get your B vitamins, and most dietary supplements are rich in this area.

2. A deficiency in vitamin A *might* cause all-the-time mucus because vitamin A is necessary for the proper functioning of all your mucus membranes. Eating one or two carrots per day might help if this is the case. Some women do better with animal sources of vitamin A—eggs and liver, and most multi-vitamin supplements have ample vitamin A.

3. Sleep-time light apparently causes some women to have a continuous mucus discharge. Darkening your bedroom might help. See the preceding section titled "Consider night light."

4. Another cause of all-the-time mucus might be "cervical erosion"— a very misleading term. This refers to a condition in which the mucus-secreting membranes *inside* the cervical canal have grown out of place and now are also on the *outside* of the cervix. In the vaginal environment these tissues secrete mucus continuously. A physician who knows what he is doing can deaden such outside tissue through a freezing process (cryotherapy), laser, or hot cautery, but a physician of lesser competence may get too

ambitious and destroy tissue in the inner cervix as well, thus creating a problem of too little mucus or none at all.

5. Infection—particularly yeast infection—is another cause of persistent vaginal discharge. Sometimes using a broad-spectrum antibiotic to cure an infection someplace else in your body can cause a vaginal yeast infection. The antibiotic kills both the "good" and the "bad" bacteria in the vagina, and sometimes the bad come back before the good. Natural yogurt and acidophilus tablets are recommended by some health writers to help restore a proper bacterial balance in the intestinal tract and the vagina.

A more confusing type of discharge is that of bacterial vaginitis (Gardnerella organism). This is treated with an appropriate oral or vaginal antibiotic.
—Konald A. Prem, M.D.

6. If you have a problem with *periodic* yeast infections, check your sexual practices. Oral-vaginal contact can re-introduce the fungus that causes the infection. (For moral aspects of such activity, see "Marital Sexuality: Moral Considerations" in "Resources.")

Couple X had a continuing problem with periodic vaginal yeast infections. They finally figured it out, stopped the oral-genital contact in their foreplay, and solved the problem.

7. Don't use tampons except when necessary for a short time, and tell this to your daughters, too. Tampons can cause urinary tract infections because the string provides easy access for bacteria to enter the urethra, the external entrance to the urinary tract. They can also cause atypical cells in the cervix.

"Monica," a non-sexually-active young woman, used tampons regularly and was having frequent urinary tract infections. Then a pap smear revealed atypical cells, and the physician scheduled a colposcopy (a further cervical exam). In the few weeks between the two examinations, Monica menstruated and stopped using tampons. The colposcopy revealed perfectly normal cells.

8. If you have periodic vaginal infections, check—or change—your laundry soap. You might be allergic to some but not to others.

"Kay" had a yeast infection that would not go away despite the advice of several doctors. Then she switched back to her previous brand of laundry soap, and her infection disappeared.

Too little mucus

If you're not finding *any* mucus or just very little, start eating the vegetables that are rich in vitamin A. It may not help you, but it certainly has helped some. We do not recommend taking Vitamin A as a supplement just by itself except with good nutritional counsel; it can be toxic in large doses.

See also pages 446-447 for nutritional helps for adequate mucus and vaginal lubrication.

One woman reported very little mucus. We suggested eating one or two raw carrots daily. Her next report: abundant mucus that was stretching five inches. Another woman reported an outstanding improvement in the quality of her mucus although the quantity remained the same.

Delayed ovulation; long cycles

We have already reviewed several factors that contribute to delayed ovulation and long cycles: stress—whether psychological or from physical sickness, nutritional deficiencies, body imbalance, and sleep-time light in some cases.

What you do about some of these is a matter of recognizing your situation and applying common sense. For example, if you start to have some cycle irregularities after you start dieting or running or doing some other extensive exercise, you have to review the appropriate sections of this chapter and make the necessary changes in your eating and exercise.

If you should experience delayed ovulation, you need to realize that sometimes this happens even though you cannot determine a cause. Be glad that you know where you are in your cycle even if it's an extended Phase II. If you were using calendar rhythm, you might be without a clue. For example, consider the experience illustrated in Figure 31.3.

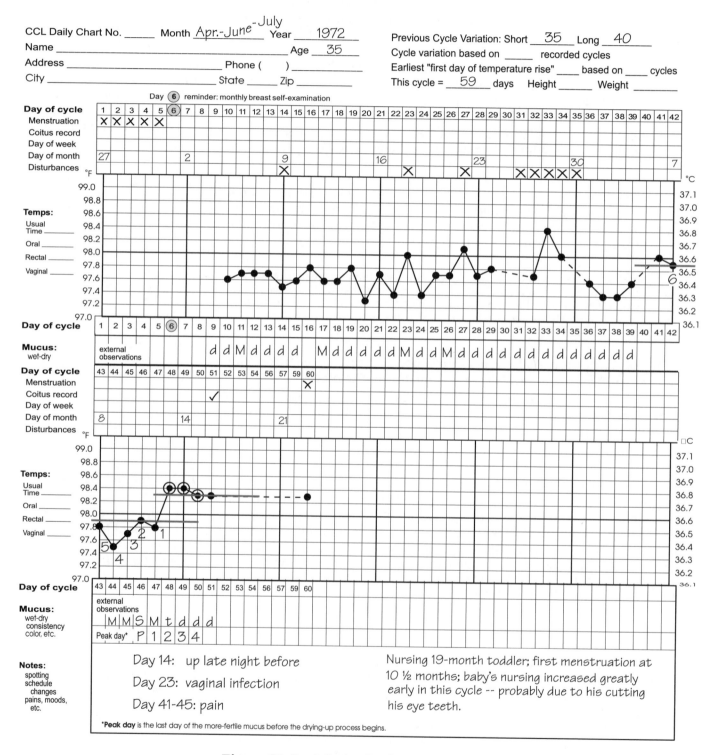

Figure 31.3   A Long Cycle and Trust

The couple who provided the charts in Figure 31.3 had been using the Sympto-Thermal Method for less than one year and had experienced previous surprise pregnancies with calendar rhythm. They had also previously assumed pregnancy if menstruation had not occurred by Day 41 which was the length of previous longest cycle.

This time they trusted what they had learned and they waited. They knew on Day 41 that they were neither pregnant nor past the fertile time. Nine days later they were in Phase III.

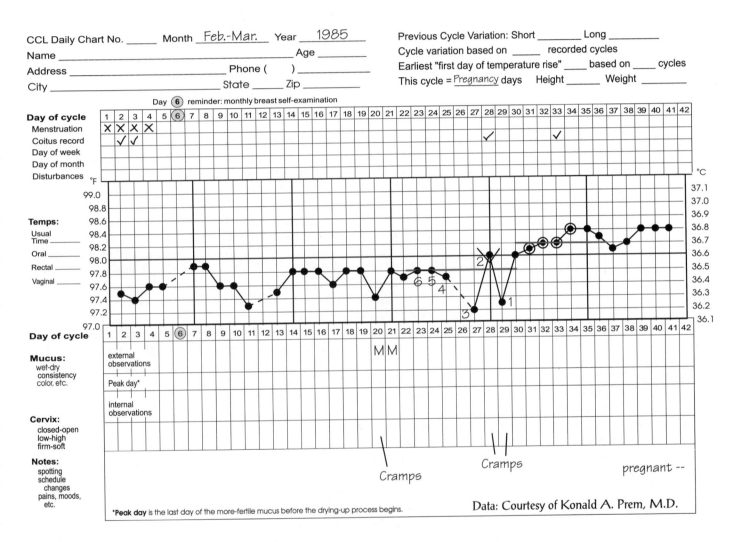

Figure 31.4   A Long Cycle and Lack of Trust

The chart in Figure 31.4 shows quite a different situation. The woman whose cycle is illustrated in Figure 31.4 normally had quite regular cycles; she was accustomed to begin her menstruation on Day 29 or 30. However, ovulation was delayed in this cycle. Although she experienced cramps on Day 20 and some mucus on Days 20 and 21, her temperature stayed low. By Day 28 she and her husband convinced themselves that she must have ovulated. They didn't trust her temperature record and figured that menstruation

Cycle Irregularities

would start on Day 29 as usual. She probably interpreted her cramps on Day 28 as pre-menstrual.

That sort of thinking is called "thinking calendar rhythm." That is, thinking that because her *usual* cycle pattern was a certain way, *every* cycle would be that way. By "thinking calendar rhythm" the couple ignored the scientific evidence that they were not yet into Phase III and had relations on Day 28. As the subsequent temperatures show, Day 28 was very close to ovulation, and it is no surprise that the couple conceived a child.

This chart illustrates two important facts of life. First, the woman who normally is quite regular may experience an occasional cycle that is significantly different from her usual pattern. In this case, with ovulation about Day 28, this cycle would have been about 42 days long instead of her customary 28 or 29 days.

Secondly, the chart illustrates why calendar rhythm simply had to "fail" in unusual cycles. Couples who have good reason to postpone pregnancy should not start to "think calendar rhythm."

Irregular cycles: an overview

Your fertility cycle is a wonderful thing, but it's not a simple thing. As you have seen, it can be affected by a number of factors. Many women rejoice in their newly discovered body-awareness which helps them to understand their fertility cycle, to notice changes in their cycle pattern—and to seek help if necessary.

In one sense, cycle irregularity doesn't make any difference to the practice of natural family planning provided you don't have a very extended mucus patch. Even in that case, you can still practice NFP with great effectiveness, but more abstinence is required. With other forms of cycle irregularity, you may be dry for an extended time between menstruation and the fertile time. Phase I will be extended, and more days will be available for the marital embrace if you use the Last Dry Day rules.

On the other hand, cycle irregularity *may* indicate that something is out of balance; or you might prefer having a cycle pattern closer to the classical average of 28 to 30 days. Therefore, you may want to know what you can do to come closer to the average cycle pattern. Therefore we will try to keep you informed.

● Anecdotes and research

We realize that our comments about the possible influence of specific vitamins and minerals on the fertility cycle are based more on anecdotes—individual stories—than upon scientific research. In addition, there are legitimate differences of opinion. For example, one of our nutrition advisors thinks that an insufficient cervical mucus discharge may be the first clinical sign of a vitamin A deficiency. On the other hand, our chief medical advisor reminds us that nothing has been scientifically demonstrated along these lines.

Two things need to be said about the lack of scientific verification of actions or nutrients that might be helpful for achieving greater cycle regularity. First, much research takes its start from anecdotal evidence. Second, most research does not find 100% results. For example, we would be totally surprised if research discovered that *every* woman with scanty mucus found an improved mucus sign by eating one medium size carrot each day, but we are convinced from anecdotal reports that *some* women find such improvement.

The bottom line for women who have irregular cycles is this: you may

The last word is far from written about temporary or persistent cycle irregularity. Some of the work borders on the comical. For example, researchers have scientifically demonstrated that a husband's underarm odors can help his wife to achieve greater cycle regularity![8,9] Underarm deodorants apparently did not interfere with this effect, but anti-perspirants would destroy any benefit from this source. We refrain from giving any advice on how to use this finding.

very well be able to bring your cycle pattern more into line with the classical average cycle pattern by using one or more of the appropriate strategies.

● Getting practical help

Besides what is in this book, you may need to read *Fertility, Cycles and Nutrition*. The Couple to Couple League publishes this book to make the practice of natural family planning easier for couples who experience more than the usual cycle irregularity. The author, Marilyn Shannon, and her husband are teachers of NFP, and Mrs. Shannon regularly teaches a university course on human anatomy and physiology. Through her counseling, she became well aware of the problems some couples experience—and how improved nutrition helped them. She wrote this book at CCL's request, and it's a winner.

If you are having any sort of cycle irregularities, including difficulties in achieving pregnancy or problems during pregnancy, you may do yourself a great favor by studying and applying the information in *Fertility, Cycles and Nutrition*. See "Resources" at the end of this manual.

● Continuing education

It seems clear to us that there is no one single practice or remedy that is going to be a panacea for every case of cycle irregularity. Still, we remain confident that among the variety of things already known and some that are yet to be discovered, there is some help for almost every case. We will continue to publish in the *CCL Family Foundations* whatever we discover. See "Resources."

Self-Test Questions: Chapter 31

1. True_____ False_____ A certain amount of cycle irregularity is normal.

2. The concern of this chapter has been cycle variations in which there is more than _____ weeks between the shortest and longest cycles.

3. List two kinds of stress that can delay ovulation:
   a) _____
   b) _____

4. Your first few postpartum cycles while still nursing are likely to be
   a) longer   b) shorter   than your usual cycle range.

5. True_____ False_____ Excessive light each night while sleeping can delay ovulation for some women.

6. True_____ False_____ A moderate amount of body fat is necessary for ovulation and cycle regularity.

7. Excessive exercise can greatly delay or suppress ovulation and menstruation. This condition is known as _____ _____.

8. Eliminating all salt from your diet may also remove your most frequent source of _____, an element necessary for the proper functioning of your _____ gland.

9. A deficiency in _____ may cause a very scanty cervical mucus pattern.

10. True_____ False_____ While cycle irregularity posed a great problem for the calendar rhythm method, the mucus-only and the sympto-thermal methods can be practiced effectively in the presence of highly irregular cycles.

Answers to self-test
1. True   2. two   3. bodily sickness . . . emotional or psychological stress   4. b) longer than your usual cycle range
5. True   6. True   7. runners' amenorrhea   8. iodine. . . thyroid   9. vitamin A   10. True

References

(1) Ann Gundlach, "Shannon book already getting results," *CCL Family Foundations,* July-August 1990, 9.

(2) Joy De Felice, *The effects of light on cervical mucus patterns in the menstrual cycle: a clinical study.* Available from the author, c/o Sacred Heart Medical Center, West 101 Eighth Ave., Spokane, WA.

(3) Shannon, 69-72.

(4) E.M. Dewan, "On the possibility of a perfect rhythm method of birth control by periodic light stimulation," *American Journal of Obstetrics and Gynecology* 99:7 (1967) 1016-1019.

(5) Louise Lacey, *Lunaception: A Feminine Odyssey into Fertility and Contraception* (New York: Coward, McCann & Geoghegan, 1974).

(6) De Felice, op cit., and in Shannon, op cit.

(7) John F. Kippley, "By the light of the silvery moon," the *CCL News* (September-October 1985) 4.

(8) George Preti, W.B. Cutler, C.M. Christensen, H. Lawley, G.R. Huggins, and C.R. Garcia, "Human axillary extracts: Analysis of compounds from samples which influence menstrual timing," *Journal of Chemical Ecology,* 13:4 (1987) 717-731.

(9) Winnifred Berg Cutler, G. Preti, A. Krieger, G.R. Huggins, C.R. Garcia, and H.J. Lawley, "Human axillary secretions influence woman's menstrual cycles: The role of donor extract from men," *Hormones and Behavior* 20 (1986) 463-473.

32

Miscarriages

Miscarriages are a mystery. Over the years we have received many questions about miscarriages. We have inquired of medical experts for answers, but we have not found much specific, practical information. However, we will share what we have learned.

A miscarriage occurs because the developing young baby dies in the uterus (*in utero*) or because something goes wrong with the mother's support system—her hormones and uterus, and/or the baby's placenta. The common estimate is that approximately 15% to 20% of all babies die through miscarriage. Some estimates run even higher.[1]

Causes in general

The causes of miscarriages in the first weeks are debated. Some say the most common cause is genetic. That means that something goes wrong very early with the process of development. It doesn't mean that the parents have transmitted a genetic defect. Others say that the most common causes of early miscarriages are related to maternal hormonal deficiencies and the fertilization of an immature egg. In either case, the newly conceived baby fails to develop, and it dies at a very early age. The remains may disintegrate, thus leaving no visible evidence of a baby's body at the time of the miscarriage.

The timing of a miscarriage lends itself to speculation about other causes. By six weeks the baby's primitive heart is beating and his brain is already sending out detectable brain waves, and by eight weeks all his organs have been formed. Developmental failures in key organs may be a major cause of miscarriage during the first nine weeks.

In most, but not all, miscarriages in the first 12 weeks, the death of the fetus occurred weeks before the miscarriage.

While genetic causes are more frequent in the first nine weeks, environmental causes become more frequent thereafter. Examples of such causes in the 9 to 12 week interval include the following:

> Thyroid disease, diabetes, immunologic factors, antiphospholipid antibodies, infections, smoking, alcohol, irradiation, and environmental toxins.[2]

During the early weeks of pregnancy, the corpus luteum is responsible for the production of progesterone. By the end of the first trimester, the placenta normally takes over completely the production of the pregnancy hormones. A developmental failure in the placenta or its poor interaction with the uterus could be major causes of miscarriages in the 12 to 14 week range.

After the first trimester, a few babies will still die in utero from fatal flaws in development, just as some full term or premature babies have such serious developmental problems that they die shortly after birth. Non-genetic causes of miscarriages are more common at this time and include anomalies of uterine development, fibroids, incompetent cervix, and intrauterine adhesions.[3]

A still more technical analysis of causes of miscarriage lists the causes as genetic, hormonal, anatomic, and due to immunologic factors, microbiologic agents, and environmental agents.[5] Since this is not a medical textbook, we will focus on environmental causes because you can have some control over these.

Please note: exercise, lifting heavy items, and running are not listed as causes of early miscarriage.

Specific environmental causes

Environmental causes include some over which you may have little or no control such as airborne pollution and viruses. They also include actions which you or others do to yourself.

Abortion can damage the uterus.

Alcohol, nicotine, aspartame (NutraSweet®), and caffeine (to some degree) are all related to an increased risk of miscarriage and/or birth defects.

Inadequate nutrition is related to miscarriages, birth defects, and low birth-weight babies.

Condoms and diaphragms may interfere with a woman's proper immune response to her husband's sperm.

Excessive pollution can affect men as well as women.

Radiation from X-rays *may* affect a woman's eggs.

Medical procedures such as chorionic villus sampling (CVS) or amniocentesis can cause miscarriages and birth defects.

Certain medications can cause miscarriages and/or birth defects.

Severe viral illnesses apparently can cause miscarriages.

There is more about most of these in *Fertility, Cycles and Nutrition* which has a whole chapter devoted to "Repeated Miscarriage and Birth Defects" including the father's role.

Prevention

The best thing you can do to prevent miscarriages is to live healthily.

● Never have an abortion.

● If you consume alcohol, if you smoke, if you consume drinks or foods sweetened with NutraSweet®, and even if you drink large quantities of caffeine, you need to make some changes.

During pregnancy, you should eliminate alcohol completely or limit it to an occasional glass of wine with a meal.

The data on **caffeine** is mixed regarding bad effects upon pregnancy. There have been conflicting reports about its effects upon low birth weight. Caffeine not only crosses the placenta but it also crosses into breastmilk. It also causes swings in a pregnant mother's blood sugar that can adversely affect feelings of morning sickness and general well-being. The prudent thing to do is this: either eliminate caffeine from your diet or reduce your consumption to one or two morning wakeup cups of coffee or tea.

Nicotine reduces the size of the baby's placenta, leading to low birth weight; it also crosses the placenta, affecting your unborn child. You should eliminate smoking entirely during pregnancy—and thereafter.

The data on the chemical **aspartame** that is marketed under the trade name NutraSweet® is less well known. The basic book on this subject is *Aspartame (NutraSweet®) Is It Safe?* by internal medicine specialist H. J. Roberts, M. D.[6] His book refers to pregnancy on pages 34, 36, 134, 181-183 and 269.

Dr. Roberts starts his 23rd chapter, "Pregnant Women; Nursing Mothers" with this advice: "IN MY OPINION, *PREGNANT women and nursing mothers should avoid aspartame-containing products*" (p. 181). He then lists five reasons of which the last is "No fetus or infant should be knowingly exposed to methyl alcohol, a poison" (p. 181). Methyl alcohol is a by-product of aspartame.

Elsewhere he explains that another by-product, phenylalanine, is harmful to brain development (pp. 34, 36). He also notes the possible connection of aspartame with infant blindness (p. 134) and the appeals of The Aspartame Consumer Safety Network to the FDA not to approve the addition of aspartame to certain food products. In this appeal, the consumer group noted that

> "many physicians are now warning their pregnant patients to stay away from aspartame during pregnancy. Dr. Louis Elsas of Emory University and Dr. William Partridge of UCLA warn that use of aspartame during pregnancy can cause mental retardation and other birth defects" (p. 269).

We acknowledge that this subject is controversial. We also acknowledge that we are much more impressed by the credentials of Dr. Roberts than we are of the G. D. Searle Company that developed NutraSweet® and was also one of the first to develop and market the Pill in 1960. Remember that the FDA gave its blessing to Searle's Pill (Enovid), and it was touted as perfectly safe, just like aspartame.

As a result of our reading of the evidence, we do not allow products containing aspartame to be used at the bi-annual CCL conference, and we do not allow such products into our home. For those of you who remain skeptical, we extend the invitation of Dr. Roberts: "Read the book, weigh the evidence, and judge for yourself" (p. 3). See "Resources."

● Regarding **nutrition**, be sure to re-read the nutrition related sections of Chapters 20 and 21 dealing with pregnancy and Chapter 31 dealing with irregular cycles. If you have any doubts at all whether your nutrition is really what it should be, be sure to read *Fertility, Cycles and Nutrition*. Make sure you are getting sufficient folic acid (400 mcg daily) for about three months before you conceive and at least until three months after you conceive.

If you use dietary supplements—vitamins and minerals—use them prudently. A good thing in proper amounts can be counter-productive in excessive amounts; this applies particularly to vitamins A and D.

Vitamin E is necessary for cell division and has been in the fertility folklore for ages; "Adelle Davis in her book *Let's Have Healthy Children* calls special attention to the role of vitamin E and folic acid in preventing miscarriage."[7] Davis points out that "vitamin E prevents the inactivation of vitamin A which is necessary to maintain a healthy uterine lining to receive the newly fertilized egg."[8] Get enough each day during pregnancy—at least 200 to 400 I. U.

If you live in an area of higher than usual pollution, you might try taking 100 to 500 milligrams of vitamin C each day because it's supposed to help as a detoxifier.

Can a bad case of the winter flu cause a miscarriage? Perhaps—some anecdotal cases point in that direction. Is there anything you can do to guard against acute gastrointestinal infections? Some people think that along with basic good nutrition and proper rest, eating one or two cups of yogurt daily can help prevent certain infections.[9]

● **Barrier methods.** In 1989 researchers at the University of North Carolina at Chapel Hill reported that women who use methods of birth control that prevent semen from reaching the uterus "are more than twice as likely to develop one of the most serious complications of pregnancy" compared to women who had been repeatedly exposed to the semen of their husbands.[10] The complication is preeclampsia or toxemia of pregnancy, and it is very serious, even life-threatening. It occurs in about seven percent of pregnancies and is twice as common in first-time pregnancies. The theory is that certain proteins in the husband's semen signal the wife's immune system not to attack the baby in her uterus, and it applies only to the husband's semen, not semen from promiscuous sex. This finding would apply to condoms, diaphragms, spermicides, and withdrawal.

Thirteen months later, a spokesman for the National Institute of Child Health and Human Development wrote that "women should feel free to use barrier contraceptives without fear of the disease."[11] In contrast to the original research of the Chapel Hill team, the latter research consisted of reviewing data from two other pregnancy studies which found no increased risk of preeclampsia from using barrier methods. Both sides agree that the matter needs further research. Our only comment is that this could be one more example that nature has the last word; in the language of American baseball, "Nature bats last."

● All your life, you should be insisting upon proper shielding of your ovaries from **X-rays**. The effect can be cumulative, and one expert believes that accumulated radiation may be a cause of Down's Syndrome. Also, watch this carefully with your children. One of our daughters had her wrist X-rayed repeatedly because of a break that wasn't set right, and we really had to raise a fuss to get her ovaries shielded. She was only eight at the time, and the doctor laughed at us, bragging about the number of healthy kids he had fathered despite his exposure to radiation. What he seemed to forget was that he has the women in his office take the X-rays from behind lead-plated walls. He also ignored the fact that a baby girl has all the ova she will ever have when she's born while the mature man produces millions of new sperm cells each day. Those lead shields exist for good reason, and it's only good common sense to do your best to protect your genetic heritage—in yourself and in your children—both female and male.

● It has been alleged that fertilization with older sperm or ova increases the risk of birth defects and miscarriages. However, nothing has ever been demonstrated about any increase in miscarriages and/or birth defects resulting from intercourse at the margins of the fertile time. In fact, one NFP researcher—Dr. Josef Roetzer—for years has had couples using the margins for seeking pregnancy, and he states that he has found no increase in birth defects or miscarriages above the averages. Furthermore, if there is any merit to the allegation, it means that everyone seeking pregnancy should practice fertility awareness and have relations at the most fertile time of the cycle. That's precisely what you do when you use your knowledge of NFP for seeking pregnancy.

This [Chapel Hill] research, whatever its value, distracts from the main cause of toxemia of pregnancy. Dr. Tom Brewer has shown conclusively that toxemia is a disease of nutrition. Adequate diet, especially protein, and adequate weight gain are the keys.

—Marilyn Shannon

• Another environmental factor may be electric blankets. "According to a study by researchers at the University of Colorado Medical School, pregnant women who sleep under electric blankets are more likely to have a miscarriage than those who don't. And turning the blanket off won't help matters."[12] We don't understand how an electric field can exist with the power off; we simply report the study. Another concern is the electromagnetic field caused by high tension wires. Does this affect pregnant women who live under or near such wires? No proof yet, but it's being studied.

• Do not allow your doctors to do an early amniocentesis or chorionic villus sampling (CVS). The only purpose of these procedures is to determine if your baby has a condition for which some parents will then tell the doctor to kill the baby. Yet these procedures themselves can kill the baby or seriously injure it. Dr. H. P. Dunn of New Zealand puts it this way:

> It cannot be stressed too much, in fact it should be written down for the patient to read in advance, that: *There is no point in having an amniocentesis unless there is a prior decision to have an abortion in the event of an unfavorable report.* If the mother is not one who goes in for abortion, it is an illogical and unnecessary risk to undertake these investigations.[13]

Researchers have reported fetal loss rates of 4.7% for amniocentesis when done by experts; for CVS, fetal loss rates of 1.2 to 14.6 percent have been reported; a large U. S. study found rates from 2.3 to 5.6 percent, and almost all of these were perfectly normal and healthy babies.[14] In addition to the death rate, there are possible injuries and ill-effects to the babies and to the pregnancy. Dr. Dunn lists a dozen such unhappy events from club feet and congenital dislocation of hips to premature rupture of membranes and premature delivery.[15]

A late amniocentesis (about 30 weeks) can have a therapeutic benefit for the baby. It is used to diagnose Rh sensitization and to plan for its treatment.[16]

• Avoid all unnecessary medications. If you *must* take a medication, be sure to discuss it with your physician, and take it only under his guidance.

Naturally, some are much worse than others. Cytotec (misoprostol), an anti-ulcer drug from G.D. Searle, is a synthetic prostaglandin[17] which is so dangerous to pregnancy that it has to be called an abortifacient.

• If you have repeated miscarriages, seek competent medical expertise in the evaluation of your hormones, physiology, and anatomy. _Natural_ progesterone therapy to prevent repeated miscarriages has become common practice among fertility physicians.

If you have a miscarriage. . .

What if you have a miscarriage? What should you do? Here we write from our own experience and from our Catholic faith. We have experienced three miscarriages—two at about 10 weeks of pregnancy and the other at 13 weeks. The first two miscarriages were between our first two full-term babies and occurred before we knew the fertility awareness you have learned; the third was a baby very consciously conceived during a time of maximum fertility.

The common signs of a possible miscarriage are cramping and spotting or bleeding. If you start having some of these signs in the early months, it's normally not necessary for you to go to a hospital. In later months when the baby is much bigger, it might be different. In our case, we phoned the doctor who told us to stay home unless hemorrhaging occurred.

Each of our three miscarriages occurred in the bathroom, and John stirred the waters and fished around in the toilet bowl looking for a baby or body for conditional baptism. In the cases of the first two miscarriages, we found nothing resembling even the tiniest human form. However, with the 13-week baby, we found the perfectly formed body of a baby boy about three inches long.

It is Catholic belief that the soul of a baptized infant who dies goes straight to heaven, not because of anything he or she has done but because of what God has done through the Sacrament of Baptism. It is also Catholic belief that the soul—the immortal spirit of life—does not or may not leave the body until some time after apparent death has occurred. That is, the person may appear to be dead but is not 100% dead yet. This very ancient belief is totally in accord with modern instances of the recovery of persons who have been declared dead according to all visible signs. These beliefs account for the practice of conditional baptism which is what we did in the case of the remains of the 13-week fetal-baby. John held the body in one hand and poured water over it with the other saying at the same time these words:

"If you are able to be baptized,
I baptize you
in the name of the Father
and of the Son and of the Holy Spirit."

We did the same thing with the remains of our two 10-week miscarriages, hoping that a baby was there.

What do you do with the remains? We entrusted the remains of the first to the local hospital that assured us that they would be treated respectfully as human tissue and buried. The second we buried very deep in the garden. With the third, we placed the body in a jar of rubbing alcohol for preservative purposes and then gave the jar to a Catholic mortician for burial. He buried the remains at the time of his next Catholic burial (hidden inside the casket) and gave us the location of the burial plot.

If you have a late-term miscarriage or stillbirth, the baby's body may be so large that it requires a separate burial. Marilyn Shannon has described her family's experience with a home funeral and burial in the local Catholic cemetery. This was after her sixth baby died in utero at five and one-half months from a cord entanglement. She also chose to wait for a natural delivery instead of having it induced.[18]

Do you need a "D & C" (dilation and curettage) after a miscarriage? There is no need for a routine D & C after every miscarriage. In this procedure, the doctor opens up (dilates) the cervix so he can scrape the lining of the uterus to remove anything left from the pregnancy. In the normal case, whatever has been built up in the uterus during the pregnancy is shed in connection with the miscarriage, and a D & C is unnecessary. The normal bloody discharge after a miscarriage is similar to that after childbirth, and it will last longer than a menstrual period. If your blood clotting factors are low, note that chlorophyll is rich in vitamin K which is necessary for proper clotting. If you think your bleeding is becoming excessively heavy, check with your physician; don't be opposed to a D & C if you are hemorrhaging.

It is normal for parents, and especially mothers, to grieve over the loss of a baby, no matter how early. In our case, Sheila deeply felt the loss of all three. John was especially affected after the third because he held the perfectly formed three-inch body in his hands.

To give fuller recognition of the child's humanity, name the baby and record the dates in your family history book.
—Joy Kondash, M.D.

The time after a miscarriage is almost always fertile. That is, you will almost always ovulate between a miscarriage and your next menstruation.

Return of fertility

Begin taking your temperature immediately. In some cases, the temperature will remain high for some time, as it was during pregnancy, before it drops down to the usual pre-ovulation levels.

If you want to postpone your next pregnancy, refrain from marital relations until your sympto-thermal signs indicate that you are in Phase III.

In the case illustrated in Figure 32.1, the woman began taking her temperatures on the third day after her miscarriage. After a while, the temperatures dropped, more-fertile mucus was obvious despite her continued spotting, ovulation occurred, and her temperature pattern rose as her mucus discharge disappeared.

Incidentally, the chart also provides an excellent example of temperatures taken at different times. The solid line temperatures are her 7:00 a.m. waking temperatures; the broken line temperatures were taken at 9:00 a.m. after she had been up for two hours.

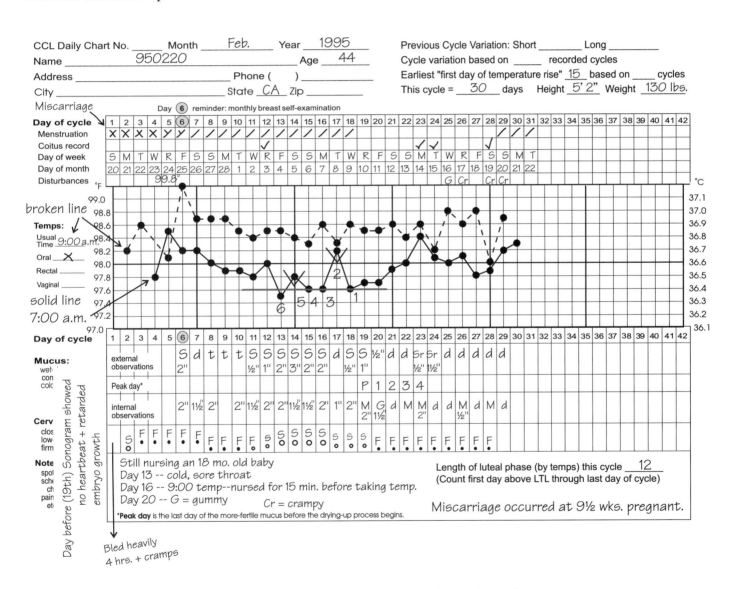

Figure 32.1 Return of Fertility after Miscarriage

Should we wait?

If you want to become pregnant as soon as you can, should you wait after a miscarriage? If so, for how long? Medical opinion is divided on this question. Some doctors routinely advise their patients to wait several months, but we know of no scientific basis for such a routine rule unless the mother had a D & C.

If you are not hemorrhaging or having any other complications, feel free to follow the advice of Dr. Konald A. Prem: "I see no reason to wait."[19]

Summary

As we said at the beginning of this chapter, miscarriages are a mystery. In our own case, a healthy mother in her mid-twenties had two successive early miscarriages and then immediately proceeded to carry her second full term baby. The third miscarriage occurred in her mid-thirties. We are not aware of any nutritional, lifestyle, or environmental factors that would be applicable. Four years later we conceived again and had a full term baby.

If you suffer a miscarriage, you may never know the cause; that was certainly our experience. There are no replacement children, but it is a common experience that the birth of another child greatly aids the healing process.

Self-Test Questions: Chapter 32

1. True____ False____ Excessive amounts of alcohol and even vitamins can interfere with your liver's ability to process your fertility hormones.

2. True____ False____ Both nicotine and high caffeine consumption are associated with higher rates of miscarriages.

3. True____ False____ According to Catholic belief, it is permissible to confer conditional baptism on the fetal body after a miscarriage if there are any signs of life or reason to believe that "visible death" was only recent and the soul may still be present.

4. True____ False____ If you start to have a miscarriage, you should always rush to a hospital.

5. After a miscarriage, you should
   a) always have a D & C.
   b) have a D & C only if there is a clear medical reason for it.

6. If you want to become pregnant right away after a miscarriage,
   a) you can try as soon as your fertility returns if you don't have a specific medical indication to postpone pregnancy.
   b) you should wait for three to six months.

Answers to self-test
1. True 2. True 3. True 4. False 5. b) have a D & C only if there is a clear medical reason for it. 6. a) you can try as soon as your fertility returns if you don't have a specific medical reason to postpone pregnancy.

References

(1) The American Fertility Society, *Recurrent Pregnancy Loss* (Birmingham, AL, 15 June 1993, 7-page pamphlet) 1.

(2) John T. Bruchalski, M.D., personal communication, 20 June 1995.

(3) Bruchalski.

(4) D. Warburton and F.C. Fraser, "Spontaneous abortion risks in man: data from reproductive histories collect in a medical genetics unit," *Am J Hum Genet* 16 (1964) 1.

B.J. Poland, J.R. Miller, D.C. Jones, et al., "Reproductive counseling in patients who have had a spontaneous abortion," *Am J Ob Gyn* 127 (1977) 685.

(5) Amer. Fert. Soc., 103.

(6) H.J. Roberts, M.D., *Aspartame (NutraSweet®) Is It Safe?* (Philadelphia: The Charles Press, 1990). A registered trademark of the NutraSweet® Co.

(7) Shannon, 101.

(8) Adelle Davis, revised by M. Mandell, M.D., 1981, *Let's Have Healthy Children* (New York: Signet, 1981) 20-21.

(9) Shannon, verbal communication, 03 May 1994.

(10) William Booth, "Pregnancy disorder tied to condoms, diaphragms: woman's immune system can attack fetus," *Washington Post,* 8 December 1989, A-3. Original source: *JAMA* 8 December 1989.

(11) Associated Press report, "No link found between condoms, pregnancy illness," *Washington Times* 4 January 1991. Original source: *JAMA* 2 January 1991.

(12) "Electric blankets linked to miscarriages," *Parents Magazine* (December 1987) 17.

(13) H.P. Dunn, M.D., *The Doctor and Christian Marriage* (New York: Alba House, 1992) 42.

(14) Dunn, 42.

(15) Dunn, 43. Here he refers to M.R.C. Working Party, "An assessment of the hazards of amniocentesis," *Brit. J. Obstet. Gynec.* 85 (1978), Supplement No. 2, 1-41.

(16) Dunn, 42.

(17) "New drug prevents NSAID-induced ulcers," *American Druggist* (February 1989) 74-76.

(18) Marilyn Shannon, "Consolation in a home funeral," *CCL Family Foundations* (September-October 1992) 20-21. Though the average waiting time is 1 to 3 weeks, Mrs. Shannon waited six weeks for a normal delivery of the body. She did this to avoid the dangers of having the cervix forced open by laminaria for the induced delivery. She wonders if this might be related to the problem of incompetent cervix which causes difficulties with subsequent pregnancies. When her clotting factors got low, she quickly brought them up with chlorophyll which is rich in vitamin K.

(19) Konald A. Prem, M.D., manuscript review, December 1994.

33

Premenopause and Natural Family Planning

Menopause is the time after you have had your last menstrual period. Your ovaries have stopped ovulating; they are in a state of permanent rest as far as your fertility is concerned. Therefore, menopause lasts the rest of your life.

Premenopause is the time of transition between your years of more or less regular cycles and menopause. *Premenopause* is the primary subject of this chapter because this is when the changes occur in your cycles. During this time of change, you may have signs or feelings you've never had before and which will disappear sometime during menopause. When some women say, "I'm going through menopause," what they really mean is, "I'm going through the 'change of life' called *premenopause*, and I'm experiencing some of its signs and feelings."

In the scientific literature, this is frequently referred to as the **menopausal transition**, a term introduced by Alan Treloar in 1982.[1] We continue to use the term premenopause because it is simpler. Others have used the term "premenopause" to designate *all* of a woman's cycle history before menopause, but that use is too broad for our purposes.

Two other terms you will find in the literature about menopause are **the climacteric** and **perimenopause**. We use "perimenopause" ("around menopause") several times in this chapter. These words refer to changes related to menopause both *before* and for at least one year *after* your very last period.[2]

● *Menopause*

Menopause is a normal occurrence for the mature woman; it is not a disease. The changes that will occur in your total sexuality including your fertility-menstrual cycle are real; they are not just in your head. On the other hand, the way you accept them can affect your outlook on life. Some researchers find that in cultures where women increase in status during menopause, it is associated with fewer troubles or no troubles at all. In cultures where women decrease in status, menopause can be more difficult.[3] Of course, all of this applies to premenopause as well.

A natural occurrence

Age

In the United States, the average age at the beginning of menopause is about 49 to 50.[4] Dr. Alan Treloar found that more than half the women in his study reached premenopause between 45 and 50. "By age 50 about half of them [in Treolar's study] had reached menopause, and by age 53 almost 90% had stopped menstruating and were menopausal.[5] About one percent reach menopause before age 40, and 25% between ages 40 and 45. In our own case, Sheila's last period occurred at 54 years and seven months.

Causes

There seems to be general agreement that the cause of menopause is that you run out of eggs to ovulate.

When you were only 8 weeks old in your mother's uterus, you had about 7,000,000 ova in their first stage of development. From then until menopause there is a continuing reduction in the number of those germ cells, mostly before you were born. At birth you still had approximately 2,000,000 of these germ cells called oocytes (oh-uh-sites), each surrounded by cells that will develop into a follicle. By puberty, you had about 300,000 oocytes, and you continue to lose them during your reproductive years. Ovulation accounts for the loss of only 400 to 500 oocytes. The few oocytes that remain after menopause do not respond to FSH and LH.

Atresia is the technical name for this process of degeneration and absorption of those oocytes. There is general agreement that the *rate* of atresia determines the age of menopause.

In Chapter 9 you learned that FSH causes a follicle and the egg within it to develop. That's true, but the actual process is much more complicated. The only reason to have a higher understanding is to understand the decreased fertility of premenopause explained below. If you find this explanation too complicated, then skip it. You certainly don't need this information to practice NFP.

When your estrogen and progesterone levels are low, this condition is sensed by your hypothalamus, the control center in your brain for the endocrine glands. The hypothalamus signals the pituitary gland to release FSH. The FSH causes a *group* of oocytes and their follicles to begin developing, and they all contribute to the production of estrogen in the form called *estradiol*. Then one becomes the *dominant* follicle; when it becomes fully mature, it releases its ovum in ovulation. Sometimes two oocytes become fully mature but rarely more than two. The other oocytes that started to develop are lost and are part of the process of atresia.

Under the influence of estradiol, the cells lining the uterus multiply very rapidly, and the uterus itself contracts rhythmically to aid sperm migration. The cervix produces mucus, and fallopian peristalsis and the hair-like cilia in the fallopian tubes act in unison to move the ovum towards the uterus.

Premenopause

1. Basic Questions

Questions about premenopause fall into five categories:

1. Basic question. What causes menopause? What causes the changes of premenopause?

2. The experience. What can I expect to experience? Is what I'm now experiencing typical? How long might it continue?

3. Alleviation of certain signs and feelings. What can I do to alleviate hot flashes or flushes if these are troublesome? What can I do to eliminate vaginal dryness?

4. Natural family planning during premenopause. Will my cycles be affected? What happens to my fertility? Should we use the same rules?

5. Entering menopause. How do I know when I'm into menopause?

● What causes premenopause?

The causes of premenopause center on reduced estradiol, the most common form of estrogen in humans. The woman over 45 who is still having regular menstrual cycles has lower levels of estradiol all during her cycle. This may be due to two factors: 1) fewer follicles to respond to FSH and produce estradiol and 2) reduced estradiol output from those follicles. Whatever the precise causes, there are several effects. The amount and the fertile qualities of cervical mucus are reduced, uterine contractions are weaker, and the peristalsis of the fallopian tubes is slower. All of these add up to reduced fertility during premenopause.

● When does premenopause start?

One researcher says the beginning of premenopause is when you start having changes in your genital bleeding.[6] Others have said that the transition time has started when you have gone three months without a period.[7] Another says it starts when you notice your first hot flash.[8]

Obviously, there is not 100% agreement on how to describe the beginning of premenopause. It seems to us that it could vary from woman to woman, just as the age at which it starts varies considerably. The bottom line is this: it doesn't make much difference when it starts except for the woman in her mid-forties who is actively seeking pregnancy. The woman who experiences an early premenopause may be infertile by the time she reaches 45. The woman who has a late start *may* still be fertile at ages 45 to 48. Very few are fertile after age 48.

● How long does premenopause last?

On the basis of his extensive research, Dr. Rudolph Vollman said that cycle irregularity associated with premenopause begins approximately 20 cycles before menopause.[9] Others put it in more general terms of one to two years. Please note: because of cycle irregularities, Dr. Vollman's 20 cycles are not the same as 20 months.

2. The Experience of Premenopause

You may experience cycles that are longer or shorter than you've ever had before; complete cycles as short as 13 days have been reported.

"Mean [i.e. average] cycle length at age 15 is 35 days, at age 25 it is 30 days, and at age 35 it is 28 days. This decrease in cycle length is due to shortening of the follicular [pre-ovulatory] phase of the cycle, with the luteal phase length remaining constant. After age 45, altered function of the aging ovary is detectable in regularly menstruating women. The mean [average] cycle length is shorter than in younger women and is attributable, in all cases, to a shortened follicular phase."[10] "In all cases" is debatable; short luteal phases are not uncommon. However, the main point remains valid: after age 45, earlier ovulation accounts for a general shortening of cycles among women who are still menstruating regularly. On the other hand, once you enter premenopause, you may ovulate less frequently and therefore you will have much longer cycles.

Your menstrual periods may be lighter or heavier than ever before. (Very low estrogen levels may cause anovulatory cycles with light periods; prolonged estrogen may cause a heavier buildup of the endometrium with a resulting heavier flow.) You may experience anovulatory cycles since they occur more frequently during premenopause. Cycle irregularities typically are the first signs that you are entering premenopause.

You may also experience hot "flashes" or flushes and night sweats; these are the two most commonly mentioned conditions, and these may continue even into menopause. The intensity of hot flashes varies considerably. Sometimes there's a very warm feeling, definitely uncomfortable. At other times the flushes can be mild, almost unnoticeable, or noticeable but causing no discomfort. Night sweats are hot flashes that happen at night, and you can get moist and clammy from these.

A common explanation is that very low estrogen levels cause the capillaries in your skin to open suddenly, especially in your "blush" areas of neck and face. These may last from a few seconds to several minutes.

There's a small litany of premenopausal conditions or symptoms that women experience less frequently, and we list them in alphabetical sequence: anxiety, depression, fatigue, insomnia, irritability, loss of concentration, loss of libido, mental imbalance, nervousness, pains in muscles and joints and bones, palpitations, shortness of breath, and urinary incontinence. Finally reduced estrogen levels reduce your vaginal and cervical secretions, and you may experience vaginal dryness and vulval irritation. Thinner and relatively dry vaginal walls can result in painful intercourse.

3. Alleviation of Symptoms

Attitude

If you review the litany of possible premenopausal symptoms, you will notice that several of them are psychological. That is not to say that they are not real. However, as we mentioned before, in cultures where a woman is held in greater honor after menopause than before, there are few complaints associated with perimenopause.

The other thing to keep in mind is this: the above litany is what some women have reported they experienced some of the time. You don't need to worry about experiencing the whole range. About 20% of women go through premenopause with almost no discomfort or signs. Most of the rest may have only the common experience of hot flushes.

Importance of nutrition

The most practical, economical, and healthy things you can do to minimize the symptoms of premenopause are to eat right and to exercise regularly. Problems caused by inadequate nutrition during your years of normal fertility may be increased during premenopause.

● An inadequate supply of **vitamin A** during your "normal" years may cause an inadequate mucus discharge. During premenopause this might get worse, and you may experience such a dry vulva and vagina that you need lubrication for intercourse.

There are several commercial products to alleviate vaginal dryness. Some doctors suggest REPLENS; its primary ingredient is not absorbed. This product also makes the vaginal environment more acidic, thus affording some protection against vaginal bacterial infection.

Dr. H.P. Dunn advises that a wife can also "apply an ordinary domestic cream to this area before intercourse."[11] Okay, but avoid creams with fragrances and be aware that other chemicals might cause irritations. Perhaps a vitamin E hand cream might be among the best. Some of them also contain vitamins A and D.

Another option has been suggested: saliva. It may sound gross and it carries the risk of transmitting infections, but it's always available. Slower lovemaking with more foreplay may also reduce the dryness of the vulva. After you reach menopause, frequency of intercourse and higher levels of androgens (produced by the wife's adrenals) appear to be related to normal vaginal moisture.[12]

The use of raw egg white has also been suggested, but caution was given about possible vaginal reactions to the foreign protein of the egg.

Topical application of an estrogen cream is a common medical treatment. However, the estrogen will be absorbed and may produce cervical mucus, so you would want to restrict your use of such creams to menopause or to Phase III during premenopause.

● The **B-complex vitamins and vitamin E** may be essential for reducing or eliminating many of the discomforts associated with premenopause. We have read enough anecdotal accounts of women getting relief from premenopausal discomforts through vitamin E that we think that women over 45 would do well to take 400 I. U. of natural source vitamin E daily, more when necessary to overcome stronger and persistent discomforts. Some think that 400 I.U. of vitamin E may help to maintain healthy vaginal walls. However, women having diabetes, high blood pressure, or rheumatic heart disease should seek competent medical advice before such supplementation.

The B-complex vitamins are also necessary for coping with depression and emotional ups and downs of the perimenopausal years. You may very well have a teenager who is giving you fits just when you're coping with the changes of premenopause. Refined flours and products made from them have lost much of what you need; this is also true about refined sugar.

Flax oil contains essential fatty acids which are very helpful to the mucus membranes and glands. Women who try 1 or 2 one-gram capsules a day will notice lighter bleeding and many of the good effects attributed to vitamin E.

—Marilyn Shannon

● As your ovaries start producing less estrogen, your **adrenal glands** are supposed to take up the slack by producing a hormone very similar to ovarian estrogen. Potassium is vital for the proper functioning of the adrenals and excessive salt in your diet causes you to lose potassium. One of the adrenal secretions is converted to estrogen *by your body fat*. White sugar overworks the adrenals.[13] The conclusion: eat fruits and vegetables rich in potassium (e.g., bananas), be moderate in your use of salt, be very moderate in your use of sugar, and if you are slim, allow yourself to put on a bit of weight and fat when you enter menopause.

On the other hand, don't eliminate iodized salt from your diet unless you get your iodine from some other source such as seafood or a daily kelp tablet.

Vitamins C and E, the B vitamins, zinc, and the essential fatty acids found in salad oils and flax oil are also important to adrenal function.

—Marilyn Shannon

Here's a more technical description. As fewer ovarian follicles (and eventually none) produce less estrogen in the form called estradiol, the adrenal glands continue to produce estrogen in a form called estrone. The amount produced directly is very small. The adrenals also produce a hormone called androstenedione that your body fat converts to estrone. Don't worry about how to pronounce "androstenedione." The important thing is this: "This conversion has been shown to correlate with body size, with heavy women having higher conversion rates and circulating estrogen levels than slender subjects."[14] Who knows?—maybe the normal slight weight gain is nature's way to keep a woman healthy during menopause.

● We recommend **not** undergoing any sort of hormone replacement therapy (HRT) during *pre*menopause. This treatment started with estrogen replacement therapy (ERT). Then when the dangers of unopposed estrogen became more clear, synthetic progesterone was added, so ERT became HRT. The estrogen in such treatment might produce a mucus discharge, and that could cause confusion and additional abstinence during premenopause.

Once you have gone six months without a period, most physicians would regard you as menopausal; once you are truly menopausal, any mucus produced by HRT would no longer be confusing.

Our recommendation is to pursue the nutrition-exercise path as much as possible for any necessary therapy.

Our reservations about hormonal treatment are based on several factors. A possible connection between HRT and an increased risk of breast cancer concerns us. The facts are admittedly confusing. In 1994, Dr. Ellen Grant, an advocate of the Pill in the Sixties, strongly opposed both the Pill and HRT on purely medical grounds.[15] In June 1995 one medical journal reported a 71% increase in the risk of breast cancer among women ages 60-64 who had been on HRT for five or more years and a 45% increase in the risk of death from breast cancer among women who had been taking estrogen for five or more years.[16] About a month later, a different medical journal carried an apparently conflicting report.[17] Obviously, the situation was not clear as we were writing this book. Our advice: be cautious.

The enthusiasm for HRT concerns us because there was this same sort of enthusiasm for the Pill in the Sixties. "Most studies on the benefits of hormone-replacement therapy have been funded by the pharmaceutical industry."[18] IUDs and silicone implants were touted as safe and harmless. Lastly, we wonder whether it's necessary for every menopausal woman (or even the 35% sometimes estimated to need HRT[19]) to be so dependent upon her doctor and pharmacy for the rest of her life.

At the same time, we recognize that many reputable physicians believe that the best way to ward off osteoporosis for some menopausal women is a combination of vitamin and mineral supplementation, sufficient exercise, and hormone replacement therapy. Research on this problem continues. For example, in mid-1995 there were reports that a non-hormonal treatment for osteoporosis might be available by early 1996. Your local library may have recent information about current theories and practices. Our bi-monthly magazine, *CCL Family Foundations*, reports on published research to keep members up-to-date.

● All of these items add up to the need to become more diet conscious during this time, not in the sense of calorie reduction but in the sense of making sure you're getting the nutrients you need. You especially need to foster the proper functioning of your adrenals. Exercise is also very important in warding off osteoporosis, and it has to be load-bearing exercise such as walking, not swimming. With proper nutrition and exercise, you will have a much easier time during your menopausal years. Balanced dietary supplements may be a big help in meeting your nutritional needs. Again, we recommend the study of *Fertility, Cycles and Nutrition* that has a brief chapter on menopause.

4. Natural Family Planning During Premenopause

Can you become pregnant during premenopause? Yes, but fertility declines during your premenopausal years even though you may have every external sign of normal fertility. You would most likely have difficulty achieving pregnancy—and staying pregnant—after age 44, and you would have even greater problems of achieving pregnancy after age 48. However, most NFP users are not seeking pregnancy at these ages; they want to continue to practice NFP up through menopause. Thus, after a description of reduced fertility, we devote most of this section to the practice of NFP during this phase of life.

The graph in Figure 33.1 and the numbers in Table I tell it all. In 1961, Louis Henry, a French demographer, published data from population groups in which there was evidence of little or no "family planning."[20] Henry's data shows a marked decline in fertility as a woman gets older, particularly after age 40. Several researchers have isolated ten groups for which the age of the wives is quite certain. A graphic display of those declining rates is quite dramatic.

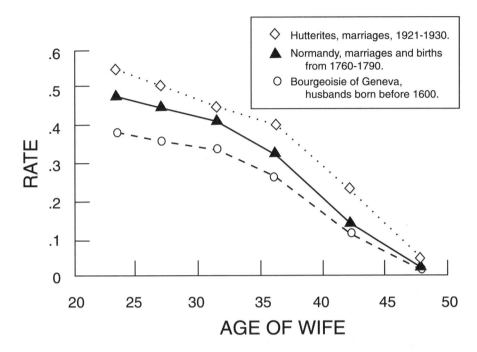

Figure 33.1 Marital Age-specific Fertility Rates
Three historical populations. Adapted from Menken and Larsen, Figure 3.
Reprinted with permission.[21]

For simplicity we are showing the detail for only three of those ten populations. The last two columns in Table I are the summary data for all ten. Fertility rates refer to births per 1000 woman-years.

Table I

Marital Age-Specific Fertility Rates in Populations with No Evidence of Fertility Limitation

Age	Population* 1	2	3	Typical age pattern	Percent decline
20-24	550	480	389	463	0
25-29	502	450	362	435	6
30-34	447	410	327	397	14
35-39	406	315	275	322	31
40-44	222	125	123	169	64
45-49	61	10	19	25	95

* (1) Hutterites, marriages, 1921-1930. (2) Normandy, marriages and births from 1760-1790.
(3) Bourgeoisie of Geneva, husbands born before 1600.

Source: Henry (1961); adapted from Table III, Menken and Larsen. Reprinted with permission.

In Table I, the next to last column on the right shows a birth rate of only 25 babies per 1000 woman-years were born to women in the 45 - 49 age group. The last column on the right indicates that is a 95% decline from the collective birth rate of those groups, ages 20-24. The 25 per 1000 is the same as 2.5 per 100 woman years, the standard measurement. That means that from 45 to 49, age alone is 97.5% effective for the avoidance of pregnancy—without any fertility awareness or deliberate abstinence.

Once you reach age 50, "women who are capable of bearing children are so rare that they appear as single cases and not in demographic rates."[22]

● Our own experience

Perhaps we are one of those rare couples. After learning this, we reviewed Sheila's charts beginning at age 48.

During year 48, she had 13 cycles, all ovulatory (as indicated by an upward thermal shift). The cycle variation was 21 to 31 days (one each) with the rest between 25 and 28 days.

During year 49: 14 cycles, all ovulatory. Range: 17 to 44 days, one of 37 days, the rest between 25 and 32 days.

During year 50: 13 cycles, 12 ovulatory, 1 without sufficient data. Range: 16 to 32 (one each) with the rest between 24 and 30.

During year 51: 9 cycles, all ovulatory. Range: 20 to 128 (2 of 20 days, 1 of 55, 1 of 128) with the rest between 21 and 38 days.

During year 52: 10 cycles and part of the eleventh, all apparently ovulatory. Range: 13 to 52 (one each), the rest between 18 and 35 days. In the 13-day cycle, the thermal shift started on Day 4.

During year 53: 9 cycles. The year started well into a 130 day ovulatory cycle. It ended 94 days into a "cycle" that was 310 days long. In between, there were 6 cycles. A 74 day cycle was anovulatory; it was the first clearly anovulatory cycle of Sheila's premenopause, and it was the last cycle before the start of the 310 day cycle.

During year 54: As mentioned already, Sheila's 54th birthday occurred 94 days into the 310 day cycle which concluded with a very weak thermal shift. Next was a 19 day ovulatory cycle. Then she had her last period which started at age 54 years, 7 months, 3 weeks and 3 days.

It looks worse on paper than it was. During these five years, Sheila continued to have quite regular cycles for the most part, but occasionally there was a very short or very long cycle. We share this for two reasons. First, everyone should be aware of the possibility of unusually short and long cycles. Second, if you reach menopause later than the average, you can know that we have shared your experience.

Phase I

In the half dozen or so years before you enter premenopause, you may experience the most regular cycles of your fertile lifetime. However, during premenopause, irregularity of cycle length is fairly common, and you may have more long cycles than short ones. However, because the short ones can be very short, we recommend a conservative approach to Phase I.

● Do not have relations during menstruation beyond Day 3. This assumes that the first three days are days of heavy flow since coitus on days of heavy flow almost never results in pregnancy. However, if you have only two days of heavy flow and a very light flow on Day 3, abstain on Day 3, and wait until you have dry days. Note well: a very short menses sometimes means a very early ovulation.

If you know from experience that you can detect the beginning of mucus on days of light flow or spotting, you may decide to use up through Day 5 or

6 on such days provided you do not have any mucus on those days. However, the normal experience will be to use a Day 3 cutoff during menstruation.

● To go beyond Day 6, you must be experiencing days that are dry in every way—no mucus and no menses.

● You can apply the 21/20 Day Rule, the Doering Rule, and the Last Dry Day Rule after Day 6 only if you have dry days after menstruation. Once you have very short cycles, the 21/20 Day Rule and the Doering Rule will not be applicable.

● Take your temperature every day during the premenopausal years. In that way, if you have a very early ovulation, you will have temperatures for a pre-shift six. Second, your thermal shift pattern is your only positive sign of being in post-ovulation infertility.

Phase III

To be more conservative for Phase III, require a **four** day thermal shift for *every* rule. That means you would require four days of thermal shift for Rules B, C, K, and R as well as for the four-day temperature-only rule.

In our opinion, which we cannot prove, adding the extra day probably raises the avoiding-pregnancy effectiveness rate from less-than-1 per 100 woman-years to less-than-1 per 1,000 woman years. The late Dr. Rudolph Vollman used to say that pregnancies simply are not observed when couples wait until the evening of the fourth day of high temperatures. We don't believe there's a 100% system, but such comments are very reassuring to the couple who have a more serious need to avoid pregnancy.

Off and on mucus

Some women experience off and on patches of mucus in long cycles during premenopause, much like you might experience during the breastfeeding transition phase. Thus the "patch guidelines" may be one option for you. (Check Chapter 25 for the breastfeeding situation.) Please note that we are talking about very long cycles—40, 50, 60 days and longer. We would not recommend using the patch guidelines if your cycle range is only from 25 to 35 days.

Obviously, the most conservative plan is to consider yourself in Phase II from the beginning of any mucus until you have a sympto-thermal start of Phase III. There's nothing wrong or unusual about such a plan, and many couples will follow that policy. However, some couples may be looking for ways to reduce abstinence, sometimes quite significantly, without greatly increasing the chances of pregnancy. This is particularly true if they have been experiencing very long cycles with delayed ovulation and long patches of mucus. What follows is written from that perspective.

In the normal cycle, ovulation will be accompanied by three or more days of mucus discharge. It would be rare for a mucus patch of only 1 or 2 days to be ovulatory.

● **Patches of three days or more**
Here we assume that ovulation may occur in a mucus patch of three or more days.

1. Begin abstinence on the first day of mucus. Consider the last day of the patch as a Peak Day, even if every day was one of less-fertile mucus.

2. Continue to abstain until the evening of the fourth (or fifth) day of drying-up past the Peak Day.

3. If your temperatures have remained low, consider yourselves back into an extended Phase I.

4. If your temperatures are rising during the drying-up, wait until you have a sympto-thermal indication of being in Phase III.

In this case, "drying-up" can refer to two situations: 1) definite dry days or 2) days of distinctly less-fertile mucus after a patch of more-fertile mucus.

This advice is admittedly conservative. We know couples who use the rules for the one or two day patches (right below) when they've had longer patches. Let's face it: once you are 48, age alone makes you highly infertile. With two days of dryness and continued low temperatures, you have little chance of achieving pregnancy, and that's particularly true if the dryness is cross-checked by a closed cervix. The choice is yours.

● **Patches of one or two days**

What if your patches are only 1 or 2 days long and you never have a full four days of dryness between them? Can you reduce the required number of dry days after such patches? Most likely yes, depending upon your recent experience.

We need to use a new term: "**ovulation patch**." That's a mucus patch which is closely followed by a thermal shift, and that combination gives you good evidence that ovulation occurred in conjunction with *that* mucus patch.

Ask yourself three questions: (The first two are similar.)

1) Have your "ovulation patches" in recent cycles been *at least* five days long? (Six or more days are better.)

2) Have your "ovulation patches" *always* been more than 2 days long?

3) Have you been having 1 or 2 day patches for long enough to say they are now a premenopausal pattern for you?

If you can answer "yes" to those questions, you can reasonably presume that your 1 and 2 day patches are not associated with ovulation. Therefore there is no need to wait additional drying-up days for an ovum to die. You also need to presume that your patch pattern will remain substantially the same. That's a reasonable assumption; it doesn't have absolute certainty, but what in life does?

With "yes" to those three questions, you may decide to follow this system with 1 and 2 day mucus patches:

1. Abstain on those mucus days and until the evening of the second dry day thereafter.

2. Consider yourself back into an extended Phase I on the evening of that second dry day after the 1 or 2 day patch.

We cannot point to any research on this to **prove** that it works. That's why we have carefully described the principles or assumptions on which it is based—1) the rarity of ovulation occurring in one or two day mucus patches, 2) your own recent history, and 3) the presumption that your pattern of ovulation patches will remain essentially the same.

We repeat: these patch guidelines are not for regular cycles; they are for use during extended times between menstruation and ovulation.

In every case—very short patches or longer patches—if your temperatures start going up just before or during the drying-up, abstain and wait for a temperature cross-check of being in Phase III.

If your temperatures stay low after the mucus has disappeared or changed from "more-fertile" to "less-fertile," then you have evidence that ovulation has not occurred and that you are still in an extended Phase I.

Also, be sure to follow the standard rules for Phase I: not in the morning, and not on consecutive days; we also recommend the internal observation for mucus.

The most difficult aspect of NFP during premenopause is the occasional appearance of a continuous mucus discharge either 1) all during the cycle or 2) between menstruation and ovulation.

Continuous mucus

● Phase III

If you have mucus all during the cycle, you can still accurately determine the start of Phase III from your temperature pattern.

If you get no help at all from changes in the mucus, use the four-day temperature-only rule.

If you notice a distinct **change** from the more-fertile to the less-fertile in combination with your thermal shift, use a sympto-thermal rule. This holds even though the less-fertile mucus may remain throughout Phase III.

● Anovulatory cycles

If you have frequent anovulatory cycles in which you have mucus from one period to the next, you may have a situation in which a competent physician might help. (There's a condition called endometrial hyperplasia that a good physician can investigate and perhaps treat.)

● Phase I

A continuous mucus discharge from menstruation until after ovulation can be a difficult situation, especially if it lasts for some time. In most cases, you will be able to distinguish the distinctly less-fertile mucus from the more-fertile mucus. Then the question arises: can you use the days of the **less**-fertile mucus as Phase I and use the days of **more**-fertile mucus to establish the start of Phase II? The answer depends mostly on your own experience.

● **Basic principles.** 1. We operate on the principle that if mucus is fluid enough to flow out of the cervix, it is also fluid enough to permit at least some sperm migration even when it is a less-fertile mucus. To us, the pregnancies resulting from relations on such days are more important than electron microscope pictures of less-fertile mucus that illustrate the difficulty of sperm migration.

2. The key is the length of your more-fertile mucus patches. If you have enough days between the start of your more-fertile mucus and ovulation, then sperm from your last intercourse on days of less-fertile mucus would not survive until ovulation.

●● If you have been experiencing only **3 or 4 days** of the more-fertile mucus including Peak Day, we think there is a small risk of pregnancy from marital relations on the pre-ovulatory days of the less-fertile mucus. We do not know how much, but we ourselves would not use any days of the less-fertile pre-ovulatory mucus in such circumstances.

●● If you have been experiencing at least **5 or 6 days** of the more-fertile mucus from start through Peak Day, we estimate that you would have only a very small chance of pregnancy, probably well under 5%, resulting from intercourse on the days of the less-fertile mucus before the start of the more-fertile mucus. This assumes that Peak Day has been occurring on or before the first day of thermal shift. We do not base that figure on actual studies but on the unlikelihood of ovulation occurring three days before Peak Day and the additional unlikelihood of extended sperm survival.

●● If you always have **7 or more days** of the more-fertile mucus from its start through Peak Day, we would estimate the odds of pregnancy from relations on the last day of the less-fertile mucus to be less than 1%, i. e., one per 100 woman-years of exposure. Again, we base that on the combined great unlikelihood of ovulation on Peak Day minus 3 and extended sperm survival.

We repeat the obvious: if you are having cycles of your typical variation, all of this is of no interest. We are trying to provide some reduction of abstinence for the couple who are having very long cycles in which there are 1) patches of mucus interspersed with dry days or 2) continuous mucus from menstruation until after ovulation.

We stress again the importance of good nutrition; it is important for you to have sufficient vitamin A and vitamin E so that your mucus will respond well to your estrogen. That is, when your estrogen level is up, you want the more-fertile mucus to tell you that you're getting near ovulation.
Elimination of night-light while sleeping may also reduce the cycle irregularities associated with premenopause.

The cervix sign

"For us, the cervix is almost the bottom line backup in the midst of confusing signs. If I can feel its firmness, it gives me great confidence. If not, we abstain."

— J.S., CCL/NFP teacher

Some women have told us that the cervix sign is the only sign that gives them confidence during the time of premenopause. Your experience may be different from that in the sidebar, but the point is this: If you gain experience and confidence in the cervix sign during your years of normal fertility, that experience may be very helpful during premenopause.

Perspective

In the last analysis, for some couples who are very serious about avoiding pregnancy during these years, there aren't any easy answers: there may be some extended abstinences, but there will usually be at least a normal Phase III and a brief Phase I.

In such times, your mutual attitudes are all important. It's very important for each spouse to be extra caring for the other, to show your love by word and deed. If a wife sends some signals that she almost enjoys the abstinence because she didn't like sex that much anyway, the signal might be interpreted by her spouse as, "She doesn't love me any more." Some men have done some very foolish things during their forties and fifties regardless of the quantity of sex. It's a time for renewed courtship.

It's also a good time to make a prayer out of any difficulties you experience. You may have teenagers when you're going through premenopause, and your teenagers will undoubtedly be experiencing sexual temptations. Offer up your own marital chastity and whatever difficulties you and your spouse may experience. Offer these sufferings in union with the sufferings of Christ as a living prayer for the spiritual welfare of your children and your fellow members of the Body of Christ. That's what the doctrine of the Communion of Saints is all about.

It also may help to keep things in perspective. The duration of premenopause is generally around 20 cycles, and most couples experience only minor difficulties during most of these cycles. Premenopause is only temporary; it's a time of transition.

Pregnancy during premenopause

If you are trying to have a baby during this time, realize ahead of time that your chances are considerably less than during your years of prime fertility. For one thing, if you start having very long cycles, that means that you're ovulating less frequently. Second, your mucus discharge may be very scant and of poor quality for sperm migration. Third, if you have very short luteal phases, implantation may not take place and miscarriage may result.

On the other hand, if you should experience an unplanned pregnancy, accept it as a baby who is very much wanted by God. Many are the couples—especially in the days of calendar rhythm—who later rejoiced in their unsought premenopausal child.

To be sure, you would probably have the well-publicized fears of bearing a child with Down's Syndrome. The pessimist sees an increased risk in the more mature years; the optimist sees a 98% chance of having a fully normal child. A Danish study considered a woman to be a high risk for birth defects if she was over 35 and if either parent had an abnormality. However the actual incidence of birth defects was 1.2% in the high risk group and 1.4% in the normal group.[23] The famed geneticist Jerome Lejeune questioned the established risk categories, noting that the often repeated statement that "older women have a greater chance of bearing a mongoloid child" may not be correct.[24] Furthermore, "upwards of 80% of Down's babies will occur to younger mothers" [under 35].[25] As Dr. and Mrs. J.C. Willke put it:

> At a maternal age of 30, 99.9% of babies do not have it;
> at a maternal age of 36, 99.6% of babies do not have it;
> at a maternal age of 40, 99.1% of babies do not have it.[26]

On the other side of the coin, there's a greater chance that your premenopausal child will be a high achiever, and with your experience from other children, you may be wiser and better parents.

Confidence

Above all, be confident. Once you have practiced the STM for years, your own fertility awareness is not going to desert you overnight. You have learned and cared for the tools to understand your fertility and infertility during this change of life, and your knowledge and experience will be very helpful during this relatively short period of change.

If the going should be a little rough, don't give up and resort to sterilization or contraception. Remember what Jesus taught:

> Enter by the narrow gate, for the gate is wide and the way is easy
> that leads to destruction, and those who enter by it are many.
> For the gate is narrow and the way is hard that leads to life, and
> those who find it are few (Mt 7:13-14).

Even from a practical viewpoint, why take such drastic measures when menopause is so near at hand? Ask for and receive God's help to remain chaste in your marriage; don't turn to a life of sin at the end of years of living virtuously.

Be not afraid. Be confident in God. Remember that He has a purpose in designing us exactly as He did, and that purpose serves our true happiness. So let the time of premenopause be a time for growth in your relationships—with God and with each other.

5. Entering Menopause

How does a couple know that the wife has entered menopause and will never be fertile again? The key ingredient is the lack of menstruation for an extended time.

In *The Menstrual Cycle,* Dr. Rudolph Vollman graphed the length of the last menstrual cycle for a group of 32 women[27] (see Figure 33.2). Of these,

22 had a last cycle of less than 100 days,
5 had last cycles of 100 to 199 days,
3 had cycles of 200 to 250 days,
1 just over 300 days
1 of 355 days.

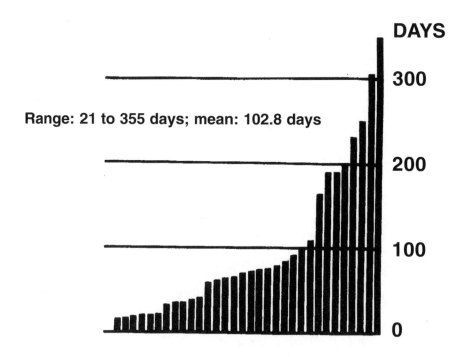

Range: 21 to 355 days; mean: 102.8 days

Figure 33.2
**Distribution of the Length of the Last Menstrual Cycle
before Menopause in 32 Women**

From Rudolph F. Vollman, M.D., *The Menstrual Cycle,* 1977 by permission
of the author and publisher, W. B. Saunders, Philadelphia PA 19105.

Thus, in this sample, once past six months of no periods, there was a 22% chance (7 out of 32) of having another menstrual period. Beyond eight months, there was a 9% chance (3 out of 32) of having another menstruation. Beyond 10 months (304 days) there was only a 3% chance (1 out of 32) of having another menstruation. Vollman showed no "last cycles" of over one year in length.

Relative infertility

The year before menopause begins is a time of greatly reduced fertility, so the chances of becoming pregnant are much less than the chances of having another menstruation.

● Practical advice

Physicians generally counsel women to regard themselves as into menopause after six months of amenorrhea. We would add this: after six months of amenorrhea, continue to chart temperatures and mucus for another six months. You will most likely be completely without any mucus sign, but if you should experience a mucus discharge during the first 12 months after a period (you never know it's your last period except by hindsight), abstain during that time and for five days of dryness afterwards. If your temperatures rise during the mucus dry-up, wait for a sympto-thermal beginning of Phase III.

Once in menopause, your temperature pattern will continue to show variation, sometimes with several days of highs and lows.

After 12 months of charting since your last menstrual period, you can assume that you are one year into menopause. Your fertile years have come to an end.

Spiritual abstinence

Once into menopause, there is no need to abstain from marital relations for reasons of avoiding pregnancy. However, there is another reason, a higher reason.

Completely voluntary, totally unselfish abstinence from marital relations for spiritual reasons is definitely a form of prayer and fasting. Couples at any time in their married life together can offer such abstinence as a form of fasting for chastity and life. For example, some couples regularly make such abstinence part of their annual Lenten prayer and sacrifice.

For menopausal couples, we are not suggesting total or heroic abstinence, but we are suggesting that through voluntary periodic abstinence menopausal couples can make a valuable contribution to the tremendous effort needed to replace the contemporary culture of death with the culture of life. Listen anew to Pope John Paul II as he calls for prayer and fasting in the conclusion of his great encyclical, *The Gospel of Life*, (*Evangelium Vitae*):

> A great prayer for life is urgently needed, a prayer which will rise up throughout the world. Through special initiatives and in daily prayer, may an impassioned plea rise to God, the Creator and lover of life, from every Christian community, from every group and association, from every family and from the heart of every believer.
>
> Jesus himself has shown us by his own example that prayer and fasting are the first and most effective weapons

against the forces of evil (cf. Mt. 4:1-11). As he taught his disciples, some demons cannot be driven out except in this way (cf. Mk. 9:29).

Let us therefore discover anew the humility and the courage to pray and fast so that power from on high will break down the walls of lies and deceit: the walls which conceal from the sight of so many of our brothers and sisters the evil of practices and laws which are hostile to life. May this same power turn their hearts to resolutions and goals inspired by the civilization of life and love.[28]

Self-Test Questions: Chapter 33

1. True_____ False_____ Menopause is the time when your ovaries permanently stop ovulating.

2. True_____ False_____ You know you are into menopause when you completely stop having periods.

3. The longest "last cycle" before menopause recorded by Dr. Rudolph Vollman was _____ days.

4. The average length of the last cycle before menopause in Dr. Vollman's study was _____ days.

5. The change-of-life time between your regular cycles and menopause is called _____.

6. This change-of-life time typically takes about _____ cycles.

7. True_____ False_____ Cycles as short as 13 or 17 days sometimes occur during premenopause.

8. True_____ False_____ Premenopause is generally a time of increased fertility.

9. The _____ glands are supposed to secrete a form of estrogen to help make up for the lack of estrogen from the ovaries around and after menopause.

10. True_____ False_____ Too much salt in your diet can reduce the potassium which is necessary for the proper functioning of your adrenal glands.

11. A completely salt-free diet may result in a deficiency of _____ (that a person can get from some other source such as seafood or kelp tablets).

12. The feasibility of using the mucus patch guidelines during long premenopausal cycles depends mostly on these two factors in your own experience:
    a. _____
    b. _____

13. A continued low temperature pattern tells you that
    a. _____
    b. _____

14. True____   False____   During premenopause there may be an increase in cycles without ovulation.

15. During premenopause, if you are avoiding pregnancy, you should not have relations beyond Day _____ during menstruation; you can apply the 21/20 Day Rule, the Last Dry Day Rule, and the Doering Rule beyond that day only if _____ days occur after menstruation.

Answers to self-test
1. True   2. True   3. 355   4. 102.8 days or 14.5 weeks   5. premenopause   6. 20   7. True   8. False   9. adrenal
10. True   11. iodine   12. a) a history of long cycles with patches of mucus b) the length of your ovulation patches
13. a) you have not ovulated b) you are not pregnant   14. True   15. three. . . dry

References

(1) Alan E. Treloar, "Predicting the close of menstrual life," in A.M. Vida, M. Dinnerstein, and S. O'Donnell, eds., *Changing perspective on menopause* (Austin: University of Texas Press, 1982) 289-304. Referred to in Ann M. Voda and Theresa George, "Menopause," Chapter 3 in *Annual Review of Nursing Research*, Vol. 4 (Springer Publishing, 1986) 65.

(2) Ann M. Voda, (see Treloar above) 64.

(3) P.A. van Keep, "The climacteric in different cultural contexts," *The Climacteric: An Update: proceedings of the 4th Jan Palfijen symposium; European conference on the menopause, Antwerp, 1-2 Sept 1983* (Boston: MTP Press, 1984) 11-18.

(4) Howard L. Judd, M.D., "Menopause and postmenopause," *Current Obstetric and Gynecologic Diagnosis and Treatment*, eds. M.L. Pernoll and R.C. Benson (Norwalk, CT: Appleton and Lanye, 1987) 959.

(5) Glen Metcalf, M.D., "The approach to the menopause," *ACNFP Newsletter* 16:3 (June-September 1991) 5.

(6) P.A. van Keep, W.H. Utian, and A. Vermeulen, eds., *The Controversial Climacteric* (Lancaster, England: M.T.P. Press, 1982). A.E. Treolar (1982). Referred to by Voda, (1986) 65.

(7) Voda (1986) 65.

(8) Voda (1986) 64.

(9) Rudolph F. Vollman, M.D., *The Menstrual Cycle* (Philadelphia: W.B. Saunders Co., 1977) 26.

(10) Judd, 960.

(11) H.P. Dunn, M.D., *The Doctor and Christian Marriage* (New York: Alba House, 1992) 27.

(12) William J. Bologna, R.Ph., "Genitourinary problems associated with menopause," *Drug Store News* (22 January 1990) IP24.

(13) Kurt W. Donsbach, Ph.D., *Menopause* (Huntington Beach, CA: Int'l Institute on Natural Health Sciences, 1979) 7-8.

(14) Judd, 962.

(15) Ellen Grant, M.D., *Sexual Chemistry: Understanding Your Hormones, the Pill and HRT* (Toronto: Reed Books Ltd., 1994). Grant believes that proper nutrition and exercise provide the best way to avoid menopausal osteoporosis.

(16) Graham A. Colditz, Susan E. Hankinson and nine others, "The use of estrogens and progestins and the risk of breast cancer in postmenopausal women," *New England Journal of Medicine*, 332:24 (June 15, 1995) 1589-1593.

(17) Janet L. Stanford, Ph.D. and five others, "Combined estrogen and progestin hormone replacement therapy in relation to risk of breast cancer in middle-aged women," *JAMA* 274:2 (12 July 1995) 137-142.

(18) "Menopause," *Newsweek*, 25 May 1992, 71.

(19) Lila Nachtigall, M.D., quoted in "Menopause" above, 81.

(20) Louis Henry, "Some data on natural fertility," *Eugenics Quarterly* (1961) 8: 81-91.

(21) Jane Menken and Ulla Larsen, "Fertility rates and aging," *Aging, Reproduction and the Climacteric*, eds. Luigi Mastroianni and Alvin Paulsen (New York: Plenum, 1986) 152.

(22) Menken and Larsen, 1986, 156.

(23) John Philip et al., "Should the indications for prenatal chromosone analysis be changed?" *British Medical Journal* (29 October 1977) 1117-1119.

(24) *Cincinnati Right to Life News*, J.C. Willke, M.D., ed., July 1978. According to Barbara Willke, R.N., Dr. Lejeune (d. 1994) who was known for his work in Down's Syndrome, was convinced that there is no correlation between the mother's age and Down's Syndrome.

(25) Adams et al., "Down's Syndrome, recent trends," *JAMA* 246:7 (14 August 1981) 758-760. Quoted in Dr. and Mrs. J.C. Willke, *Abortion: Questions and Answers*, 1988 revision, (Hayes: Cincinnati, 1988) 213.

(26) Willke, 213.

(27) Vollman, 24.

(28) John Paul II, *Evangelium Vitae* (St. Peter's in Rome, 25 March 1995) n. 100.

34

Pre-menstrual Syndrome and Natural Family Planning

We make no claims that we are any sort of experts about Pre-Menstrual Syndrome (PMS), sometimes called Pre-Menstrual Tension Syndrome (PMTS). However, there is a body of common knowledge we can share.

PMS or PMTS is divided into four classes of symptoms.

PMT-A: Nervous tension, mood swings, irritability, and anxiety.

PMT-B: Weight gain, swelling of extremities, breast tenderness, and abdominal bloating.

PMT-C: Increased appetite, craving for sweets, fatigue, headache, heart pounding, and dizziness.

PMT-D: Depression, forgetfulness, crying, confusion and insomnia.

What PMS is

In *Fertility, Cycles and Nutrition*, Marilyn Shannon explains six possible causes of PMS:[1]

1. Abnormal luteal function
2. Abnormal fluid retention
3. Hypoglycemia
4. Elevated levels of the hormone prolactin
5. Vitamin E deficiency
6. Caffeine consumption.

What causes PMS?

None of those six possible causes of PMS "just happens." There are underlying causes for each one of those. What you eat and what you don't eat are implicated in each of these causes of PMS. The hopeful element is that you can most likely reduce your PMS symptoms without having to take pharmaceutical products.

How to reduce PMS symptoms

● **The Abraham approach**

Dr. Guy Abraham has adopted a twofold nutritional strategy for reducing PMS symptoms—eating guidelines and a dietary supplement. Dr. Abraham summarizes his dietary guidelines as follows:

Dr. Abraham's Dietary Guidelines for PMS:

- Limit consumption of refined sugar (5 Tbs/day), salt (3 grams/day), red meat (3 oz/day), alcohol (1 oz/day), coffee, tea and chocolate. (Note: one gram = about 1/30 of 1 ounce by weight.)

- Limit tobacco use.

- Limit intake of protein to 1 gram per kilogram of body weight per day. [One gram per 2.2 pounds.]

- Rely more on fish, poultry, whole grains and legumes as sources of protein and less on red meat and dairy products.

- Limit intake of dairy products to 2 servings per day.

- Limit intake of fats, mainly saturated and cooked (less than 20% of calories).

- Increase intake of complex carbohydrates (60 - 70% of calories).

- Increase intake of green leafy vegetables, legumes, whole grains and cereals.

- Increase intake of cis-linoleic acid containing foods (safflower oil is an excellent source). [1 - 2 tablespoons per day of unheated, unrefined oil on your salad —Shannon.][2]

Doctor Abraham has also formulated a dietary supplement—Optivite—which contains the balance of vitamins and minerals he considers necessary to help your reproductive system function normally. Does this two-prong attack work? Says Shannon:

> Not infrequently one of my natural family planning clients or university students will mention that she's recently tried Optivite and dietary measures and has noticed a definite improvement in both her moods and her energy level—within a month![3]

● Other approaches

Dr. Abraham's free booklet on PMS and Optivite gets into exercise as well (see "Resources"). We've also seen (but cannot recall the source) a four-step program that includes exercise as well as diet. We aren't sure how a mother with small children is going to take a lazy bath, but we pass on the information for whatever it may be worth.

1. Half an hour of aerobic exercise twice each day, not just during the symptoms;
2. Relaxing during the symptoms—a lazy bath or a walk;
3. Six small meals a day during the symptoms;
4. Natural source vitamin E daily and vitamin B6 during the symptoms.

Other researchers have found that natural source vitamin E helps relieve three of the four classes of symptoms—A, C, and D. They suggest taking 300 to 400 I.U. of natural source vitamin E daily and 100 milligrams of vitamin B6 during the symptoms.

There's a debate about vitamin E—natural source or synthetic. The letters "dl" on the label indicate synthetic ingredients. We cannot solve the debate whether the synthetics are inferior in nutrition. You can make up your own mind based on your further study on the subject, your pocketbook, and perhaps your own experience.

One thing is clear. What you do or don't eat and drink can affect your overall health, fertility, and PMS symptoms. Even physicians who take a largely pharmaceutical approach also tell their patients to stop their intake of caffeine.

A second thing is clear to us. If you have PMS symptoms, you should study the nutritional approach further with the help of *Fertility, Cycles and Nutrition.*

The Dalton approach

The name of Dr. Katherina Dalton is famous for her pioneering work in treating PMS with natural progesterone vaginal suppositories starting back in the 1950s. To pursue study of that approach, read her book, *Once a Month*.[4] We limit ourselves to the following brief comments.

1. Natural progesterone therapy runs from expensive to very expensive.

2. This therapy is controversial; other researchers have not been able to duplicate her results. Interest in it has died almost completely.

3. If you do take this therapy, do not start the therapy each cycle until you have three days of elevated temperature readings. The progesterone from the suppository will cause your body temperature to rise, so you want three unaffected temperature readings for your sympto-thermal indication of being in Phase III.

4. By waiting until the third day of natural thermal shift, you accomplish two objectives: 1) you start taking it only when you need it to supplement a weak output from your corpus luteum, and 2) you eliminate any possible abortifacient effect of taking the progesterone before ovulation occurs. In other words, if a woman blindly followed advice such as "Start taking this on Day 15," she would be taking it *before* ovulation in cycles with delayed ovulation.

In our opinion, women ought to exhaust the diet and exercise strategies before resorting to an expensive pharmaceutical therapy.

NFP and PMS

Every woman who has any of the symptoms of PMS should use the Sympto-Thermal Method. Such fertility cycle awareness is essential for an educated understanding of where you are in your cycle each day, what hormones are dominant during that part of the cycle, and why you feel the way you do today.

We have emphasized repeatedly in this manual that nutrition can make a big difference in your cycle patterns. Everything we have seen about PMS indicates that proper nutrition and sufficient exercise are the best ways to reduce or eliminate the unpleasant symptoms called PMS.

We also repeat the need to keep things in balance. For example, water retention during the luteal phase is blamed for part of the PMS; elimination or greatly reduced intake of both salt and sugar are recommended for reducing water retention. However, if you completely reduce your intake of iodized salt, you need another source of iodine so you won't experience a thyroid deficiency and increased cycle irregularity. Seafood and kelp tablets are such sources.

PMS is no fun, but your knowledge of your own cycle and the need for proper nutrition and exercise puts you miles ahead of the woman who has no idea why she is feeling the way she does—or what she can do about it.

There is no self-test for this chapter.

References

(1) Shannon, 48-51.

(2) Guy Abraham, M.D., "Nutritional factors in the etiology of the premenstrual tension syndromes, *Journal of Reproductive Medicine* 28 (1983) 458. Quoted in Shannon, 51-52.

(3) Shannon, 53.

(4) Katherina Dalton, M.D., *Once a Month* 4th U.S. edition (Claremont, CA: Hunter House, 1990).

35

Pharmaceutical Products and NFP

by Paul F. Weckenbrock, R. Ph.

Numerous pharmaceutical products can affect a woman's fertility. This chapter summarizes the actions of specific drugs and how these drug actions could potentially alter the physical signs a woman observes in the practice of NFP.

It is your responsibility to learn all you can about the medical condition being treated and the drugs used to treat this condition. For persons interested in learning more about a drug they are taking, the *Physicians' Desk Reference*, available at most public libraries, contains information on widely prescribed drugs. Patients can also ask their physician or pharmacist for a copy of the manufacturer's package insert, which is the literature accompanying each container of medication.

Unfortunately, the drug companies do not report effects on a woman's fertility signs, other than the obvious changes in menstruation and/or other vaginal bleeding. Consequently, drug effects on the fertility signs observed in the practice of NFP must be inferred from a drug's mechanism of action, the listing of adverse effects in the manufacturer's package insert, or from the medical literature. Specific "warnings," "adverse effects" and "mechanism of action" sections in the package insert with respect to the endocrine and genitourinary system provide clues to the drug effects on NFP.

A women practicing NFP should always note on her fertility chart when she is taking medication, which includes medications prescribed by a physician, or purchased without a prescription. Notes on the chart should include the name and purpose of the drug, when it was taken, and any unusual changes in the fertility signs.

If a woman experiences a drug side effect listed in the manufacturer's literature, it may not be necessary to stop or change the drug as long as the woman knows that the drug caused the effect. Also, just because the manufacturer lists a drug effect, it does not mean that every person will experience the effect.

How to use this chapter

We do not suggest reading this chapter word for word. Instead, it is a reference that NFP users may find helpful when they are taking a medication which might affect their fertility or menstrual cycle.

This chapter has been divided into thirteen common classes of drugs. Questions about drug effects on fertility received by CCL involve mainly those affecting the woman. However, some drugs can affect male fertility, for example, those causing impotence.

The 13 drug classes listed in this chapter are:
1. Acne relief agents
2. Analgesics
3. Anti-anxiety agents
4. Antibiotics
5. Antidepressants
6. Antihistamines
7. Antipsychotics
8. Antivertigo agents
9. Diuretics
10. Expectorants
11. Gastrointestinal agents
12. Hormones
13. Steroids (non-hormonal)

Each class includes a discussion of individual drugs, the *trade names* appearing first in *italics*, with the generic name following in parenthesis. A list of the common U.S. government approved uses, the drug's mechanism of action, effects on the fertility cycle, and some adverse effects may also be included.

Prevention

"An ounce of prevention is worth a pound of cure." This old maxim is still true. Improved nutrition and lifestyles are more important in improving one's health than drugs, many of which only mask symptoms. In addition, deep religious faith can reduce the anxieties, depression and tensions that sometimes arise from a family life or job situation that is far from what you would like it to be.

A healthy low fat, high fiber diet combined with exercise can reduce the risk of heart disease. Men sometimes take their good health for granted until it's too late. Perhaps some husbands will take nutrition more seriously if they realize that impotency is a common side effect of medicines for high blood pressure. There are excellent reasons for both husbands and wives to eat right and to exercise sensibly.

Medications Which Generally Affect Fertility

1. Acne relief agents

Trade and generic names
Accutane (Isotretinoin)

Accutane is used in severe cases of acne called recalcitrant cystic acne. It is a drug which is chemically related to vitamin A.

There is an extremely high incidence of birth defects with this drug; therefore it is **not recommended for sexually active women of childbearing years.** If *Accutane* is used, very strict adherence to the most conservative interpretation of the fertility charts must be observed. CCL recommends no coitus in Phase I or Phase II and using a conservative Rule C interpretation for Phase III.

The manufacturer's literature specifically warns against taking additional vitamin A products because of the chemical similarity between vitamin A and *Accutane*.

● **Common effects on fertility cycle**

Most likely will dry up the cervical mucus sign, since this drug is designed to dry mucus membranes. Up to 80% of patients taking *Accutane* will experience a drying effect on mucus membranes, possibly eliminating the cervical mucus sign.

● ● ●

Non Steroidal Anti-Inflammatory Agents (NSAID)

The purpose of analgesics is to reduce pain. There are many types of analgesics, most of which do not interfere with the signs of fertility. For example, aspirin and acetaminophen (*Tylenol*, and others) are the most widely used analgesics but have no known effects on the fertility cycle.

In contrast, the nonsteroidal anti-inflammatory agents (NSAIDs), which are some of the more widely advertised and prescribed pain-relief medications, can affect the fertility cycle by inhibiting prostaglandins.

Instead of using the above drugs for menstrual cramps, many women and teenage girls have obtained quick and excellent relief by taking magnesium obtainable at the vitamin section of grocery, drug or health food stores. Refer to *Fertility, Cycles and Nutrition* by Marilyn Shannon for a further explanation of the benefits of magnesium for this and other fertility-related problems (see "Resources").

● **Common effects on fertility cycle**

May cause menstrual bleeding changes, probably due to their effect on the uterus and the inhibition of prostaglandins.

May cause scanty mucus sign.

May cause a delay in ovulation and temperature shift.

May cause breast changes.

Miscellaneous
● **Common effects on fertility cycle**

May delay ovulation. If so, the temperature shift will be delayed.

May cause a drying effect on the cervical mucus as evidenced by the tendency of this drug to cause a dry mouth.

May cause menopausal symptoms or breast changes due to its potential to elevate the prolactin level.

● ● ●

Benzodiazepines
● **Common effects on the fertility cycle**

Benzodiazepines,(e.g., *Valium*), are the most common class of drug in this category. They do not generally create problems with observing and interpreting the signs of fertility. There has been some indication of delayed ovulation and correspondingly delayed menstruation, but this effect does not seem to be significant.

2. Analgesics

***Trade* and generic names**

Motrin, Rufen, Advil, Nuprin, Midol 200, Pamprin IB (Ibuprofen);

Naprosyn, Anaprox Aleve (Naproxen);

Nalfon (Fenoprofen);

Ansaid (Flurbiprofen);

Relafen (Nabumetone);

Orudis (Ketoprofen);

Feldene (Piroxicam);

Indocin (Indomethacin);

Clinoril (Sulindac);

Tolectin (Tolmetin);

Meclomen (Meclofenamate);

Ponstel (Mefenamic Acid);

Lodine (Etodolac);

Toradol (Ketorolac Tromethamine);

Cataflam, Voltaren (Diclofenac);

Daypro (Oxaprozin)

***Trade* and generic names**

Ultram (Tramadol)

3. Anti-anxiety agents

Trade and generic names
BuSpar (Buspirone)

Non-benzodiazepine products

BuSpar affects the blood levels of the neurotransmitters serotonin and dopamine. This may raise the prolactin level which can affect the fertility cycle.

● Common effects on fertility cycle

May delay ovulation and therefore the onset of the flow of cervical mucus.

May also delay the basal temperature shift, and hence, the next menstruation.

May cause lactation or adversely affect the thyroid gland.

May cause spotting and, in rare cases, amenorrhea.

● ● ●

4. Antibiotics

Classes of Antibiotics
Penicillins, tetracyclines, cephalosporins, macrolides(e.g. erythromycin), and other classes.

Too numerous to list all of the proprietary and generic names of antibiotics.

If a woman has a tendency towards yeast infections, antibiotics—especially the "broad spectrum" type—can often bring on this type of infection because the antibiotic kills the "healthy" bacteria which are normally present in the vagina. This allows for an overgrowth of the yeast. Eating yogurt with an active culture or taking acidophilus tablets while on antibiotic therapy may help prevent this problem.

● Common effects on fertility cycle

The drugs in this class do not directly affect the fertility cycle. However, they may produce a secondary vaginal infection[1].

Discharge from a vaginal infection may conceal normal cervical mucus making it difficult to ascertain the mucus sign.

● ● ●

5. Antidepressants

● Commentary

There are three basic classes of antidepressant drugs: Selective Serotonin Reuptake Inhibitors (SSRI); Tricyclic and Tetracyclic; and others grouped under Miscellaneous. All antidepressants can interfere with a woman's fertility cycle. These drugs affect the neurotransmitters in the central nervous system, often the same neurotransmitters that stimulate the hypothalamus and pituitary glands which are directly involved with fertility. Therefore, antidepressants can delay ovulation which results in longer cycles. These drugs can also cause higher prolactin levels. Elevated prolactin levels can affect the luteal phase, the temperature shift, the mucus sign, the menstrual bleeding pattern, and in more extreme cases cause the production of breastmilk. Elevated prolactin (while not breastfeeding) is also associated with premenstrual syndrome and infertility.[2]

Taking antidepressants does not prohibit the observation of the signs of fertility in NFP; these signs can still be interpreted to determine the Phases of fertility. However, it may cause some temporary confusion until your body adjusts to the drug and/or you adjust to the new patterns of fertility. **CCL strongly encourages couples to use the more conservative rules for NFP if the wife is taking antidepressant drugs, at least until you become familiar with the effects of the drug on the signs of fertility and ovulation.**

Selective Serotonin Reuptake Inhibitors(SSRI)

This is the most popular category of antidepressants at the time of this writing. These drugs are most active in interfering with the signs of fertility. A woman should expect some adverse effect on her fertility system since these drugs are potent inhibitors of the reuptake of the neurotransmitter, serotonin, that results in higher blood levels of serotonin. This often affects the pituitary gland thereby elevating prolactin in the blood and, at times, affecting thyroid function.

● Common effects on fertility cycle

May delay ovulation and cause a slow or weak temperature rise when ovulation occurs.

May produce a drying effect on the cervical mucus or a constant less-fertile type of mucus with few days of the more-fertile type.

May produce breast pain, breast enlargement, and lactation due to elevated prolactin levels.

May cause menstrual irregularities, e. g., delayed ovulation and menstruation, amenorrhea, and bleeding without a previous ovulation (breakthrough bleeding or anovulatory cycles). Verify ovulation with basal temperatures since the cervical mucus may disappear without ovulation occurring, and bleeding may occur without a previous temperature shift to indicate ovulation.

May cause hypothyroidism, which can also adversely affect fertility by causing a delayed ovulation and a confused pattern of the less-fertile type mucus.

Tricyclics and Tetracyclics

Tricyclics and tetracyclics are commonly prescribed for depression. They may affect fertility due to their involvment with neurotransmitters, one of which is serotonin. Usually the effect on the fertility cycle is not to the degree that is experienced with the SSRI drugs.

● Common effects on fertility cycle

May delay ovulation and cause a slow or weak temperature rise when ovulation occurs.

May have a drying effect on cervical mucus or cause a scant mucus pattern, generally of the less-fertile or tacky type mucus with few days of the more-fertile slippery, stretchy type of mucus.

May cause menstrual irregularity, breast enlargement, breast pain, amenorrhea and irregular shedding.

May cause breakthrough bleeding in prolonged cycles. Verify ovulation with the basal temperatures since the cervical mucus may disappear without ovulation occurring, and bleeding may occur without a previous temperature shift to indicate ovulation.

Subclassifications of antidepressants

Trade and generic names

Zoloft (Sertraline);
Paxil (Paroxetine);
Prozac (Fluoxetine);
Luvox (Fluvoxamine)

Trade and generic names
Tricyclics:

Elavil, Endep (Amitriptyline);
Pamelor, Aventyl (Nortriptyline);
Tofranil (Imipramine);
Sinequan, Adapin (Doxepin);
Surmontil (Trimipramine);
Asendin (Amoxapine);
Norpamin (Desipramine);
Vivactil (Protriptyline);
Anafranil (Clomipramine).
Combination products:
Triavil, Etrafon (Perphenazine/Amitriptyline).

Tetracyclics:
Ludiomil (Maprotiline)

Trade and generic names
Desyrel (Trazodone);
Wellbutrin (Bupropion);
Effexor (Venlafaxine);
Serzone (Nefazodone)

Miscellaneous

There are several drugs which are not classified as SSRI agents, tricyclics or tetracyclics; they stand alone as antidepressants. These drugs affect the same neurotransmitters as other antidepressants, and they can produce effects similar to those of tricyclics and tetracyclic drugs but in varying degrees. The potential for these same effects varies from drug to drug but generally is the same as for the tricyclics and tetracyclics.

● Common effects on fertility cycle

See tricyclic and tetracyclic profile.

● ● ●

6.
Antihistamines

**Trade and generic names
(standard actions)**
Benadryl (Diphenhydramine);
Tavist (Clemastine);
Clistin (Carbinoxamine);
PBZ (Tripelennamine);
Chlor-Trimeton, Teldrin (Chlorpheniramine);
Polaramine (Dexchlorpheniramine);
Dimetane (Brompheniramine);
Phenergan (Promethazine);
Temaril (Trimeprazine);
Tacaryl (Methdilazine). Other generic antihistamines usually found in combination products: Pyrilamine, Triprolidine.

An antihistamine is a drug that is used in cough and cold preparations to dry nasal mucus secretions. It is also used for various allergic reactions and in over-the-counter sleep aids. Due to its drying effect on secretions from mucus membranes, a woman may notice a similar effect with her cervical mucus. Generally the mucus may become less stretchy, and less in quantity than what she was accustomed to in the past. Rarely would it dry the mucus totally unless the mucus pattern was normally scanty prior to antihistamine therapy.

Numerous antihistamines are sold either over-the-counter or by prescription. They are available either as a single drug by itself or in a combination product for colds or allergies. Antihistamines are also used in sleep-aid products which are sold over-the-counter.

Look closely at the label of ingredients on all cough, cold, and allergy-type products. Often an antihistamine is in combination with several other drugs in the various products. Ask the pharmacist or physician for help to determine the contents.

● Common effects on fertility cycle

May produce a drying or thickening effect on the cervical mucus. If the woman is experiencing a dry mouth, the chances are that it is producing a similar effect on the cervical mucus membranes also.

Should have no effect on the temperature sign.

**Trade and generic names
(antiserotonin action)**
Periactin (Cyproheptadine);
Seldane (Terfenadine);
Optimine (Azatadine);
Claritin (Loratadine)

Antihistamines with antiserotonin action

A few antihistamines have antiserotonin activity. Serotonin increases prolactin levels. This in turn can affect the fertility cycle and the breast as well. (See the discussion under antidepressants regarding neurotransmitters and the effect on prolactin.)

● Common effects on fertility cycle

May cause a delay in ovulation and some changes in the menstrual flow along with painful menstruation. If ovulation is delayed then the appearance of cervical mucus and the temperature shift would also be delayed.

May cause breast tenderness or pain.

May cause galactorrhea, the production of breastmilk in non-nursing mothers.

● ● ●

Drugs in this category generally act to depress or diminish conditional behavioral responses, to reduce the effects of stimuli to the brain, and they have a limited ability to induce generalized sedation. These drugs commonly cause the patient to lack initiative and to lose interest in his or her environment.

Antipsychotic agents affect dopamine which is a neurotransmitter. This chemical in turn affects the levels of the neurotransmitter, serotonin, and also the function of numerous glands, systems and organs in the body.[3] The effects of interest for natural family planning observations involve basal metabolism, hormonal balance, and body temperature.

A rise in the serotonin level can cause an elevated prolactin level. With elevated prolactin it is not surprising to see side effects involving the breast, lactation, the menstrual cycle and the ability to ovulate.

Ovulation is not generally suppressed, and the temperature shift should continue to occur. However, antipsychotic agents may raise a woman's temperature throughout the entire cycle. Therefore, the woman must also chart the date when she started the medication and when she makes any changes in the dosages. With good records, she will not confuse a drug-stimulated rise in her temperature with the postovulation thermal shift. Once her body stabilizes with the new drug or dosage, she should easily become familiar with the new temperature levels.

CCL recommends abstinence in the cycles in which a woman starts or changes an antipsychotic drug of this sort.

● Common effects on fertility cycle

May cause changes in the menstrual cycle with delayed ovulation or a total suppression of ovulation. May cause longer cycles. If ovulation is delayed, then the appearance of cervical mucus and the temperature shift would also be delayed.

May cause an overall rise in the basal temperature pattern.

May cause a drying effect on cervical mucus since it is common to experience dryness in other mucus membranes, i.e., mouth and eye. Drugs of this category should not totally eliminate the cervical mucus sign, but it may have less stretch, less quantity, and a less watery consistency than in unaffected cycles.

May cause moderate breast engorgement, breast pain, and/or varying degrees of lactation(from a few drops of milk to full lactation).

Lithium

Lithium affects the neurotransmitters through a different mechanism than other agents in this class. Lithium may either increase or decrease the thyroid function, depending on the individual, and this can cause some changes in a woman's fertility signs. This effect is more likely in long term therapy, yet it is relatively infrequent.

Lithium has also been associated with severe birth defects.

● Common effects on fertility cycle

May change the overall temperature levels, both the Low Temperature Level as well as the High Temperature Level if the thyroid gland is affected. If thyroid function slows, then the temperature levels will lower. If thyroid function increases, then the overall temperature levels will rise.

7. Antipsychotic agents

Trade **and generic names**

Thorazine (Chlorpromazine);
Sparine (Promazine);
Vesprin (Triflupromazine);
Mellaril (Thioridazine);
Serentil (Mesoridazine);
Stelazine (Trifluoperazine);
Trilafon (Perphenazine);
Tindal (Acetophenazine);
Compazine (Prochlorperazine);
Prolixin, Permitil (Fluphenazine);
Taractan (Chlorprothixene);
Navane (Thiothixene);
Haldol (Haloperidol);
Moban (Molindone);
Loxitane (Loxapine);
Resperdal (Risperidone);
Clozaril (Clozapine).

May cause a change in the cervical mucus pattern. Some women with hypothyroidism (low thyroid) may experience an all-the-time mucus pattern that is followed by a more-fertile mucus patch.

● ● ●

8. Antivertigo agents (motion sickness drugs)

Trade and generic names
Antivert, Bonine (Meclizine);
Bucladin-S (Buclazine);
Benadryl (Diphenhydramine);
Dramamine
 (Dimenhydrinate);
Marezine (Cyclizine);
Transderm-Scop (Scopola-
 mine-Transdermal)

These agents have a strong tendency to cause dryness of mouth, and they may dry up the cervical mucus as well. This is due to the general drying effect on mucus membranes. If you take these drugs for more than one day, the cervical mucus sign may not provide sufficient warning of approaching ovulation.

● Common effects on fertility cycle
May decrease but not eliminate the normal secretion of cervical mucus. Therefore the mucus sign may not provide sufficient warning of approaching ovulation. This will depend upon the length of time taking this medication. If only for a dose or two the effect may be minimal and only last a day or two. If for a prolonged period, then the effects may be more noticeable.

● ● ●

9. Diuretics

Trade and generic names
Lozol (Indapamide);
Zaroxolyn (Metolazone);
Midamor (Amiloride);
Metahydrin, Naqua
 (Trichlormethiazide);
Bumex (Bumetanide)

A few diuretics have a slight tendency to cause a dry mouth. If a woman experiences a dry mouth, she should assume that the medication may have a similar effect on her cervical mucus.

● Common effects on fertility cycle
May cause a drying effect on the cervical mucus if a woman experiences a dry mouth from the drug. This is due to the drying effect that these drugs can have on mucus membranes It should not eliminate the mucus, only decrease the quantity and quality.

Trade and generic names
Aldactone (Spironolactone).
Also contained in the combi-
nation drug Aldactazide
(Spironolactone/
Hydrochlorothiazide).

Another diuretic
Aldactone interferes with the production of testosterone. (Women produce testosterone in their ovaries and adrenal glands.) It may increase the conversion of testosterone to estradiol, and thus can cause cycle irregularities due to an increase in estrogen.

● Common effects on the fertility cycle
May cause amenorrhea.

If cycles become irregular due to a delay in ovulation, the temperature shift will also be delayed

May delay the onset or prolong the development of the cervical mucus pattern due to a delay in ovulation.

● ● ●

Drugs in this class primarily work by thinning bronchial mucus. They can have a similar effect on cervical mucus, making it more stretchy or watery and thus more conducive to sperm migration. Guaifenesin (gway-fén-e-sin) is, or should be, routine infertility therapy if there is a cervical mucus problem (see Chapter 21). This is especially true for women taking the fertility drug, clomiphene (*Clomid* or *Seraphene*), because clomiphene usually has a pronounced drying effect on cervical mucus.

Theoretically the following less-used products can produce similar effects:
Organidin (Iodinated Glycerol), and other iodine products; and terpin hydrate.

● ● ●

Reglan is used to facilitate gastric emptying time to reduce reflux into the esophagus. It also raises prolactin levels due to its antagonistic effect on dopamine, a neurotransmitter that ultimately affects the pituitary release of prolactin. Some doctors use it occasionally to increase prolactin levels and lactation in nursing mothers.

● **Common effects on the fertility cycle**
May delay ovulation which in turn will delay the temperature shift.
May cause scanty or ambiguous cervical mucus with patches of more-fertile mucus. The length of the uncertain pattern of mucus will depend upon how long ovulation is delayed.
May cause lactation, nipple tenderness, reversible amenorrhea, and breast pain, tenderness or swelling.

● ● ●

It will come as no surprise that hormones will affect fertility signs. This is obvious for estrogen and progesterone, but it also applies to the others in this class. Synthetic estrogens and progesterones are widely used in hormonal birth control and hormone replacement therapy. The safety of such use is also widely debated. Except in some rare emergency cases, there is usually plenty of time to consider the wisdom of taking hormonal medication. A woman should know *why* it is being prescribed and what side effects she may encounter—long-term as well as short-term. Ask the physician to write down the "indication" for which it is being prescribed. A pharmacist can provide a copy of the manufacturer's "package insert" which includes a listing of the government approved indications and warnings.
Ask for and read the patient information brochure.
Because so many inquiries have dealt with just a few hormonal products, our commentary will focus on them, but the comments apply in general to all drugs in this class.

10. Expectorants

Trade and generic names
Robitussin Plain,
Breonesin (Guaifenesin).
There are many other products containing guaifenesin; look closely at the label.

11. Gastro-intestinal agent

Trade and generic name
Reglan (Metoclopramide)

12. Hormones

Estrogen

Premarin is a popular conjugated estrogen and is one of several agents that are available. A woman is exposed to the same risks of side effects as with the various estrogens which are contained in the variety of birth control pills, although *Premarin* is generally a weaker potency than those contained in the birth control pill.

CCL encourages women to eliminate other possible causes of menstrual or fertility problems before taking estrogen. For example, before taking estrogen, the doctor should rule out nutritional deficiencies, polycystic ovaries, adrenal problems, and a thyroid imbalance.

A woman who is taking estrogen for premenopausal symptoms should expect some changes in the cervical mucus pattern besides the increased risk of breast cancer and other side effects. CCL encourages women to seek alternative, more natural approaches to relieving these symptoms(refer to the book *Fertility, Cycles and Nutrition*).

● **Birth defects.** When taking estrogen, a woman in her fertile years should consider herself in Phase II and abstain until she is past ovulation as determined by the basal temperature shift. There is a higher risk of birth defects in children conceived while taking estrogen products. Read the entire **"Warning"** section under the individual estrogen products in the *Physician's Desk Reference* (PDR) or other reference books available at pharmacies, public libraries or bookstores.

Once a woman is into menopause, the concern over birth defects is no longer an issue. However, the risks of cancer and other side effects continue to be a concern.

● **Common effects on the fertility cycle**

May slightly lower the basal body temperature levels.

May produce signs of mucus, possibly the more-fertile type, especially if applied vaginally.

May cause the cervix to change, i.e., open, rise, and soften, especially with vaginal preparations. (This is in theory at this time since there have been no reports to CCL headquarters of this experience.)

Other possible effects: breakthrough bleeding, spotting, change in menstrual flow, PMS, amenorrhea during and after treatment, dysmenorrhea, breast tenderness with enlargement or possible breastmilk secretion, and changes in libido; cancer, blood clots and gall bladder disease are other possible side effects from estrogen therapy.

Progesterone

The progesterone question comes most frequently from women who have been advised to take this drug either to 1) bring on a period because she has some form of secondary amenorrhea (absence of menstruation after puberty) or 2) to stop excessive bleeding.

Provera has been the more commonly known form of progestin and has been the source of many inquiries. It is Upjohn's trade name for the generic medroxyprogesterone acetate which is available from non-Upjohn sources. (Pharmacia-Upjohn is an American drug company that produces a drug whose *only* government-approved use is for abortion. It also produces other hormonal products for birth control which can work by causing an early abortion rather than preventing conception. CCL supports the right-to-life boycott of Upjohn products.)

***Trade* and generic names**
   Oral: *Premarin* (Conjugated estrogens);
   Estrace (Estradiol);
   Ogen (Estropipate);
   Estratab, Menest (Esterfied estrogens).
   Vaginal creams: *Premarin, Ogen, Estrace, Ortho Dienestrol.*
   Skin patch: *Estraderm, Climara* (Estradiol).

Progesterone therapy to stop excessive bleeding is good treatment if the bleeding is due to endometrial hyperplasia, but hyperplasia must be diagnosed first by endometrial biopsy.
   — Konald A. Prem, M.D.

● U.S. Government approved "indications"

There are only two U.S. government approved indications for progestin therapy: 1) secondary amenorrhea (absence of periods), as a test to determine if estrogen is being produced; 2) abnormal uterine bleeding due to hormonal imbalance in the absence of organic pathology such as fibroids or uterine cancer. Note: **Progestin** is a synthetic form of progesterone.

Progestins are also used in birth control products and for hormone replacement therapy.

Trade **and generic names**

Provera, Amen, Cycrin (Medroxyprogesterone); *Norlutin* (Norethindrone); *Norlutate, Aygestin* (Norethindrone acetate); and additional generic products.

● Contraindications and warnings

Be sure to read the Patient Insert. There are seven contraindications which may be a cause of concern. Progestins, such as *Provera*, should not be used in the first four months of pregnancy. They are not effective in preventing miscarriage and may harm the baby. The cause of miscarriage is usually a defective ovum which these agents could not be expected to influence. In fact, progestins have a uterine relaxant property which may actually delay the miscarriage. These agents have been linked to genital abnormalities in babies who were exposed to progestins in the first trimester of pregnancy. (The case may be different with *natural* progesterone.) The benefit of the drug should outweigh the risk if used during pregnancy.

● Common effects on the fertility cycle

Progesterone will elevate the basal body temperature usually producing an elevated flat level which looks much like a post-ovulatory temperature shift. It would be difficult to detect ovulation if it should occur.

Will have a drying effect on cervical mucus, producing a thick, tacky mucus if any at all, similar to a post-ovulatory type of mucus..

Will probably have a similar effect on the cervix—closing, lowering and firming.

When taking progestin to control excessive bleeding, it will make it difficult to know if and when ovulation will occur. With the physician's approval, consider beginning the drug only after ovulation has occurred as demonstrated by the temperature sign and take it only during the true luteal phase of the cycle.

● Other adverse effects

"Possible adverse reactions" listed in the Patient Insert include (in alphabetical sequence): amenorrhea, breakthrough bleeding, changes in cervical erosion and cervical secretions, changes in menstrual flow, mental depression, and spotting.

Hormonal birth control agents

There are many various forms which usually contain the combination of estrogen and progestin but sometimes are progestin-only. The combination drugs affect fertility adversely by suppressing ovulation, thickening cervical mucus, and preventing the normal development of the inner lining of the uterus, thus preventing implantation.

The progestin-only drug seems to have a lesser effect on ovulation than the combination pills. Its primary effectiveness appears to come from its prevention of implantation. The effect on implantation makes these, as well as the combination pills, abortifacients, which means they have the ability to cause an abortion. It is possible with any given cycle which is controlled by this powerful drug.

Trade **and generic names**

These products include oral tablets generically referred to as "the Pill," implants (e.g. *Norplant*) and injections (e.g. *Depo-Provera*). The list of product names is too long to include for the purposes of this chapter.

If you have to take the birth control pill for a medical reason, please review the section on "medical-moral abstinence" in Chapter 17.

● U.S. Government approved use

The only approved use of these agents is for birth control except for *Depo-Provera* which includes the additional indication of use in endometrial and renal cancer.

● Other uses

Physicians will sometimes prescribe one of the hormonal birth control agents for a short time to control endometriosis and ovarian cysts. When taken for legitimate medical reasons, these drugs still retain all their potential for adverse effects; they also retain their potential to cause early abortions if the woman continues to ovulate.

● Common effects on fertility cycle

These products are incompatible with the observation of the fertility signs, producing an elevated flat basal body temperature pattern, little if any cervical mucus, and most likely an unchanging cervix.

● Other adverse effects

The authoritative drug reference, *Facts and Comparisons*, lists 78 side effects.[4] The package insert for any particular brand will list a similar number, if not identical.

Among the principal risks are blood clotting defects and increased risk of cancers, especially breast cancer. Among those with the potential to complicate life after the Pill are prolonged amenorrhea upon discontinuation, elevated prolactin levels, and vaginal yeast infections. For more information, reread in Chapter 1, the sections, "Why not use the Pill?" and "Why not use Norplant and Depo-Provera?" Read also *The Pill: How does it work? Is it safe?*, a pamphlet published by CCL (see "Resources").

Thyroid hormone

Drugs in this class are used to replace a deficiency of naturally occurring thyroid hormones.

Trade and generic names
Synthroid, Levothroid (Levothyroxine);
Armour Thyroid (Thyroid desiccated);
Proloid (Thyroglobulin);
Cytomel (Liothyronine);
Euthroid, Thyrolar (Liotrix).

● Common effects on fertility cycle

Generally will improve the fertility signs as the thyroid gland functions more normally.

Should cause an overall upward shift in the Low Temperature Level and High Temperature Level.

Should generally improve the mucus sign.

● ●

Ovulation Stimulants
Clomiphene

Trade and generic names
Clomid, Serophene, Milophene (Clomiphene)

Clomiphene acts as an anti-estrogen agent to make the body think it needs more FSH. FSH is necessary to develop a follicle. It is generally taken for five days beginning on day three or five of the cycle to stimulate the development of a follicle.

● Common effects on the fertility cycle

Clomiphene most likely will cause a drying effect on the cervical mucus because of its anti-estrogen properties, especially if the woman takes the drug for more than one cycle. Taking guaifenesin may help to counter this effect and to produce sufficient mucus for sperm migration.

Also, the cervix will most likely *not* show the normal changes you would expect during a cycle not influenced by this drug.

Clomiphene should not affect the basal body temperature, and you should easily identify the upward shift in temperatures after ovulation.

Other possible effects: abdominal discomfort due to ovarian enlargement; "hot flushes" similar to menopause, and multiple births.

Urofollitropin

Urofollitropin is given on successive days leading up to ovulation to promote follicular development.

● Common effects on fertility cycle

Urofollitropin should not adversely affect the basal temperature pattern, cervical mucus or cervix. In fact, it may cause greater development of the cervical mucus.

Trade **and generic name**
Metrodin (Urofollitropin) injection.

Gonadotropins

Menotropins are from a natural source (not synthetic) of FSH and LH that is given on successive days leading up to ovulation to promote follicular development.

● Common effects on fertility cycle

Pergonal should not adversely affect the basal temperature, cervical mucus or cervix. It may enhance the cervical mucus.

Other possible effects: Ovarian enlargement, multiple births.

Trade **and generic names**
Pergonal, Humegon (Menotropins) injection

Chorionic Gonadotropin (HCG)

HCG products stimulate ovulation in the same manner as LH.

● Common effects on fertility cycle

Stimulates ovulation of an already developed follicle.

Trade **and generic names**
A.P.L., Profasi HP (Human Chorionic Gonadotropin) and others

● ●

Anti-endometriosis

Two drugs, Danazol and Leuprolide, are used in the treatment of endometriosis; however, Leuprolide has largely replaced the former.

● Common effects on fertility cycle

Both will completely suppress fertility in most women and place them into temporary menopause.

Both will suppress the signs of fertility since ovulation is suppressed. However, if cervical mucus should appear while taking these drugs, consider it a sign of fertility and abstain. They may cause birth defects. Leuprolide and Danazol may produce androgenic effects in a baby, and Leuprolide may also

Trade **and generic names**
Danocrine (Danazol); Lupron Depot (Leuprolide).

cause an early abortion. Therefore, CCL recommends complete abstinence through at least the first cycle or during the first 30 days of therapy, if the menstrual period does not appear.

The endometriosis itself makes pregnancy unlikely because of its effects on the fertility organs.

● Other adverse effects

Hot flushes, masculinization effects such as facial hair (much worse with Danazol) which are generally reversible, vaginitis and bleeding discharges, and breast tenderness.

● ● ●

13. Steroids

Trade **and generic names**
Cortisone-Generic;
Deltasone, Orasone (Prednisone);
Medrol, Depo-Medrol (Methylprednisolone);
Celestone (Betamethasone);
Decadron, Hexadrol (Dexamethasone);
Cortef (Hydrocortisone);
Delta-Cortef (Prednisolone);
Aristocort, Kenacort (Triamcinolone)

This class of drugs is frequently referred to by the single generic name of cortisone. Steroid hormones are different in function from the sex hormones but are similar in chemical structure. They also are administered orally, by injection, and topically, that is, by creams, ointments, and oral and nasal inhalers. Topical applications are least likely to cause adverse effects on fertility; oral and injectable products have a greater tendency to cause a disturbance in the fertility cycle.

● Common effects on fertility cycle

May significantly delay ovulation, sometimes causing extended amenorrhea. Therefore, the mucus sign may not appear until later than usual. The temperature shift will be correspondingly delayed but will provide a positive sign that ovulation has occurred.

May cause menstrual bleeding irregularities and post-menopausal bleeding possibly associated with a stimulation of estrogen production.

Caution: This class of drugs has an interrelationship with the pituitary and thyroid glands, and there is speculation that these drugs may prolong the fertile time further into the temperature shift. Therefore, if the wife is taking any form of steroid medication, CCL suggests that the couple should add at least two days to the most conservative Phase III interpretation.

● ● ●

A closing note

The pharmaceutical industry continues to research and market new products. A book such as this cannot keep current.

If your physician prescribes a medication, don't be afraid to ask both him and the pharmacist a very simple question: "Will this affect my fertility or my menstrual cycle?" "If I become pregnant, how will this affect my baby?" Ask for and read the package insert that comes with all prescription medications. Carefully read the label of non-prescription medications.

In short, don't take a drug unless you really need it. When you have such a need, become an informed consumer.

References

1. Shannon, 85-89.
2. Shannon, 59-60.
3. Shannon, 71-72.
4. *Facts and Comparisons* "Oral Contraceptives, Adverse reactions," (St. Louis: Facts and Comparison: 1996 and continually updated) 107i.

Part VII: Helping Others

Up to this point, the focus of this book has been on **you**—*your* signs of fertility and *your* response to the Lord in living a chaste and generous marriage.

At this point you may realize that Natural Family Planning is one of the best kept "secrets" of the modern world despite the efforts of CCL and other organizations to make it known. Perhaps you may feel like one of those servants in the biblical parable of the talents (Mt 25: 14-30) whose master entrusted to his stewardship a certain treasure . You want to do something to put your new talent to work. You want to share it with others so that you too can hear some day: "Well done, good and faithful servant; you have been faithful over a little, I will set you over much; enter the joy of your Master" (Mt 25: 21). The three chapters in this part of the book are about sharing with **others** what others have shared with you.

36

Educating Your Doctor and Your Friends

If you expect your doctor to know much about Natural Family Planning, you may be surprised. The same holds true for many other health care professionals including nurses and physician assistants. Why? There are several obvious reasons, and all of them—or none of them—may apply to your own doctor and his staff.

1. Education. Most medical and nursing schools have no course on natural family planning, not even a visiting lecturer for one or two hours. What gets attention? Disease, drugs, physical therapy or surgery, and other forms of patient care. However, NFP is not a disease; it requires no drugs; it needs no physical therapy or surgery; and as an NFP user, you are hardly a "patient." NFP doesn't get lost in the shuffle; it never gets into the deck!

Then there's the problem of faulty education. If NFP is mentioned, it may be based on experiences of wrong-way calendar rhythm or statistics from a group of couples who had no serious motivation to avoid pregnancy. If enough people in any study decide to take chances, the statistics are going to show a high rate of "user unplanned pregnancies."

2. Attitudes. Many doctors believe that men will not accept any abstinence. No doubt some doctors have listened to harried wives complain about husbands who won't leave them alone and who ask for something—anything!—to keep from getting pregnant while their husbands use them day and night. From this can come the view that a husband has as much sexual self-control as a bull in the presence of an estrous (in-heat) cow. With such a view, the doctor who admits that NFP works very well as a method won't believe that you and your husband are capable of making it work. Or he may think that you are an elite couple but that ordinary couples won't accept the abstinence of NFP.

3. Time. Education in Natural Family Planning takes some time—several hours at least—and time normally costs money. The only reason CCL can give its NFP class instruction so cheaply is that our professionally trained Teaching Couples volunteer their time. Instruction during normal working hours by doctors or their staff would be quite expensive.

4. Money. We hope this doesn't apply to your physician, but it may apply to some: there's no money for the doctor in promoting NFP. There are no diaphragms to be fitted and refitted, no IUDs to be inserted and removed, no Pills to be prescribed and re-prescribed, no checkups to make sure the Pill isn't harming you, no sterilization surgery, no infected uterus or sterilization complications to treat. Note also that it usually costs more—sometimes much more—to *remove* an implant such as Norplant than to insert it.

Consider the birth control history of a typical modern woman—and the money it costs. She starts taking the Pill six months before she's married, probably sooner if she's fornicating. She has to keep going in every six months for a medical checkup and probably switches brands at least once. Then she gets worried about the Pill so she gets fitted with a diaphragm and buys the necessary creams or jellies. Wanting to be really safe, her husband uses condoms also. Then they decide to have their two children. After her second child, she has a tubal ligation. There's about a one-in-three chance that within a few years she will experience some unhappy effects called Tubal Ligation Syndrome. She may start having much heavier and more painful periods so she needs more medical treatment. If the problems continue, she may have a hysterectomy. If her doctor removes her ovaries as well, then she's a candidate for hormone replacement therapy for years and years.

The last part of that scenario applies only to a minority, but the first part is all too typical. Furthermore, the scenario omits the infertility that sometimes results from the Pill or from pre-marital sex; it also omits treatment for the sexually transmitted diseases of many young women—single and married.

Add it all up. The modern lifestyle that rejects sexual self-control both before marriage and within marriage is costly.

We and you would like to think that your doctor is not prejudiced against NFP because there's no money in it for him or her. Unfortunately, in a culture in which some physicians murder unborn children by the thousands and are not ostracized by their medical associations, questions are raised that would not have been entertained for a moment in the 1950s.

On the other hand, if there is a physician in your area who is NFP-only, he will be grateful for your support—emotional and financial. He doesn't generate a practice from providing unnatural forms of birth control, and he will understand your concerns.

5. Personal experience. The birth control practices of your physician and his or her spouse may well affect the doctor's thinking. The odds are very heavy that if they are in their fertile years, they're using unnatural methods of birth control, and so it's likely that your doctor may have a bias towards unnatural methods and against NFP.

Educating the professionals

1. Materials. Simple ignorance may be the major cause of your physician's bias regarding Natural Family Planning. An easy way to break down prejudice based on ignorance is to give your doctor good educational materials.

—*Dear Healthcare Provider* is a short brochure written by Dr. John Bruchalski, a specialist in obstetrics and gynecology. In it he explains why he recommends only NFP for family planning and why "without a doubt, the women who choose to study the Sympto-Thermal Method will become your best [informed] patients."

—*A Healthcare Provider's Reference* was written for doctors and other health care professionals with the help of Dr. Konald A. Prem when he was a professor of obstetrics and gynecology at the University of Minnesota Medical

School. Every doctor will recognize the higher level of language used in this leaflet. Most doctors appreciate the simplified explanations we use in *The Art of Natural Family Planning*.

—*The Effectiveness of Natural Family Planning* reviews and refutes the biased statistics sometimes carried in popular magazines. Such factual information will help any fair-minded person recognize the high effectiveness of NFP.

—If your doctor will take the time to read it, give, loan or sell him a copy of this manual, *The Art of Natural Family Planning*.

—Ask your physician to review the ten-minute video, *NFP: Safe Healthy and Effective*. Perhaps he will make it available to other patients.

If your physician is Catholic, consider giving him a copy of "In obedience to Christ: A pastoral letter to Catholic couples and physicians on the issue of contraception" by Bishop Glennon P. Flavin.[1] It's brief and to the point; it has helped some doctors immensely.

2. Your experience. Educate your doctor (or midwife) with your own experience. When you want to achieve pregnancy, let him know by way of a note or phone call. When you achieve pregnancy, you can save yourself a pregnancy test and a needless visit. (Prenatal visits usually don't start until eight or ten weeks past conception, so you can save most of the cost of your NFP training by avoiding an unnecessary visit and pregnancy test.) When your temperature has been up for 22 days, calculate your "due date" using Dr. Prem's formula, and immediately notify your doctor about your anticipated delivery date. Send him a neatly done copy of your chart.

Since you know you are pregnant, be sure to check with your doctor if you think you need any sort of medication, even aspirin. Of course, both you and your spouse should avoid smoking and alcohol, ideally for three months before pregnancy as well as during it.

Follow the nutrition rules in Chapter 20; make sure you are consuming sufficient folic acid both before and during pregnancy.

If your physician refuses to acknowledge the merits of NFP after all of this, you should question his competence because one factor of competence is openness to new knowledge.

CCL's weekend seminars for physicians provide an excellent introduction to NFP and related issues. Twice a year. Contact CCL headquarters for information, or check ***www.ccli.org***.

"No physician should refuse to teach the best methods of calculating the fertile period to patients requesting the instruction."

—*Carl Hartman, M.D.,*[2]

Educating your friends

Educating your friends is a different matter. Many women have a low opinion of their husbands. We've heard many times, "My Jimmie—he'd never go for anything that required abstinence." Maybe so. But if he loves his wife and would like to increase his own self-respect, he will. However, if Jimmie has a truly pathological addiction to sex, he will probably need good counseling, prayer and study, and the grace of the Sacraments to achieve sexual freedom— the freedom to say no to his compulsive urges.

● A misinterpretation

Some of your Christian friends may be suffering under an erroneous interpretation of one-half of one verse in the Bible. The half-verse reads this way: ". . . so let wives also be subject in everything to their husbands" (Ephesians 5:24b).

Some have taken that half verse out of context and used it to "justify" an unholy master-slave relationship in which the husband can tell his wife to do anything—even seriously immoral acts—and she submissively does it as her "Christian duty." That's not only nonsense; it's anti-Christian. The text must be interpreted in the context of the immediate sentences and the overall passage. The *whole* sentence and the first part of the next sentence form the immediate context:

> As the Church is subject to Christ, so let wives also be subject in everything to their husbands. Husbands, love your wives, as Christ loved the Church and gave Himself up for her, that He might sanctify her (Ephesians 5:24-26a).

Thus, wifely submission is in the context of a self-sacrificing husband who is willing to suffer in order to help her grow in holiness. Therefore, no husband can use Scripture as an authorization to order his wife to use contraceptives, to masturbate him, or to perform acts of marital sodomy—either fellatio (oral copulation) or anal copulation. It's just the opposite. He must be willing to practice the periodic abstinence of natural family planning by accepting the self-control that is one of the fruits of the Spirit (Galatians 5:22-25).

● The practical aspects

With all your friends you can emphasize several practical ways in which NFP works well.

- It works for achieving pregnancy.
- It works for avoiding pregnancy.
- It works for your marriage.
- It works for your own self-worth and for your husband's self respect.
- It's health enhancing.
- It's safe, and you're not worried about the effects of chemical birth control and the IUD. You might also tell how chemical birth control and the IUD really work. Share with one and all the CCL brochure, "The Pill: How does it Work? Is it Safe?"

With your Christian friends, share the booklet, *Birth Control and Christian Discipleship.* It reviews the historical and religious aspects of birth control and looks at the issue in a Christian perspective. We have heard reports of some remarkable changes taking place after truth-seeking folks have read this brief publication.

Your efforts to share what you have found in NFP may not change the world, but they may lead someone you love to be grateful to you now and for eternity.

Additional reading

"Dear Healthcare Provider"
"The Effectiveness of Natural Family Planning"
"A Healthcare Provider's Reference"

Self-Test Questions: Chapter 36

1. Doctor John Bruchalski's introductory NFP brochure for physicians is titled _____
    _____.

2. A brochure about NFP written in more technical language for doctors is titled

    _____.

3. A review of NFP effectiveness studies is contained in a pamphlet titled

    _____.

4. A booklet that reviews the historical aspects of the birth control issue and puts it in a
    Christian perspective is titled _____.

5. The NFP video that can be purchased to lend is titled _____.

Answers to self-test
1. "Dear Doctor"   2. "A Physician's Reference to Natural Family Planning"   3. "The Effectiveness of Natural Family Planning"   4. *Birth Control and Christian Discipleship*   5. *NFP: Safe Healthy Effective*

References

(1) Bishop Glennon P. Flavin, "In obedience to Christ: A pastoral letter to Catholic couples and physicians on the issue of contraception," *The Southwestern Nebraska Register*, 11 October 1991. Bishop Flavin was bishop of Lincoln, Nebraska at the time. Reprints are available through CCL.

(2) Carl Hartman, *Science and the Safe Period: A Compendium of Human Reproduction* (Baltimore: Williams and Wilkins, 1962) viii.

37

Educating Your Clergy

After you have completed the CCL course of NFP instruction—either in classes or through the CCL *Home Study Course*—and have practiced NFP for three cycles, you know more about Natural Family Planning than:
>—98% of physicians, nurses and other health care providers
>—97% of ministers, priests, and rabbis
>—95% of married couples.

Of course, those are estimates, but they give you a fairly accurate picture of the great ignorance about NFP that is still common today.

Why the ignorance?

Now that you have finished a course of NFP instruction, it may seem very simple to you. That's because NFP in essence **IS** simple. Once you understand the basics of NFP and its vocabulary, you could write the rules *you* use on a wallet-size business card as we did in the "Introduction."

So you may wonder: if NFP is so easy to understand, why don't doctors, nurses and health care providers know more about it? Since the Catholic Church teaches that unnatural methods of birth control are always and everywhere immoral for married couples, why aren't all the priests and religious educators well informed? And what about the other Christian clergy whose churches were strongly opposed to unnatural forms of birth control before 1930?

In Chapter 36 we offered some ideas about educating your doctor and your friends, and the same thing holds true for your clergy. On the whole, they have not learned about NFP in their seminary training except in some very rare cases. They are generally ignorant about NFP, and many share one of the fruits of ignorance—prejudice. They think that either NFP doesn't work or that making it work requires a level of virtue that they could never sell to the members of their congregations.

The result is that the vast majority of their congregations' fertile-age couples are using unnatural methods, frequently those with abortifacient properties. They suffer the physical, marital and spiritual consequences of acting contrary to God's plan for married love. They also miss the many blessings that come from the right practice of natural family planning. Consequently, all society suffers, including the congregations.

If you are lucky, your clergyman is already sold on NFP; maybe he convinced you to take the NFP course. If so, **please thank him**. He needs to know that he's helped you and that you're grateful.

Materials

In the more typical case, your clergyman is as ignorant about NFP as your doctor, and you can help—if you *want* to. Assuming that you do, where do you start?

We suggest that you do *not* unload everything at once. Since your clergyman is most likely busy, the more you give him at one time, the less likely he is to read it. So first give him just three brochures or pamphlets and lend him one ten-minute video:
—"Dear Father"
—"NFP: Safe Healthy Effective"
—"The Pill: Is It Safe? How Does It Work?"
—*NFP: Safe Healthy Effective* is a 10 minute educational video that explains the scientific basis for NFP. It was designed for use in a doctor's office so it does not get into the moral and religious dimensions of birth control. Still, it is an excellent and brief introduction to NFP.

Two weeks later, stop back to pick up the video and give him six more brochures:
—"From Contraception to Abortion to Columbine"
—"The Legacy of Margaret Sanger"
—"Tubal Ligation: Some Questions and Answers"
—"Vasectomy: Some Questions and Answers"
—"The Effectiveness of Natural Family Planning"
—*Birth Control and Christian Discipleship*

Consider donating the course as part of your tithe.
— Mary Durbin

Wait another two weeks and ask him if he's ready to start *The Art of Natural Family Planning*. If so, ask him to start with Part III, "Does God Care about Birth Control?" Of course, if he's a married Protestant minister, he and his spouse may want to learn the method for their own personal use. In that case, explain how they can take the course locally or through the *CCL Home Study Course*.

If your clergyman shows an interest in the moral and religious aspects of the whole sexuality issue at stake in birth control, get a copy of *Sex and the Marriage Covenant* into his hands. After that, he may be interested in further study and would find Prof. Janet Smith's two books very helpful—*Humanae Vitae: A Generation Later* and *Why Humanae Vitae Was Right: A Reader* (see "Resources").

Your experience

At this point, you've done what you can with prepared materials. The next and continuing step is sharing experience—yours and that of others. Both your doctor and your clergyman need to hear that NFP is livable and that it works—for conception control and for marriages.

Call your clergyman to ask if you can make an appointment for 20 minutes some Saturday morning or early weekday evening to share how you learned about NFP and how it has helped you. Be honest; don't glamorize your sharing, but share simply and directly. Give him an opportunity to ask questions, and thank him for his time.

Besides your own experience, another excellent way to bring regular witness is to give him a membership in CCL. Every other month he will receive *CCL Family Foundations* with its important and helpful information plus the experience of user couples.

If your clergyman becomes convinced and enthusiastic about Natural Family Planning, he may want his engaged and married couples to share his convictions and enthusiasm. Perhaps he may see the benefits of having all his engaged couples take the CCL/NFP course as part of their preparation for marriage. We believe that the combination of the full CCL course and *Marriage Is for Keeps* provides an excellent preparation for marriage (see "Resources").

In addition to our books, brochures, and the video, CCL has another item that can help him as an educator and preacher. *Last Supper Themes Applied to Love and Marriage* is a series of seven homilies. Each develops something that Jesus said or did at the Last Supper and then applies it to the birth control issue. Each refers to a different brochure, which is to be attached to the church bulletin, for teaching the necessary details. Probably few pastors would use these word for word, but the homilies can serve as a springboard for a pastor's own ideas.

Prayer

Those who successfully share materials and their own experience with others always prepare with prayer. They also ask their close spiritual friends to pray for them *while they are meeting* with the clergyman or doctor. Then they are able to go with a deep sense of peace and humility, knowing that God is in charge. If they are rebuffed, they are able to forgive more easily and to continue praying.

Perseverance in prayer is important. Sometimes it takes years for doors to open.

Here the saying holds true, 'One sows and another reaps,' (Jn 4:37).

If you educate your clergyman and your doctor about the merits of natural family planning, you have educated the two most important opinion shapers in the area of birth control. Be assured that other ministers, priests, and physicians have been educated out of a stage of ignorance, prejudice, and antagonism to acceptance and then advocacy of NFP! It doesn't happen overnight, but it's happening now and will continue to happen in the future.

We know physicians who formerly prescribed the Pill and barrier contraceptives but have changed completely. Now they will not prescribe any form of contraception, and they either teach NFP or make referrals to certified Teaching Couples. Grass roots education of the "professionals" is at the heart of it.

Additional reading

Birth Control and Christian Discipleship
"Dear Father"
"From Contraception to Abortion Columbine"
"The Legacy of Margaret Sanger"
"NFP: Safe, Healthy, Effective"
"Tubal Ligation: Some Questions and Answers"
"Vasectomy: Some Questions and Answers"

There are no self-test questions for this chapter.

38

Sharing the Gifts

The Western world is reeling under the onslaught of the sexual revolution. The United States provides a clear and unhappy case history of the effects of the sexual revolution.

The sexual revolution did not start in 1960. It started some 140 years previously in the 1820s in England where the neo-Malthusians began to promote marital contraception in the face of universal Christian teaching to the contrary. For the first time in Christian history, there was an organized group of more or less respectable people openly calling the traditional Christian teaching erroneous and outdated. This was the first organized effort urging married couples to break apart the divinely established connection between "making love" and "making babies." This was truly revolutionary.

The American Comstock laws of 1873 represented a reaction against the neo-Malthusian doctrines, and they undoubtedly helped to maintain the Christian tradition against contraception. However, the evil genius of Margaret Sanger prevailed.

● In 1913-1914 she established her National Birth Control League.

● In 1930-1931 much of Protestantism accepted contraception.

● In the mid-Thirties the Supreme Court took note of the dominant religious trend in the country and began limiting the application of the Comstock laws.

● In 1939 Sanger established Planned Parenthood.

● In 1965 and 1972 the U. S. Supreme Court struck down the last of the Comstock laws.

● In 1973 the same court made the absurd ruling that all laws *prohibiting* abortion were unconstitutional. The United States went from banning condoms in 1873 to accepting abortion for birth control in 1973.

● In 1993 the U. S. Supreme Court ruled that abortion was so much a part of the American culture that it was protected by the Constitution.

The effects of the sexual revolution are everywhere. The American divorce-marriage ratio was one divorce for every 11 marriages in 1910. That was the year of the last national census before Sanger promoted the sexual revolution with her National Birth Control League. The divorce-marriage ratio rose steadily as more and more couples accepted contraception. By the late Seventies, there was one divorce for every two marriages, and that ratio has held steady. That's a 550% increase from 1910! Note well that since 1910 the propaganda for contraception has told people that if they used contraception, they could have unlimited sex, very small families and *therefore* happier marriages! It sounds plausible, but it was and is simply contrary to God's plan

The sexual revolution

for marriage and sex. Therefore, it cannot work for the true good of the family or society. (See Chapter 17, "Your marriage and NFP," for low divorce rate among users of natural family planning.)

The negative effects of the contraceptive sexual revolution continue to spread. Pope Paul VI was ridiculed in 1968 when he predicted that widespread contraception would lead to a general lowering of morality (*Humanae Vitae*, n. 17). Twenty-five years later, newspapers would report a high school game in which the boys earned points for each act of seduction and intercourse with younger girls. As the game was played in Cincinnati, additional points were given for impregnating the girl and more yet if she didn't kill the baby through abortion. This is in spite of the fact that Planned Parenthood and its fellow travelers in the media and education have been preaching tirelessly for 25 years that teenagers should use condoms to be "responsible."

In the United States, the greatest source of poverty is the family headed by a mother without a husband. In 1960, 6% of American white babies and 22% of black babies were born out-of-wedlock. In 1994, 22% of white babies and 68% of black babies were born out-of-wedlock. In June 1995 headlines screamed, "Out-of-wedlock births surge by 54%" from 1980 to 1992.[1] The report noted that the white out-of-wedlock rate rose 94 percent from 1980 to 1992, while the black rate rose by only seven percent.

With no husband to support the family, the mothers have to work or go on welfare. Babies of all colors and cultures need fathers. When so many children are being raised by part-time mothers and no fathers, how can anyone be surprised at the high crime rate in the ghettos of the fatherless poor?

Abortion has likewise increased dramatically. About 1.5 million unborn babies are killed each year in the United States alone through surgical abortion. Abortifacient chemical birth control (The Pill, Norplant, Depo-Provera, etc.) may kill a similar number.

● **Close to home**

The national statistics about the effects of the sexual revolution sometimes numb us or leave us somewhat indifferent because they are about people "out there." So look around.

1. What mature family do you know that has not been affected and afflicted by the sexual revolution?

2. Can you honestly say that none of your parents, your own children, your brothers and sisters and *their* children have been afflicted by the sexual revolution?

3. Do you believe that the "health" or "sex education" curriculum in your school system—whether private or public—has not been influenced by the materials and/or philosophy of Planned Parenthood?

If you can answer "none" to the first question and "yes" to the second and third questions, you are either living in a wonderful ghetto or you are not aware of what's going on around you—and maybe right in your own extended family and neighborhood schools.

The time from the Malthusians of the 1860s to the Sangerites of the present has amply demonstrated that the promises of the sexual revolution are lies. Unfortunately, they're lies that many want to believe. At one point, Margaret Sanger advised her 16 year old granddaughter that sex with anyone was permissible if it was sincere, and that three times a day was about the right amount.[2] Contraceptive sex education programs in schools around the world differ only quantitatively from the Sangerian philosophy. Sanger's personal life was an adulterous disaster, and yet she remains the most influential American woman of the 20th century, and her influence is still bringing disaster to the United States and to every country influenced by its economic power. It's time for a change.

A plan

What the world needs are people who will remain faithful to their marriage covenant—freely, fully, fruitfully and joyfully—who will respect and not misuse the gift of sex within marriage. The world needs people who are chaste. The world needs people who, if they fall into sins of unchastity, call their sins "sins," repent, and resolve to continue the struggle for chastity. The world today needs people who are willing to stand up and be counted for NFP and chastity. "The world" is vague. All of this applies right in your own community and neighborhood.

1. The Couple to Couple League has a very simple plan for bringing the **blessings of NFP** to the people: a network of volunteer Teaching Couples who regularly teach the CCL classes on Natural Family Planning. Cities need three to four Teaching Couples for every 100,000 total population, roughly one for each major neighborhood. Rural areas need at least one Teaching Couple for every populated county. Rural teachers may not have many couples to teach, but to make the service practical, classes need to be held within reasonable distances.

Some couples cannot attend classes because of their schedules or because there are no teachers nearby. The Couple to Couple League has developed the *CCL Home Study Course* to serve these couples. Both forms of education use *The Art of Natural Family Planning*. That means that anyone in the English-speaking world who can read at the normal level of a 16 year old can learn natural family planning.

2. Your community—large or small—also needs consistent **teaching of chastity** and related virtues from childhood through adulthood. The Couple to Couple League has formed another organization, The Foundation for the Family, Inc., to develop and promote education in chastity. The Foundation also publishes *Marriage Is for Keeps*, a small book to assist engaged couples to prepare for lifelong holy matrimony. (See "Resources.")

How you can help

These efforts are low budget. Their success depends upon self-sacrificing love as shown in three ways: the offering of prayer and acts of self-denial, the offering of funds, and the offering of time by volunteers who promote and teach chastity and natural family planning.

● **Prayer.** The life of chastity is the life of applied love. We cannot be chaste without the help of God who is Love, and we need to pray for that help. We need to pray for each other, so we ask you to pray for the total welfare of each family which is part of the CCL family. We ask you to pray for a rebirth of chastity throughout Christianity and the world at large. We ask you to pray specifically for the work of the Couple to Couple League and the Foundation for the Family. Even a brief prayer takes thought and time. Please make that sacrifice frequently.

● **Funds.** Free-will contributions are the lifeblood of CCL and the Foundation for the Family. Although CCL's front line teaching is done by volunteers, there has to be a full-time staff to train and support them, to publish a support magazine and other materials, and to assist NFP efforts internationally, especially in developing countries and Eastern Europe. A small annual contribution confers all membership benefits including the bi-monthly *CCL Family Foundations.* However, free-will gifts beyond the low membership contribution are what make the works of these organizations possible. Many couples use a part of their tithe money to support CCL because they view it as doing an important work of the Lord. We ask for your prayerful generosity.

● **Volunteers.** The crucial work of promoting and teaching Natural Family Planning is done by volunteers who want to share what they have received. Did you learn NFP completely "on your own," so to speak? If you learned it from CCL materials, you received it from others who freely donated funds so that those materials could be written, printed, and distributed.

The volunteer teachers and promoters who make up the CCL team are some of the greatest people in the world. They range in education from high school graduates to graduates in all the professions. For the most part, they are family people with all the time-consuming obligations of ordinary family life. Yet they have volunteered their time and effort to share their knowledge of NFP with others through the standardized teaching program of the League.

If you share the convictions and the principles of the League, and if you are willing to participate in an important community service, perhaps you may be ready to promote or teach Natural Family Planning. Review the following questions.

1. Do you believe the traditional Christian teaching that it is morally wrong to use unnatural forms of birth control?

2. Do you believe that couples who have sufficiently serious reason to postpone pregnancy *should* be able to learn and practice NFP?

3. Do you think that the CCL program of value-oriented NFP instruction should be readily available in *your* county or your part of town?

4. Can you spend one night a week—at home—studying to become NFP teachers and then two evenings a month—out of your house— promoting and teaching NFP?

5. Each CCL/NFP course is a series of four two-hour classes spaced a month apart. Would you be willing to teach two or three such series of classes each year as a community service? (Three series would involve teaching one night a month.)

6. Do you share the CCL philosophy about ecological breastfeeding, natural mothering, and the need of young children for full-time mothering?

7. Do you want to help couples and their families grow in the life of virtue which makes life richer, more meaningful, and ultimately happier?

Teaching NFP. If you and your spouse can answer "yes" to those seven questions, then write CCL Headquarters in Cincinnati for an application and other information about becoming a certified CCL Teaching Couple.

Promoting NFP. If your spouse cannot get involved in teaching for one reason or another, or if you greatly prefer promotion to teaching, then send for information about becoming a CCL Promoter. The work of Promoters is just as important as teaching. In some ways it is even more important because without adequate promotion, there's no one to teach. The chastity promotion can be done just as well by Promoters as by Teachers.

The League provides a special Home Study program to train NFP teachers. You can complete it in six months, and that counts all the back and forth mailing time, etc. Because of inevitable interruptions and distractions, most couples take about nine months to complete it—the same time it takes to have a baby.

Once you have completed the regular CCL/NFP course—either by classes or through the *CCL Home Study Course*, you will have no problem with the certification program. You know the basics. Teacher training consists largely of sharpening your skills for things beyond the basics.

The pro-chastity, pro-family, pro-life apostolate of the League has its share of difficulties almost everywhere. That's why it is needed so much. This apostolate is vitally important for rebuilding respect for chastity and sound family life. It works with ordinary people who are willing to let the Lord do some extraordinary things through them. Please pray about filling this need in *your* community. If you are ready and willing to help, please write us today. It only takes a one sentence letter to identify your interest. Then we'll send you the appropriate materials.

CCL • Box 111184 • Cincinnati OH 45211

"What Can the Couple to Couple League Do for My Community?"   *Additional reading*

Chapter 38: Questions for Reflection

1. Is God calling me to share what I have learned? _____
   If so, how? _____

2. Is God calling us as a couple to share what we have learned? _____
   If so, how? _____

3. Is God calling me to support the Couple to Couple League in prayer? _____
   If so, how? _____

References

(1) Christopher Connel, Associated Press report, "Out-of-wedlock births surge by 54%," *Cincinnati Enquirer*, 7 June 1995, A-2.

(2) Elasah Drogin, *Margaret Sanger: Father of Modern Society* (New Hope, KY: CUF Publications, 1989) 90.

Part VIII

End of the Book Stuff

Glossary of Terms

Abortion. The destruction of a human life at any time between fertilization/conception and birth. An abortion is called spontaneous when it occurs solely from natural causes; it is called induced when it results from human interference with the normal development of the unborn baby through the use of procedures, drugs, or devices designed to kill it.

Abortifacient. A device or drug that causes an abortion.

Abstinence. In the context of sexuality, abstinence means refraining from sexual intercourse. Chaste abstinence means refraining from all activities that cause orgasm or cause one to become excessively aroused.

Amenorrhea. Prolonged absence of menstrual periods.

Anovulatory. Without ovulation; a menstrual cycle in which no ovulation occurs is anovulatory.

Artificial birth control. Unnatural forms of birth control using artifacts such as devices and drugs; sometimes used to mean all unnatural forms of birth control. See unnatural birth control.

Basal temperatures. The temperature of the human body at rest, unaffected by activity, food, or drink.

Billings Method. See mucus-only method.

Breastfeeding. Abr: BF. Feeding a baby at a mother's breast. See "cultural bf.," "ecological bf.," and "total bf."

Calendar rhythm. A system of estimating female fertility based on previous cycle lengths.

Cervical cap. A contraceptive device fitted over the cervix to prevent normal sperm migration.

Cervical erosion. Better called "cervical eversion." An extension of the inner membrane or "skin" of the cervix to the outside of the cervix where the glands frequently secrete cervical mucus constantly.

Cervical mucus. A fluid secreted by glands in the cervix; it becomes watery and stretchy before and at the time of ovulation.

Cervix. The lower, narrow part of the uterus extending slightly into the vagina.

Climacteric. The time of hormonal changes preceding a woman's last menstruation before menopause.

Coitus. A term, from Latin, for sexual intercourse.

Coitus interruptus. Withdrawal from intercourse resulting in ejaculation outside the vagina. See Onanism.

Coitus reservatus. Sexual intercourse controlled so that neither party experiences orgasm.

Conception. The creation of a new human life through the union of sperm and ovum; the process of becoming pregnant; fertilization.

Condom. A contraceptive device put over the penis to prevent sperm from entering the vagina. The female condom is a somewhat similar device used by a female to prevent sperm from being deposited in the vagina.

Continence. In the context of sexuality, another term for abstinence.

Contraception. The practice of using behaviors, devices or drugs intended to prevent conception resulting from intercourse; unnatural forms of birth control.

Contraceptives. Devices and drugs used in the practice of contraception.

Corpus luteum. The name given to an ovarian follicle after it has released its ovum; as a gland it secretes progesterone for about ten to fourteen days after ovulation.

Cultural breastfeeding. A form of breastfeeding in which a mother uses bottles, pacifiers and practices which reduce her baby's suckling at the breast. For contrast, see ecological breastfeeding.

Diaphragm. A contraceptive device inserted into the vagina to cover the cervix to prevent sperm from entering it.

Douche. A stream of water directed into the vagina to cleanse, medicate, or act as a spermicidal contraceptive.

Dysmenorrhea. Very painful menstrual periods.

EBF. Abbreviation for ecological breastfeeding.

Ecological breastfeeding. The type of nursing that fosters mother-baby togetherness and frequent suckling; characterized by 1) nursing as often as the baby wants; 2) no supplements or solids during the first six months; 3) baby-led weaning; and 4) the absence of bottles, pacifiers, babysitters, and other mothering substitutes. EBF provides, on the average, about 14 months of postpartum infertility.

Ectopic pregnancy. See tubal pregnancy.

Ejaculation. The spasmodic expulsion of semen from the penis.

Endocrine glands. Glands that secrete substances into the bloodstream for the purpose of controlling metabolism and other bodily functions.

Endometrium. The inner lining of the uterus that builds up in each cycle and then is discharged in menstruation if pregnancy has not occurred.

Episiotomy. An incision made to enlarge the vaginal opening at birth.

Estrogen. A hormone that causes the cervix to undergo physical changes, to secrete mucus, and also causes the endometrium to develop.

F. Abbreviation for Fahrenheit, a scale for measuring temperatures.

Fallopian tubes. The pair of tubes that conduct eggs from either ovary to the uterus.

Fertile, fertility. In human reproduction, the state of the woman being able to conceive or of the man's sperm being able to fertilize the ovum.

Fertility awareness. Being aware of a woman's fertility through systematic observation of her normal bodily signs.

Fertility, Cycles and Nutrition. A book dealing with the effects of nutrition on the fertility cycle; see "Resources."

Follicle. Any one of thousands of tiny ovarian containers which each hold one ovum; upon release of its ovum, it becomes a gland called the corpus luteum. See FSH.

Foremilk. The first portion of the milk received at a breastfeeding session.

FSH. Abbreviation for follicle stimulating hormone, a substance secreted by the pituitary gland to stimulate the maturation of ovarian follicles.

Full thermal shift. Three or more waking temperatures on consecutive days at a level .4 (4/10) of 1 degree F. above the Low Temperature Level.

Gynecologist. A medical doctor who specializes in the treatment of female reproductive organs.

High Temperature Level. The temperature level which is .4 (4/10) of 1° F. above the Low Temperature Level. See also full thermal shift.

Hindmilk. The last portion of the milk received when the baby empties a breast.

Hormone. A glandular secretion that influences the action of cells and organs in another part of the body.

Hormone Replacement Therapy. The somewhat controversial practice of taking estrogen or estrogen and progestin during the climacteric and during menopause. Abbreviation: HRT.

HRT. Abbreviation for Hormone Replacement Therapy.

HTL. Abbreviation for High Temperature Level.

Implantation. The process of a newly conceived life embedding in the lining of the uterus.

Impotence. The inability to sustain an erection for coitus.

Infertility. The state of a woman being unable to conceive or of a man being unable to fertilize an ovum.

IUD. Abbreviation for intrauterine device, a device placed within the uterus to destroy human life prior to implantation.

Labia. The lips, both inner and outer, of the vulva; the outermost parts of the female genital sex organs.

Lactation. The process of producing and yielding milk from the mammary glands.

LH. Abbreviation for luteinizing hormone.

Libido. Feelings of sexual desire.

Lochia. A postpartum discharge, usually bloody and usually lasting several weeks.

Low Temperature Level. The lower level from which the thermal shift is measured; usually determined by normal high readings among the pre-shift six temperatures.

LTL. Abbreviation for Low Temperature Level.

Luteal phase. The postovulation phase of the menstrual cycle under the influence of progesterone secreted from the corpus luteum. As measured by temperatures, it starts on the first day of the sustained thermal shift. As measured by mucus, it starts on Peak Day + 1.

Luteinizing hormone. A pituitary hormone that helps to cause ovulation.

Mammary glands. The glands in the breast that secrete milk.

Masturbation. Deliberate stimulation of the genital organs for sexual pleasure and orgasm apart from sexual intercourse. Generally refers to self-stimulation. Stimulation of another person for such purposes is called mutual masturbation.

Mcg. Abbreviation for microgram (1/1000 of one milligram or one-millionth of one gram).

Menarche. A young woman's first menstruation.

Menopause. The natural cessation of menstruation and ovarian activity at the end of a woman's fertile years.

Menses. Synonym for menstruation.

Menstruation. A vaginal bloody discharge caused by the sloughing off of the outer layers of the endometrium.

Mg. Abbreviation for milligram (1/1000 of one gram).

Minipill. A low-dosage oral contraceptive; a less powerful version of the Pill. It probably acts more often as an abortifacient than as a contraceptive.

Miscarriage. The loss of a pregnancy due to natural causes; sometimes called a spontaneous or natural abortion.

Mittelschmerz. A German term meaning "pain in the middle"; a feeling sometimes associated with ovulation.

Montgomery glands. Small, raised glands in the areolar tissues (the pigmented area surrounding the nipple).

Mucus. A watery, slippery substance secreted by various mucus glands. See cervical mucus.

Mucus-only method. A system of NFP which uses only the mucus sign and menstruation to determine the fertile and infertile times.

Mucus patch. The duration of a cervical mucus discharge from its start through Peak Day. Secondary meaning: any occurrence of mucus days from the first day through the last day.

Natural Family Planning. Refers to "systematic" NFP and ecological breastfeeding. Systematic NFP refers to using one or more of a woman's common bodily signs to determine the fertile and infertile times of the cycle so the couple can plan intercourse according to their desire to achieve or avoid pregnancy. See also "ecological breastfeeding."

NFP. Abbreviation for natural family planning.

Nocturnal emission. An involuntary and unconscious nighttime ejaculation of excess semen.

Obstetrician. A medical doctor who specializes in the delivery of babies and in pre-and postnatal care of the mother.

Onanism. The traditional theological name for the contraceptive behavior of withdrawal; by extension it refers to all contraceptive behaviors; from the sin of Onan described in Genesis 38:6-10. See "withdrawal."

Orgasm. The climax of sexual excitement.

Os. The opening of the cervix; from the Latin word for mouth.

Ovary. The female reproductive organ containing the ova, or eggs.

Overall thermal shift. A thermal shift pattern in which there are at least three valid temperatures above the LTL, in an overall rising or elevated pattern, with at least one reaching a level 4/10 (or more) of 1° F. above the LTL.

Ovulation. The process of an ovarian follicle releasing its ovum, thus making the woman fertile and able to become pregnant.

Ovulation patch. A mucus patch that is closely followed by a thermal shift.

Ovum. (plural: ova) The woman's egg.

Patch. See mucus patch.

Peak Day. The last day of more-fertile mucus before the drying-up process begins.

Pediatrician. A medical doctor who specializes in the treatment of children.

Penis. The male sexual organ used for coitus and urination.

Perimenopausal. Refers to the months before and after a woman's last period when she enters menopause, especially the 20 cycles before the onset of menopause and the year after her last period.

Phase I. The time of pre-ovulation infertility.

Phase II. The fertile time.

Phase III. The time of postovulation infertility.

Pill. Capitalized, it refers to all the various birth control pills whether they act as abortifacients or contraceptives.

Pituitary gland. A gland located at the base of the brain that releases various hormones which control the functions of other organs.

POB. Abbreviation for pre-ovulation base, an older term for the Low Temperature Level.

Postovulation infertility. The infertile time starting several days after ovulation and continuing until the next menstruation.

Postpartum. After childbirth.

Premenopause. The transition stage in life between the years of normal fertility and menopause.

Pre-ovulation infertility. The infertile time starting with menstruation. The end of this infertile time is determined in several ways.

Pre-shift base. An older term for the Low Temperature Level.

Pre-shift six. The six valid temperatures immediately before the first three rising temperatures that make up the thermal shift. These temperatures are used to set the Low Temperature Level.

Pre-shift spike. One or two much higher temperatures among the pre-shift six temperatures.

Progesterone. A female hormone secreted by the corpus luteum.

Progestin, progestogen. Names for synthetic progesterone.

Prolactin. A hormone that stimulates the secretion of milk in the breastfeeding mother and helps her to bond with her baby. In the non-nursing woman, elevated levels of prolactin are sometimes associated with PMS.

Prostate gland. A male sexual organ that provides a fluid which mixes with sperm to produce semen.
PSB. Abbreviation for pre-shift base, an older term for the Low Temperature Level.

Rhythm method. See "calendar rhythm."

Scrotum. The sac below the penis that contains the testicles.
Shaving. In the context of NFP, the process of lowering one or two temperatures among the pre-shift six to the next highest level.
Sperm. The male cells that unite with the female ovum to cause conception.
Split dry-up. An unusual drying-up pattern after Peak Day. See Chapter 27 for details.
Split peak. An unusual drying-up pattern after Peak Day. See Chapter 27 for details.
Sterilization. The process of rendering either male or female sterile, i.e., incapable of becoming pregnant or causing pregnancy.
Strong thermal shift. A thermal shift pattern in which three consecutive temperatures are all at least 2/10 of 1° F. above the Low Temperature Level and the last temperature is at or above the High Temperature Level.
Sympto-thermal method. A natural family planning system making use of all the signs of fertility and infertility.

Testicles. The male sexual organs contained in the scrotum and producing sperm.
Thermal shift. The postovulation rise in temperatures sustained in an overall rising or elevated pattern for at least three days, reaching and staying at a level usually .4 (4/10) of 1° F. above the Low Temperature Level. See also "full thermal shift," "overall thermal shift," and "strong thermal shift."
Thermal shift level. See High Temperature Level.
Total breastfeeding. The practice in which a mother's breastmilk is the only food or drink given her baby; not the same as ecological breastfeeding.
Tubal ligation. A contraceptive sterilization procedure consisting of tying the Fallopian tubes to prevent sperm from meeting ova.
Tubal pregnancy. Ectopic pregnancy; a pregnancy in which implantation occurs within the Fallopian tube rather than the uterus.

Unnatural birth control. All forms of birth control contrary to God's order of creation; includes artificial birth control such as devices and drugs, both contraceptive and abortifacient, and contraceptive behaviors such as withdrawal and heterosexual sodomy. "Unnatural means" is the term that was used by the Church of England in its debate about birth control after World War I and culminating in 1930.
Uterus. The female organ in which the baby grows during the nine months of pregnancy; frequently called the womb.

Vagina. The female genital canal extending from the uterus to the vulva.
Vaginal foams and jellies. Chemical contraceptive products made to be inserted in the vagina before coitus to kill sperm.
Vasectomy. A male sterilization procedure that prevents sperm from becoming part of the semen.
Vulva. The external parts of the vagina including the labia.

Waking temperatures. The temperatures taken upon waking from the longest and best sleep of the 24 hour day; usually upon waking in the morning.
Withdrawal. The contraceptive practice of withdrawing the penis so that ejaculation occurs outside the vagina; coitus interruptus; Onanism.
Womb. The uterus.

Glossary of Terms

Resources

This section lists the books published by The Couple to Couple League, a few other books available through the League, some CCL brochures, and several organizations. For a complete listing of all the books, brochures, and tapes available from CCL, send for the CCL Catalog. Our resource list is alphabetical by category.

How to order

- Request a Catalog from CCL Headquarters.
- Send check with order by mail.
- Or, order by phone with VISA, MasterCard, or Discover. (The minimum order by credit card is listed in the current catalog.)

Address:
CCL Order Department
P.O. Box 111184
Cincinnati, OH 45211-1184
Phone for orders only: (800) 745-8252. (Eastern time zone)

Internet Orders—
Order any of CCL's NFP materials or catalog items directly on-line at the League's website, ***www.ccli.org***.

Additional readings

Breastfeeding

- *Additional Readings Packet.* This packet contains all the brochures and booklets referred to at the end of the various chapters in this manual.

- *Breastfeeding and Natural Child Spacing: How Ecological Breastfeeding Spaces Babies* by Sheila Matgen Kippley (197 pages). Ecological breastfeeding calls for mother-baby togetherness. The trouble is, much in Western culture is oriented to mother-baby separation. Sheila Kippley shows how you and your baby can enjoy the close relationship of ecological breastfeeding without becoming a social dropout.

- *La Leche League*, P.O. Box 4079, Schaumburg, IL 60168-4079; (847) 519-7730 or (800) LA LECHE. This organization helps women to breastfeed their babies successfully.

- *Nighttime Parenting* by William Sears, M.D. (203 pages). Pediatrician William Sears follows a natural approach to solving problems associated with nighttime parenting including sleeping disorders, night-waking, and even ways to reduce the risk of SIDS.

● *The Womanly Art of Breastfeeding* by La Leche League (465 pages). The standard book on how to breastfeed and overcome nursing problems.

Continuing education

● *CCL Family Foundations* is the official magazine of The Couple to Couple League. Usually 32 pages, six issues per year. A standard benefit to all CCL members. Provides support for every aspect of NFP.

Fathering

● *St. Joseph's Covenant Keepers* newsletter (Family Life Center International, P.O. Box 6060, Port Charlotte FL 33949). This is published six times per year and is edited by Steve Wood. It aims to help husbands to become better fathers and husbands. A unique publication.

Fertility and infertility

● *Fertility, Cycles and Nutrition* by Marilyn M. Shannon (3rd edition, 180 pages). The only book we know of which relates infertility to nutrition in the context of informed fertility awareness. Has chapters on female infertility, male infertility, and repeated miscarriages and birth defects. Shows how improved nutrition can enhance marginal fertility and reduce the risk of certain birth defects.

● *Practical Helps for Seeking Pregnancy* by John F. Kippley (6 panel brochure). Lists a number of low-tech things you can do to enhance your mutual fertility. A brief review of many of the things described in Chapter 21 of the book in your hands. Handy for sharing an introduction to the natural approach but unnecessary for anyone owning *The Art of Natural Family Planning*, 4th edition.

Marriage

● *Creative Abstinence* by Oscar and Susan Staudt (6 panel brochure). Describes how to overcome difficulties with abstinence and how to use such times for building your marriage.

● *Marriage Is for Keeps: Foundations for Christian Marriage* by John F. Kippley (113 pages). The Wedding Edition contains the Readings and the Rite of Marriage (178 pages). Every couple can benefit from this small book intended to help Catholic engaged couples prepare for making the commitment of holy marriage. A combination of using this text and attending the CCL course on NFP is one of the best ways to prepare for Christian marriage. Couples married some years can benefit equally. If the glow has gone, your mutual study of this thought-provoking book can help you to recover it.

● *"Until Death Do Us Part"* by John F. Kippley (8 panel brochure). Succinctly reviews the biblical teaching about the permanence of marriage.

Morality/ theology

● *Sex and the Marriage Covenant: A Basis for Morality* by John F. Kippley (400 pages). Shows how a covenant theology of sex explains and upholds biblical teachings on sexuality. Written to be readable by the general reader. Janet Smith says that its "basic thesis on the meaning of sexuality is rather dazzling for its clarity and simplicity (and in its ability to be applied to a wide range of sexual moral issues)."

● *Why Humanae Vitae Was Right: A Reader* edited by Janet E. Smith (591 pages). Contains selections from 20 different authors on a wide range of issues raised by the 1968 encyclical which reaffirmed the traditional Christian teaching against all unnatural forms of birth control.

● *Birth Control and Christian Discipleship* by John F. Kippley (2nd ed., 45 pages). Describes how the social and liberal-religious acceptance of contraception led to the sexual revolution and the acceptance of abortion. Also: the arithmetic of Pill-caused abortions; NFP; the Bible and birth control; birth control in the light of Christian discipleship.

● *Marital Sexuality: Moral Considerations* (8 panel brochure). Evaluates the meaning of various sexual practices. Obtainable separately or as part of the *Additional Readings Packet*.

● *Birth Control: What does the Catholic Church really teach?* by John F. Kippley (16 panel brochure). Describes authentic Catholic teaching on birth control in a succinct question-answer format.

Nutrition

● American Pro-Life Enterprises (P. O. Box 1281, Powell OH 43065-1281, USA. Information: (614) 881-5520. Orders: (800) 227-8359. Mention CCL and receive a discount. This organization handles the Optivite dietary supplement recommended by M. Shannon and the Professional Prenatal Formula developed according to her recommendations. It also handles competitive brands and a wide variety of other dietary supplements.

● *Fertility, Cycles and Nutrition* by Marilyn M. Shannon. Everyone agrees that what you eat affects the state of your health. This book is unique because it applies the same principle to a particular aspect of health—normal fertility. Irregular cycles, painful and extremely heavy periods, some luteal phase defects, PMS—all of these problems and more can be alleviated by optimum nutrition. We publish and recommend this book because we think it makes good sense to exhaust the low-tech, low cost nutritional approach before turning to the much more expensive pharmaceutical methods.

● Optimox Corporation (P.O. Box 3378, Torrance, CA 90510). Telephone: 800-223-1601. Website: www.optimox.com. Optimox markets the Optivite dietary supplement. Offers a free booklet on PMS and Optivite.

Parenting

● *CCL Family Foundations* supports you in your practice of NFP and in your efforts to be good parents to your children (see "Continuing education").

The Pill

● *Breast Cancer, Its Link with Abortion and the Birth Control Pill* by Chris Kahlenborn, M.D. (397 pages). Analyzes the studies to demonstrate the links.

● *The Pill: How does it Work? Is it Safe?* by Paul Weckenbrock (12 panel brochure). Documents the effects of the birth control pill.

Postabortion counseling

● WEBA (Women Exploited By Abortion, Inc.) 3400 Werk Road, Cincinnati OH 45211, (513) 921-9322. This organization assists women who have had abortions to seek forgiveness and spiritual reconciliation with God.

Thermometers, charts, etc.

● For prices on thermometers, charts, books and other materials, obtain a CCL Catalog or visit the online store at **www.ccli.org**.

Index

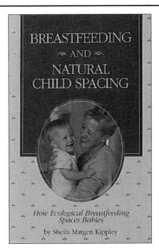
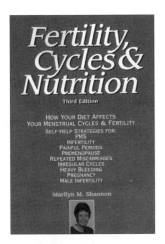